Autism and Child Psychopathology Series

Series Editor

Johnny L. Matson, Baton Rouge, LA, USA

More information about this series at http://www.springer.com/series/8665

Justin B. Leaf
Editor

Handbook of Social Skills and Autism Spectrum Disorder

Assessment, Curricula, and Intervention

Springer

Editor
Justin B. Leaf
Director of Research
Autism Partnership Foundation
Seal Beach, CA, USA

ISSN 2192-922X ISSN 2192-9238 (electronic)
Autism and Child Psychopathology Series
ISBN 978-3-319-62994-0 ISBN 978-3-319-62995-7 (eBook)
DOI 10.1007/978-3-319-62995-7

Library of Congress Control Number: 2017953963

Printed on acid-free paper

This Springer imprint is published by Springer Nature
The registered company is Springer International Publishing AG
The registered company address is: Gewerbestrasse 11, 6330 Cham, Switzerland

This book is dedicated to my amazing advisors who I have had the privilege of working with and learning from.

Thank you:
Alan Harchik, James Sherman, Jan Sheldon, John McEachin, Mitchell Taubman, and Ronald Leaf

This book is also dedicated to my loving, caring, supportive, and fun family.

Thank you:
Fay, Carol (Nana), and Edward (Papa)
Jeremy and Cole
Debbie (Mom), Jamie, and Ron (Dad)
Alexander and Jackson
Misty

Preface

Deficits in social behavior are a hallmark characteristic of autism spectrum disorder (ASD). There are currently numerous studies that have evaluated social behavior, various social assessments, and multiple procedures to improve the social behaviors of individuals diagnosed with ASD. Today, many individuals diagnosed with ASD receive intervention to help improve their social behavior. It was important to compose a book that brought well-respected professionals together to write chapters on the social lives of individuals diagnosed with ASD, including assessments that can be used to identify strengths, weaknesses, and potential social behavior targets, and chapters on various interventions to improve social behavior. It is my hope that bringing these experts together resulted in a useful handbook for any professional who works with individuals diagnosed with ASD and for any family member who lives with an individual diagnosed with ASD.

The handbook is separated into four distinct sections. The first section includes chapters that review social deficits that are commonly observed with individuals diagnosed with ASD. The second section is composed of chapters that review various behavioral and curriculum assessments used to identify social strengths and deficits of individuals diagnosed with ASD. The third section includes numerous chapters, each dedicated to evaluating interventions which have been empirically evaluated and/or implemented to improve the social behavior of individuals diagnosed with ASD. The fourth and final section includes two chapters that provide suggestions for future research on social behavior and future clinical directions for teaching social behavior.

This book is the result of many top professionals who were willing to write chapters for this handbook. I would like to personally and publicly thank each of the contributing authors for their dedication to this handbook, but, more importantly, for their dedication to improving the lives of individuals diagnosed with ASD. I also want to thank my loving, brilliant, and supportive wife, Misty, who helped me through the entire process. Finally, this book would not have happened without the tireless work of two future stars in the field of ASD and behavior analysis. Thank you Julia L. Ferguson and Joseph H. Cihon for all of your tireless and hard work on this project and for making this handbook a reality.

Seal Beach, CA, USA — Justin B. Leaf
May 2017

Contents

Contributors

Shahla Ala'i-Rosales College of Health and Public Service, University of North Texas, Denton, TX, USA

Kevin M. Ayres School of Education, The University of Georgia, Athens, GA, USA

Nirit Bauminger-Zviely School of Education, Bar-Ilan University, Ramat-Gan, Israel

Courtney Bolton Semel Institute for Neuroscience, University of California Los Angeles, Los Angeles, CA, USA

Denys Brand Department of Applied Behavioral Science, University of Kansas, Lawrence, KS, USA

Rachel Cagliani School of Education, The University of Georgia, Athens, GA, USA

Karis A. Casagrande Department of Psychology, Michigan State University, East Lansing, MI, USA

Joseph H. Cihon Autism Partnership Foundation, Seal Beach, CA, USA

Endicott College, Beverly, MA, USA

Pegeen Cronin Clinical Psychologist, Cronin Assessment, Los Angeles, CA, USA

Robert Didden Behavioural Science Institute, Radboud University, Nijmegen, The Netherlands

Florence D. DiGennaro Reed Department of Applied Behavioral Science, University of Kansas, Lawrence, KS, USA

Ruth Ellingsen Semel Institute for Neuroscience, University of California Los Angeles, Los Angeles, CA, USA

Julia L. Ferguson Autism Partnership Foundation, Seal Beach, CA, USA

B.J. Freeman Medical Psychology, UCLA School of Medicine, Los Angeles, CA, USA

Linda Heitzman-Powell University of Kansas Medical Center, Kansas City, KS, USA

Amy J. Henley Department of Applied Behavioral Science, University of Kansas, Lawrence, KS, USA

Thomas S. Higbee Department of Special Education & Rehabilitation, Utah State University, Logan, UT, USA

Jennifer Hilton Endicott College, Beverly, MA, USA

Brooke R. Ingersoll Department of Psychology, Michigan State University, East Lansing, MI, USA

Debra M. Kamps Juniper Gardens Children's Project, University of Kansas, Kansas City, KS, USA

Yael Kimhi Levinsky College of Education, Tel Aviv, Israel

Elizabeth Laugeson Semel Institute for Neuroscience, University of California Los Angeles, Los Angeles, CA, USA

Justin B. Leaf Director of Research, Autism Partnership Foundation, Seal Beach, CA, USA

Cynthia P. Livingston University of South Florida, Tampa, FL, USA

Rose Mason Assistant Professor, Department of Educational Studies, College of Education, Purdue University, Kansas City, KS, USA

Mary E. McDonald Department of Specialized Programs in Education, Hofstra University, Hempstead, NY, USA

Gail G. McGee Department of Psychiatry and Behavioral Sciences, Emory University School of Medicine, Atlanta, GA, USA

Raymond G. Miltenberger University of South Florida, Tampa, FL, USA

Hannah Morton Institute for Child Development, Binghamton University, Binghamton, NY, USA

Matthew D. Novak Department of Applied Behavioral Science, University of Kansas, Lawrence, KS, USA

Marissa Novotny University of South Florida, Tampa, FL, USA

Misty Oppenheim-Leaf Autism Partnership Foundation, Seal Beach, CA, USA

Marie Rocha UC Davis MIND Institute, University of California, Sacramento, CA, USA

Sally J. Rogers UC Davis MIND Institute, University of California, Sacramento, CA, USA

Raymond G. Romanczyk Institute for Child Development, Binghamton University, Binghamton, NY, USA

Robert K. Ross Beacon ABA Services, Inc., Milford, MA, USA

Samantha Russo Endicott College, Beverly, MA, USA

Ron Scholte Behavioural Science Institute, Radboud University, Nijmegen, The Netherlands

Tyra P. Sellers Department of Special Education & Rehabilitation, Utah State University, Logan, UT, USA

Sally B. Shepley College of Education, University of Kentucky, Lexington, KY, USA

Peter Sturmey The Graduate Center and Queens College, City University of New York, New York, NY, USA

Mitchell Taubman Autism Partnership Foundation, Seal Beach, CA, USA

Karen A. Toussaint Department of Behavior Analysis, College of Health and Public Service, University of North Texas, Denton, TX, USA

Jason Travers Department of Special Education, The University of Kansas, Lawrence, KS, USA

Andrea Trubanova Wieckowski Department of Psychology, Virginia Tech, Blacksburg, VA, USA

Ty Vernon The Gevirtz School, University of California, Santa Barbara, CA, USA

Giacomo Vivanti Drexel Autism Institute, Drexel University, Philadelphia, PA, USA

Fred R. Volkmar Yale University School of Medicine, New Haven, CT, USA

Sara M. Weinkauf JBA Institute, Torrance, CA, USA

Mary Jane Weiss Endicott College, Beverly, MA, USA

Susan W. White Department of Psychology, Virginia Tech, Blacksburg, VA, USA

Kaylie Wiseman Institute for Child Development, Binghamton University, Binghamton, NY, USA

Brent Van der Wyk Yale University School of Medicine, New Haven, CT, USA

Heather M. Zerger University of South Florida, Tampa, FL, USA

Inge Zweers Department of Developmental Psychology, Utrecht University, Utrecht, The Netherlands

About the Editor

Justin B. Leaf, PhD, BCBA-D is the director of research and training for the Autism Partnership Foundation (APF) and for the Center for the Advancement of Behavior Analysis™ (CABA). Dr. Leaf is also an adjunct professor at Endicott College. Dr. Leaf received his doctorate degree in behavioral psychology from the Department of Applied Behavioral Science at the University of Kansas. He worked under the mentorship of Drs. James Sherman and Jan Sheldon. Currently, he leads the research team at APF and conducts research projects nationally and internationally. His research interests include examining methods to improve social behaviors and, more importantly, develop meaningful friendships for children and adolescents diagnosed with autism spectrum disorder (ASD), comparing different teaching methodologies, evaluating parameters of reinforcement, and evaluating long-term outcomes for individuals diagnosed with ASD. Dr. Leaf has over 50 publications in peer-reviewed journals or book chapters and has presented at national and international professional conferences and invited events. He is an associate editor for the *Review Journal of Autism and Developmental Disorders* and serves on the editorial boards for the *Journal of Autism and Developmental Disorders*, *Education and Training in Autism and Developmental Disabilities*, and the *Journal of Applied Behavior Analysis*.

An Introduction to the Handbook

1

Justin B. Leaf

In 1943, Leo Kanner wrote a paper describing 11 individuals exhibiting behaviors we now know are distinctive features of a diagnosis of autism spectrum disorder (ASD). Within his description, Kanner (1943) outlined social deficits that were commonly displayed by the 11 individuals whom he was observing. For several years, ASD has been included in the *Diagnostic and Statistical Manual of Mental Disorders* (currently in its fifth edition; DSM-5, American Psychiatric Association [APA], 1980, 2000, 2013). Although there have been changes to the diagnostic criterion of ASD over time, a consistent hallmark of the diagnosis has been a lack of appropriate social behavior (e.g., APA, 1980, 2000, 2013; Yaylaci & Miral, 2017). Furthermore, some professionals have stated that the lack of appropriate social behavior is the primary diagnostic feature (e.g., Soto-Icaza, Aboitiz, & Billeke, 2015).

What is known today is there is a wide range of deficits observed in social behavior for individuals diagnosed with ASD (APA, 2013). These deficits include social language (Tager-Flusberg, 1981), emotional behavior (Baron-Cohen & Wheelwright, 2004), play skills (Taubman, Leaf, & McEachin, 2011), and a failure to develop meaningful friendships and prosocial relationships (Bauminger & Shulman, 2003). It is also known that there is an increasing prevalence in the number of individuals who will be diagnosed with ASD (Centers for Disease Control and Prevention [CDC], 2006; Newschaffer, Falb, & Gurney, 2005). This increasing prevalence makes it even more important for researchers to conduct studies which evaluate social deficits, identify the best ways to assess social behavior, and evaluate efficacious intervention strategies to improve social behavior of individuals diagnosed with ASD. The increasing prevalence of ASD will also make it imperative for practitioners to implement the most effective interventions to help improve the social behavior of individuals diagnosed with ASD.

For several years, my colleagues and I have strived to disseminate the importance of teaching social skills for individuals diagnosed with ASD and conduct research on social behavior as it relates to individuals diagnosed with ASD (e.g., Cheung, Schulze, Leaf, & Rudrud, 2016; Kassardjian et al., 2013; Oppenheim-Leaf, Leaf, Dozier, Sheldon, & Sherman, 2012). We have accomplished this through conducting workshops (e.g., Leaf & Streff, 2009; Taubman, Leaf, McEachin, & Leaf, 2012), presenting at conferences (e.g., Leaf, 2015; Milne, Leaf, Townley-Cochran, Leaf, & Oppenheim-Leaf, 2015), and authoring curriculum books (e.g., Taubman et al., 2011).

J.B. Leaf (✉)
Director of Research, Autism Partnership Foundation, Seal Beach, CA, USA
e-mail: jblautpar@aol.com

J.B. Leaf (ed.), *Handbook of Social Skills and Autism Spectrum Disorder*, Autism and Child Psychopathology Series, DOI 10.1007/978-3-319-62995-7_1

Unfortunately, we have encountered resistance from parents and professionals for prioritizing social skills interventions as part of a comprehensive curriculum for individuals diagnosed with ASD. A common statement we typically hear is, "students with autism are not social." In my clinical and research experience, it is not that individuals diagnosed with ASD are not social or that individuals diagnosed with ASD do not desire to be social with their peers. Rather, it is that individuals diagnosed with ASD do not display appropriate social behavior (e.g., Leaf et al., 2016), and these deficits should be specifically targeted as part of comprehensive intervention.

Another reason we have found that social behavior is commonly not prioritized as part of comprehensive intervention is a heavy focus on other skills such as language development (Sundberg & Michael, 2001), reduction of aberrant behavior (Wunderlich & Vollmer, 2015), and academic priorities (e.g., Stasolla et al., 2016). Within many clinical settings, one of the primary goals is determining the function of an individual's aberrant behavior and reducing these aberrant behaviors (e.g., Santiago, Hanley, Moore, & Jin, 2016). Although we agree that interventionists should address aberrant behavior as part of comprehensive program, especially when aberrant behavior interferes with learning (Koegel, Firestone, Kramme, & Dunlap, 1974) or will result in missed opportunities for social interaction (Taubman et al., 2011), this should not preclude teaching social behavior. Within many clinical settings, another common target is improving language. Although we agree that it is important to improve language for individuals diagnosed with ASD, this also should not impede teaching social behavior.

We commonly encountered the desire for professionals, and sometimes parents, to teach academic skills (e.g., math facts) at the expense of teaching social behavior. The tendency to focus on other skills (e.g., language, aberrant behavior, and academic skills) in clinical settings parallels the trends observed within the research. For example, research on functional behavioral assessment/functional analysis and reducing aberrant behavior is one of the most commonly studied methodologies today (e.g., Hanley, Iwata, & McCord, 2003). There is also a tremendous amount of research on developing and improving language (e.g., Johnson, Kohler, & Ross, 2017). Finally, there are several studies that have focused on improving academic behaviors (e.g., Kelly, Axe, & Allen, 2015). Although there has been an increase in the number of studies teaching and evaluating social behavior as it relates to ASD (e.g., Matson, Matson, & Rivet, 2007), the amount of studies are far fewer compared with the areas mentioned above.

My colleagues and I understand the parental desire for their children to learn the language and academic skills that their peers are learning. We also understand the tremendous pressure that teachers and school administrators are under to ensure that students meet individual educational plan objectives and state standards. However, it remains unclear why these skills are consistently prioritized within interventions over social behavior. In our opinion, social behavior can lead to meaningful outcomes, and it is unclear if prioritizing academic goals will lead to the same meaningful outcomes (Ayres, Lowrey, Douglas, & Sievers, 2011). As Dr. Peter Gerhardt commonly informs professionals, we have to ensure that we teach functional skills that will lead to meaningful outcomes for individuals diagnosed with ASD, especially as they become adults (Gerhardt, 2016).

Another common argument for not targeting social behavior for individuals diagnosed with ASD is the potential to destroy that student's individuality (Devita-Raeburn, 2016). Many believe that by teaching social behavior, we minimize uniqueness, alter personalities, and force conformation of societal norms (Devita-Raeburn, 2016). We acknowledge that every individual is unique and we want them to grow up to be comfortable with who they are; however, this does not mitigate the need to teach social behavior.

Ultimately, individuals diagnosed with ASD often do not realize what opportunities they may miss through a lack of social skills. Moreover, individuals diagnosed with ASD often cannot provide assent for the direction of programming. As such, a parent or guardian provides consent.

Deciding not to prioritize and develop social skills can lead to life-altering negative consequences. Alternatively, learning these social skills can lead to life-altering positive consequences. Without being able to make an informed choice, it could be deemed unethical for a professional to not teach important social behaviors. Once an individual can provide assent, that individual may determine if he or she should engage in the appropriate social behavior.

Another rationale we commonly encounter for not targeting social behavior is parents saying, "We are not social ourselves. Why does our child have to be?" Often, when I hear this type of excuse I think, "Well, you are social enough to be in a relationship" and "You were social enough to have a child." Although I would not recommend saying this to a parent, it does illustrate that parents can assent to electing to not be social, while sometimes individuals diagnosed with ASD cannot. If a parent elects to stay at home and watch TV as opposed to inviting others over to her/his house, they can identify the missed social opportunities. Parents also know the positive and negative side effects that occur by choosing not to engage in these social opportunities. As stated above, individuals diagnosed with ASD often cannot provide assent. Thus, this excuse should not be a reason why we do not teach social behavior to individuals diagnosed with ASD.

Ultimately, one of the main reasons social behavior may not be a priority is teaching appropriate social skills is very difficult. Social behaviors are nuanced with many variables that an individual must respond to within a social interaction. For example, when teaching someone to join into an ongoing game, the individual must identify which game and with what peers to join, ask to join into that game in a way that will lead to acceptance by their peers, identify how to respond if their peers accept them into the game, and how to respond if the peers do not accept them into the game. As evident from this one example, there are a multitude of variables to consider even within a basic social skill. The amount of variables multiply with more complicated skills, such as friendship development. This can be highlighted by Jim Parson's character, Dr. Sheldon Cooper, attempting to make friends in the "Friendship Algorithm" episode of *The Big Bang Theory* (Lorre, Molaro, & Cendrowski, 2009).

Simply put, teaching social behavior is very complex, especially compared with teaching less complex skills like requesting (e.g., Brodheard, Higbee, Gerencser, & Akers, 2016), matching (e.g., Farber, Dube, & Dickson, 2016), or receptive labeling (e.g., Grow & Van Der Hijde, 2017). The complexity of teaching social behavior makes evaluating interventions to improve social behavior more difficult within research, as it could result in less functional/experimental control. This difficulty could also result in professionals and parents departing from teaching social behavior within clinical settings.

Regardless of how difficult teaching social behaviors can be, or the reasons why social skills are not made a priority, it is imperative to teach social behaviors to individuals diagnosed with ASD for several reasons. For one, teaching social behavior may promote more natural language. When we make teaching social behavior with individuals diagnosed with ASD a priority, it increases the likelihood of fostering appropriate social interaction, and, therefore, could lead to more opportunities to communicate with their peers. In our clinical practice, we have seen that by teaching social behavior we simultaneously promote natural language.

Another rationale for teaching social behavior with individuals diagnosed with ASD is that research has shown that when students have positive social relationships, they enjoy and do better in school (Ladd, Birch, & Buhs, 1999). Thus, by teaching social behavior, the individuals we serve may gain collateral skills with no additional time or cost. If the argument is that academic skills or language development must be made a priority over social skills, it would be inconsistent with the research on the benefits of teaching social behavior.

Teaching social behavior may lead to higher rates of peer approval for individuals diagnosed with ASD as well as the development of meaningful friendships. We do not teach social behaviors such as joint attention (e.g., Taylor &

Hoch, 2008), observational learning (DeQuinzio & Taylor, 2015), joining in (e.g., Leaf et al., 2012), or winning graciously (e.g., Leaf et al., 2012) just so that the individual can display these skills. We teach these skills, and other social behaviors, to increase the likelihood that the individual has positive, prosocial relationships and friendships (Bauminger & Shulman, 2003).

When an individual, with or without a diagnosis of ASD, does not engage in appropriate social behavior, it may lead to a lack of meaningful friendships or prosocial relationships. Unfortunately, this can lead to serious negative consequences such as loneliness (Bauminger, Shulman, & Agam, 2003), depression (e.g., Hurley, 2008), and thoughts of suicide or attempting/committing suicide (Dodd, Doherty, & Guerin, 2016; Mayes, Gorman, Hillwig-Garcia, & Syed, 2013). Research shows that individuals diagnosed with ASD are more susceptible to these negative outcomes (Mayes et al., 2013). The potential for these negative consequences solidifies the rationale for why teaching social behaviors to individuals diagnosed with ASD should be prioritized.

Ultimately, the reason why it is imperative to teach social behavior is to improve the quality of life for individuals diagnosed with ASD (Taubman et al., 2011). If you were to ask most, if not all, parents what they would want for their child it would be for them to have a high quality of life. If you were to ask most professionals why they went into the human service field or why they decided to work with individuals diagnosed with ASD, one would hope their answer would include to help improve the lives of those they serve. In reality, most individuals diagnosed with ASD can live high quality of lives without knowing advanced math facts, all of the U.S. presidents, or cursive handwriting. However, it is my and my colleagues' contention that you cannot have a high quality of life if you do not have meaningful friendships. Therefore, teaching social behaviors with individuals diagnosed with ASD *MUST* be made a priority.

Given the importance of teaching social behavior to individuals diagnosed with ASD and the growing literature on social behavior (Matson et al., 2007), it is imperative for professionals to have a resource dedicated to social behavior as it relates to individuals diagnosed with ASD. It is for these reasons that this handbook was created. The handbook should be used as a tool for professionals, academics, practitioners, as well as parents and family members. My goal for editing this book is that consumers have a useful resource that can guide them through the literature on social assessment, social behavior, and interventions to teach social behavior for individuals diagnosed with ASD. By having this book as a guide, it is my hope that this handbook can help practitioners in their everyday work with individuals diagnosed with ASD.

To help write this book, top professionals and leaders in the field of ASD and behavior analysis were recruited to write chapters on their area of expertise. All authors have many years of research and clinical experience. It is without a doubt that the authors of each chapter are recognized as experts on the subject matter provided within each of the chapters. It is my hope that having so many experts contributing to this handbook will result in an important informational guide for researchers, academics, students, clinicians, and parents.

1.1 Four Sections of This Book

1.1.1 Section One: Social Skills Deficits

The first section is meant to inform consumers of the social behaviors and social deficits commonly displayed by individuals diagnosed with ASD. The second chapter of this handbook was written by Volkmar and Vander Wyk, who describe the social nature of individuals diagnosed with ASD, specifically reviewing the clinical manifestations and the neuroscience of the social deficits. The third chapter was written by Sturmey who outlines perilous behaviors commonly displayed by individuals diagnosed with ASD including symptoms of depression, anxiety, loneliness, and suicide. The fourth chapter, written by Zweers, Scholte, and Didden, provide information on the serious issue of bullying as it pertains to individuals diagnosed with ASD.

This chapter specifically discusses the prevalence of bullying, role of the environment, causes, and prevention/intervention. The fifth chapter of this handbook was written by Bauminger-Zviely and Kimhi, and it describes friendships as they pertain to individuals with ASD. Specifically, the chapter describes the characteristics of friendships, how friendships are displayed across the life span, and future directions.

1.1.2 Section Two: Assessment

The second section of this book provides information on various ways to assess social behavior for individuals with ASD. The sixth chapter of the book written by Freeman and Cronin describes various social skills assessments that can be used to evaluate social behavior. This chapter describes the assessments, the strengths of various assessments, and the limitations of various assessments. The next chapter was written by Cronin and Freeman and describes assessments used to evaluate adaptive behavior. In this chapter, the authors describe methodological concerns when measuring adaptive behavior as well as commonly used assessments such as the Vineland Adaptive Behavior Scales (Sparrow, Cicchetti, & Saulnier, 2016) and the Behavior Assessment System for Children (Reynolds & Kamphaus, 2015). The eighth chapter, written by Romanczyk, Wiseman, and Morton, describes curriculum-based assessments and how these assessments can be used to help with selecting appropriate social targets for individuals diagnosed with ASD. Within this chapter, the authors describe various assessments such as the Assessment of Basic Language and Learning Skills (Partington, 2006) and the Hawaii Early Learning Profile (Wheat & Baker, 2010).

1.1.3 Section Three: Social Skills Interventions

The bulk of this handbook is dedicated to the third section, which describes various interventions that can be used to help improve the social behavior of individuals diagnosed with ASD. The section begins with a chapter written by DiGennaro Reed, Novak, Henley, and Brand. The authors discuss the importance of evidence-based interventions. This chapter is critical to the handbook as it can help consumers identify what constitutes evidence-based interventions. This is important because there are numerous pseudoscientific, antiscientific, nonevidence-based, and not scientifically supported procedures promoted for individuals diagnosed with ASD. The tenth chapter was written by Weiss, Hilton, and Russo who describe how discrete trial teaching can be used to teach social behavior. Weiss and colleagues describe how discrete trial teaching can be used to teach more than just simple skills (e.g., matching, imitation, receptive labeling). The next chapter, written by Ala'i-Rosales, Toussiant, and McGee, provides an overview of incidental teaching procedures and how they can be used to make meaningful social gains for individuals diagnosed with ASD. The authors of this chapter provide detailed examples of how the procedures can be implemented effectively.

The next chapter of the book, written by Vernon, describes pivotal response training (PRT) and how it can be effectively used to improve social behavior. Throughout the chapter, Vernon describes the key components to PRT and how they can be used to improve social behavior. This chapter is followed by a description of another comprehensive program to improve the overall quality of individuals diagnosed with ASD known as the Early Start Denver Model (ESDM). This chapter, written by Rogers, Vivanti, and Rocha, describes the ESDM model as well as the research supporting that model to teach social behavior.

This topic is followed by a chapter written by Ayres, Travers, Shepley, and Cagliani who describe video-based instruction. In this chapter, the authors provide a rationale for using video-based instruction to improve social behavior, considerations for using video-based instruction, how video-based instruction can be used to teach a wide variety of skills, and areas for future research. The next chapter of the book, written by Higbee and Sellers, focuses on visual learning strategies (e.g., activity schedules and social scripts). This chapter provides a thorough description of the procedures, clinical implications, and research implications of visual learning strategies.

Kamps, Mason, and Heitzman-Powell provide a chapter on peer-mediated interventions. The authors define what constitutes peer-mediated interventions and provide a key summary of the research. This is followed by a chapter written by Casagrande and Ingersoll describing parent-mediated interventions. In this chapter, the authors provide a detailed description of the various research procedures and a discussion of future areas of research.

The next two chapters are dedicated to interventions that use demonstration and role-playing as part of the intervention to teach social behavior. In a chapter written by Cihon, Weinkauf, and Taubman, the authors describe the teaching interaction procedure (TIP). Within the chapter, the authors describe the historical roots of the TIP and how the procedure has an emerging literature base demonstrating its effectiveness for teaching social behavior for individuals diagnosed with ASD. Miltenberger, Zerger, Novotny, and Livingston describe a similar procedure known as behavioral skills training (BST). Within this chapter, the authors describe the various components of BST as well as the research demonstrating the effectiveness of the procedure.

Ellingsen, Bolton, and Laugeson's chapter describes the benefits of social skills groups for teaching social behaviors to individuals diagnosed with ASD. So often, interventions are implemented in a one-to-one instructional format, and it is critical to ensure that teaching also occurs within a group instructional format. This chapter describes the importance of and how to implement social skills groups.

The next chapter, written by Ross, describes how matrix training procedures can be used to improve social behavior for individuals diagnosed with ASD. In this chapter, the author thoroughly describes matrix training and how it can be applied in a clinical setting.

This is followed by a chapter written by Leaf and Ferguson, which reviews a commonly implemented procedure, Social Stories™. In this chapter, the authors describe the guidelines of Social Stories™, describe the variations of Social Stories™, and provide a critical analysis of the research on Social Stories™. The final chapter in this section was written by Wieckowski and White. In this chapter, the authors describe various interventions that have an emerging research base but may be implemented with individuals diagnosed with ASD. It may be the case that in 5–10 years some of these procedures may have a robust amount of research available and would no longer be considered emerging interventions.

1.1.4 Section Four: Future Directions

The final section of the handbook looks to the future of teaching social behavior as it relates to ASD. Leaf, Oppenheim-Leaf, and Weiss write about future directions as it pertains to research evaluating social behavior, social assessment(s), and interventions to help improve social behavior. The authors provide numerous suggestions that future researchers should consider when conducting future methodological evaluations. Taubman and Ferguson provide the final chapter that describes how clinicians should proceed when teaching social behavior to individuals diagnosed with ASD. Within this final chapter the authors describe a progressive approach for teaching social behavior.

1.2 Conclusion

This handbook covers a wide variety of topics as they relate to social behavior and individuals diagnosed with ASD. From deficits, to assessment, to interventions, and to future directions, this handbook can be used as a guide for any person (professional or nonprofessional) working or living with individuals diagnosed with ASD. We hope that this handbook will help guide clinical practice, will be used as a resource to gain knowledge about areas related to social behavior for individuals diagnosed with ASD, and help guide future research. If these goals can be reached, it will no doubt improve social behavior and the lives of individuals diagnosed with ASD.

References

American Psychiatric Association. (2013). *Diagnostic and statistical manual of mental disorders* (5th ed.). Arlington, VA: American Psychiatric Publishing.

American Psychiatric Association. (2000). *Diagnostic and statistical manual of mental disorders: DSM-IV-TR*. Washington, DC: American Psychiatric Association.

American Psychiatric Association. (1980). *Diagnostic and statistical manual of mental disorders* (3rd ed.). Washington, DC: Author.

Ayres, K., Lowrey, K., Douglas, K., & Sievers, C. (2011). I can identify saturn but I can't brush my teeth: What happens when the curricular focus for students with severe disabilities shifts. *Education and Training in Autism and Developmental Disabilities*, *46*(1), 11–21.

Baron-Cohen, S., & Wheelwright, S. (2004). The empathy quotient: An investigation of adults with Asperger syndrome or high functioning autism, and normal sex differences. *Journal of Autism and Developmental Disorders*, *34*(2), 163–175.

Bauminger, N., & Shulman, C. (2003). The development and maintenance of friendship in high functioning children with autism, maternal perceptions. *Autism*, *7*(1), 81–97.

Bauminger, N., Shulman, C., & Agam, G. (2003). Peer interaction and loneliness in high-functioning children with autism. *Journal of Autism and Developmental Disorders*, *33*(5), 489–507.

Brodheard, M. T., Higbee, T. S., Gerencser, K. R., & Akers, J. S. (2016). The use of a discrimination-training procedure to teach mand variabliity to children with autism. *Journal of Applied Behavior Analysis*, *49*(1), 34–48.

Centers for Disease Control and Prevention. (2006). Mental health in the United States: Parental report of diagnosed autism in children aged 4–17 years- United States, 2003–2004. Surveliance summaries, May 5, 2006. *Morbidity and Mortality Weekly Report*, *17*, 481–486.

Cheung, Y., Schulze, K. A., Leaf, J. B., & Rudrud, E. (2016). Teaching community skills to two young children with autism using a digital self-managed activity schedule. *Exceptionality*, *24*(4), 241–250.

DeQuinzio, J. A., & Taylor, B. A. (2015). Teaching children with autism to discriminate the reinforcered and nonreinforced respones of others: Implications for observational learning. *Journal of Applied Behavior Analysis*, *48*(1), 38–51.

Devita-Raeburn, E. (2016). The controversy over autism's most common therapy. *Spectrum News*. Retrieved from: https://spectrumnews.org/features/deep-dive/controversy-autisms-common-therapy/

Dodd, P., Doherty, A., & Guerin, S. (2016). A systematic review of suicidality in people with intellectual disabilities. *Harvard Review of Psychiatry*, *24*(3), 202–213.

Farber, R. S., Dube, W. V., & Dickson, C. A. (2016). A sorting-to-matching method to teach *compound* matching to sample. *Journal of Applied Behavior Analysis*, *49*(2), 294–307.

Gerhardt, P. F. (2016). *Is behavior analysis meeting our obligation to adults with ASD?* Invited paper presented at the meeting of the California Association of Behavior Analysis, Santa Clara, CA.

Grow, L. L., & Van Der Hijde, R. (2017). A comparison of procedures for teaching receptive labeling of sight words to a child with autism spectrum disorder. *Behavior Analysis in Practice*, *10*(1), 62–66.

Hanley, G. P., Iwata, B. A., & McCord, B. E. (2003). Functional analysis of problem behavior: A review. *Journal of Applied Behavior Analysis*, *36*(2), 147–185.

Hurley, A. D. N. (2008). Depression in adults with intellectual disability: Symptoms and challenging behavior. *Journal of Intellectual Disabilities Research*, *52*(11), 905–916.

Johnson, G., Kohler, K., & Ross, D. (2017). Contributions of Skinner's theory of verbal behaviour to langauge intervnetions for children with autism spectrum disorders. *Early Child Development and Care*, *187*(3–4), 436–446.

Kanner, L. (1943). Autistic disturbances of affective contact. *Nervous Child*, *2*, 217–250.

Kassardjian, A., Taubman, M., Rudrud, E., Leaf, J. B., Edwards, A., McEachin, J, …, & Schulze, K. (2013). Utilizing teaching interactions to facilitate social skills in the natural environment. *Education and Training in Autism and Developmental Disabilities, 48*(2), 245–257.

Kelly, A. N., Axe, J. B., & Allen, R. F. (2015). Effects of presession pairing on the challenging behavior and academic responding of children with autism. *Behavioral Interventions*, *30*(2), 135–156.

Koegel, R. L., Firestone, P. B., Kramme, K. W., & Dunlap, G. (1974). Increasing spontaneous play by suppressing self-stimulation in autistic children. *Journal of Applied Behavior Analysis*, *7*(4), 521–528.

Ladd, G. W., Birch, S. H., & Buhs, E. S. (1999). Children social and scholastic lives in kindergarten: Related spheres of influence? *Child Development*, *70*(6), 1373–1400.

Leaf, J. B. (2015). *A preliminary evaluation of a behaviorally based social skills group for young children diagnosed with autism spectrum disorder: A randomized control trial*. Paper presented at Massachusetts Association for Behavior Analysis.

Leaf, J. B., Leaf, J. A., Milne, C., Taubman, M., Oppenheim-Leaf, M., Torres, N., …, & Yoder, P. (2016). An evaluation of a behaviorally based social skills group for individuals diagnosed with autism spectrum disorder. *Journal of Autism and Developmental Disorders, 47*(2), 243–259.

Leaf, J. B., Oppenheim-Leaf, M. L., Call, N. A., Sheldon, J. B., Sherman, J. A., Taubman, M., …, & Leaf, R. (2012). Comparing the teaching interaction procedure to social stories for people with autism. *Journal of Applied Behavior Analysis, 45*(2), 281–298.

Leaf, J. B. & Streff, T. (2009). *Teaching social skills using the teaching interaction procedure*. Workshop to the Northwest Missouri Conference on Autism, St. Joseph, MO.

Lorre, C., Molaro, S. (Writer), & Cendrowski, M. (Director). (2009). Friendship algorithm [Television series episode]. In C. Lorre (Producer), *The big bang theory.* Los Angeles, CA: Warner Brothers Television.

Matson, J. L., Matson, M. L., & Rivet, T. T. (2007). Social-skills treatments for children with autism spectrum disorders: An overview. *Behavior Modification, 31*(5), 682–707.

Mayes, S. D., Gorman, A. A., Hillwig-Garcia, J., & Syed, E. (2013). Suicide ideation and attempts in children with autism. *Research in Autism Spectrum Disorders, 7*(1), 109–119.

Milne, C., Leaf, J. A., Townley-Cochran, D., Leaf, J. B., & Oppenheim-Leaf, M. (2015). *Teaching social behaviors to individuals with autism: Within the context of a social skills group*. Paper presented at the meeting of the Association of Behavior Analysis, San Antonio, TX.

Newschaffer, C. J., Falb, M. D., & Gurney, J. G. (2005). National autism prevalence trends from United States special education data. *Pediatrics, 115*(3), e277–e282.

Oppenheim-Leaf, M. L., Leaf, J. B., Dozier, C., Sheldon, J. B., & Sherman, J. A. (2012). Teaching typically developing children to promote social play with their siblings with autism. *Research in Autism Spectrum Disorders, 6*(2), 777–791.

Partington, J. W. (2006). *Assessment of basic language and learning skills-revised (The ABLLS-R): An assessment, curriculum guide, and skills tracking system for children with autism or other developmental disabilities*. Pleasant Hill, CA: Behavior Analysts.

Reynolds, C. R., & Kamphaus, R. W. (2015). *Behavior assessment system for children* (3rd ed.). San Antonio, TX: The Psychological Corporation.

Santiago, J. L., Hanley, G. P., Moore, K., & Jin, S. C. (2016). The generality of interview-informed functional analyses: Systematic replications in school and home. *Journal of Autism and Developmental Disorders, 46*(3), 797–811.

Sparrow, S. S., Cicchetti, D. V., & Saulnier, C. A. (2016). *Vineland adaptive behavior scales* (3rd ed.). Bloomington, MN: NCS Pearson, Inc.

Stasolla, F., Perilli, V., Boccasini, A., Caffo, A. O., Damiani, R., & Albano, V. (2016). Enhancing academic performance of three boys with autism spectrum disorders and intellectual disabilities through a computer-based program. *Life Span and Disability, 19*(2), 153–183.

Soto-Icaza, P., Aboitiz, F., & Billeke, P. (2015). Development of social skills in children: Neural and behavioral evidence for the elaboration of cognitive models. *Frontiers in Neuroscience, 9*, 333.

Sundberg, M. L., & Michael, J. (2001). The benefits of Skinner's analysis of verbal behavior for children with autism. *Behavior Modification, 25*(5), 698–724.

Tager-Flusberg, H. (1981). On the nature of linguistic functioning in early infantile autism. *Journal of Autism and Developmental Disorders, 11*(1), 45–56.

Taylor, B. A., & Hoch, H. (2008). Teaching children with autism to respond to an initiate bids for joint attention. *Journal of Applied Behavior Analysis, 41*(3), 377–391.

Taubman, M., Leaf, R., & McEachin, J. (2011). *Crafting connections: Contemporary applied behavior analysis for enriching the social lives of person with autism spectrum disorder*. New York: DRL Books.

Taubman, M. T., Leaf, R. B., McEachin, J. & Leaf, J. B. (2012) *Teaching social skills that change lives: Developing meaningful relationships for people diagnosed with autism*. Workshop to the International Association of Applied Behavior Analysis, Seattle, WA.

Wheat, J., & Baker, T. (2010). HELP 3-6 assessment manual (2nd Ed.). P. Teaford (Ed.), Retrieved from http://www.vort.com/HELP-3-6-Assessment-Manual-2nd-Ed.html

Wunderlich, K. L., & Vollmer, T. R. (2015). Data analysis of response interruption and redirection as treatment for vocal stereotypy. *Journal of Applied Behavior Analysis, 48*(4), 749–764.

Yaylaci, F., & Miral, S. (2017). A comparison of DSM-IV-TR and DSM-5 diagnostic classifications in the clinical diganosis of autistic spectrum disorder. *Journal of Autism and Developmental Disorders, 47*(1), 101–109.

Part I

Social Skills Deficits

2 Understanding the Social Nature of Autism: From Clinical Manifestations to Brain Mechanisms

Fred R. Volkmar and Brent van der Wyk

Beginning in the 1800s, reports of "wild" or feral children and other children we might now recognize as having autism began to appear (Donvan & Zucker, 2016), but it was not until the 1940s in reports by Leo Kanner (1943) and Hans Asperger (1944) that autism spectrum disorder (ASD) began to be clearly recognized. In their papers, Asperger and Kanner both used the word "autism" to suggest a special difficulty of social interaction exhibited in the cases they observed. As time has gone on, the unusual social nature of autism has been more clearly recognized, and much progress has been made in understanding, at the basic science level, potential mechanisms and best approaches to treatment (McPartland, Tillman, Yang, Bernier, & Pelphrey, 2014; Reichow & Barton, 2014; Voos et al., 2013).

Early controversy on the nature of autism began to shift in the 1970s, as it became clear that autism was a brain-based disorder (given the high rates of seizure disorders children exhibited in adolescence; Volkmar & Nelson, 1990) and had a very strong genetic basis given the much higher concordance rates in monozygotic twins (Folstein & Rutter, 1977). It also became clear that autism responded more positively to structured interventions rather than unstructured psychotherapy (Bartak & Rutter, 1976). Since the official recognition of autism in 1980 (DSM III APA, 1980), research has exploded. With earlier detection and intervention, many individuals with autism and related conditions are now functioning independently in community settings (Howlin, Moss, Savage, Bolton, & Rutter, 2015) and indeed sometimes, as adults, appearing to no longer exhibit the condition (strictly defined; Fein et al., 2013).

In this chapter, we selectively review some aspects of this unique constellation of social difficulties noted in autism and related ASD both as they manifest clinically and as they may be related to brain mechanisms. In summarizing these results, we argue for a new conceptualization of autism that emphasizes these social learning problems as central. We should note that it is a testament to the field that this review cannot aim, in the space available, to be anything but selective, highlighting those aspects of social difficulties that appear to us most salient in terms of clinical or research relevance.

2.1 Autism as a Central Feature of the Condition

In his 1943 report, Kanner emphasized that autism (lack of interest in others) was one of two cardinal features of the condition (resistance to change and oversensitivity to the nonsocial

F.R. Volkmar, MD (✉) • B. van der Wyk, PhD
Yale University School of Medicine,
New Haven, CT, USA
e-mail: fred.volkmar@yale.edu

J.B. Leaf (ed.), *Handbook of Social Skills and Autism Spectrum Disorder*, Autism and Child Psychopathology Series, DOI 10.1007/978-3-319-62995-7_2

environment being the other). His insightful description served as the basis for subsequent refinements of the concept (Volkmar & Reichow, 2014). Kanner emphasized that the social disability in autism was marked and profound, and impacted the child's ability to understand and learn from others. This core disability helps us understand the impact of ASD on aspects of learning, communication, multitasking, and behavior.

Attempts to define autistic social dysfunction have evolved over time. In his very influential synthesis of Kanner's original report and subsequent work, Rutter (1978) emphasized delayed and deviant social development NOT simply the functioning of overall developmental delay. Other early investigators similarly identified social difficulties as a central diagnostic feature (Wing & Gould, 1979). This tradition continued in the DSM-III (Diagnostic and Statistical Manual 3rd Ed.) and its various successors (see Volkmar & McPartland, 2014).

Although there is general agreement that "autism" – that is the serious social disability – is the defining feature of ASD (Grossman, Carter, & Volkmar, 1997), attempts at more detailed characterization have been complicated. The complications arise given changes with age and developmental level, as well as major differences in approaches (e.g., should social problem be assessed relative to normative development or should specific abnormal features by identified). Quantification of social problems plagued the field for many years. On one side, attempts to estimate levels of severity are reflected in screening and diagnostic instruments looking at the "severity" of autism (e.g., on instruments like the ADOS (Autism Diagnostic Observation Scale) or CARS (Childhood Autism Rating Scale); see Lord, Corsello, & Grzadzinski, 2014). On the other hand, there are some approaches that assess social levels based on normative social processes such as normed tasks of memory for faces (Klin et al., 1999) or assess socialization skills based on instruments like the Vineland Adaptive Behavior Scales (Volkmar et al., 1987). As we note subsequently, a series of innovative measures have now been developed as part of the study of brain processing social information and may offer alternative approaches. For example, work from the initial eye tracking studies conducted at Yale (Klin, Jones, Schultz, Volkmar, & Cohen, 2002) revealed major differences in the way more cognitively able individuals with autism viewed the social "panorama," as measured by infrared cameras, during observation of short clips from the movie classic *Who's Afraid of Virginia Wolff*. In that initial study, there was essentially no overlap between the groups in terms of focusing on eyes in the scenes (with a Cohen's *d* of 3.6) (Fig. 2.1).

Progress has also been made in the area of genetics. It has become clear that many genes are potentially involved with a broader autism phenotype likely exhibiting some, but not all, of the features of those individuals with more classic autism (Ingersoll et al., 2014; Rutter & Thapar, 2014). Although the relationship between social vulnerabilities to genetic vulnerabilities remains to be specified, work using more precise and sophisticated animal models is now underway (Thirtamara Rajamani, 2015).

2.2 A Selective Review of Specific Areas of Social Disturbance

2.2.1 Attachment

The process of attachment serves to give the developing infant opportunities for bonding and to develop complex social relationships with primary caregivers. In typically developing children, this process is quite robust, and while life long, becomes particularly noteworthy around 9–10 months as infants become quite comfortable with parents and quite wary of strangers. Attachment is manifested through a number of behaviors that include maintenance of proximity to caregivers as well as strong affective connections (Rutter, 2008). Early impressions of an absence of parental attachment in autism proved to be incorrect as a series of studies indicated some attachment to parents – albeit sometimes in atypical ways (Rogers, Ozonoff, & Maslin-Cole, 1991, 1993).

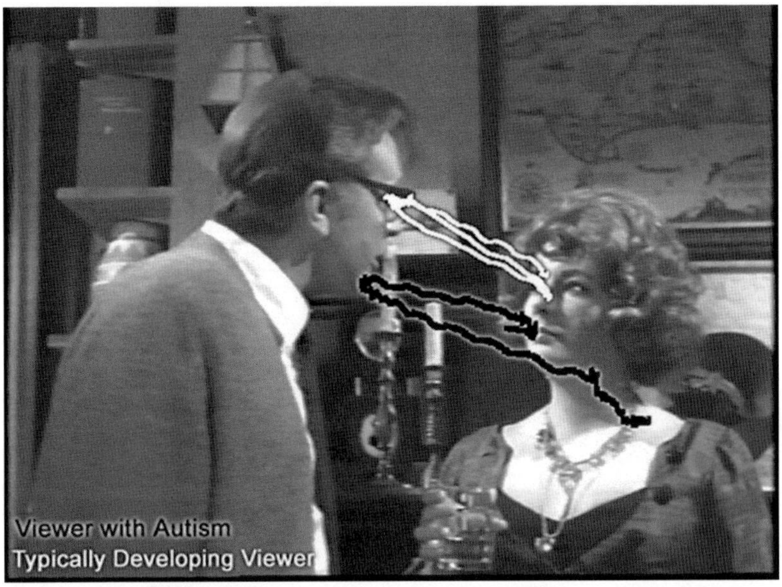

Fig. 2.1 Visual focus of a typically developing adult (top line) and a high functioning man with autism (bottom line) while moving a short movie clip from the class film *Who's Afraid of Virginia Woolf?* The typically developing individual focuses on the top portion of the face while observing the interaction. The individual with autism focuses on the mouth region (losing much of the social–emotional information; Reprinted, with permission, from Klin et al., 2002).

For example, young children with autism are apparently more likely to exhibit disorganized patterns of attachment than typically developing children (Claussen, Mundy, Mallik, & Willoughby, 2002). In addition, they may exhibit unusual attachments to inanimate objects (i.e., in contrast to the usual "transitional objects" of children, typically soft and intensely specific) and to hard objects (bundles of twigs, cereal boxes, and toy trains); it is the category of objects rather than the special objects that is of paramount importance (Volkmar et al., 1994).

2.2.2 Perception of Faces

Faces have special salience for a newborn child. The ability to look at faces and derive meaning and information from facial expression is an important prerequisite for many other social skills. Clearly, there are alternate pathways, for example, blind infants usually develop social skills in typical ways albeit with understandable delays in some areas such as joint attention (Bigelow, 2003). The interest in faces appears to be innate in a typically developing child with a very early preference for looking at faces or face-like stimuli, relatively rapid recognition of parent's faces, use of the top half of the face as a source of greater information (Farah, Wilson, Drain, & Tanaka, 1998), and activation of a specific areas of the brain (the fusiform gyrus) for aspects of facial recognition (Kanwisher, McDermott, & Chun, 1997). Sophistication in facial recognition and face processing continues to develop at a rapid pace during the first year of life. By the first birthday, the typically developing child is exquisitely sensitive to familiar and unfamiliar faces and has difficulties processing faces if the latter are presented upside down (the facial inversion effect). Face processing is smooth and rapid by this time and continues to develop over the next years of life (Fabio Falck-Ytter, 2008).

A substantial body of work now exists on difficulties in facial perception in individuals with ASD. This work uses various methods, based on behavioral responses, neurophysiological correlates (electroencephalogram [EEG]), and neuroanatomy (e.g., functional magnetic resonance imaging [fMRI]). These difficulties (some of which are discussed in greater detail in subsequent portions of the chapter) manifest clinically by the early onset of difficulties with gaze, difficulty using the face to regulate and derive meaning in social interaction, and lack of eye contact (Chawarska et al., 2014a; Chawarska, Macari, Volkmar, Kim, and Shic, 2014b). Behaviorally, these difficulties are also expressed in diminished social–emotional responses to others. These impairments include reduced eye contact, joint attention, social orienting, deficits in the imitation of faces and in the face recognition, attenuated responses to emotional displays of others and in gaze behaviors (McPartland, Webb, Keehn, & Dawson, 2011), and may have implications for imitation in general (Rogers, Cook, & Meryl, 2014).

Some of the earliest work with young children relied on retrospective analysis of videotapes (e.g., made at the child's first birthday – often a rather social event albeit one in a familiar environmental context). For example, Osterling and Dawson (1994) revealed that children subsequently diagnosed with ASD paid significantly less attention to faces than typically developing controls. Other work with older individuals has used a range of methods. For example, behavioral studies have revealed difficulties with tasks that involve face processing (Dawson, Webb, & McPartland, 2005), some differences in processing inverted faces (Fabio Falck-Ytter, 2008), and lack of some of the usual early markers of evolved facial perception such as the lack of the facial inversion effect in autism as well as facial memory (Klin et al., 1999). These difficulties also involve problems with the use of emotional information provided by the face to guide accurate perception and awareness of others (Tanaka et al., 2012). Studies have also shown differences in the process of face recognition. For example, typically developing children employ a piecemeal processing strategy in looking at objects, but not at faces. While in ASD, face processing is more like that of a typical child in looking at objects (Chawarska & Shic, 2009).

As we discuss subsequently, a growing body of work has used EEG and fMRI methods to clarify neurophysiological and neuroanatomical correlates of these abilities, and new experimental procedures (e.g., eye tracking) have been used to clarify, in much greater detail, specific differences in processes such as face perception. As a practical matter for the developing child with autism, the nonsocial world has much greater salience (relative to the typically developing children) – a phenomenon strongly emphasized by Kanner (1943) in his original report on the condition.

2.2.3 Gaze Behavior and Eye Contact

Unusual aspects of gaze and limited or poor eye contact are frequently noted by parents as some of the first signs of autism. These processes are intimately related to other aspects of social development including facial processing (Chawarska et al., 2014a, 2014b). The ability to engage in mutual gaze is important for both perception of feelings and attentional focus of others, as well as the ability to engage in the back and forth of communication in social interactions (Mundy, 2016). As with face processing, the interest in others is expressed early on in the typically developing infants ability to focus on the parent, while in infants with ASD, reduced levels of mutual gaze are striking (McPartland et al., 2011). Data are somewhat conflicting on the age at which this can first be demonstrated, with some evidence suggesting it can be observed as early as 6 months and other work suggesting this is less clear until about 18 months (Chawarska, Volkmar, & Klin, 2010; Ozonoff & South, 2001; Young, Merin, Rogers, & Ozonoff, 2009). In this and other studies, differences in methods are likely critical. Data from eye tracking have been, perhaps, the most convincing demonstration of early differences (Chawarska, Macari, & Shic, 2013).

2.2.4 Imitation

The desire to imitate emerges very early in typical development. Imitation is important in laying the foundation for many other skills including communication. A considerable amount of research on the emergence of imitation in autism has revealed substantial impairments in imitation, in all its various forms, and these difficulties are interrelated with other core social abilities such as joint attention, play, and emerging communication abilities (for a review, see Rogers, 2014). It has been argued that difficulties in this area are a core aspect of autism (Rogers & Pennington, 1991). Although this issue remains a topic of theoretical debate, there is widespread agreement that intervention focused on enhancing imitation and social attention is essential for young children with autism (Rogers et al., 2006).

Intervention for imitation difficulties has focused on the various forms of imitative activities, for example, object imitation (Ingersoll, Lewis, & Kroman, 2007), motor imitation (Ingersoll & Schreibman, 2006), gestural imitation (Ingersoll et al., 2007; Ingersoll & Schreibman, 2006), and overall imitation (Ozonoff & Cathcart, 1998). Although it is generally assumed that enhanced abilities in imitation will be related to gains in other areas, few studies have directly addressed the issue, but the work available suggests important gains in related skills such as communication, play, joint attention, and overall cognitive abilities (Ozonoff & Cathcart, 1998; Rogers & Vismara, 2014). A number of the model programs developed for young children with autism target imitation as a critical developmental skill, for example, the Early Start Denver Model of Rogers, Dawson, and Vismara (2012), Pivotal Response Training (Koegel & Frea, 1993), and applied behavior analytic models (Ingersoll et al., 2007). Fostering imitation is also naturally involved in interventions targeting other abilities such as joint attention and play (Kasari, Freeman, & Paparella, 2001; Kasari, Huynh, & Gulsrud, 2011).

2.2.5 Play Skills

Although difficult to define, play is a central activity of childhood. It involves important cognitive, motor, and social aspects and becomes symbolic, an important foundation for other skills (Piaget, 1952). Play begins with simple object manipulation (sensorimotor play) and then progresses to functional play (e.g., using materials in conventional ways) and finally becomes much more symbolic and complex play (where the activity of play is much less constrained by the actual materials present). For example, a small cup might be used initially for banging or smelling, but then becomes used for functional play such as feeding a doll, to then becoming rather unconstrained so that the cup might assume any number of symbolic functions. There are important cultural and contextual factors in understanding play, and play is a central focus of children's lives during preschool (and beyond) and serves as a practice ground both for pretense and as a pleasurable shared joint experience with parents, siblings, and with peers. Piaget (1952) emphasized the importance of play for cognitive development.

Difficulties in symbolic play in ASD have been well documented since the 1970s (Ricks & Wing, 1975). Subsequent work confirmed the lack of symbolic play in young children with autism (Wing, Gould, Yeates, & Brierley, 1977) with play tending to be stereotypic and repetitive with difficulties extending to both nonsymbolic and symbolic play (Ungerer & Sigman, 1981). These difficulties extend to the easiest forms of play so that both sensorimotor and functional play skills are delayed and/or deviant in their development even when overall cognitive ability is controlled.

Intervention studies have shown that a range of methods can be used to improve play skills. These include both direct, as well as, more naturalistic teaching and the use of peers (particularly in the preschool period) to facilitate play abilities (Kasari, Freeman, & Paparella, 2006; Rogers, 2005).

2.3 Neural Aspects of Social Information Processing

2.3.1 Early Studies of Social Cognition

Social and affective processing has been, until recently, a rather neglected branch of cognitive psychology. The prevailing attitude was that complex social behaviors could be explained as the aggregation of simpler and more foundational cognitive components: attention, memory, etc. However, concerted research efforts during the 1970s and 1980s led to a set of findings that challenged this established view and argued for dedicated cognitive mechanisms for social information processing. Behavioral studies of face processing (Valentine, 1988; Yin, 1969) and biological motion (Johansson, 1973; Kozlowski & Cutting, 1977) suggested specialized mechanisms for this kind of social perception. Similarly, Cosmides and Tooby (1992) pursued a research program that argued convincingly for specialized mechanisms for social reasoning. At the time, investigation of the neural bases of such function in healthy subjects was beyond the ability of science, but studies of patients with brain damage, developmental disorders, and electrophysiological studies of nonhuman primates all began to point to dedicated neural mechanisms for a number of social processes (Bauer, 1984; Brothers, 1990; Signer, 1987). This work came together in a seminal article by Brothers (2002), in which the term "social brain" was coined. Brothers argued that the evidence suggested that not only were there good reasons to suspect that specializations for social information processing is evolutionarily adaptive, but that by the evidentiary standards of the day, social processing was a cognitive module – an innately specialized and encapsulated neurocognitive mechanism (Fodor, 1986). The elevation of social cognition to "modular" status placed it on par with language in the pantheon of cognitive psychology and jump started a research program that continues to this day into the neural bases of social cognition.

At the time, the awareness that ASD was primarily a disorder of social cognition led researchers to study the condition. Indeed, the field of social cognition has benefited from the growing awareness of and attention to ASD and lifted it from a niche research area to one with profound public health significance. This work also benefited from coincident developments in human brain imaging methods, most notably, fMRI.

fMRI uses powerful magnetic fields to image regional changes in blood oxygenation. These changes are thought to be driven by the metabolic needs of neurons that fluctuate as a function of their activity. A standard strategy in an fMRI experiment is to present stimuli to individuals and measure the resulting blood oxygenation-dependent signal (BOLD). Differences in the BOLD signal, as a function of stimuli or task, are interpreted as differences in the underlying brain activation to those signals. As fMRI is noninvasive, it provided the opportunity to study aspects of brain function in healthy controls. An advantage that fMRI had over other noninvasive methods, such EEG and ERP, was an incredibly high degree of spatial accuracy. It was this spatial resolution that was particularly attractive to researchers interested in finding and cataloging the neural correlates of various modules of cognition, and in this respect, social cognition was no different.

2.3.2 Key Nodes of Social Cognition in Healthy Individuals

Brothers (1990, 2002) identified several cortical and subcortical nodes of the social brain, namely the orbitofrontal cortex, the temporal cortex, and the amygdala, (Kling & Brothers, 1992; Perrett, Hietanen, Oram, Benson, & Rolls, 1992; Raleigh & Steklis, 1981). Much of the evidence implicating these regions came from the study of nonhuman primates, using electrophysiology and experimentally induced lesions. In humans, early fMRI studies supported the initial delineation of the social brain with only minor revisions. In a set of early studies of face processing, two subsets of the temporal cortex were identified on the fusiform gyrus and the super temporal sulcus (Haxby, Hoffman, & Gobbini, 2000; Kanwisher et al., 1997; McCarthy, Puce, Gore, & Allison, 1997). Simple contrasts of static face versus nonface stimuli activated a region on the fusiform gyrus on the ventral surface of the temporal lobe, termed the fusiform face area (FFA). More complex facial stimuli, which captured dynamic aspects of a face in motion, tended to activate a lateral and posterior surface of the temporal lobe in the superior temporal sulcus (STS; Beauchamp, Lee, Haxby, & Martin, 2003; Pelphrey, Singerman, Allison, & McCarthy, 2003b). Emotion in faces, especially negative affect, tended to activate the amygdala, consistent with social brain theory (Breiter et al., 1996). The orbitofrontal cortex, extending dorsally along the medial surface of the prefrontal cortex and the dorsal medial prefrontal cortex (dmPFC), was associated with mentalization (Happe et al., 1996) and affective arousal (Ketter, George, Kimbrell, Benson, & Post, 1996).

However, new regions and functions were also being discovered. For example, while fearful faces activated the amygdala, in addition to the FFA, disgusted faces activated the insula that was also activated during the experience of disgust (Phillips et al., 1997). The perception of bodies and actions also required the extension of initial theory. Regions in the posterior temporal cortex were activated by the perception of bodies (Chan, Peelen, & Downing, 2004; Downing, Jiang, Shuman, & Kanwisher, 2001). The STS itself was also found to be active to the perceptions of bodily movement (Bonda, Petrides, Ostry, & Evans, 1996; Carter & Pelphrey, 2006; Pelphrey et al., 2003; Puce & Perrett, 2003) and were modulated by the social and mental significance of those actions (Beauchamp et al., 2003; Vander Wyk, Hudac, Carter, Sobel, & Pelphrey, 2009; Vander Wyk, Voos, & Pelphrey, 2012). Finally, with respect to mentalization and theory of mind, regions in the temporoparietal junction (TPJ) were activated during such tasks (Castelli, Happé, Frith, & Frith, 2000; Gallagher & Frith, 2003; Saxe & Kanwisher, 2003; Völlm et al., 2006) and have spawned a lively and ongoing debate as to how functional roles are partitioned across these regions (Buccino et al., 2007; see also Farah et al., 1998).

A surprising addition to the set of social regions came from electrophysiological studies in nonhuman primates. While studying the response properties of motor neurons, researchers identified neurons, now dubbed "mirror neurons," that fired in response to both the performance and observation of specific actions (Rizzolatti, Fogassi, & Gallese, 2001). The response properties of mirror neurons are intriguing because they might represent a mechanism by which the affective or cognitive state, which is hidden from direct observation, could be related to detailed knowledge about one's own affect and cognition. For example, during action perception, merely representing the ongoing details of a bodily motion misses a great deal of useful and predictive information about why the action was being taken. Thus, the additional computational challenge for the observer is to decode from those actions potential motivating goals, beliefs, and affect. As mirror neurons appeared to play a role in the self-generation of actions, they were proposed to have a more direct association with the goals, beliefs, and actions that the observer themselves would have when activating that action plan (Rizzolatti, 2005; Uddin, Iacoboni, Lange, & Keenan, 2007). Their activation during observation, thus, would permit the activation of mental states that the observer could infer the actor as having (Meltzoff & Brooks, 2001). The evidence for a mirror neuron system in human neuroimaging is complex. Many studies reported mirror neuron-like patterns of activation (e.g., Gazzola & Keysers, 2009; Lacoboni et al., 1999). But other studies note, or have argued, that any cognitive inferences from action to underlying mental intention can be performed without reference to mirror neurons (Kilner & Frith, 2008; Lingnau, Gesierich, & Caramazza, 2009; Turella, Pierno, Tubaldi, & Castiello, 2009).

Nevertheless, the notion of social representations of others rising out of self-representation has a long history in developmental and social psychology (Lacoboni, 2009; Meltzoff, 1990). For example, physical imitation, which can be observed even in very young infants (Meltzoff & Moore, 1977), was thought to be a precursor to more sophisticated social learning and even abstract social cognitive phenomena divorced from purely physical embodiment, such as empathy and theory of mind (Bandura, 1962). Mirror neurons presented as potential mechanism for at least the early stages of this development and their discovery energized the investigation into the neural bases of these relatively high-level social phenomena (Gallese, 2001; Kaplan & Lacoboni, 2006; Lacoboni, 2009; Lacoboni et al., 1999; Molnar-Szakacs & Overy, 2006; Williams, Whiten, Suddendorf, & Perrett, 2001). As with many efforts in social cognitive neuroscience, from a relatively circumscribed list, the number of potential regions identified as part of the "mirror neuron system" has expanded (for a review, see Molenberghs, Cunnington, & Mattingley, 2012).

2.3.3 Social Neuroscience of ASDs

ASDs have been at the heart of many discussions in social neuroscience from the very beginning. In Brothers' (1990) article, autism was presented as evidence for the modularity of the social processing system. Since then, virtually every aspect of social cognition has been examined in ASD samples in some way or another (for a recent review, see Philip et al., 2012). With respect to social perception and face/body motion perception, differences in brain activation between individuals on the spectrum and healthy controls observed are generally consistent with behavioral difficulties seen in these individuals. For example, early studies report less selective activation of the fusiform in ASD relative to healthy controls during face processing (Schultz et al., 2000; Wang, Dapretto, Hariri, Sigman, & Bookheimer, 2004; although for other perspectives, see Hadjikhani et al., 2004; Hadjikhani, Joseph, Snyder, & Tager-Flusberg, 2007) as well as in the STS during action perception (Ahmed & Vander Wyk, 2013; Blake, Turner, Smoski, Pozdol, & Stone, 2003; Freitag et al., 2008). Similarly, both the dmPFC and the TPJ showed a similar lack of selective activation during mentalization tasks in individuals with ASD (Happe et al., 1996; Lombardo, Chakrabarti, Bullmore, Baron-Cohen, & Consortium, 2011; Silani et al., 2008). Similar findings can be found in other domains of social cognition. Thus, one of the most consistent results from this work has been a relative lack of specialization in the core circuits for social cognition. However, other findings are also worth considering, and here we take the ongoing study of face processing as an example.

Even in the early fMRI studies of face processing, there were hints that there was more than simply a lack of specialization in the ASD samples. Studies found that individuals on the spectrum recruited other brain regions outside of the fusiform to a greater degree than healthy controls (Pierce, Müller, Ambrose, Allen, & Courchesne, 2001; Schultz et al., 2000). This suggests two, not necessarily distinct, possibilities. First, it may be that ASD is associated with an intrinsically large-scale reorganization of cortical circuitry, which includes both regional increases and decreases in activation during social cognition tasks. Recent studies of large-scale cortical networks are consistent with this account showing a relatively broad difference in the pattern of connectivity in ASD (Minshew & Williams, 2007; Monk et al., 2009). These data are often collected while the individual is at rest, reducing the chances that the differences are due to differences in explicit strategies.

A second possibility is that individuals with ASD selectively or strategically engage with social tasks differently than typically developing controls. For instance, individuals with ASD tend not to look directly at eyes when looking at faces (Pelphrey et al., 2002). This differential engagement would be expected to have consequences for the resulting brain activation. In one study, input selectivity was experimentally manipulated by having controls and individuals with ASD attend to locations on a face that corresponded to greater or lesser amounts of eye contact (Perlman, Hudac, Pegors, Minshew, & Pelphrey, 2011). In high eye contact conditions, individuals with ASD showed relatively normal levels of fusiform activation. Results such as these suggest preserved function in socially selective regions that may be accessible through top-down strategic manipulation of behaviors. However, it remains to be seen whether such findings are robust or predict social function in individuals.

2.3.4 Key Limitations in Research

The study of the brain function in ASD extends well-beyond face processing, but this subset of the literature is illustrative of key strengths and limitations of neuroimaging applied to the study of ASD. First, few results have been consistently replicated. For example, studies have found hypo-, hyper-, and normal activation in the fusiform gyrus during different face processing tasks in individuals with ASD relative to typically developing individuals. This variability is due in part to the enormous heterogeneity intrinsic to the disorder. But it is also due to the small sample sizes typical of neuroimaging studies and methodological variation across labs in the choice of task and condition contrast.

2.3.5 Theoretical Models

A number of different overarching theoretical models have been proposed to account for the social difficulties in autism. At the more global level, these have posited deficits in theory of mind (Baron-Cohen, Leslie, & Frith, 1985), difficulties in executive functioning (Corbett, Constantine, Hendren, Rocke, & Ozonoff, 2009), central coherence (Happe, Briskman, & Frith, 2001), the extreme male brain (Baron-Cohen, 2002), and enactive mind (Klin, Jones, Schultz, & Volkmar, 2014). As a practical matter, these theories have been helpful in stimulating research, even though they have their limitations and often significantly overlap to some degree (South, Ozonoff, & McMahon, 2007; for a comprehensive review, see Chown, 2016).

At a more granulate theoretical level, a range of models have been proposed. Understanding differences in face perception and eye gaze has been a central focus of this effort with a number of competing models proposed. For example, (1) it has been proposed that eye contact and gaze are actively avoided because it is experienced as aversive (Hutt, Hutt, Lee, & Ounsted, 1964), or (2) that due to hypoactivation of structures, like the amygdala, eye contact is not associated with a positive social experience (Shultz, Klin, & Jones, 2011), or (3) that eye contact is much less salient and thus interferes with social communication (Senju, Southgate, White, & Frith, 2009), or (4) that it is disturbance related to difficulties in subcortical and cortical brain systems pathways that process social information (Kliemann, Dziobek, Hatri, Baudewig, & Heekeren, 2012).

2.3.6 Implications for Treatment

It has long been recognized that the social learning problems of autism were rightly a major focus of treatment. The highly influential report from the National Research Council on Educating Young Children with Autism (2001) highlighted the importance of enhanced social engagement for learning and developmental progress. Over time, a number of different approaches for enhancing social skills in general, and relative to specific social processes in particular, have been made (for a comprehensive review of evidence-based approaches, see Ferraioli & Harris, 2011).

Overall, methods for teaching social skills take several forms. At the more general level, approaches for enhancing social skills, vary somewhat, with age. For example, peer inclusion (with some degree of peer training) is helpful particularly in preschool and early school aged children. As children become older, social skills groups (of various types) are used, and with adolescence and adulthood, individual work becomes more common. Various evidence-based methods have been developed for processes as diverse as joint attention, video modeling, imitation, theory of mind skills, etc. and have been utilized with a growing body of work. Some comprehensive models (e.g., the Early Start Denver Model and Pivotal Response Training) emphasize acquisition of important social skills.

The advances made are important, but unfortunately so are the limitations of the available research. Peer inclusion models, adoptions of existent treatment approaches (e.g., like cognitive behavioral therapy), and individualized approaches to teaching social skills and social communication skills continue to be important. Unfortunately, the available literature relative to adolescents and adults (where social differences are often acutely experienced) remains quite limited indeed.

2.4 Summary

Researchers have demonstrated that ASD is an early onset neurodevelopmental disorder characterized from the beginning by a profound social disability; this impacts the developing child's motivation and ability to undemand others and develop truly reciprocal relationships. It has far reaching impact on styles of learning and information processing. Although progress has been made in identifying potential neural mechanisms, the brain basis of the condition remains complex and relatively poorly understood. On the other hand, the work available has demonstrated some of the potential "downstream" impacts of this social disability. In some respects, it may, perhaps, be better to regard autism and related conditions as disorders of social learning. From a practical standpoint, it is clear that the fundamental principles of treatment are to minimize negative aspects of autism and their impact on learning, and maximize, to the extent possible, both more normative developmental processes and alternative pathways to social leaning. As with basic research on brain mechanisms, a body of intervention research has now developed (Reichow & Barton, 2014; Reichow, Doehring, Cicchetti, & Volkmar, 2011) and, for many, but sadly not all, individual outcome appears to be improving (Fein et al., 2013). In this chapter, we have reviewed the clinical manifestations of social dysfunction in autism as well as potential neural mechanisms. We have also summarized some aspects of intervention and theory as they relate to this issue. Clearly, a major theme of this entire body of work has been to more precisely delineate what is likely to be a highly heterogeneous social phenotype. Hopefully, with changes in improved methods of characterization and the use of more ecologically valid methods for examining specific mechanisms of social dysfunction, progress will continue and lead to more truly comprehensive theories. Future work must be truly interdisciplinary and transdisciplinary for this to be achieved.

References

Ahmed, A. A., & Vander Wyk, B. C. (2013). Neural processing of intentional biological motion in unaffected siblings of children with autism spectrum disorder: An fMRI study. *Brain and Cognition, 83*(3), 297–306. doi:10.1016/j.bandc.2013.09.007

Amrican Psuyhiatric Association. (1980). *Diagnostic and statistical manual*. Washington, DC: APA Press.

Asperger, H. (1944). Die "autistichen Psychopathen" im Kindersalter. *Archive furpsychiatrie und Nervenkrankheiten, 117*, 76–136.

Bandura, A. (1962). Social learning through imitation. In M. R. Jones (Ed.), *Nebraska symposium on motivation*. Lincoln, NE: University of Nebraska Press.

Baron-Cohen, S. (2002). The extreme male brain theory of autism. *Trends in Cognitive Sciences, 6*, 248–254.

Baron-Cohen, S., Leslie, A. M., & Frith, U. (1985). Does the autistic child have a "theory of mind?". *Cognition, 21*(1), 37–46.

Bartak, L., & Rutter, M. (1976). Differences between mentally retarded and normally intelligent autistic children. *Journal of Autism and Childhood Schizophrenia, 6*(2), 109–120.

Bauer, R. M. (1984). Autonomic recognition of names and faces in prosopagnosia: A neuropsychological application of the guilty knowledge test. *Neuropsychologia, 22*(4), 457–469.

Beauchamp, M. S., Lee, K. E., Haxby, J. V., & Martin, A. (2003). FMRI responses to video and point-light displays of moving humans and manipulable objects. *Journal of Cognitive Neuroscience, 15*(7), 991–1001.

Bigelow, A. E. (2003). The development of joint attention in blind infants. *Development and Psychopathology, 15*(2), 259–275.

Blake, R., Turner, L. M., Smoski, M. J., Pozdol, S. L., & Stone, W. L. (2003). Visual recognition of biological motion is impaired in children with autism. *Psychological Science, 14*(2), 151–157.

Bonda, E., Petrides, M., Ostry, D., & Evans, A. (1996). Specific involvement of human parietal systems and the amygdala in the perception of biological motion. *The Journal of Neuroscience, 16*(11), 3737–3744.

Breiter, H. C., Etcoff, N. L., Whalen, P. J., Kennedy, W. A., Rauch, S. L., Buckner, R. L., & Rosen, B. R. (1996). Response and habituation of the human amygdala during visual processing of facial expression. *Neuron, 17*(5), 875–887.

Brothers, L. (1990). The neural basis of primate social communication. *Motivation and Emotion, 14*(2), 81–91.

Brothers, L. (2002). The social brain: A project for integrating primate behavior and neurophysiology in a new domain. In J. T. Cacioppo (Ed.), *Foundations in social neuroscience* (pp. 367–385). Cambridge: MIT Press.

Buccino, G., Binkofski, F., Fink, G. R., Fadiga, L., Fogassi, L., Gallese, V., … Henson, R. N. (2007).

Separate coding of different gaze directions in the superior temporal sulcus and inferior parietal lobule. *Current Biology*, *17*(1), 20–25.

Carter, E. J., & Pelphrey, K. A. (2006). School-aged children exhibit domain-specific responses to biological motion. *Social Neuroscience*, *1*(3–4), 396–411.

Castelli, F., Happé, F., Frith, U., & Frith, C. (2000). Movement and mind: A functional imaging study of perception and interpretation of complex intentional movement patterns. *NeuroImage*, *12*(3), 314–325.

Chan, A. W., Peelen, M. V., & Downing, P. E. (2004). The effect of viewpoint on body representation in the extrastriate body area. *Neuroreport*, *15*(15), 2407–2410.

Chawarska, K., Macari, S., & Shic, F. (2013). Decreased spontaneous attention to social scenes in 6-month-old infants later diagnosed with autism spectrum disorders. *Biological Psychiatry*, *74*(3), 195–203.

Chawarska, K., Macari, S., Volkmar, F. R., Kim, S. H., & Shic, F. (2014a). ASD in infants and toddlers. In *Handbook of autism and pervasive developmental disorders, Volume 1: Diagnosis, development, and brain mechanisms* (pp. 121–147). Hoboken, NJ: John Wiley & Sons Inc.

Chawarska, K., Macari, S. L., Volkmar, F. R., Kim, S. H., Shic, F., Paul, R., … Pelphrey, K. A. (2014b). ASD in infants and toddlers. In *Handbook of autism and pervasive developmental disorders* (4th ed.). Hoboken, NJ: John Wiley & Sons, Inc.

Chawarska, K., & Shic, F. (2009). Looking but not seeing: Atypical visual scanning and recognition of faces in 2 and 4-year-old children with autism spectrum disorder. *Journal of Autism and Developmental Disorders*, *39*(12), 1663–1672.

Chawarska, K., Volkmar, F. R., & Klin, A. (2010). Limited attentional bias for faces in toddlers with autism spectrum. *Archives of General Psychiatry*, *67*(2), 178–185.

Chown, N. (2016). *Understanding and evaluating autism theory*. London, UK: Jessica Kingsley.

Claussen, A. H., Mundy, P. C., Mallik, S. A., & Willoughby, J. C. (2002). Joint attention and disorganized attachment status in infants at risk. *Development and Psychopathology*, *14*(2), 279–291.

Corbett, B. A., Constantine, L. J., Hendren, R., Rocke, D., & Ozonoff, S. (2009). Examining executive functioning in children with autism spectrum disorder, attention deficit hyperactivity disorder and typical development. *Psychiatry Research*, *166*(2–3), 210–222.

Cosmides, L., & Tooby, J. (1992). Cognitive adaptations for social exchange. In J. H. Barkow, L. Cosmides, & J. Tooby (Eds.), *The adapted mind: Evolutionary psychology and the generation of culture* (pp. 163–228). Oxford: Oxford University Press.

Dawson, G., Webb, S. J., & McPartland, J. (2005). Understanding the nature of face processing impairment in autism: Insights from behavioral and electrophysiological studies. *Developmental Neuropsychology*, *27*(3), 403–424.

Donvan, J., & Zucker, K. (2016). *In a different key: The story of autism*. New York, NY: Penguin.

Downing, P. E., Jiang, Y., Shuman, M., & Kanwisher, N. (2001). A cortical area selective for visual processing of the human body. *Science*, *293*(5539), 2470–2473.

Fabio Falck-Ytter, T. (2008). Face inversion effects in autism: A combined looking time and pupillometric study. *Autism Research: Official Journal of the International Society for Autism Research*, *1*(5), 297–306.

Farah, M. J., Wilson, K. D., Drain, M., & Tanaka, J. N. (1998). What is "special" about face perception? *Psychological Review*, *105*(3), 482–498.

Fein, D., Barton, M., Eigsti, I. M., Kelley, E., Naigles, L., Schultz, R. T., … Tyson, K. (2013). Optimal outcome in individuals with a history of autism. *Journal of Child Psychology and Psychiatry*, *54*(2), 195–205.

Ferraioli, B., & Harris, S. (2011). Treatments to increase social awareness and social skills. In B. Reichow, P. Doehring, D. Cicchetti, & F. R. Volkmar (Eds.), *Evidence-based practices and treatments for children with autism* (pp. 171–196). New York, NY: Springer.

Fodor, J. A. (1986). *The modularity of mind*. Cambridge, MA: MIT press.

Folstein, S., & Rutter, M. (1977). Infantile autism: A genetic study of 21 twin pairs. *Journal of Child Psychology and Psychiatry, and Allied Disciplines*, *18*(4), 297–321.

Freitag, C. M., Konrad, C., Häberlen, M., Kleser, C., von Gontard, A., Reith, W., … Krick, C. (2008). Perception of biological motion in autism spectrum disorders. *Neuropsychologia*, *46*(5), 1480–1494.

Gallagher, H. L., & Frith, C. D. (2003). Functional imaging of 'theory of mind'. *Trends in Cognitive Sciences*, *7*(2), 77–83.

Gallese, V. (2001). The shared manifold hypothesis. From mirror neurons to empathy. *Journal of Consciousness Studies*, *8*(5–6), 33–50.

Gazzola, V., & Keysers, C. (2009). The observation and execution of actions share motor and somatosensory voxels in all tested subjects: Single-subject analyses of unsmoothed fMRI data. *Cerebral Cortex*, *19*(6), 1239–1255.

Grossman, J. B., Carter, A., & Volkmar, F. R. (1997). Social behavior in autism. *Annals of the New York Academy of Sciences*, *807*, 440–454.

Hadjikhani, N., Joseph, R. M., Snyder, J., Chabris, C. F., Clark, J., Steele, S., … Feczko, E. (2004). Activation of the fusiform gyrus when individuals with autism spectrum disorder view faces. *NeuroImage*, *22*(3), 1141–1150.

Hadjikhani, N., Joseph, R. M., Snyder, J., & Tager-Flusberg, H. (2007). Abnormal activation of the social brain during face perception in autism. *Human Brain Mapping*, *28*(5), 441–449.

Happe, F., Briskman, J., & Frith, U. (2001). Exploring the cognitive phenotype of autism: Weak "central coherence" in parents and siblings of children with autism: I. Experimental tests. *Journal of Child Psychology and Psychiatry, and Allied Disciplines*, *42*(3), 299–307.

Happe, F., Ehlers, S., Fletcher, P., Frith, U., Johansson, M., Gillberg, C., … Frith, C. (1996). Theory of mind in the brain. Evidence from a PET scan study of Asperger syndrome. *Neuroreport*, *8*(1), 197–201.

Haxby, J. V., Hoffman, E. A., & Gobbini, M. I. (2000). The distributed human neural system for face perception. *Trends in Cognitive Sciences*, *4*(6), 223–233.

Howlin, P., Moss, P., Savage, S., Bolton, P., & Rutter, M. (2015). Outcomes in adult life among siblings of individuals with autism. *Journal of Autism and Developmental Disorders*, *45*(3), 707–718.

Hutt, C., Hutt, S. J., Lee, D., & Ounsted, C. (1964). Arousal and childhood autism. *Nature*, *204*, 908–909.

Ingersoll, B., Lewis, E., & Kroman, E. (2007). Teaching the imitation and spontaneous use of descriptive gestures in young children with autism using a naturalistic behavioral intervention. *Journal of Autism and Developmental Disorders*, *37*(8), 1446–1456.

Ingersoll, B., & Schreibman, L. (2006). Teaching reciprocal imitation skills to young children with autism using a naturalistic behavioral approach: Effects on language, pretend play, and joint attention. *Journal of Autism and Developmental Disorders*, *36*(4), 487–505.

Ingersoll, B., Wainer, A., Volkmar, F. R., Paul, R., Rogers, S. J., & Pelphrey, K. A. (2014). The broader autism phenotype. In *Handbook of autism and pervasive developmental disorders* (4th ed.). Hoboken, NJ: John Wiley & Sons.

Johansson, G. (1973). Visual perception of biological motion and a model for its analysis. *Perception & Psychophysics*, *14*(2), 201–211.

Kanner, L. (1943). Autistic disturbances of affective contact. *The Nervous Child*, *2*, 217–250.

Kanwisher, N., McDermott, J., & Chun, M. M. (1997). The fusiform face area: A module in human extrastriate cortex specialized for face perception. *The Journal of Neuroscience*, *17*(11), 4302–4311.

Kaplan, J. T., & Lacoboni, M. (2006). Getting a grip on other minds: Mirror neurons, intention understanding, and cognitive empathy. *Social Neuroscience*, *1*(3–4), 175–183.

Kasari, C., Freeman, S., & Paparella, T. (2006). Joint attention and symbolic play in young children with autism: A randomized controlled intervention study. *Journal of Child Psychology and Psychiatry, and Allied Disciplines*, *47*(6), 611–620.

Kasari, C., Freeman, S. F. N., & Paparella, T. (2001). Early intervention in autism: Joint attention and symbolic play. *International Review of Research in Mental Retardation: Autism*, *23*, 207–237.

Kasari, C., Huynh, L., & Gulsrud, A. C. (2011). Play interventions for children with autism. In S. W. Russ & L. Niec (Eds.), *Play in clinical practice: Evidence-based approaches* (pp. 201–217). New York, NY: Guilford Press.

Ketter, T. A., George, M. S., Kimbrell, T. A., Benson, B. E., & Post, R. M. (1996). Functional brain imaging, limbic function, and affective disorders. *The Neuroscientist*, *2*(1), 55–65.

Kilner, J. M., & Frith, C. D. (2008). Action observation: Inferring intentions without mirror neurons. *Current Biology*, *18*(1), R32–R33.

Kliemann, D., Dziobek, I., Hatri, A., Baudewig, J., & Heekeren, H. R. (2012). The role of the amygdala in atypical gaze on emotional faces in autism spectrum disorders. *The Journal of Neuroscience*, *32*(28), 9469–9476.

Klin, A., Jones, W., Schultz, R. T., & Volkmar, F. R. (2014). The enactive mind-from actions to cognition: Lessons from autism. In F. R. Volkmar, S. J. Rogers, R. Paul, & K. A. Pelphrey (Eds.), *Handbook of autism and pervasive developmental disorders* (vol. 1, pp. 682–703). Hoboken, NJ: Wiley.

Klin, A., Jones, W., Schultz, R. T., Volkmar, F. R., & Cohen, D. (2002). Defining and quantifying the social phenotype in autism. *American Journal of Psychiatry*, *159*(6), 895–908.

Klin, A., Sparrow, S. S., de Bildt, A., Cicchetti, D. V., Cohen, D. J., & Volkmar, F. R. (1999). A normed study of face recognition in autism and related disorders. *Journal of Autism and Developmental Disorders*, *29*(6), 499–508.

Klin, A., Volkmar, F. R., & Sparrow, S. S. (1992). Autistic social dysfunction: Some limitations of the theory of mind hypothesis. *Journal of Child Psychology & Psychiatry & Allied Disciplines*, *33*(5), 861–876.

Kling, A. S., & Brothers, L. A. (1992). The amygdala and social behavior. In J. P. Aggleton (Ed.), *The amygdala : Neurobiological aspects of emotion, memory and mental dysfunction* (pp. 353–378). New York, NY: Wiley-Liss.

Koegel, R. L., & Frea, W. D. (1993). Treatment of social behavior in autism through the modification of pivotal social skills. *Journal of Applied Behavior Analysis*, *26*(3), 369–377.

Kozlowski, L. T., & Cutting, J. E. (1977). Recognizing the sex of a walker from a dynamic point-light display. *Perception & Psychophysics*, *21*(6), 575–580.

Lacoboni, M. (2009). Imitation, empathy, and mirror neurons. *Annual Review of Psychology*, *60*, 653–670.

Lacoboni, M., Woods, R. P., Brass, M., Bekkering, H., Mazziotta, J. C., & Rizzolatti, G. (1999). Cortical mechanisms of human imitation. *Science*, *286*(5449), 2526–2528.

Lingnau, A., Gesierich, B., & Caramazza, A. (2009). Asymmetric fMRI adaptation reveals no evidence for mirror neurons in humans. *Proceedings of the National Academy of Sciences*, *106*(24), 9925–9930.

Lombardo, M. V., Chakrabarti, B., Bullmore, E. T., Baron-Cohen, S., & Consortium, M. A. (2011). Specialization of right temporo-parietal junction for mentalizing and its relation to social impairments in autism. *NeuroImage*, *56*(3), 1832–1838.

Lord, C., Corsello, C., & Grzadzinski, R. (2014). Diagnostic instruments in autistic spectrum disorders. In F. Volkmar, R. Pauls, S. Rogers, & K. Pelphrye (Eds.), *Handbook of autism and pervasive developmental disorders* (4th ed.pp. 609–660). Hoboken, NJ: John Wiley & Sons.

McCarthy, G., Puce, A., Gore, J. C., & Allison, T. (1997). Face-specific processing in the human fusiform gyrus. *Journal of Cognitive Neuroscience*, *9*(5), 605–610.

McPartland, J. C., Tillman, R. M., Yang, D. Y. J., Bernier, R. A., & Pelphrey, K. A. (2014). The social neuroscience of autism spectrum disorder. In *Handbook of autism and pervasive developmental disorders, Volume 1: Diagnosis, development, and brain mechanisms* (pp. 482–496). Hoboken, NJ: John Wiley & Sons Inc.

McPartland, J. C., Webb, S. J., Keehn, B., & Dawson, G. (2011). Patterns of visual attention to faces and objects in autism spectrum disorder. *Journal of Autism and Developmental Disorders, 41*(2), 148–157.

Meltzoff, A. N. (1990). Foundations for developing a concept of self: The role of imitation in relating self to other and the value of social mirroring, social modeling, and self practice in infancy. In D. Cicchetti & M. Beeghly (Eds.), *The self in transition: Infancy to childhood* (pp. 139–164). Chicago, IL: University of Chicago Press.

Meltzoff, A. N., & Brooks, R. (2001). "like me" as a building block for understanding other minds: Bodily acts, attention, and intention.n. In B. Malle, L. J. Moses, & D. Baldwin (Eds.), *Intentions and intentionality: Foundations of social cognition* (pp. 171–191). Cambridge: MIT Press.

Meltzoff, A. N., & Moore, M. K. (1977). Imitation of facial and manual gestures by human neonates. *Science, 198*(4312), 75–78.

Minshew, N. J., & Williams, D. L. (2007). The new neurobiology of autism: Cortex, connectivity, and neuronal organization. *Archives of Neurology, 64*(7), 945–950.

Molenberghs, P., Cunnington, R., & Mattingley, J. B. (2012). Brain regions with mirror properties: A meta-analysis of 125 human fMRI studies. *Neuroscience and Biobehavioral Reviews, 36*(1), 341–349.

Molnar-Szakacs, I., & Overy, K. (2006). Music and mirror neurons: From motion to 'e'motion. *Social Cognitive and Affective Neuroscience, 1*(3), 235–241.

Monk, C. S., Peltier, S. J., Wiggins, J. L., Weng, S. J., Carrasco, M., Risi, S., & Lord, C. (2009). Abnormalities of intrinsic functional connectivity in autism spectrum disorders. *NeuroImage, 47*(2), 764–772.

Mundy, P. (2016). *Autism and joint attention: Development, neurosience, and clinical fundamentals*. New York: Guilford Press.

National Research Council (NRC). (2001). *Educating young children with autism*. Washington, D.C: National Academy Press.

Osterling, J., & Dawson, G. (1994). Early recognition of children with autism: A study of first birthday home videotapes. *Journal of Autism and Developmental Disorders, 24*(3), 247–257.

Ozonoff, S., & Cathcart, K. (1998). Effectiveness of a home program intervention for young children with autism. *Journal of Autism and Developmental Disorders, 28*(1), 25–32.

Ozonoff, S., & South, M. (2001). Early social development in young children with autism: Theoretical and clinical implications. In G. Bremner & A. Fogel (Eds.), *Blackwell handbook of infant development handbooks of developmental psychology* (pp. 565–588). Malden, MA: Blackwell Publishers.

Pelphrey, K. A., Mitchell, T. V., McKeown, M. J., Goldstein, J., Allison, T., & McCarthy, G. (2003). Brain activity evoked by the perception of human walking: Controlling for meaningful coherent motion. *Journal of Neuroscience, 23*(17), 6819–6825.

Pelphrey, K. A., Sasson, N. J., Reznick, J. S., Paul, G., Goldman, B. D., & Piven, J. (2002). Visual scanning of faces in autism. *Journal of Autism and Developmental Disorders, 32*(4), 249–261.

Pelphrey, K. A., Singerman, J. D., Allison, T., & McCarthy, G. (2003). Brain activation evoked by perception of gaze shifts: The influence of context. *Neuropsychologia, 41*(2), 156–170.

Perlman, S. B., Hudac, C. M., Pegors, T., Minshew, N. J., & Pelphrey, K. A. (2011). Experimental manipulation of face-evoked activity in the fusiform gyrus of individuals with autism. *Social Neuroscience, 6*(1), 22–30.

Perrett, D. I., Hietanen, J. K., Oram, M. W., Benson, P. J., & Rolls, E. (1992). Organization and functions of cells responsive to faces in the temporal cortex [and discussion]. *Philosophical Transactions of the Royal Society of London B: Biological Sciences, 335*(1273), 23–30.

Philip, R. C., Dauvermann, M. R., Whalley, H. C., Baynham, K., Lawrie, S. M., & Stanfield, A. C. (2012). A systematic review and meta-analysis of the fMRI investigation of autism spectrum disorders. *Neuroscience and Biobehavioral Reviews, 36*(2), 901–942.

Phillips, M. L., Young, A. W., Senior, C., Brammer, M., Andrew, C., Calder, A. J., … Williams, S. (1997). A specific neural substrate for perceiving facial expressions of disgust. *Nature, 389*(6650), 495–498.

Piaget, J. (1952). *Play, dreams and imitation in childhood*. London, UK: Routledge.

Pierce, K., Müller, R.-A., Ambrose, J., Allen, G., & Courchesne, E. (2001). Face processing occurs outside the fusiform 'face area' in autism: Evidence from functional MRI. *Brain, 124*(10), 2059–2073.

Puce, A., & Perrett, D. (2003). Electrophysiology and brain imaging of biological motion. *Philosophical Transactions of the Royal Society of London. Series B: Biological Sciences, 358*(1431), 435–445.

Raleigh, M. J., & Steklis, H. D. (1981). Effects of orbitofrontal and temporal neocortical lesions on the affiliative behavior of vervet monkeys (Cercopithecus Aethiops Sabaeus). *Experimental Neurology, 73*(2), 378–389.

Reichow, B., & Barton, E. E. (2014). Evidence-based psychosocial interventions for individuals with autism spectrum disorders. In *Handbook of autism and pervasive developmental disorders, Volume 2: Assessment, interventions, and policy* (pp. 969–992). Hoboken, NJ: John Wiley & Sons Inc.

Reichow, B., Doehring, P., Cicchetti, D., & Volkmar, F. R. (Eds.). (2011). *Evidence-based practices and treatments for children with autism*. New York, NY: Springer.

Ricks, D. M., & Wing, L. (1975). Language, communication, and the use of symbols in normal and autistic children. *Journal of Autism and Childhood Schizophrenia*, *5*(3), 191–221.

Rizzolatti, G. (2005). The mirror neuron system and its function in humans. *Anatomy and Embryology*, *210*(5), 419–421.

Rizzolatti, G., Fogassi, L., & Gallese, V. (2001). Neurophysiological mechanisms underlying the understanding and imitation of action. *Nature Reviews Neuroscience*, *2*(9), 661–670.

Rogers, S. J. (2005). Play interventions for young children with autism spectrum disorders. In L. Reddy, T. Files-Hall, & Schaefer (Eds.), *Empirically based play interventions for children* (pp. 215–239). Washington, DC: American Psychological Association.

Rogers, S. J., Cook, I., & Meryl, A. (2014). Imitation and play in autism. In F. R. Volkmar, S. J. Rogers, R. Paul, & K. A. Pelphrey (Eds.), *Handbook of autism and pervasive developmental disorders* (vol. 1, pp. 382–405). Hoboken, NJ: Wiley.

Rogers, S. J., Dawson, G., & Vismara, L. A. (2012). *An early start for your child with autism: Using everyday activities to help kids connect, communicate, and learn*. New York, NY: Guilford Press.

Rogers, S. J., Hayden, D., Hepburn, S., Charlifue-Smith, R., Hall, T., & Hayes, A. (2006). Teaching young nonverbal children with autism useful speech: A pilot study of the Denver model and PROMPT interventions. *Journal of Autism and Developmental Disorders*, *36*(8), 1007–1024.

Rogers, S. J., Ozonoff, S., & Maslin-Cole, C. (1991). A comparative study of attachment behavior in young children with autism or other psychiatric disorders. *Journal of the American Academy of Child and Adolescent Psychiatry*, *30*(3), 483–488.

Rogers, S. J., Ozonoff, S., & Maslin-Cole, C. (1993). Developmental aspects of attachment behavior in young children with pervasive developmental disorders. *Journal of the American Academy of Child and Adolescent Psychiatry*, *32*(6), 1274–1282.

Rogers, S. J., & Pennington, B. F. (1991). A theoretical approach to the deficits in infantile autism. *Development and Psychopathology*, *3*(2), 137–162.

Rogers, S. J., & Vismara, L. (2014). Interventions for infants and toddlers at risk for autism spectrum disorder. In *Handbook of autism and pervasive developmental disorders, Volume 2: Assessment, interventions, and policy* (pp. 739–769). Hoboken, NJ: John Wiley & Sons Inc.

Rutter, M. (1978). Diagnosis and definitions of childhood autism. *Journal of Autism and Developmental Disorders*, *8*(2), 139–161.

Rutter, M. (2008). Implications of attachment theory and research for child care policies. In *Handbook of attachment: Theory, research, and clinical applications* (2nd ed.pp. 958–974). New York, NY: Guilford Press.

Rutter, M., & Thapar, A. (2014). Genetics of autism spectrum disorders. In *Handbook of autism and pervasive developmental disorders, Volume 1: Diagnosis, development, and brain mechanisms* (pp. 411–423). Hoboken, NJ: John Wiley & Sons Inc.

Saxe, R., & Kanwisher, N. (2003). People thinking about thinking people: The role of the temporo-parietal junction in "theory of mind". *NeuroImage*, *19*(4), 1835–1842.

Schultz, R. T., Gauthier, I., Klin, A., Fulbright, R. K., Anderson, A. W., Volkmar, F., … Gore, J. C. (2000). Abnormal ventral temporal cortical activity during face discrimination among individuals with autism and Asperger syndrome. *Archives of General Psychiatry*, *57*(4), 331–340.

Senju, A., Southgate, V., White, S., & Frith, U. (2009). Mindblind eyes: An absence of spontaneous theory of mind in Asperger syndrome. *Science*, *325*(5942), 883–885.

Shultz, S., Klin, A., & Jones, W. (2011). Inhibition of eye blinking reveals subjective perceptions of stimulus salience. *PNAS Proceedings of the National Academy of Sciences of the United States of America*, *108*(52), 21270–21275.

Signer, S. F. (1987). Capgras' syndrome: The delusion of substitution. *Journal of Clinical Psychiatry*, *15*, 402–440.

Silani, G., Bird, G., Brindley, R., Singer, T., Frith, C., & Frith, U. (2008). Levels of emotional awareness and autism: An fMRI study. Social Neuroscience, 3(2), 97–112. 15:402-440.

South, M., Ozonoff, S., & McMahon, W. M. (2007). The relationship between executive functioning, central coherence, and repetitive behaviors in the high-functioning autism spectrum. *Autism*, *11*(5), 437–451.

Tanaka, J. W., Wolf, J. M., Klaiman, C., Koenig, K., Cockburn, J., Herlihy, L., … Schultz, R. T. (2012). The perception and identification of facial emotions in individuals with autism spectrum disorders using the let's face it! Emotion skills battery. *Journal of Child Psychology and Psychiatry*, *53*(12), 1259–1267.

Thirtamara Rajamani, K. K. (2015). Animal models of drug addiction and autism spectrum disorders. *Dissertation Abstracts International: Section B: The Sciences and Engineering, 76*(5-B(E)), No Pagination Specified.

Turella, L., Pierno, A. C., Tubaldi, F., & Castiello, U. (2009). Mirror neurons in humans: Consisting or confounding evidence? *Brain and Language*, *108*(1), 10–21.

Uddin, L. Q., Iacoboni, M., Lange, C., & Keenan, J. P. (2007). The self and social cognition: The role of cortical midline structures and mirror neurons. *Trends in Cognitive Sciences*, *11*(4), 153–157.

Ungerer, J. A., & Sigman, M. (1981). Symbolic play and language comprehension in autistic children. *Journal of the American Academy of Child Psychiatry*, *20*(2), 318–337.

Valentine, T. (1988). Upside-down faces: A review of the effect of inversion upon face recognition. *British Journal of Psychology*, *79*(4), 471–491.

Vander Wyk, B. C., Hudac, C. M., Carter, E. J., Sobel, D. M., & Pelphrey, K. A. (2009). Action understanding

in the superior temporal sulcus region. *Psychological Science*, *20*(6), 771–777.
Vander Wyk, B. C., Voos, A., & Pelphrey, K. A. (2012). Action representation in the superior temporal sulcus in children and adults: An fMRI study. *Developmental Cognitive Neuroscience*, 2(4), 409–416. doi:10.1016/j.dcn.2012.04.004
Volkmar, F. R., Klin, A., Siegel, B., Szatmari, P., Lord, C., Campbell, M., . . . et al. (1994). Field trial for autistic disorder in DSM-IV. American Journal of Psychiatry, 151(9), 13611367.
Volkmar, F. R., & McPartland, J. C. (2014). From Kanner to DSM-5: Autism as an evolvingdiagnostic concept. *Annual Review of Clinical Psychology*, *10*, 193–212.
Volkmar, F. R., & Nelson, D. S. (1990). Seizure disorders in autism. *Journal of the American Academy of Child and Adolescent Psychiatry*, *29*(1), 127–129.
Volkmar, F. R., & Reichow, B. (2014). The evolution of autism as a diagnostic concept: From Kanner to DSM-5: A commentary. In *Handbook of autism and anxiety* (pp. 217–230). Cham, Switzerland: Springer International Publishing.
Volkmar, F. R., Sparrow, S. S., Goudreau, D., Cicchetti, D. V., Paul, R., & Cohen, D. J. (1987). Social deficits in autism: An operational approach using the vineland adaptive behavior scales. *Journal of the American Academy of Child and Adolescent Psychiatry*, *26*(2), 156–161.
Völlm, B. A., Taylor, A. N., Richardson, P., Corcoran, R., Stirling, J., McKie, S., … Elliott, R. (2006). Neuronal correlates of theory of mind and empathy: A functional magnetic resonance imaging study in a nonverbal task. *NeuroImage*, *29*(1), 90–98.
Voos, A. C., Pelphrey, K. A., Tirrell, J., Bolling, D. Z., Vander Wyk, B., Kaiser, M. D., … Ventola, P. (2013). Neural mechanisms of improvements in social motivation after pivotal response treatment: Two case studies. *Journal of Autism and Developmental Disorders*, *43*(1), 1–10.
Wang, A. T., Dapretto, M., Hariri, A. R., Sigman, M., & Bookheimer, S. Y. (2004). Neural correlates of facial affect processing in children and adolescents with autism spectrum disorder. *Journal of the American Academy of Child and Adolescent Psychiatry*, *43*(4), 481–490.
Williams, J. H., Whiten, A., Suddendorf, T., & Perrett, D. I. (2001). Imitation, mirror neurons and autism. *Neuroscience and Biobehavioral Reviews*, *25*(4), 287–295.
Wing, L., & Gould, J. (1979). Severe impairments of social interaction and associated abnormalities in children: Epidemiology and classification. *Journal of Autism and Developmental Disorders*, *9*(1), 11–29.
Wing, L., Gould, J., Yeates, S. R., & Brierley, L. M. (1977). Symbolic play in severely mentally retarded and in autistic children. *Journal of Child Psychology and Psychiatry, and Allied Disciplines*, *18*(2), 167–178.
Yin, R. K. (1969). Looking at upside-down faces. *Journal of Experimental Psychology*, *81*(1), 141.
Young, G. S., Merin, N., Rogers, S. J., & Ozonoff, S. (2009). Gaze behavior and affect at 6 months: Predicting clinical outcomes and language development in typically developing infants and infants at risk for autism. *Developmental Science*, *12*(5), 798–814.

3 Have a Happy, Fun, Assertive Life! (Avoid Depression, Anxiety, Loneliness, and Suicide!)

Peter Sturmey

3.1 Skinner and Mental Health

Skinner's (1953) *Science and Human Behavior* paints a broad picture of behavior analytic approaches to behavior that included sections on mental health. Skinner's argument was that society – in the form of parental practices, government, religion, and education – controls our behavior relating to primary reinforcers mostly through punishment. Parents effectively stop a child stealing food by spanking them and sending them to bed without any supper; the teacher stops their children through reprimands, paddling, and suspensions; and religions threaten eternal damnation and remove the possibility of eternal life by threats of excommunication, shunning, and other forms of time-out from religious participation. Such contingencies are effective in terminating unwanted behavior and may contribute to the survival of a culture but come at a heavy price (Sidman, 1989). People may learn to avoid the punisher, related stimuli, and the punishment through avoidance, lying, and dissimulation; or emit pain-elicited aggression (Ulrich, Hutchinson, & Azrin, 1965) and operant aggression to terminate future punishment (Azrin, Hutchinson, & Sallery, 1964). Discriminative stimuli for punishment also come to suppress other ongoing operant behavior (Estes & Skinner, 1941) and eventually we learn to only exhibit sufficient behavior to avoid future punishment, but no more. We may become the passive person who barely complies, but does no more. Punishment also elicits emotional behavior that interferes with ongoing operant, adaptive behavior and that is distressful for the person concerned. Some people learn to minimize such distress through abuse of alcohol, prescribed medication, and illicit substances, practices that further cascade into unhappy and potentially dangerous lives. Some forms of punishment produce physical injuries. Finally, in some situations, the addictive nature of punishment for the punisher results in social situations that are harmful to everyone. For example, the couple who live in separate parts of the same house without talking to each other, except for escalating arguments and fights and the behavior support plan that involves escalating degrees of punishment without implementing effective positive alternatives in barren, neglectful, and disrespectful environments.

Skinner (1953) pointed out that many people manage this situation quite well by using strategies described in the previous paragraph in an unsystematic manner. Skinner advises that if you have a problem with your landlord, go to see him to address the problem or move! By implication, staying in an apartment with no heating, dealing with the emotional side effects of the situation through distraction, smoking, drinking, and complaining about it is a personal mistake.

P. Sturmey (✉)
The Graduate Center and Queens College, City University of New York, New York, NY, USA
e-mail: psturmey@gmail.com

J.B. Leaf (ed.), *Handbook of Social Skills and Autism Spectrum Disorder*, Autism and Child Psychopathology Series, DOI 10.1007/978-3-319-62995-7_3

Skinner (1953) described self-management as the deliberate application of strategies to modify one's own behavior and included a controlling behavior that altered the future probability of a controlled behavior. One learns to set the alarm clock on Sunday (i.e., the controlling behavior) to ensure one gets up on time the rest of the week (i.e., the controlled behavior). In so doing, one not only gets up on time, but, perhaps even more importantly, enjoys a leisurely, pleasant breakfast, and arrives at work relaxed and in a good frame of mind, but also avoids rushing and becoming too irritated in traffic only to arrive at work in a bad mood. Skinner used these strategies with himself to have a happy, healthy, and productive life into his 90s (Epstein, 1997). Skinner identified seven strategies for self-management. First, people use physical restraint. For example, we fold our hands to ensure not fidgeting or walk away from an embarrassing situation and successfully avoid the associated social disapproval and guilt in both cases. Second, we alter discriminative stimuli to change future behavior, by removing discriminative stimuli for competing behavior, for example, by giving tempting desserts to our willing friends. We also present discriminative stimuli for the behavior we want to engage in, for example, by making appointments with friends to go to the gym and writing reminders for ourselves. Third, we sometimes use reinforcer deprivation and satiation. We skip snacking on poor-quality food so later we really enjoy a good meal and we drink a bottle of water before the office party to avoid eating and drinking too much and embarrassing ourselves. Fourth, we manipulate emotional states by removing stimuli that elicit undesirable emotional states. We put away photographs of dead family members and display wedding photographs, rather than pictures of corpses on the mantel piece. We avoid the negative effects of anger by taking a couple of deep breaths before replying to an insult. Fifth, we deliberately arrange aversive consequences for our own behavior we want to reduce when we self-record and have to look at an incomplete to do list at the end of a lazy, disorganized day. Sixth, we change our future behavior and emotional states with drugs when we take a stiff drink before we go face the music. Finally, we go do something else to avoid doing something unpleasant by looking away, changing the topic of conversation, or being especially nice to people we dislike in order to avoid a fight. We can view self-management as a choice between engaging in some impulsive behavior (e.g., snapping at someone irritating us and immediately terminating their aversive behavior) and engaging in controlled behavior (e.g., making an excuse to terminate other people's irritating conversation and avoid later embarrassment).

Skinner (1972) went on to analyze mental health issues, such as depression, in behavior analytic terms. In a generic behavioral case formulation (Skinner, 1953, 1972), he gives the example of a student who graduates from college whose former behavior is useless in his new job. The student feels unsure and frustrated because his behavior is undergoing operant extinction with its accompanying negative emotional side effects. He feels anxious and unsure because he does not know how to avoid punishment in his new job. He has no sense of accomplishment because his behavior is no longer reinforced and feels guilty and ashamed, because, in the past, lazy and ineffective behavior has been punished.

When faced with people in this situation, it is tempting to give them good advice. After bereavement, we tell other people, "Don't make any major decisions straight away." Skinner (1953) advised therapists to avoid doing this, first because the other person may reject our advice and second because it does not foster the other person's independence and self-management. Rather, Skinner advises that the therapist's job is to induce a generalized repertoire of self-management to deal with life's adversities. Although Skinner avoided recommending specific treatment strategies, he did suggest the use of self-recording so the client themselves might begin to change their behavior and discriminate the relationship between the environment and their behavior. Hence, after a week of self-recording behavior and mood, the student who graduated from college might say, "It's odd, but I had a good time on Thursday afternoon when I walked past the pet store and just loved the animals in there." Rather than instructing him to go buy a puppy, the therapist might ask the person, "What do you make of that?" or "What might you do next week to be a bit happier?" This analysis prefigures subsequent work on behavioral case formulation (Sturmey, 1996, 1997, 2007a, 2008; Turkat, 1985) and behavioral activation for depression (Jacobson, Martell, & Dimidjian, 2001; Sturmey, 2009a).

3.2 Happiness, Depression, and Loneliness

In Beckett's (2012) play *Happy Days*, Winnie talks endlessly about very little while occasionally playing with a gun from her sole available possession, her purse. Winnie is almost successful in not facing the dreadful situation she is in – stuck in a heap of life's literal and metaphorical rubble, first up to her waste in Act One and then up to her neck in Act Two, as her body gradually disappears into the ground that will inevitably swallow us all up one day. What is remarkable is that even buried up to her neck she has no problem in continuing to talk. Skinner (1959) used high-rate verbal behavior as an everyday example of avoidance of things even more painful than the trivia so many of us constantly talk about. In a similar manner, Bennett's (2007) lonely protagonists, in the television show *Talking Heads,* endlessly engage in monologues and fight off their inevitably deteriorating situations. In the show, a middle-aged widow and mother abandoned by her callous thieving son and facing up to her daughter's incestuous relationship with her late husband are all part of life's challenges. Bennett's (2007) protagonists manage their own painful behavior by "taking a tablet," talking endlessly to no-one but themselves to avoid their own emotional pain.

People with intellectual and developmental disabilities (IDD) face similar challenges to the rest of us, but often they face them with more limited personal resources, including weaker social and self-management skills and fewer resources. Like everyone, individuals with IDD experience stressful life events, which often include losses, histories of punishment – such as stigmatization, bullying, and abuse – and extinction of their adaptive behavior, such as when people ignore and avoid them. Many individuals with mild IDD are also overly socially responsive or "externally directed" and hence may be more vulnerable to social contingencies including extinction (Zigler & Balla, 1982).

Earlier reviews have documented a growing literature on depression focused on establishing the fact that individuals with IDD could present with depression, leading to the development of screening and diagnostic assessment instruments and early behavioral and pharmacological treatment studies for individuals with IDD (Došen, 1984; Dosen & Menolascino, 1993; Matson, 1982a, 1983a, 1983b; Sturmey, 2005). Over the last 20 years, there has been an explosion of research, including reviews of specific disabilities such as Down syndrome (Walker, Dosen, Buitelaar, & Janzing, 2011), ASD (Autism Spectrum Disorders) (Matson & Williams, 2014; Stewart, Barnard, Pearson, Hasan, & O'Brien, 2006), and older adults (Prasher, 2003). Thus, this section will only illustrate general trends rather than attempt a comprehensive review of this literature.

3.2.1 Prevalence and Risk Factors

The prevalence of depression in individuals with IDD ranges from 3 to 6% (Cooper, 1997; Cooper, Smiley, Morrison, Williamson, & Allan, 2007; Hurley, 2008) and may be as high as approximately 7–9% in adults aged over 50 years (Hermans, Beekman, & Evenhuis, 2013). These figures vary widely, reflecting problems with case finding, case definition, modification of diagnostic criteria, including the use of alleged behavioral equivalents of depression, the accuracy of self versus proxy reports of mental health (Emerson, Felce, & Stancliffe, 2013), and definitions and sampling of populations.

Research has explored the risk factors for depression in the general population extensively within specific contexts such as late life, numerous chronic health conditions, pregnancy, and disability. Hence, the common risk factors for depression are well known and include stressful life events, especially those involving losses, weak social support, weak social skills, aversive life circumstances, including chronic medical and life-threatening conditions, and conditions restricting mobility. Among studies of risk factors for depression in individuals with IDDs, the following risk factors have been found: (a) weak social support (Meins, 1993) and amount of negative social support (McGillivray & McCabe, 2007); (b) deficits in social skills (Helsel & Matson, 1988; Matson, Lott, Mayville, Swender, & Moscow, 2006) – including excessive seeking of reassurance and negative social interactions from others (Hartley, Lickel, & MacLean, 2008) – and nonverbal social skills (Hartley & Birgenheir, 2008); (c) greater sensitivity to criticism than people without IDD (Esdale, Jahoda, & Pert, 2015); (d) quality and frequency of social support (McGillivray & McCabe, 2007); (e) social strain (Lunsky & Benson, 2001); (f) stressful life events – including losses (especially loss of relatives), illness, bullying – and number and intensity of life events (Hove, Assmus, & Havik, 2016), disruptive life events (McGillivray & McCabe, 2007), and victimization (Ung et al., 2016); and (g) cognitive variables – such as automatic negative thoughts, self-esteem, feelings of hopelessness, rates of self-reinforcement, amount of negative social support (McGillivray & McCabe, 2007; Nezu, Nezu, Rothenberg, DelliCarpini, & Groag, 1995), and hopelessness (Esbensen & Benson, 2005). Determining the relative magnitude of these variables, both generally and on a case-by-case basis, is difficult as many of these variables covary and interact. For example, weak social skills, lack of social support, negative social interactions, and social strain may all covary, but determining the causal relationships between them is difficult. A positive feature of this literature, however, is that, unlike structural features such as age, gender, and degree of IDD, these variables can be included in clinical case formulations (Sturmey, 2009b) and are susceptible to change. Thus, if a client or practitioner can identify the controlling variables and arrange the environment to change those variables, they may be able to promote happiness and reduce their depressed behavior (LeJuez, Hall Brown, & Hopko, 2009).

3.2.2 Assessment and Functional Analysis

Assessment serves several different functions including screening, diagnosis, prognosis, communication among professionals, explanation of presenting problems, determination of service eligibility, prediction of effective and ineffective treatment, and evaluation of response to treatment (Sturmey, 2007b). Several authors have reported screening for depression in individuals with IDD. An interesting example comes from Chaplin et al. (2013), who evaluated a self-assessment screening tool for anxiety and depression in adults with mild and moderate IDD. The authors found that the majority of individuals referred for self-assessment could complete the procedure with acceptable concurrent validity with existing psychometric measures of anxiety and depression. A second example comes from Brown, Jacobstein, Yoon, and Bullock (2016) who, as part of a settlement agreement in a class action deinstitutionalization federal lawsuit, implemented a district-wide strategy to proactively monitor the health of individuals including screening for depression. They reported that only 59% of the sample had completed screens for depression. In response, Brown et al. developed and used a modified Glasgow Depression Scale (Cuthill, Espie, & Cooper, 2003), made it available to nurses, and posted it on the web to increase accessibility. There are now numerous psychometric measures of depression for individuals with IDD including screening items and depression scales within longer measures of psychopathology and standalone scales to assess depression and semi-structured diagnostic interviews (Finlay, 2005; Finlay & Lyons, 2001; Ross & Oliver, 2003). These measures are also sometimes used for diagnosis and to measure changes in individual clinical work and clinical trials.

Literal application of unmodified Diagnostic and Statistical Manual for Mental Disorders (DSM) or International Classification of Diseases criteria would probably preclude diagnosis of mood disorders in most individuals with IDD because of requirements of self-report of symptoms

(Sturmey, 1993, 2005). There have been two responses to this problem. First, authors have modified diagnostic criteria, such as removing criteria deemed to be less applicable to individuals with IDD, such as diminished sexual functioning, rewording criteria, and/or changing cut-off scores. Second, the inclusion of challenging behavior as behavioral equivalents (Cooper, Melville, & Einfeld, 2003; Cooper, Barnhill, & Fletcher, 2016).

A final aspect of assessment is case formulation and functional assessment and analysis. Although traditionally associated with challenging behavior, such as aggression, practitioners and researchers have used functional assessment and analysis to understand and guide treatment of depression. For example, McKnight, Nelson, Hayes, and Jarrett (1984) conducted functional assessments based on observations of social interactions and self-reports of thinking to identify women with depression who had only social skills deficits and women who had only irrational cognitions. When McKnight et al. implemented social skills training or cognitive treatment in a multielement design with each woman, they each responded best to the treatment that matched the function of their depressed behavior on measures of mood and cognition. Recently, Johansson et al. (2012) compared standardized online cognitive behavior therapy (CBT), individualized CBT, and an active treatment control for depression. CBT consists of both cognitive strategies, such as identifying and changing maladaptive patterns of thinking etc., and behavioral strategies, such as goal setting and self-recording etc. Participants were 121 adults with mostly acute depression, the majority of whom had comorbid conditions and were taking or had taken psychotropic medication. Both CBT groups received online modules of training for depression that had previously been shown to be effective, but the individualized group also received an individualized treatment plan developed by researchers based on the available diagnostic and self-report data. Outcomes generally favored individualized treatments, especially for more severe depression, which resulted in better outcomes than the standardized treatment on measures of depression and quality of life. Thus, the ideas and methods of functional assessment and analysis can be used to guide individual, function-based treatment of depression in the general population.

3.2.3 Prevention and Treatment

3.2.3.1 Promoting Happiness

The best way to treat depression is to prevent it in the first place. One way to do this is to have a happy life. Several applied behavior analytic studies have addressed this.

Green and Reid (1996) operationalized and reliably observed behavioral indices of happiness and unhappiness in five adults with profound IDD. Happy behaviors included smiling and unhappy behaviors included crying and turning away. They found that the behavioral indices for mood were reliable. Both familiar and unfamiliar people agreed when these individuals appeared happy or unhappy and the raters agreed with the behavioral indices. They then conducted preferences assessments and observed changes in behavioral indices of mood as a function of the presence of preferred and nonpreferred stimuli. Such procedures, while having certain limitations, are quite robust in increasing behavioral indices of happiness (Dillon & Carr, 2007; Lancioni, Singh, O'Reilly, Oliva, & Basili, 2005).

Carr, Magito McLaughlin, Giacobbe-Grieco, and Smith (2003) expanded on this work, when they used activities selected to induce positive affective behavior and ratings of positive and negative mood in adults living in group homes. They then modified affective behavior by introducing positive mood inducing activities, such as preferred leisure activities, which resulted in reduced challenging behavior. Further, this was true even when provocative stimuli that evoked challenging behavior, such as demands, were presented.

This is an interesting approach to understanding affective behavior and in promoting happiness. It should not be dismissed as merely a procedure that can be used with individuals with severe or profound IDD as it parallels behavioral activation procedures in the general population and with individuals with borderline and mild IDD (see later). One notable difference is that, in this approach, caregivers present different preferred and nonpreferred stimuli, whereas in behavioral activation, the person self-manages using procedures such as goal setting, self-recording, and scheduling. Future research might evaluate the effects of such self-management procedures on behavioral indices of mood.

Promoting happiness and prevention of depression in people with IDD are more than presenting the right stimuli. It is equally important that the individual with IDD has a program or lifestyle of activities that are valuable to them personally and that engaging in these activities is easy and occurs frequently. The individual must also have a healthy lifestyle, including a good diet and exercise, and appropriate and prompt medical care to eliminate discomfort and promote health. The services and family members must also reduce aversive stimulation, whether it is nagging, coercive interactions, violence, aggression in the home, or abuse. Aversive stimulation cannot be completely eliminated from any of our lives and it may not even be desirable to do so as aversive stimulation provides the opportunity to learn resilience skills. So, in addition to managing aversive stimulation, caregivers should also provide teaching opportunities to learn how to manage aversive stimulation. Although these processes and outcomes can be achieved primarily through caregiver behavior, this is not the most desirable approach. Rather, promoting autonomy by teaching a generalized repertoire of self-management is preferable as is releases the person from social control of their own behavior (Skinner, 1953). Learning this behavioral repertoire is a lifetime activity that begins early in life but continues throughout the lifespan.

3.2.3.2 Treating Depression

The literature on the treatment of depression has grown considerably over the last 40 years. Early behavioral studies evaluated social skills training in cases studies (Matson, Dettling, & Senatore, 1979) and some small *N* experiments (Lindauer, DeLeon, & Fisher, 1999; Matson, 1982a), although these studies were limited with respect to demonstrating response and stimulus generalization and maintenance. A recent review of social skills training groups with individuals with ASD (Hotton & Coles, 2016) found evidence from two studies, one pre–post test design (Hillier, Fish, Siegel, & Beversdorf, 2011) and one randomized control trial (RCT; Yoo et al., 2014) that social skills may reduce depression, anxiety, and stress, but the participants in both studies had average intelligence quotients. In a similar vein, Lindauer et al. (1999) reported a functional analysis and treatment of depression-related behavior in a woman with IDD and mood disorder. Previously, her mood disorder had only partially responded to psychotropic medication. Lindauer et al. reported a small *N* experiment, which showed that negative affective behavior and self-injury were reduced by the availability of preferred leisure materials.

As noted earlier, CBT includes both cognitive and behavioral treatment strategies. CBT for depression includes behavioral activation, which includes values clarification, goal setting, self-recording, and progressive activation in line with one's values. Research has shown that behavioral activation is the active component of CBT for depression and largely equivalent to the CBT package (Jacobson et al., 1996; Sturmey, 2009). Further, depression is readily subject to a functional assessment (Kanter, Cautilli, Busch, & Baruch, 2005) and even functional analysis (McKnight et al., 1984). Thus, behavioral activation has been extended to treat depression in people with IDD. In a feasibility pilot study, Jahoda et al. (2015) demonstrated that behavioral activation could be used to treat subclinical and clinical depression in individuals with IDD, and several nonexperimental case studies have also demonstrated the application of behavioral activation to treat depression (Green, 2016; Stuart, Graham, & Butler, 2014). A controlled trial is currently underway (Jahoda, Melville, Cooper et al., 2015). Further evidence of the effectiveness of behavioral activation comes from a component analysis of the CBT package. McGillivray and Kershaw (2015) compared the outcomes of predominantly cognitive strategies, predominantly behavioral strategies, and combined cognitive and behavioral strategies on depressed mood for 70 individuals with mild IDD and varying degrees of subclinical and clinical depression. Participants in all three groups improved and there were few differences between the groups. The significant differences that were observed were of small magnitude. For example, the participants who received predominantly cognitive strategies reported a greater reduction in automatic negative thoughts. Thus, there is now accumulating evidence that behavioral activation may be effective for individuals with IDD. Although the quantity of evidence with individuals with IDD is not yet substantial, it is consistent with a much larger literature on behavioral activation in the general population (Chan, Sun, Tam, Tsoi, & Wong, 2017; Ekers et al., 2014).

Several group design studies have evaluated CBT for depression in individuals with IDD. The application of CBT to this population has almost always been modified in various ways including slower paced sessions, more repetition, simplified spoken and written language, more concrete presentation, inclusion of caregivers in sessions and participating in homework assignments, use of visual supports, and take home booklets at the end of a course of treatment that document accomplishments and which implicitly include reminders to use treatment (Walters, Loades, & Russell, 2016). For example, Unwin, Tsimopoulou, Kroese, and Azmi (2016) reported a systematic review of CBT for depression or anxiety in individuals with IDDs and identified four RCTs for depression, three for anxiety, and four for mixed depression/anxiety, some of which reported outcome data on depression separately. Generally, there was evidence for reduction in self- and other-reported depression and automatic negative thoughts in these trials, although data on maintenance were mixed, with some studies reporting posttreatment regression. A recent systematic review and meta-analysis (Koslowski et al., 2016) identified 12 studies but found no significant effect on behavioral problems, depression, anxiety, quality of life, functioning, and a moderate, but nonsignificant Cohen's *d* of 0.49 for depression. The authors commented that studies were of moderately high but variable quality. Despite the limitations of this literature, these two systematic reviews document the feasibility of implementation of CBT for depression, which may be effective in some cases (particularly useful for practitioners are various treatment manuals that are now available, such as those by McGillvery's group).

There are several notable recent trends in this literature. These include outcome studies that address treatment of depression in individuals with ASD (McGillivray & Evert, 2014; Santomauro, Sheffield, & Sofronoff, 2016). Additionally, there are reports of other types of therapy, such as mindfulness (Cachia, Anderson, & Moore, 2016; Spek, Van Ham, & Nyklíček, 2013), an ongoing trial of light therapy (Hamers, Evenhuis, & Hermans, 2017) and electroconvulsive therapy for a variety of problems including mood disorders (Reinblatt, Rifkin, & Freeman, 2004). Some studies have implemented transdiagnostic group CBT (i.e., treatment of both depression and anxiety; Lindsay et al., 2015; Willner et al., 2013). Finally, greater attention has been given to programs that can be administered by regular staff (McGillivray & Kershaw, 2013; McGillivray, McCabe, & Kershaw, 2008; Willner et al., 2013). Thus, the literature on treatment of depression in individuals with IDD has grown considerably.

3.3 Anxiety

Many of us fear rejection, criticism, social failure, and the unknown from time to time, and all of us should fear threatening dangers, injury, pain, and death (Fredrikson, Annas, Fischer, & Wik, 1996; Lane & Gullone, 1999) to mobilize ourselves to action to protect ourselves. Some fear is highly adaptive, and to be brave in the face of danger is useful and sometimes highly regarded. To have no fear is often considered unusual or even pathological. Some individuals with IDD may have increased exposure to social criticism and discrimination, overly protective caregivers that limit the opportunities to learn to be brave, and may have reduced personal and material resources to cope with such stressors and conditioning events (Dagnan & Jahoda, 2006).

3.3.1 Prevalence and Risk Factors

Estimates of the prevalence of anxiety disorders in people with IDD and ASD have varied considerably. For example, in a large cohort of approximately 1000 adults with IDD, Cooper and colleagues (2007) found a point prevalence of approximately 2–3% for anxiety disorders and approximately 0.2–0.7% for obsessive compulsive disorder (OCD). There is some evidence that children with IDD are at a somewhat higher risk for anxiety disorders than other children. For example, Emerson (2003), conducted a secondary analysis of a large national child and adolescent mental health dataset. They calculated odds ratios (OR), which is a measure of the risk of anxiety in a particular subset of the data compared with all participants. They found that 8.7% of children with IDD and 3.6% of children without IDD had some anxiety disorder (OR = 2.4). Although specific forms of anxiety disorders were relatively rare, children with IDD were at greater risk of posttraumatic stress disorder (OR = 4.8), agoraphobia (OR = 6.4), and separation anxiety (OR = 3.7). Similar differences have been observed in other studies (Ramirez & Kratochwill, 1997) including older adults with and without IDD (Axmon, Björne, Nylander, & Ahlström, 2017; Hermans, Beekman, & Evenhuis, 2014).

Anxiety disorders are quite common among individuals with ASD. In a very large cohort of approximately 57,000 children with ASD, Simonoff et al. (2008) reported the prevalence of any anxiety/phobic disorder to be 41.9%. The prevalence of specific anxiety disorders were generalized anxiety disorders (13.4%), separation anxiety disorder (0.5%), panic disorder (10.1%), agoraphobia (7.9%), social anxiety disorder (29.2%), simple phobia (8.5%), and OCD (8.2%). In a similar study, Kim, Szatmari, Bryson, Streiner, & Wilson, (2000) found that the prevalence of overanxious behavior and separation anxiety were 13.6% and 8.5%, respectively, which were considerably higher than with children and adolescents in the general population. These illustrative studies suggest that anxiety disorders are more common in individuals with IDD and ASD than those without IDD and ASD. Second, individuals with anxiety disorders are even more common among individuals with ASD than individuals with IDD alone.

3.3.2 Assessment and Functional Analysis

It is useful to distinguish between three aspects of fear and anxiety: (1) observable fearful behavior; (2) physiological responses; and (3) covert fearful behavior. Observable fearful behavior can include motor avoidance (e.g., turning away and covering up a feared item) and avoidant verbal behavior (e.g., asking others to remove or not present the feared object). Some individuals also minimize exposure to unpleasant physiological aspects of fear by using alcohol and legal and illegal drugs. Fear can also inhibit performance of ongoing adaptive behavior (Estes & Skinner, 1941) as when someone is so scared they freeze and cannot move. Physiological aspects of fear and anxiety include autonomic arousal, such as sweating, heart racing, muscle tension and postures typical of tension, flushing, redistribution of blood to large muscle groups and skin, and gastrointestinal mobility. Sometimes such physiological aspects of anxiety and fear are overt behavior. Finally, covert anxious and fearful behavior includes a wide range of thoughts related to disastrous consequences (e.g., "I am scared," "I can't cope," "I am going to die," etc.) and emotional states and feelings, such as a sense of apprehension, foreboding, or doom. These three aspects of fear may not always covary, as when an individual behaves bravely, but remains physiologically aroused during early parts of flooding sessions.

There are many psychometric measures of fear and anxiety including use and/or modifications of existing measures from the general population and measures developed specifically for individuals with IDD/ASD (Hermans, van der Pas, & Evenhuis, 2011). An illustrative example is the *Glasgow Anxiety Scale for People with an Intellectual Disability* (GASID; Mindham & Espie, 2003), a 27-item scale. The GASID was specifically developed for use with people with IDD and discriminates between individuals with anxiety and correlates well with other psychometric and physiological measures of anxiety. Hermans and colleagues' (2011) review identified 14 similar measures and concluded that the GASID was the best available measure because of superior psychometric properties. This review also noted that the Anxiety, Depression, and Mood Scale (Esbensen, Rojahn, Aman, & Ruedrich, 2003) was also a promising measure, but with perhaps somewhat less impressive psychometric properties to assess anxiety.

Observational measures have been used extensively in behavioral assessment and treatment of anxiety. Such observational measures have included distance between the person and the feared object (Ricciardi, Luiselli, & Camare, 2006), steps of an exposure hierarchy completed successfully and fearful vocalizations (Love, Matson, & West, 1990), time spent with or near a feared object (Leitenberg, Agras, Thompson, & Wright, 1968; Matson, 1981), increasing adaptive behavior such as increased social initiations in socially avoidant children (O'Connor, 1969), improving academic performance in the presence of fearful stimuli (Jones & Friman, 1999), increases in nonfearful speech to a stranger (Matson, 1981), and holding an arm out without moving while receiving an injection (Shabani & Fisher, 2006). Sometimes these measures have also been accompanied by social validity ratings such as ratings of apparent fearfulness (Love et al., 1990), as many individuals with IDD or ASD may demonstrate idiosyncratic behavioral signs of anxiety. Thus, some researchers have defined behavioral markers of anxiety such as seeking reassurance from caregivers and perseveration on certain topics (Moskowitz et al., 2013).

Physiological measures of anxiety are commonly used in research, dating back to the 1970s (Porges, 2013; Porges & Humphrey, 1977), but they have received less attention with individuals with IDD or ASD and within clinical practice. Common research measures include heart rate variability and change, skin temperature and conductance, and hormone levels (MacNeil, Lopes, & Minnes, 2009). Exceptions to this generalization include the use of pulse oximetry as part of the validation of the GASID (Mindham & Espie, 2003) and work on heart rate change (Goodwin et al., 2006). As telemetric physiological measures become more readily available, such measures might be used more readily and conveniently in practice.

Although there is a relatively extensive literature on behavioral treatment of fear and anxiety, much less attention has been paid to functional analyses. A straightforward example of this comes from Jones and Friman (1999) who compared the effects of three conditions on the insect phobic behavior of Mike, a 14-year-old boy. The three conditions were (a) having live bugs in the classroom, (b) removing bugs from the classroom and saying, "there are no bugs anywhere in this room," and (c) saying, "There are no bugs anywhere in this room." The measure of phobic behavior was the number of math problems completed. As expected, Mike completed the fewest math problems in the first condition and the most in the last condition. The authors showed experimental control of phobic behavior using a multielement design.

The relationship between anxiety/arousal and challenging behavior has frequently been commented upon. For example, arousal might be an establishing operation (EO; e.g., increasing motivation for escape in the presence of relevant discriminative stimuli). Hence, arousal may interact with other variables, for example, arousal (EO) with a discriminative stimulus, such as a demand, might result in challenging behavior and escape, but arousal or demand alone might not. Moskowitz et al. (2013) demonstrated this empirically in three children aged 6–9 years with ASD and a DSM anxiety disorder. A notable feature of this study was the use of multimodal assessment of anxiety in that the authors used ratings, behavioral observation, and psychophysiological measures. For each child, the authors identified naturally occurring low- and high-anxiety situations presented in their natural context. They found that intervals with anxious behavior were consistently rated as very anxious. Further, two of three individuals showed higher heart rates in high anxiety situations. Additionally, challenging behavior was consistently higher in high anxiety contexts for all three children. Hence, manipulation of anxiety as an EO controlled problem behavior.

These studies show that fearful behavior can be subjected to a functional analysis using child-specific antecedents and manipulation of arousal with high fear situations. These studies also imply that practitioners should use the same basic methods of functional assessment and analysis of behavior to understand fearful and phobic behavior in individuals with IDD/ASD to design idiographic, function-based behavior support plans.

3.3.3 Prevention and Treatment

3.3.3.1 Becoming Assertive and Brave

One solution to fear is to be brave in the face of adversity. When Estes and Skinner's (1941) warning signal (a tone) interrupts ongoing operant behavior, should we freeze, abuse anxiolytic drugs, or act bravely and assertively in the face of potential imminent danger? Wolpe's (1958) answer was clear – act in a relaxed, brave, and assertive fashion around the conditioned stimuli and expose yourself to those stimuli.

One approach to becoming brave is to learn assertive skills. Bates (1980) taught 16 adults with mild–moderate IDD to introduce themselves, make small talk, ask for help, disagree with others, and respond to criticism. These skills were taught using instruction, modeling, rehearsal, feedback, and coaching scheduled during 3 weekly group meetings over 4 weeks. Using a combined multiple baseline and independent groups design, Bates showed the assertiveness training was effective in teaching assertive skills to these participants. Similarly, Sievert, Cuvo, and Davis (1988) used similar procedures to teach assertive responses to rights violation situations such as maintaining privacy of medical records to eight adults with mild IDD. Thus, teaching assertive, confident social skills might be a part of fear prevention. Another part of this might be systematic exposure to challenges throughout the lifespan to provide opportunities to acquire and maintain such skills.

3.3.3.2 Treating Anxiety

Systematic reviews of fears and phobias in individuals with IDD/ASD have reached broadly similar conclusions, namely treatment packages of exposure, modeling, and reinforcement for approach behavior are effective. For example, Jennet and Hagopian (2008) identified 13 studies treating phobias in individuals with IDD and found that treatment was highly successful, meeting American Psychiatric Association's (APA) criteria for an empirically supported treatment. A similar systematic review of treatment of fears and phobias in individuals with ASD (Lydon, Healy, O'Callaghan, Mulhern, & Holloway, 2015) and lower functioning individuals with autism (Rosen, Connell, & Kerns, 2016) have reached broadly similar conclusions. This approach has also been extended to functional analysis and treatment of OCD (Vause, Neil, Jaksic, Jackiewicz, & Feldman, 2015; Wolff, Hupp, & Symons, 2013). At this time, there are no other treatments with sufficient evidence to reach the criteria for evidence-based practices for these populations.

Lang, Regester, Lauderdale, Ashbaugh, and Haring (2010) conducted a systematic review of the evidence for CBT for anxiety disorders in individuals with ASD. They found nine studies with a total of 110 participants with ASD aged 9–23 years. Seventy-five participants were diagnosed with Asperger syndrome and 9 out of 20 individuals diagnosed with ASD were identified as "high functioning." All studies, except one single case study, used psychometric measures of anxiety. Every study reported at least one positive outcome, but only one RCT was deemed to be of high quality allowing confidence in its conclusion. Thus, although there is evidence from multiple studies of the effectiveness of CBT for anxiety disorders in individuals with Asperger syndrome, that evidence is limited by poor-quality studies and lack of studies with individuals with autism. In addition, Lang et al. noted that these CBT studies all included and emphasized behavioral aspects of CBT, such as teaching social and other adaptive skills, over strategies requiring introspection. A limitation to all such treatment studies is they have focused on simple phobias rather than agoraphobia and social anxiety.

3.4 Suicide

Skinner (1953) noted that one sure way to change the future probability of behavior was suicide. The example is not at all facetious; rather, it points us to consider suicide as an example of self-control and to consider self-control as an approach to change suicidal behavior. Work by Linehan and colleagues (2006) on dialectic behavior therapy uses behavioral notions in a vernacular way that is useful. The notion of a "chain analysis," or more technically, a stimulus response chain (Cooper, Heron, & Heward, 2007) suggests that sometimes suicidal behavior is a terminal response in a stimulus-response chain and that, as in other stimulus-response chains, intervention early in the response chain is an efficient way to change the terminal behavior. Additionally, choice of self-controlling responses over impulsive responses early in the stimulus-response chain is a useful way to identify and change behavior.

Historically, it was assumed that IDD was a protective factor against suicidality (ASD was not generally considered at that time in the context of suicidal behavior). Thus, it was assumed that individuals with IDD were relatively insensitive to precipitating factors (Kaminer, Feinstein, & Barrett, 1987); subsequent empirical research has shown this to be untrue. There is only a limited literature on suicide and IDD although there are now a number of reviews of this topic (Dodd, Doherty, & Guerin, 2016; Hannon & Taylor, 2013; Ludi et al., 2012; Mayes, Gorman, Hillwig-Garcia, & Syed, 2013; Merrick, Merrick, Lunsky, & Kandel, 2006; Ontario Center of Excellence for Child and Youth Mental health, 2014). For example, Dodd and colleagues' (2016) recent systematic review identified only 24 studies, which generally were of weak quality, most of which focused on risk factors such as concurrent mental health diagnoses. When thinking about cases and reading the literature, it is useful to distinguish between suicidal ideation, threats, attempts, and completion as well as deliberate self-harm, such as self-cutting and self-injury. Estimates of the prevalence of suicidal behavior are generally similar to the general population. For example, in a prospective, 35-year study of a nationally representative sample in Finland, Patja, Iicvanainen, Raitasio, and Loonquist (2001) found rates of suicide were similar to the general population in women with IDD, and for men with IDD, the rates were only one-third of the rates for men in the general population. The rates of suicide were 13.0 and 19.3 per 100,000 person years for women and men with IDD compared with 13.2 and 52.9 per 100,000 person years for men and women in the general population. Of the 10 suicides, nine involved people with mild IDD and one individual with moderate IDD. Most killed themselves using drowning and hanging, and only one example involved alcohol. Most were either in their 30s or 60s. Other studies have made similar observations on the rates of suicidal thoughts and behavior, noting that rates are lower than some other mental disorders, such as depression and certain personality disorders (Chesney, Goodwin, & Fazel, 2014; Jonsson, Alexanderson, Kjeldgård, & Mittendorfer-Rutz, 2014; Jonsson, Alexanderson, Kjeldgård, Westerlund, & Mittendorfer-Rutz, 2013).

In contrast, suicidal thoughts and threats are quite common in specialized services and individuals with multiple risk factors. For example, Lunsky (2004), in a study of 98 adults with IDD, found that about half were service users in a community clinic, reported that about a third of the sample had thought "life was not worth living," and reported 11% had suicide attempts. Waters, Barrett, Knapp, and Borden (1995) reported that 21% of 90 consecutive admissions to an inpatient unit had suicidal behavior, and Burge et al. (2002) reported that nearly half of inpatient admissions for individuals with IDD involve suicidal thoughts and behavior. These latter observations are quite important, as practitioners in these units should be familiar with identification, screening, evaluating, and treating this problem effectively.

Rates of suicidal thoughts and behavior are higher in individuals with IDD with multiple risk factors. For example, Mayes et al. (2013) in a sample of 791 individuals with autism aged 1–16 years found that, using maternal report data, 14% of the sample had suicidal thoughts or actions "sometimes" or "very often," which was 28 times higher than for typically developing children (i.e., 0.5%). Demographic risk factors included being 10 years or older, black or Hispanic, male, and having a lower socioeconomic status. Of those individuals with all four risk factors, 71% engaged in suicidal thoughts or actions. Some (e.g., Hannon & Taylor, 2014; Mayes et al., 2013) but not all (e.g., Chesney et al., 2014) studies have also reported somewhat elevated rates of suicidal thoughts and behavior in individuals with ASD, including Asperger syndrome (Paquette-Smith, Weiss, & Lunsky, 2014). Some studies have also reported stressful life events, such as loss of family through death, adoption or out of home placement, physical and sexual abuse, less family and social support, poorer quality of relationships, rejection, comorbid physical health problems, stress isolation, and loneliness (Ludi et al., 2012). Similarly, Paquette-Smith et al. (2014) found that among a sample of 50 individuals with Asperger syndrome, of whom 18 had a history of suicidal attempts, those who had attempted suicide were more likely to have a history of depression, more severe autism symptoms, weaker social skills, and problems shifting attention compared with those who had not attempted suicide.

Given the limited quantity of literature, there is little guidance for practitioners as how to proceed. When reviewing screening procedures, Ludi et al. (2010) noted that some dual diagnosis instruments included one or two items related to self-harm that might be useful in screening, but there was no specific instrument or procedure for assessing suicide risk in people with IDD; and existing instruments for other populations were too complex in terms of text, readability, and use of abstract language. Thus, future research should develop such procedures.

There are few reports of treatment for suicide among individuals with IDD and no evidence-base to guide treatment. Hence, practitioners must use existing literature from other populations and careful evaluation of implementation of individual treatment. Sturmey (1994) reported a case description on the treatment of suicidal threats in a man with mild IDD, which had resulted in multiple admissions to a distant inpatient program and considerable disruption to the man's life. A functional assessment indicated that suicidal threats and attempts were not related to depression, but, rather, appeared to be maintained by admission to the inpatient unit and inadvertent attention from medical and nursing staff. Therefore, intervention consisted of periods of approximately 24 h, supervised isolation contingent upon suicide threats or attempts, to keep him safe, which reduced suicidal threats, attempts, and admissions to inpatient services. The intervention was effective over a 7-month period.

Other approaches to treatment to consider might include teaching self-management skills based on Linehan et al.'s (2006) dialective behavior therapy, which has an extensive evidence-base on reducing self-harm and suicide when applied with other populations (Hawton et al., 2016; Valentine, Bankoff, Poulin, Reidler, & Pantalone, 2015). Several studies have reported modification of dialective behavior therapy with individuals with IDD (Brown, Brown, & Dibiasio, 2013; Lew, Matta, Tripp-Tebo, & Watts, 2006; McNair, Woodrow, & Hare, 2015; Sakdalan, Shaw, & Collier, 2010), which practitioners could use as treatment models.

3.5 Conclusion

Are you depressed, lonely, anxious, or suicidal? Have a great day instead! We can all do this using Skinnerian approaches to self-management. This can be done early during life to establish a generalized repertoire of self-management as a better way to live and as a strategy to prevent a wide range of life's problems, including depression and anxiety. In addition, behavioral self-management is a good treatment option for those with subclinical and clinical depression, depression, anxiety, and suicidal behavior and may be the effective mechanism underlying many evidence-based practices.

References

Axmon, A., Björne, P., Nylander, L., & Ahlström, G. (2017). Psychiatric diagnoses in older people with intellectual disability in comparison with the general population: A register study. *Epidemiology and Psychiatric Sciences*, 1–13.

Azrin, N. H., Hutchinson, R. R., & Sallery, R. D. (1964). Pain-aggression toward inanimate objects. *Journal of the Experimental Analysis of Behavior*, *7*, 223–228.

Bates, P. (1980). The effectiveness of interpersonal skills training on the social skill acquisition of moderately and mildly retarded adults. *Journal of Applied Behavior Analysis*, *13*, 237–248.

Beckett, S. (2012). *The complete dramatic works of Samuel Beckett*. London, UK: Faber & Faber.

Bennett, A. (2007). *Talking Heads*. London, UK: Random House.

Brown, J. F., Brown, M. Z., & Dibiasio, P. (2013). Treating individuals with intellectual disabilities and challenging behaviors with adapted dialectical behavior therapy. *Journal of Mental Health Research in Intellectual Disabilities*, *6*, 280–303.

Brown, M., Jacobstein, D., Yoon, I. S., Anthony, B., & Bullock, K. (2016). System-wide initiative documents robust health screening for adults with intellectual disability. *Intellectual and Developmental Disabilities*, *54*, 354–365.

Burge, P., Ouellette-Kuntz, H., Saeed, H., McCreary, B., Paquette, D., & Sim, F. (2002). Acute psychiatric inpatient care for people with a dual diagnosis: Patient profiles and lengths of stay. *The Canadian Journal of Psychiatry*, *47*, 243–249.

Cachia, R. L., Anderson, A., & Moore, D. W. (2016). Mindfulness in individuals with autism spectrum disorder: A systematic review and narrative analysis. *Review Journal of Autism and Developmental Disorders*, *3*, 1–14.

Carr, E. G., Magito McLaughlin, D., Giacobbe-Grieco, T., & Smith, C. E. (2003). Using mood ratings and mood induction in assessment and intervention for severe problem behavior. *American Journal on Mental Retardation*, *108*, 32–55.

Chan, A. T., Sun, G. Y., Tam, W. W., Tsoi, K. K., & Wong, S. Y. (2017). The effectiveness of group-based behavioral activation in the treatment of depression: An updated meta-analysis of randomized controlled trial. *Journal of Affective Disorders*, *208*, 345–354.

Chaplin, E., Chester, R., Tsakanikos, E., McCarthy, J., Craig, T., & Bouras, N. (2013). Reliability and validity of the SAINT: A guided self-help tool for people with intellectual disabilities. *Journal of Mental Health Research in Intellectual Disabilities*, *6*, 245–253.

Chesney, E., Goodwin, G. M., & Fazel, S. (2014). Risks of all cause and suicide mortality in mental disorders: A meta review. *World Psychiatry*, *13*, 153–160.

Cooper, J. O., Heron, T. E., & Heward, W. L. (2007). *Applied behavior analysis* (2nd ed.). London, UK: Prentice-Hall.

Cooper, S. A. (1997). Epidemiology of psychiatric disorders in elderly compared with younger adults with learning disabilities. *The British Journal of Psychiatry*, *170*, 375–380.

Cooper, S. A., Melville, C. A., & Einfeld, S. L. (2003). Psychiatric diagnosis, intellectual disabilities and diagnostic criteria for psychiatric disorders for use with adults with learning disabilities/mental retardation (DCLD). *Journal of Intellectual Disability Research*, *47*, 3–15.

Cooper, S. A., Smiley, E., Morrison, J., Williamson, A., & Allan, L. (2007). Mental ill-health in adults with intellectual disabilities: Prevalence and associated factors. *The British Journal of Psychiatry*, *190*, 27–35.

Cooper, S. A., Barnhill, J., & Fletcher, R. (2016). An overview of the development of the diagnostic manual–intellectual disabilities 2. *Journal of Intellectual Disability Research*, *60*, 652.

Cuthill, F. M., Espie, C. A., & Cooper, S. A. (2003). Development and psychometric properties of the Glasgow depression scale for people with a learning disability. *The British Journal of Psychiatry*, *182*, 347–353.

Dagnan, D., & Jahoda, A. (2006). Cognitive–behavioural intervention for people with intellectual disability and anxiety disorders. *Journal of Applied Research in Intellectual Disabilities*, *19*, 91–97.

Dillon, C. M., & Carr, J. E. (2007). Assessing indices of happiness and unhappiness in individuals with developmental disabilities: A review. *Behavioral Interventions*, *22*, 229–244.

Dodd, P., Doherty, A., & Guerin, S. (2016). A systematic review of suicidality in people with intellectual disabilities. *Harvard Review of Psychiatry*, *24*, 202–213.

Došen, A. (1984). Depression conditions in mentally handicapped children. *Acta Paedopsychiatrica: International Journal of Child & Adolescent Psychiatry*, *50*, 29–40.

Dosen, A., & Menolascino, F. J. (Eds.). (1993). *Depression in mentally retarded children and adults*. Leiden, Netherlands: Logon.

Ekers, D., Webster, L., Van Straten, A., Cuijpers, P., Richards, D., & Gilbody, S. (2014). Behavioural activation for depression; an update of meta-analysis of effectiveness and sub group analysis. *PloS One*, *9*(6), e100100.

Emerson, E. (2003). Prevalence of psychiatric disorders in children and adolescents with and without intellectual disability. *Journal of Intellectual Disability Research*, *47*, 51–58.

Emerson, E., Felce, D., & Stancliffe, R. J. (2013). Issues concerning self-report data and population-based data sets involving people with intellectual disabilities. *Intellectual and Developmental Disabilities*, *51*, 333–348.

Epstein, R. (1997). Skinner as self-manager. *Journal of Applied Behavior Analysis*, *30*, 545–568.

Esbensen, A. J., & Benson, B. A. (2005). Cognitive variables and depressed mood in adults with intellectual disability. *Journal of Intellectual Disability Research*, *49*, 481–489.

Esbensen, A. J., Rojahn, J., Aman, M. G., & Ruedrich, S. (2003). Reliability and validity of an assessment instrument for anxiety, depression, and mood among individuals with mental retardation. *Journal of Autism and Developmental Disorders*, *33*, 617–629.

Esdale, L., Jahoda, A., & Pert, C. (2015). Coping with criticism and praise. *American Journal on Intellectual and Developmental Disabilities*, *120*, 258–268.

Estes, W. K., & Skinner, B. F. (1941). Some quantitative properties of anxiety. *Journal of Experimental Psychology*, *29*, 390–400.

Finlay, W. M. L. (2005). Psychometric assessment of mood disorders in people with intellectual disabilities. In P. Sturmey (Ed.), *Mood disorders in people with mental retardation* (pp. 67–88). Kingston, NY: NADD Press.

Finlay, W. M., & Lyons, E. (2001). Methodological issues in interviewing and using self-report questionnaires with people with mental retardation. *Psychological Assessment*, *13*, 319–335.

Fredrikson, M., Annas, P., Fischer, H., & Wik, G. (1996). Gender and age differences in the prevalence of specific fears and phobias. *Behaviour Research and Therapy*, *34*, 33–39.

Green, C. W., & Reid, D. H. (1996). Defining, validating, and increasing indices of happiness among people with profound multiple disabilities. *Journal of Applied Behavior Analysis*, *29*, 67–78.

Green, P. (2016). A behavioural approach to helping an older adult with a learning disability and mild cognitive impairment overcome depression. *British Journal of Learning Disabilities*, *45*, 81–88.

Goodwin, M. S., Groden, J., Velicer, W. F., Lipsitt, L. P., Baron, M. G., Hofmann, S. G., & Groden, G. (2006). Cardiovascular arousal in individuals with autism. *Focus on Autism and Other Developmental Disabilities*, *21*, 100–123.

Hamers, P. C., Evenhuis, H. M., & Hermans, H. (2017). A multicenter randomized controlled trial for bright light therapy in adults with intellectual disabilities and depression: Study protocol and obstacle management. *Research in Developmental Disabilities*, *60*, 96–106.

Hannon, G., & Taylor, E. P. (2013). Suicidal behaviour in adolescents and young adults with ASD: Findings from a systematic review. *Clinical Psychology Review*, *33*, 1197–1204.

Hartley, S. L., & Birgenheir, D. G. (2008). Nonverbal social skills of adults with mild intellectual disability diagnosed with depression. *Journal of Mental Health Research in Intellectual Disabilities*, *2*, 11–28.

Hartley, S. L., Lickel, A. H., & MacLean, W. E., Jr. (2008). Reassurance seeking and depression in adults with mild intellectual disability. *Journal of Intellectual Disability Research*, *52*, 917–929.

Hawton, K., Witt, K. G., Salisbury, T. L. T., Arensman, E., Gunnell, D., Hazell, P., … van Heeringen, K. (2016). Psychosocial interventions following self-harm in adults: A systematic review and meta-analysis. *The Lancet Psychiatry*, *3*, 740–750.

Hillier, A. J., Fish, T., Siegel, J. H., & Beversdorf, D. Q. (2011). Social and vocational skills training reduces self-reported anxiety and depression among young adults on the autism spectrum. *Journal of Developmental and Physical Disabilities*, *23*, 267–276.

Hermans, H., Beekman, A. T., & Evenhuis, H. M. (2013). Prevalence of depression and anxiety in older users of formal Dutch intellectual disability services. *Journal of Affective Disorders*, *144*, 94–100.

Hermans, H., van der Pas, F. H., & Evenhuis, H. M. (2011). Instruments assessing anxiety in adults with intellectual disabilities: A systematic review. *Research in Developmental Disabilities*, *32*, 861–870.

Helsel, W. J., . Matson, J. L. (1988). The relationship of depression to social skills and intellectual functioning in mentally retarded adults. Journal of Intellectual Disability Research, 32, 411–418.

Hotton, M., & Coles, S. (2016). The effectiveness of social skills training groups for individuals with autism spectrum disorder. *Review Journal of Autism and Developmental Disorders*, *3*, 68–81.

Hove, O., Assmus, J., & Havik, O. E. (2016). Type and intensity of negative life events are associated with depression in adults with intellectual disabilities. *American Journal on Intellectual and Developmental Disabilities*, *121*, 419–431.

Hurley, A. D. N. (2008). Depression in adults with intellectual disability: Symptoms and challenging behavior. *Journal of Intellectual Disabilities Research*, *52*, 905–916.

Jacobson, N. S., Martell, C. R., & Dimidjian, S. (2001). Behavioral activation treatment for depression: Returning to contextual roots. *Clinical Psychology: Science and Practice*, *8*, 255–270.

Jacobson, N. S., Dobson, K. S., Truax, P. A., Addis, M. E., Koerner, K., Gollan, J. K., … Prince, S. E. (1996). A component analysis of cognitive-behavioral treatment for depression. *Journal of Consulting and Clinical Psychology*, *64*, 295–304.

Jahoda, A., Melville, C. A., Pert, C., Cooper, S. A., Lynn, H., Williams, C., & Davidson, C. (2015). A feasibility study of behavioural activation for depressive symptoms in adults with intellectual disabilities. *Journal of Intellectual Disability Research*, *59*, 1010–1021.

Jahoda, A., Melville, C., Cooper, S. A., Hastings, R., Briggs, A., Dagnan, D., … Jones, R. S. (2015). BEAT-IT: Comparing a behavioural activation treatment for depression in adults with intellectual disabilities with an attention control: Study protocol for a randomised controlled trial. *Trials*, *16*, 595. doi:10.1186/s13063-015-1103-5

Jennett, H. K., & Hagopian, L. P. (2008). Identifying empirically supported treatments for phobic avoidance in individuals with intellectual disabilities. *Behavior Therapy*, *39*, 151–161.

Johansson, R., Sjöberg, E., Sjögren, M., Johnsson, E., Carlbring, P., Andersson, T., … Andersson, G. (2012). Tailored vs. standardized internet-based cognitive behavior therapy for depression and comorbid symptoms: A randomized controlled trial. *PloS One*, *7*(5), e36905.

Jones, K. M., & Friman, P. C. (1999). A case study of behavioral assessment and treatment insect phobia. *Journal of Applied Behavior Analysis*, *32*, 95–98.

Jonsson, U., Alexanderson, K., Kjeldgård, L., Westerlund, H., & Mittendorfer-Rutz, E. (2013). Diagnosis-specific disability pension predicts suicidal behaviour and mortality in young adults: A nationwide prospective cohort study. *BMJ Open, 3*, e002286.

Jonsson, U., Alexanderson, K., Kjeldgård, L., & Mittendorfer-Rutz, E. (2014). Psychiatric diagnoses and risk of suicidal behaviour in young disability pensioners: Prospective cohort studies of all 19-23 year olds in Sweden in 1995, 2000, and 2005, respectively. *PloS One, 9*(11), e111618.

Kanter, J. W., Cautilli, J. D., Busch, A. M., & Baruch, D. E. (2005). Toward a comprehensive functional analysis of depressive behavior: Five environmental factors and a possible sixth and seventh. *The Behavior Analyst Today, 6*, 65–81.

Kaminer, Y., Feinstein, C., & Barrett, R. P. (1987). Suicidal behavior in mentally retarded adolescents: An overlooked problem. *Child Psychiatry and Human Development, 18*, 82–86.

Kim, J. A., Szatmari, P., Bryson, S. E., Streiner, D. L., & Wilson, F. J. (2000). The prevalence of anxiety and mood problems among children with autism and Asperger syndrome. *Autism, 4*, 117–132.

Koslowski, N., Klein, K., Arnold, K., Kösters, M., Schützwohl, M., Salize, H. J., & Puschner, B. (2016). Effectiveness of interventions for adults with mild to moderate intellectual disabilities and mental health problems: Systematic review and meta-analysis. *The British Journal of Psychiatry, 209*, 469–474.

Lang, R., Regester, A., Lauderdale, S., Ashbaugh, K., & Haring, A. (2010). Treatment of anxiety in autism spectrum disorders using cognitive behaviour therapy: A systematic review. *Developmental Neurorehabilitation, 13*, 53–63.

Lancioni, G. E., Singh, N. N., O'Reilly, M. F., Oliva, D., & Basili, G. (2005). An overview of research on increasing indices of happiness of people with severe/profound intellectual and multiple disabilities. *Disability and Rehabilitation, 27*, 83–93.

Lane, B., & Gullone, E. (1999). Common fears: A comparison of adolescents' self-generated and fear survey schedule generated fears. *The Journal of Genetic Psychology, 160*, 194–204.

Leitenberg, H., Agras, W. S., Thompson, L. E., & Wright, D. E. (1968). Feedback in behavior modification: An experimental analysis in two phobic cases. *Journal of Applied Behavior Analysis, 1*, 131–137.

LeJuez, C. W., Hall Brown, T. S., & Hopko, D. R. (2009). Behavioral formulation of depression: The case of Sally. In P. Sturmey (Ed.), *Case formulation: Varieties of approaches* (pp. 57–78). Chichester, UK: Wiley.

Lew, M., Matta, C., Tripp-Tebo, C., & Watts, D. (2006). Dialectical behavior therapy (DBT) for individuals with intellectual disabilities: A program description. *Mental Health Aspects of Developmental Disabilities, 9*, 1–13.

Lindauer, S. E., DeLeon, I. G., & Fisher, W. W. (1999). Decreasing signs of negative affect and correlated self-injury in an individual with mental retardation and mood disturbances. *Journal of Applied Behavior Analysis, 32*, 103–106.

Linehan, M. M., Comtois, K. A., Murray, A. M., Brown, M. Z., Gallop, R. J., Heard, H. L., … Lindenboim, N. (2006). Two-year randomized controlled trial and follow-up of dialectical behavior therapy vs therapy by experts for suicidal behaviors and borderline personality disorder. *Archives of General Psychiatry, 63*, 757–766.

Lindsay, W. R., Tinsley, S., Beail, N., Hastings, R. P., Jahoda, A., Taylor, J. L., & Hatton, C. (2015). A preliminary controlled trial of a transdiagnostic programe for cognitive behaviour therapy with adults with intellectual disability. *Journal of Intellectual Disability Research, 59*, 360–369.

Love, S. R., Matson, J. L., & West, D. (1990). Mothers as effective therapists for autistic children's phobias. *Journal of Applied Behavior Analysis, 23*, 379–385. http://doi.org/10.1901/jaba.1990.23-379

Ludi, E., Ballard, E. D., Greenbaum, R., Bridge, J., Reynolds, W., & Horowitz, L. (2012). Suicide risk in youth with intellectual disability: The challenges of screening. *Journal of Developmental and Behavioral Pediatrics: JDBP, 33*, 43–440.

Lunsky, Y. (2004). Suicidality in a clinical and community sample of adults with mental retardation. *Research in Developmental Disabilities, 25*, 231–243.

Lunsky, Y., & Benson, B. A. (2001). Association between perceived social support and strain, and positive and negative outcome for adults with mild intellectual disability. *Journal of Intellectual Disability Research, 45*, 106–114.

Lydon, S., Healy, O., O'Callaghan, O., Mulhern, T., & Holloway, J. (2015). A systematic review of the treatment of fears and phobias among children with autism spectrum disorders. *Review Journal of Autism and Developmental Disorders, 2*, 141–154.

Matson, J. L. (1981). Assessment and treatment of clinical fears in mentally retarded children. *Journal of Applied Behavior Analysis, 14*, 287–294. http://doi.org/10.1901/jaba.1981.14-287

Matson, J. L. (1982a). The treatment of behavioral characteristics of depression in the mentally retarded. *Behavior Therapy, 13*, 209–218.

Matson, J. L. (1983a). Depression in the mentally retarded: Toward a conceptual analysis of diagnosis. *Progress in Behavior Modification, 15*, 57–79.

Matson, J. L. (1983b). Depression in mentally retarded persons: Research findings and future directions. Australia and New Zealand Journal of Developmental Disabilities, 9, 185–190.

Matson, J. L., Dettling, J., & Senatore, V. (1979). Treating depression of a mentally retarded adult. *British Journal of Mental Subnormality, 16*, 86–88.

Matson, J. L., Lott, J. D., Mayville, S. B., Swender, S. L., & Moscow, S. (2006). Depression and social skills among individuals with severe and profound mental retardation. *Journal of Developmental and Physical Disabilities, 18*, 393–400.

Matson, J. L., & Williams, L. W. (2014). Depression and mood disorders among persons with autism spectrum disorders. *Research in Developmental Disabilities, 35*, 2003–2007.

Mayes, S. D., Gorman, A. A., Hillwig-Garcia, J., & Syed, E. (2013). Suicide ideation and attempts in children with autism. *Research in Autism Spectrum Disorders, 7*, 109–119.

Merrick, J., Merrick, E., Lunsky, Y., & Kandel, I. (2006). A review of suicidality in persons with intellectual disability. *The Israel Journal of Psychiatry and Related Sciences*, *43*, 258.

MacNeil, B. M., Lopes, V. A., & Minnes, P. M. (2009). Anxiety in children and adolescents with autism spectrum disorders. *Research in Autism Spectrum Disorders*, *3*, 1–21.

McGillivray, J. A., & Evert, H. T. (2014). Group cognitive behavioural therapy program shows potential in reducing symptoms of depression and stress among young people with ASD. *Journal of Autism and Developmental Disorders*, *44*, 2041–2051.

McGillivray, J. A., & Kershaw, M. M. (2013). The impact of staff initiated referral and intervention protocols on symptoms of depression in people with mild intellectual disability. *Research in Developmental Disabilities*, *34*, 730–738.

McGillivray, J. A., & Kershaw, M. (2015). Do we need both cognitive and behavioural components in interventions for depressed mood in people with mild intellectual disability? *Journal of Intellectual Disability Research*, *59*, 105–115.

McGillivray, J. A., & McCabe, M. P. (2007). Early detection of depression and associated risk factors in adults with mild/moderate intellectual disability. *Research in Developmental Disabilities*, *28*, 59–70.

McGillivray, J. A., McCabe, M. P., & Kershaw, M. M. (2008). Depression in people with intellectual disability: An evaluation of a staff-administered treatment program. *Research in Developmental Disabilities*, *29*, 524–536.

McKnight, D. L., Nelson, R. O., Hayes, S. C., & Jarrett, R. B. (1984). Importance of treating individually assessed response classes in the amelioration of depression. *Behavior Therapy*, *15*, 315–335.

McNair, L., Woodrow, C., & Hare, D. (2015). Using repertory grid techniques to measure change following dialectical behaviour therapy with adults with learning disabilities: Two case studies. *British Journal of Learning Disabilities*, *44*, 247–256.

Meins, W. (1993). Prevalence and risk factors for depressive disorders in adults with intellectual disability. *Australia and New Zealand Journal of Developmental Disabilities*, *18*, 147–156.

Mindham, J., & Espie, C. A. (2003). Glasgow anxiety scale for people with an intellectual disability (GASID): Development and psychometric properties of a new measure for use with people with mild intellectual disability. *Journal of Intellectual Disability Research*, *47*, 22–30.

Moskowitz, L. J., Mulder, E., Walsh, C. E., McLaughlin, D. M., Zarcone, J. R., Proudfit, G. H., & Carr, E. G. (2013). A multimethod assessment of anxiety and problem behavior in children with autism spectrum disorders and intellectual disability. *American Journal on Intellectual and Developmental Disabilities*, *118*, 419–434.

Nezu, C. M., Nezu, A. M., Rothenberg, J. L., DelliCarpini, L., & Groag, I. (1995). Depression in adults with mild mental retardation: Are cognitive variables involved? *Cognitive Therapy and Research*, *19*, 227–239.

Paquette-Smith, M., Weiss, J., & Lunsky, Y. (2014). History of suicide attempts in adults with Asperger syndrome. *Crisis*, *35*, 273–277.

Porges, S. W. (2013). A psychophysiology of developmental disabilities: A personal and historical perspective. *American Journal on Intellectual and Developmental Disabilities*, *118*, 416–418.

Porges, S. W., & Humphrey, M. M. (1977). Cardiac and respiratory responses during visual search in nonretarded children and retarded adolescents. *American Journal of Mental Deficiency*, *82*, 162–169.

O'Connor, R. D. (1969). Modification of social withdrawal through symbolic modeling. *Journal of Applied Behavior Analysis*, *2*, 15–22.

Ontario Center of Excellence for Child and Youth Mental health. (2014). *Evidence in-sight summary: Suicide in adolescents with developmental disabilities*. ON, Canada: Evidence insight.

Patja, K., Iivanainen, M., Raitasuo, S., & Lönnqvist, J. (2001). Suicide mortality in mental retardation: A 35 year follow up study. *Acta Psychiatrica Scandinavica*, *103*, 307–311.

Prasher, V. J. (2003). Depression in aging individuals with intellectual disabilities. In P. W. Davidson, V. J. Prasher, & M. P. Jamicki (Eds.), *Mental health, intellectual disabilities and the aging process* (pp. 51–66). Oxford, UK: Blackwell.

Ramirez, S. Z., & Kratochwill, T. R. (1997). Self-reported fears in children with and without mental retardation. *Mental Retardation*, *35*, 83–92.

Reinblatt, S. P., Rifkin, A., & Freeman, J. (2004). The efficacy of ECT in adults with mental retardation experiencing psychiatric disorders. *The Journal of ECT*, *20*, 208–212.

Ricciardi, J. N., Luiselli, J. K., & Camare, M. (2006). Shaping approach responses as intervention for specific phobia in a child with autism. *Journal of Applied Behavior Analysis*, *39*, 445–448.

Rosen, T. E., Connell, J. E., & Kerns, C. M. (2016). A review of behavioral interventions for anxiety related behaviors in lower-functioning individuals with autism. *Behavioral Interventions*, *31*, 120–143.

Ross, E., & Oliver, C. (2003). The assessment of mood in adults who have severe or profound mental retardation. *Clinical Psychology Review*, *23*, 225–245.

Sakdalan, J. A., Shaw, J., & Collier, V. (2010). Staying in the here andnow: A pilot study on the use of dialectical behaviour therapy group skills training for forensic clients with intellectual disability. *Journal of Intellectual Disability Research*, *54*, 568–572.

Santomauro, D., Sheffield, J., & Sofronoff, K. (2016). Depression in adolescents with ASD: A pilot RCT of a group intervention. *Journal of Autism and Developmental Disorders*, *46*, 572–588.

Sievert, A. L., Cuvo, A. J., & Davis, P. K. (1988). Training self-advocacy skills to adults with mild handicaps. *Journal of Applied Behavior Analysis*, *21*, 299–309.

Shabani, D. B., & Fisher, W. W. (2006). Stimulus fading and differential reinforcement for the treatment of needle phobia in a youth with autism. *Journal of*

Applied Behavior Analysis, *39*, 449–452. http://doi.org/10.1901/jaba.2006.30-05

Sidman, M. (1989). *Coercion and its fallout*. Boston, MA: Authors cooperative.

Simonoff, E., Pickles, A., Charman, T., Chandler, S., Loucas, T., & Baird, G. (2008). Psychiatric disorders in children with autism spectrum disorders: Prevalence, comorbidity, and associated factors in a population-derived sample. *Journal of the American Academy of Child and Adolescent Psychiatry*, *47*, 921–929.

Skinner, B. F. (1953). *Science and human behavior*. Boston, MA: Simon and Schuster.

Skinner, B. F. (1972). *Beyond freedom and dignity*. New York, NY: Bantam Books.

Spek, A. A., Van Ham, N. C., & Nyklíček, I. (2013). Mindfulness-based therapy in adults with an autism spectrum disorder: A randomized controlled trial. *Research in Developmental Disabilities*, *34*, 246–253.

Stewart, M. E., Barnard, L., Pearson, J., Hasan, R., & O'Brien, G. (2006). Presentation of depression in autism and Asperger syndrome. A review. *Autism*, *10*, 103–116.

Stuart, S., Graham, C. D., & Butler, S. (2014). Doing more, feeling better: A behavioural approach to helping a woman overcome low mood and anxiety. *British Journal of Learning Disabilities*, *42*, 328–335.

Sturmey, P. (1993). The use of ICD and DSM criteria in people with mental retardation: A review. *The Journal of Nervous and Mental Disease*, *181*, 39–42.

Sturmey, P. (1994). Suicidal threats and behavior in a person with developmental disabilities: Effective psychiatric monitoring based on a fundamental assessment. *Behavioral Interventions*, *9*, 235–245.

Sturmey, P. (1996). *Functional analysis in clinical Psychology*. London, UK: Wiley.

Sturmey, P. (Ed.). (2005). *Mood disorders in people with mental retardation*. Kingston, NY: NADD Press.

Sturmey, P. (Ed.). (2007a). *Functional analysis in clinical treatment*. New York, NY: Academic Press.

Sturmey, P. (2007b). Psychosocial and mental status assessment. In J. W. Jacobson, J. A. Mulick, & J. Rojahn (Eds.), *Handbook of intellectual and developmental disabilities* (pp. 295–316). New York, NY: Springer.

Sturmey, P. (2008). *Behavioral case formulation and intervention. A functional analytic approach*. Chichester, UK: Wiley-Blackwell.

Sturmey, P. (2009a). Behavioral activation is an evidence-based treatment of depression. *Behavior Modification*, *33*, 818–829.

Sturmey, P. (2009b). *Case formulation. Varieties of approaches*. Chichester, UK: Wiley.

Turkat, I. D. (1985). *Behavioral case formulation*. New York, NY: Plenum.

Ulrich, R. E., Hutchinson, R. R., & Azrin, N. H. (1965). Pain-elicited aggression. *The Psychological Record*, *15*, 111–126.

Ung, D., McBride, N., Collier, A., Selles, R., Small, B., Phares, V., & Storch, E. (2016). The relationship between peer victimization and the psychological characteristics of youth with autism spectrum disorder. *Research in Autism Spectrum Disorders*, *32*, 7079.

Unwin, G., Tsimopoulou, I., Kroese, B. S., & Azmi, S. (2016). Effectiveness of cognitive behavioural therapy (CBT) programmes for anxiety or depression in adults with intellectual disabilities: A review of the literature. *Research in Developmental Disabilities*, *51*, 60–75.

Valentine, S. E., Bankoff, S. M., Poulin, R. M., Reidler, E. B., & Pantalone, D. W. (2015). The use of dialectical behavior therapy skills training as stand-alone treatment: A systematic review of the treatment outcome literature. *Journal of Clinical Psychology*, *71*, 1–20.

Vause, T., Neil, N., Jaksic, H., Jackiewicz, G., & Feldman, M. (2015). Preliminary randomized trial of function-based cognitive-behavioral therapy to treat obsessive compulsive behavior in children with autism Spectrum disorder. *Focus on Autism and Other Developmental Disabilities*. doi:10.1177/1088357615588517

Walker, J. C., Dosen, A., Buitelaar, J. K., & Janzing, J. G. E. (2011). Depression in down syndrome: A review of the literature. *Research in Developmental Disabilities*, *32*, 1432–1440.

Walters, A. S., Barrett, R. P., Knapp, L. G., & Borden, M. C. (1995). Suicidal behavior in children and adolescents with mental retardation. *Research in Developmental Disabilities*, *16*, 85–96.

Walters, S., Loades, M., & Russell, A. (2016). A systematic review of effective modifications to cognitive behavioural therapy for young people with autism Spectrum disorders. *Review Journal of Autism and Developmental Disorders*, *3*, 137–153.

Willner, P., Rose, J., Jahoda, A., Kroese, B. S., Felce, D., Cohen, D., ... & Shead, J. (2013). Group-based cognitive-behavioural anger management for people with mild to moderate intellectual disabilities: Cluster randomised controlled trial. The British Journal of Psychiatry, 203, 288., bjp-bp.

Wolff, J. J., Hupp, S. C., & Symons, F. J. (2013). Brief report: Avoidance extinction as treatment for compulsive and ritual behavior in autism. *Journal of Autism and Developmental Disorders*, *43*, 1741–1746.

Wolpe, J. (1958). *Psychotherapy by reciprocal inhibition*. Stanford, CA: Stanford University Pres.

Yoo, H. J., Bahn, G., Cho, I. H., Kim, E. K., Kim, J. H., Min, J. W., … Cho, S. (2014). Randomized controlled trial of the Korean version of the PEERS® parent-assisted social skills training program for teens with ASD. *Autism Research*, *7*, 145–161.

Zigler, E., & Balla, D. (Eds.). (1982). *Mental retardation: The developmental- controversy*. Routledge. Abington, United Kingdom

Bullying Among Youth with Autism Spectrum Disorders

4

Inge Zweers, Ron Scholte, and Robert Didden

4.1 Introduction

Students with disabilities and/or autism spectrum disorders (ASD) are particularly vulnerable to be involved in bullying compared to their peers without ASD. Studies have found that students with ASD are at higher risk to be involved in bullying as a bully (i.e., perpetrator of bullying), a victim (i.e., victim of bullying), or bully-victim (i.e., both perpetrator and victim of bullying) (see Cappadocia, Weiss, & Pepler, 2012; Humphrey & Hebron, 2014; Maïano, Norman, Salvas, Moullec, & Aimé, 2015; Schroeder, Cappadocia, Bebko, Pepler, & Weiss, 2014). However, due to the nature of their disability (e.g., difficulties in understanding others' feelings and intentions, nonverbal behaviors, and nonliteral speech), it is unclear whether youth with ASD[1] construe bullying and victimization in similar ways as typically developing youth. Researchers generally agree that bullying is characterized by three defining criteria – (1) negative actions, (2) carried out repeatedly and over time, and (3) in an interpersonal relationship characterized by a power imbalance (Smith, Cowie, Olafsson, & Liefooghe, 2002). Different forms of bullying exist: *physical bullying* (e.g., hitting, kicking, and damage to property), *verbal bullying* (e.g., name-calling, insulting, and making fun of another person), and *relational bullying* (e.g., exclusion, ignoring, and spreading rumors) (see an overview by Stassen Berger, 2007). More recent forms of bullying include *cyberbullying* (e.g., hurtful text messaging or emailing, and posting hurtful messages/objectionable content on websites and social networking sites).

Because of the impairments in social understanding, interaction, and communication and difficulties with generalization in youth with ASD (American Psychiatric Association, DSM-5, 2013; Baron-Cohen, 2000; Heerey, Capps, Keltner, & Kring, 2005), many researchers have questioned the ability of youth with ASD to reliably and validly perceive and report on bullying and victimization (e.g., Fisher & Lounds Taylor, 2016; Kloosterman, Kelley, Craig, Parker, & Javier, 2013; Nowell, Brewton, & Goin-Kochel, 2014; Schroeder et al., 2014; Sreckovic, Brunsting, & Able, 2014; Zeedyk, Rodriguez, & Tipton, 2014). For instance, Nowell et al. (2014) collected qualitative data from 50 verbally fluent children with ASD to examine

[1] The research included in this chapter encompassed elementary and secondary school students in regular and special education, with ages varying from 5 to 21. In order to be clear and concise, throughout the chapter we consistently use the term youth with ASD when addressing children and adolescents with ASD in general, despite varying ages.

I. Zweers
Department of Developmental Psychology, Utrecht University, Utrecht, The Netherlands

R. Scholte • R. Didden (✉)
Behavioural Science Institute, Radboud University, Nijmegen, The Netherlands
e-mail: didden.robert@gmail.com

J.B. Leaf (ed.), *Handbook of Social Skills and Autism Spectrum Disorder*, Autism and Child Psychopathology Series, DOI 10.1007/978-3-319-62995-7_4

their understanding of bullying. Of the 20 children who responded to have been bullied, only half of them could provide an example that demonstrated a clear description/understanding of being bullied (e.g., "Most people hate me 'cause they always tease me. About how I watch those stupid kids' shows but I don't"; Nowell et al., 2014, p. 199). The authors suggest that some children with ASD inaccurately perceive what constitutes bullying. Similar findings have been reported by other studies (e.g., Fisher & Lounds Taylor, 2016). Given that individuals with ASD often have difficulties with abstract thought and generalization, the authors stress that adolescents with ASD might not "be able to abstractly relate their unique bullying experiences to examples provided on questionnaires" (Fisher & Lounds Taylor, 2016, p. 407). Therefore, specific incidences of bullying that have not been specified as examples in survey research might not get reported by students with ASD.

It can also be argued, however, that youth with ASD are in fact able to perceive and report on bullying and victimization (see studies by Adams, Fredstrom, Duncan, Holleb, & Bishop, 2014; Begeer, Fink, Van der Meijden, Goossens, & Olthof, 2016; Bitsika & Sharpley, 2014; Chen & Schwartz, 2012; Rieffe, Camodeca, Pouw, Lange, & Stockmann, 2012; van Roekel, Scholte, & Didden, 2010). For example, adolescents with ASD were as able as their regular developing peers to correctly perceive bullying in video fragments of social interactions (van Roekel et al., 2010). Also, boys with high-functioning ASD demonstrated an understanding of bullying, which was consistent with the wider literature (Bitsika & Sharpley, 2014). Moreover, research also shows that self-reports of adolescents with ASD on bullying and victimization are comparable to self-reports of regular developing adolescents. They show high internal consistency (e.g., Adams et al., 2014; Rieffe et al., 2012), correspond with reports of parents (Adams et al., 2014; Chen & Schwartz, 2012), teachers (Chen & Schwartz, 2012), and peers (Begeer et al., 2016), and are similarly correlated with other variables known to be correlated with bullying and victimization from research with typically developing youth (e.g., Adams et al., 2014; Begeer et al., 2016).

Although the literature generally suggests that youth with ASD reliably and validly perceive and report on bullying and victimization, specific impairments common among individuals with ASD might influence their understanding of bullying and victimization. More research is needed to provide insight into how youth with ASD understand, perceive, and report on bullying. When taking on an observer's role, adolescents with ASD were equally able to perceive and report on bullying in video fragments as typically developing adolescents (van Roekel et al., 2010). However, it is unknown whether youth with ASD are equally able to perceive and report on bullying situations when they themselves are involved in these situations. Investigating how youth with ASD perceive and report on bullying in real-life situations (e.g., by combining self-reports with observations) would therefore be an interesting topic for future research. Furthermore, boys with high-functioning ASD as a sample demonstrated an understanding of bullying which was consistent with definitions held in the wider community and literature (Bitsika & Sharpley, 2014). Future research would benefit from a more in-depth examination of youth's, with ASD, spontaneous definitions of bullying and the influence of providing youth with a definition of bullying when soliciting self-reports and from considering possible variations as a function of age and sex.

4.2 Prevalence

Prevalence estimates of bullying and victimization among youth with ASD are difficult to generate, because studies largely vary in sample characteristics (e.g., age, sex, IQ, sizes, countries/locations, context, and diagnoses and comorbid disorders of participants) and data collection methods (e.g., questionnaires, providing a definition or not, informants, and assessment time frame). However, numerous studies and reviews consistently indicate that youth with ASD report higher rates of victimization than their typically developing peers or peers with other special needs (e.g., Bear, Mantz, Glutting, Yang, & Boyer, 2015; Humphrey & Hebron, 2014; Maïano et al., 2015; Rose, Monda-Amaya, & Espelage, 2011; Rose et al., 2015; Schroeder et al., 2014), both in general and special education settings. Recent meta-analyses indicate that youth with ASD are at risk of general victimization up to three times more than typically developing peers across studies (see a meta-analysis of Maïano et al., 2015). Research on bullying perpetration suggests that youth with ASD are equally likely to bully classmates as compared to their typically developing peers (Rieffe et al., 2012; Rose et al., 2015; Sterzing, Shattuck, Narendorf, Wagner, & Cooper, 2012; Twyman, Saylor, Saia, Macias, & Taylor, 2010; van Roekel et al., 2010; Zablotsky, Bradshaw, Anderson, & Law, 2014). A prevalence of around 10% was found across studies (Maïano et al., 2015).

Very few studies have examined to what extent youth with ASD are involved in bullying, both as a perpetrator and a victim, the so-called bully-victims. The studies that do exist suggest there are no substantial differences between adolescents with ASD and typically developing peers in terms of prevalence of bully-victims (Rose et al., 2015; Sterzing et al., 2012; Zablotsky et al., 2014). This suggests that youth with ASD are neither more nor less likely to be involved in bullying as a bully-victim. Overall prevalence rates are estimated at 16% (Maïano et al., 2015).

Although studies have suggested that youth with ASD are vulnerable to bullying and being involved in bullying both as victim and perpetrator (e.g., Rose et al., 2011; van Roekel et al., 2010), the previously mentioned studies show that youth with ASD are particularly vulnerable to being victimized (e.g., Maïano et al., 2015; Sreckovic et al., 2014), while the risk of being involved in bullying as a bully or a bully-victim appears to be similar to typically developing peers (e.g., Maïano et al., 2015; Rose et al., 2015; Sterzing et al., 2012; Zablotsky et al., 2014). This indicates that although bullying and victimization constitutes a major problem among the general population, it constitutes an even larger problem among youth with ASD. Given that victimization is strongly linked to emotional problems (Arseneault, Bowes, & Shakoor, 2010; Due et al., 2005; Stassen Berger, 2007), there is absolute reason for concern in this respect.

Prevalence of Various Forms of Bullying and Victimization As previously described, bullying can take various forms, such as physical, verbal, and relational bullying. All of these forms are common among typically developing youth (Wang, Ianotti, & Nansel, 2009). Yet, although all forms have also been reported among youth with ASD (e.g., Adams et al., 2014; Fisher & Lounds Taylor, 2016; Humphrey & Symes, 2010a), research on the type of bullying and victimization among this population is limited (Sreckovic et al., 2014).

With respect to physical bullying among youth with ASD, Maïano et al. (2015) reported an overall prevalence estimate of 16% for physical bullying perpetration and an overall prevalence estimate of 33% for physical victimization. Compared with typically developing youth, youth with ASD do not seem to be more at risk for involvement in physical bullying, neither as perpetrator nor as victim (Maïano et al., 2015).

Regarding verbal bullying, Kloosterman et al. (2013) estimated the prevalence of perpetration at 8% (varying from 4.2% to 16.7% between individual items assessing verbal bullying), and Maïano et al. (2015) found an overall prevalence estimate of 50% for verbal victimization across six studies. While youth with ASD do not seem to be more at risk of perpetrating verbal bullying than typically developing peers, they have been estimated to be two times more at risk of being verbally victimized (Maïano et al., 2015).

With respect to relational bullying among youth with ASD, Maïano et al. (2015) reported an overall estimate of 18% for relational bullying perpetration across two studies and an overall prevalence estimate of 31% for relational victimization across seven studies. Compared with typically developing youth, youth with ASD do not seem to be more at risk for involvement in either relational bullying perpetration or victimization (Maïano et al., 2015).

Research suggests that it is not only bullying and victimization in general that constitutes a major problem among youth with ASD, but that – in this population – bullying comes in various forms, as has been established among typically developing youth. A better understanding of the involvement of youth with ASD in various forms of bullying as bullies, victims, and bully-victims seems necessary for several reasons. First, the existing studies are mainly conducted among young adolescents and adolescents with ASD, while studies among typically developing youth have shown that the use of specific forms of bullying differs with increasing age (e.g., younger children are more involved in physical bullying, whereas with increasing social understanding, older youth are more involved in verbal and relational bullying). Given the noted impairments in social understanding characteristic in youth with ASD, involvement in various forms of bullying and victimization might differ related to age. In addition, the difficulties that youth with ASD face in social understanding might be particularly relevant to the more subtle forms of relational bullying. This could suggest that involvement in relational bullying in particular would differ between typically developing youth and youth with ASD. Moreover, research among typically developing youth has shown that involvement in various forms of bullying differs with sex (e.g., boys are more involved in direct physical and verbal bullying, whereas girls are more involved in relational bullying). With diagnoses of ASD being more prevalent among boys than girls (Fombonne, 2005), the influence of sex in the involvement in various types of bullying and victimization might therefore differ between typically developing youth and those with ASD. More insight into the nature and extent of these different forms of bullying and victimization among youth with ASD would help to develop prevention and intervention efforts specifically tailored for this special population at risk.

4.2.1 Prevalence of Cyberbullying

A specific form of bullying and victimization that has become more salient over the years is cyberbullying. Studies among typically developing youth have shown that approximately 16% and 15% of children are involved in cyberbullying as perpetrator or victim, respectively (Zych, Ortega-Ruiz, & Del Rey, 2015). Given that a high percentage of youth with ASD are making use of technology for learning, socializing, and entertainment, similar to that of typically developing youth (e.g., Bannon, McGlynn, McKenzie, & Quayle, 2015; Didden et al., 2009), examining cyberbullying among this special population becomes more and more important. Nevertheless, research on this topic is limited.

A few studies have examined cyberbullying among individuals with various additional support needs, including individuals with ASD. Didden et al. (2009) conducted a study examining the prevalence of cyberbullying among Dutch children with intellectual and developmental disabilities visiting special schools. They found that between 4% and 9% of youth reported cyberbullying or victimization at least once a week. Furthermore, Kowalski and Fedina (2011) found that 21% of the children reported that they had been victims of cyberbullying and 6% reported that they had perpetrated cyberbullying at least once within the past 2 months. In another sample, Cross, Piggin, Douglas, and Vonkaenel-Flatt (2012) found that 16% of a UK sample of young individuals with disabilities were found to be at risk of persistent cyberbullying over a prolonged period. Lastly, Cappadocia et al. (2012) examined cyberbullying among youth with ASD in a predominantly Canadian sample. The youths' parents reported 6% to be cyberbullied two to three times a month, with 2% experiencing cybervictimization once a week or more.

Although Didden et al. (2009) suggest that, in general, students with developmental disabilities seem to have a somewhat lower probability to be involved in cyberbullying and/or cybervictimization, cross-study comparisons with research among typically developing youth suggest a similar risk for involvement in cyberbullying for youth with ASD and typically developing peers (Schroeder et al., 2014; Zych et al., 2015). Increased risk for youth with ASD, however, has also been suggested (e.g., Bannon et al., 2015; Kowalski & Fedina, 2011). A possible reason for this may be the youth's, with ASD, difficulties with social understanding and generalization, their lack of considering long-term consequences of their behavior, and their deficits in executive functioning (e.g., Bannon et al., 2015; Kloosterman, Kelley, Parker, & Craig, 2014) – characteristics that make youth with ASD more vulnerable to being involved in bullying in the real world – might also lead to higher vulnerability of being involved in cyberbullying (Kowalski & Fedina, 2011). Future research is needed to shed more light on the nature and extent of cyberbullying among youth with ASD and to be able to compare their experiences with those of their typically developing counterparts.

4.2.2 Reporters

When examining prevalence estimates of bullying and victimization, discrepancies in estimates arise from differences in reporters. While older studies predominantly relied on teacher and parent reports (e.g., Carter, 2009; Little, 2002; Montes & Halterman, 2007; Reid & Batten, 2006; Shtayermman, 2007), more recent research also collected self-reported data from youth with ASD (e.g., Adams et al., 2014; Chen & Schwartz, 2012; Rowley et al., 2012; van Roekel et al., 2010; Zeedyk et al., 2014). Studies comparing the prevalence estimates of multiple reporters have found mixed results. Some studies have found that teachers and parents tend to report higher rates of bullying than youth with ASD themselves (Adams et al., 2014; van Roekel et al., 2010), with parents reporting higher levels of victimization than teachers (Nowell et al., 2014) and teachers reporting higher levels of bullying perpetration than parents (Chen & Schwartz, 2012). Generally, however, it seems that peers report lower prevalence estimates for bullying and victimization of youth with ASD than teachers, parents, and youth with ASD themselves, both in mainstream educational settings (Maïano et al., 2015) and in special education settings (van Roekel et al., 2010), while the latter three informants seem to considerably agree on their reports of bullying and victimization (Bitsika & Sharpley, 2014; Chen & Schwartz, 2012; Kloosterman et al., 2013; Maïano et al., 2015; Rowley et al., 2012; Zeedyk et al., 2014). This contrasts with research among typically developing youth, in which youth (i.e., self and peers) generally report higher estimates of bullying and victimization than teachers and parents (Bradshaw, Sawyer, & O'Brennan, 2007; Monks, Smith, & Swettenham, 2003).

Among typically developing youth, teachers and parents are suggested to underestimate bullying and victimization among youth, especially among (young) adolescents (e.g., Bradshaw et al., 2007). Possible explanations for this phenomenon are that parents and teachers usually are not present in situations in which bullying occurs, while peers have been found to be present during the majority of bullying episodes (Atlas & Pepler, 1998; Hawkins, Pepler, & Craig, 2001); teachers often fail to identify the more covert and subtle forms of bullying (Craig, Henderson, & Murphey, 2000); and students often do not report incidences of bullying to adults (Whitney & Smith, 1993).

Among youth with ASD, in contrast, different processes might be at work due to their condition-related difficulties (e.g., impaired social understanding, communication difficulties, and having fewer friends). Parents and teachers might be more attentive to negative social experiences of vulnerable youth (Kloosterman et al., 2013). They might, for instance, monitor vulnerable youth like those with ASD more closely, while typically developing peers are regularly left in unsupervised situations. Consequently, parents and teachers might be able to observe more incidences of bullying among youth with ASD than among typically developing youth. Another explanation might be that, while typically developing youth might refrain from reporting incidences of bullying to adults, youth with ASD are more likely to confide in their parents and teachers (Humphrey & Symes, 2010b; Kloosterman et al., 2013). While typically developing youth tend to share more information with friends, especially with increasing age, youth with ASD report having fewer, if any, friends with whom to share information (Cappadocia et al., 2012; Humphrey & Symes, 2010b). In addition, parents and teachers of youth with ASD might interact more regularly about the youth's development and experiences. Consequently, parents and teachers would be more aware of youth's bullying and victimization experiences (Chen & Schwartz, 2012).

It is important to note that no conclusions can be drawn about who is the best reporter of bullying and victimization. Instead, as among typically developing youth (Juvonen, Nishina, & Graham, 2001), reports of different informants are suggested to be complementary. For instance, self-views – subjective experiences from the child's own perspective – provide a unique insight in youth with ASD's internal experiences (Adams et al., 2014). In contrast, peer reports – that reflect agreement among peers about the relative standing of an individual – provide unique insights in youth with ASD's social reputation. Both reports are differentially associated with social adjustment. That is, self-reported bullying and victimization is more strongly associated with self-reported adjustment measures such as internalizing problems (Adams et al., 2014; Juvonen et al., 2001), while peer-reports are more strongly associated with peer-reported adjustment measures such as peer acceptance and perceived popularity (Juvonen et al., 2001). Furthermore, parent and teacher reports are considered especially useful because data about youth across the full spectrum of functioning can be collected (Fisher & Lounds Taylor, 2016). Specifically, teachers and parents are able to provide information on experiences of low-functioning youth with ASD who are not able to participate themselves. In addition, teachers and parents can provide information on bullying and victimization in various contexts (i.e., school and home/community; Nowell et al., 2014). Hence, the different reports may represent different aspects of bullying and victimization, particularly among youth with ASD.

4.3 The Role of the Social Environment

Given that bullying has recently been considered a group process (Salmivalli, 2010), it becomes more and more important to consider the role of the social environment in bullying and victimization research. Peers are present in 85% to 88% of all bullying episodes (Atlas & Pepler, 1998; Hawkins et al., 2001) and appear to play specific roles – called participant roles (Goossens, Olthof, & Dekker, 2006; Salmivalli, Lagerspetz, Björkqvist, Österman, & Kaukiainen, 1996; Sutton & Smith, 1999) – that either maintain bullying and victimization or put it to an end. The participant roles that have been identified among typically developing youth include (Salmivalli et al., 1996; Salmivalli, Lappalainen, & Lagerspetz, 1998):

- *Bullies* show active, initiative-taking, leader-like bullying behavior.
- *Assistants* eagerly join in the bullying and show follower-like bullying behavior. They actively support the bully in attacking the victim.
- *Reinforcers* provide positive feedback to the bully by laughing, cheering, inciting, and/or providing an audience for the bully.
- *Outsiders* stay away from the bullying situation and do not take sides with either party. However, by "doing nothing" they may also encourage bullying by sending a silent message that bullying behavior is acceptable.
- *Defenders* take sides with the victim by standing up for the victim and actively trying to stop the bullying situation and/or by supporting and consoling the victim.
- *Victims* are the targets of attacks and are unable to defend themselves.

Prevalence estimates for these participant roles among typically developing youth (across sexes) are 4–14% for bullies, 6–13% for assistants, 15–20% for reinforcers, 8–32% for outsiders, 5–20% for defenders, and 5–14% for victims (Goossens et al., 2006; Salmivalli, 1999; Salmivalli et al., 1996; Salmivalli et al., 1998).

More recently, these participant roles have also been identified among homogeneous groups of youth with ASD in special education (e.g., Begeer et al., 2016; Schrooten, Scholte, Cillessen, & Hymel, 2016). Schrooten et al. (2016) found prevalence estimates of 3–7% for bullies, 8–11% for followers (i.e., assistants and reinforcers combined), 30–42% for outsiders, 16–19% for defenders, and 13–14% for victims across sexes. Based on these results, the authors suggest that the social difficulties of youth with ASD do not prevent them from taking on various participant roles in bullying situations.

While Begeer et al. (2016) did not find any differences in the rates of peer-reported bullying, victimization, and defending between youth with ASD in special education and typically developing peers in regular education, Schrooten et al. (2016) did find such differences. That is, Schrooten et al. found more outsiders and defenders, and fewer followers among boys with ASD in special education than among typically developing boys in regular education. The authors suggested that boys with ASD in special education were more inclined to stay away from bullying situations or stand up for the victim than typically developing boys in regular education, who often fail to support the victim (Atlas & Pepler, 1998; Hawkins et al., 2001). The possible explanations the authors provided include that youth with ASD in special education are more likely to adopt the defender and outsider role because prosocial behavior is more explicitly valued in special education (Rodkin et al., 2006), or that differences in role distributions are the result of the social difficulties that youth with ASD face. That is, the outsider role may be adopted more often by youth with ASD who do not know how to act, even though they want to (Bauminger, Shulman, & Agam, 2003), and the defender role may be adopted more often by youth with ASD who do not anticipate that helping a victim might increase the likelihood that they will become victimized themselves (Bannon et al., 2015). In contrast to the encouraging results that boys with ASD in special education seem somewhat less actively involved in bullying than typically developing boys in regular education, Schrooten et al. also found that girls with ASD in special education were more often victims than typically developing girls in regular education. A possible explanation the authors provide is that girls with ASD are more vulnerable to victimization because they compose a minority group in special education (Schumann, Craig, & Rosu, 2013). Yet, victimization rates of both boys and girls with ASD in special education were lower than those reported among youth with ASD in regular education (Carter, 2009; Little, 2002; Rose et al., 2011).

4.4 Educational Setting

In addition to the participant roles that peers play in bullying episodes, the wider context (e.g., peer group) is important to consider as well. Much research on bullying is conducted in schools because youth spend a fairly large amount of time in school settings. The composition of the peer group in school settings differs to a considerable extent between regular and special education settings. That is, in regular education settings, the peer group consists of typically developing peers who generally do not experience substantial difficulties in their development, whereas in special education settings, the peer group consists of peers who all face substantial difficulties leading to additional support needs. Whether youth with ASD attend special education as opposed to general education might therefore influence their involvement in bullying and victimization.

Findings related to the effects of educational settings on bullying and victimization, however, have been inconsistent. Whereas Rose et al. (2011) found in their review that students with disabilities educated in segregated classrooms or schools were victimized more often than students with and without disabilities in regular education, other studies found no significant differences in the rates of bullying or victimization across youth with ASD in special education and typically developing youth in regular education (Begeer et al., 2016; van Roekel et al., 2010). Yet, the majority of studies found that students with ASD who were educated in regular education classrooms or mainstream schools were more likely to be victimized than students who were educated in segregated settings (Hebron & Humphrey, 2014; Maïano et al., 2015; Rowley et al., 2012; Sterzing et al., 2012; Zablotsky et al., 2014). The main explanation for these findings is that, in educational settings in which youth with ASD have more social interactions with typically developing peers, they face a higher likelihood of being victimized, simply because they stand out for being different (Schroeder et al., 2014). In addition, the social and emotional difficulties that youth with ASD face (e.g., lack of understanding others' intentions, feelings, and nonliteral speech, and emotional dysregulation) may be a cause of misinterpretation between youth with ASD and their typically developing counterparts. In special education settings, students with ASD may be less likely to stand out from their peers, because – despite the heterogeneity in specific difficulties that they show – all students in special education settings have additional support needs (Begeer et al., 2016; Hebron & Humphrey, 2014; van Roekel et al., 2010).

The explanation of standing out for clearly being different can, in contrast, also serve as a protective factor. Researchers have shown that students with more severe additional support needs (either social or cognitive in nature) were less likely to be bullied, regardless of educational setting (Rowley et al., 2012; Shtayermman, 2007; Zablotsky et al., 2014). This could provide evidence that youth who are more noticeably different – that is, those who have more obvious disabilities visible to their peers – are being protected from victimization (Kasari, Locke, Gulsrud, & Rotheram-Fuller, 2011, as cited in Sreckovic et al., 2014). Another explanation might be that youth with more severe ASD are just less likely to be socially involved with their peers and therefore less likely to experience victimization (Rowley et al., 2012). Furthermore, the more severely affected youth with ASD could be better monitored by teachers (Nowell et al., 2014; Shtayermman, 2007) or other adults in their environment, which protects them from experiencing victimization.

School factors that vary across educational settings (e.g., smaller classrooms, amount of adult supervision, structure and routine organization, and teachers trained in additional support needs) complicate the comparisons made even more. Some researchers have posited that smaller class sizes and more adult supervision in special education might decrease the risk for youth with ASD to become victimized in school (Hebron & Humphrey, 2014; Sterzing et al., 2012). Interestingly, however, parents of children with ASD included in regular education reported that their schools more effectively dealt with bullying incidences than parents of children with ASD in special education settings (Reid & Batten, 2006).

All in all, these studies seem to suggest that especially youth with high-functioning ASD, who are more often included in regular education, are at increased risk for experiencing victimization (Nowell et al., 2014; Zablotsky et al., 2014). The higher skills of these youth may mask the pervasive (social) difficulties that they face (Shtayermman, 2007), leaving them less protected and vulnerable to peer victimization in settings in which there is not much adult supervision (Zablotsky et al., 2014). Humphrey and Symes (2011) explained the underlying mechanism causing this increased risk for victimization (i.e., a social outcome for included students with ASD) in their "Reciprocal Effects Peer Interaction Model" (REPIM; Humphrey & Symes, 2011, pp. 400–401). That is, the noted impairments characteristic of youth with ASD (e.g., difficulties in social understanding and a lack of social skills) combined with characteristics of their typically developing peers (e.g., lack of awareness and understanding of ASD, low acceptance of differences and atypical behavior) lead to reduced quality and frequency of peer interactions. This in turn leads to a limited social network and lower levels of support, which makes youth with ASD more vulnerable to victimization. These processes appear to follow a vicious cycle in which the negative social experiences of youth with ASD lead them to be less motivated for future social interactions with peers. The subsequent avoidant and solitary behaviors of youth with ASD causes even less awareness and understanding among their typically developing peers (Humphrey & Hebron, 2014; Humphrey & Symes, 2011). In contrast, youth with ASD who are educated in segregated settings for special education and who are surrounded by peers with additional support needs, do not seem to differ from typically developing peers in regular education with respect to their involvement in bullying and victimization (Begeer et al., 2016; van Roekel et al., 2010). This preliminary evidence is particularly important considering that increasing numbers of students with disabilities, including students with ASD, participate in regular education classrooms for at least part of their school day. Even students with ASD who are in special education classrooms are increasingly included in regular education schools in which they have opportunities to interact with their typically developing peers (Chen & Schwartz, 2012).

Of additional interest in future research would be efforts to distinguish individual (personal) and contextual (school) factors in understanding the social experiences of students with ASD. Large variability exists in the extent to which students with ASD have the opportunity to interact with typically developing peers and peers with other psychological and/or behavioral needs when educated in various settings (regular education, special needs classroom in regular education, specialist ASD classroom in regular education, special needs classroom in segregated special school, etc.). Thus, examining the perpetration and victimization of youth with ASD attending different educational settings is an interesting and relevant topic for future research. Furthermore, despite the relatively homogeneous composition of classrooms in segregated specialist ASD schools (e.g., Begeer et al., 2016; Schrooten et al., in press; van Roekel et al., 2010), comparable rates of bullying and victimization were found in youth with ASD and their typically developing counterparts in regular education. Investigating which characteristics of youth with ASD lead to increased risk of bullying and victimization is another fruitful area of further research.

4.5 Causes and Consequences

There is a growing literature on risk and protective factors for bullying and victimization of youth with ASD. Studies to date have provided preliminary evidence for differences and similarities in risk and protective factors among youth with ASD and typically developing youth (Hebron & Humphrey, 2014; Humphrey & Hebron, 2014; Sreckovic et al., 2014). Youth with ASD tend to exhibit risk factors for bullying and victimization that reflect characteristics or behaviors associated with the diagnosis of ASD, and in addition, they tend to lack protective factors that are associated with decreased risk of victimization among typically developing youth (Schroeder et al., 2014). Yet, much of the work in this area has relied on cross-sectional, regression-based, or qualitative methods: caution in interpretation is thus required. Although directions of effects have been suggested, we cannot infer *causality* from these studies; in fact, many associations have the potential to be bidirectional. To this end, we discuss *correlates* of bullying and victimization that might act as risk or protective factors: when high rates of a particular factor are associated with an increased risk of victimization (i.e., considered as a risk factor), lower rates of that factor are associated with a decreased risk (i.e., considered as a protective factor), and the other way around.

Correlates of Victimization Several studies on the association between victimization and autistic symptomatology, such as impaired social skills, social vulnerability, communication difficulties, and stereotypic behaviors, have shown mixed results. On the one hand, youth with ASD who show higher levels of autistic symptoms have been found to be more at risk for victimization (Cappadocia et al., 2012; Sofronoff, Dark, & Stone, 2011; Zablotsky et al., 2014), which is consistent with research among typically developing peers that shows that youth who have difficulties in these areas are more at risk for victimization. On the other hand, youth with ASD who show less severe autistic symptoms (Rowley et al., 2012; Shtayermman, 2007; Sterzing et al., 2012) have been found to be more at risk for victimization, which seems to reflect a difference in risk factors with typically developing youth. Two different mechanisms might be at work here. First, it seems that the context determines to a certain extent whether the level of autistic symptoms is a risk factor. That is, when youth with ASD are surrounded by typically developing peers, they stand out for being different because of their autistic behavior (Schroeder et al., 2014; Wainscot, Naylor, Sutcliffe, Tantam, & Williams, 2008). When youth with ASD are surrounded by peers with additional support needs (e.g., in special classrooms or segregated special education), they may be less likely to stand out from their peers due to their autistic behavior, because – despite the heterogeneity in specific difficulties – all youth show certain difficulties (Begeer et al., 2016; Hebron & Humphrey, 2014; van Roekel et al., 2010). Second, instead of clearly showing that either higher or lower levels of autistic symptomatology are associated with victimization, autistic symptomatology seems to show a curvilinear relationship with victimization. That is, the more youth with ASD are perceived as deviating from peer group norms due to their socially incongruent behavior, the more rejected/neglected they are among peers and the more at risk they are for victimization. This would explain why, in some studies, higher levels of autistic symptomatology are associated with increased risk of victimization (Cappadocia et al., 2012; Sofronoff et al., 2011; Zablotsky et al., 2014). When autistic symptomatology becomes more and more severe, however – to such an extent that the disabilities of youth with ASD are clearly visible to their peers – the risk of victimization seems to decrease, and sometimes youth with ASD are even protected from victimization (Kasari et al., 2011). This would explain why, in other studies, lower levels of autistic symptomatology are associated with increased risk of victimization (Rowley et al., 2012; Shtayermman, 2007; Sterzing et al., 2012).

Other aspects related to the condition of ASD, such as comorbid disorders, difficulties with emotions, and behavioral problems, have more consistently been shown to play a role in the likelihood that youth with ASD are victimized. Higher levels of both externalizing (Cappadocia et al., 2012; Hebron & Humphrey, 2014) and internalizing behavior problems (Adams et al., 2014; Cappadocia et al., 2012; Didden et al., 2009; Hebron & Humphrey, 2014; Kowalski & Fedina, 2011; Zeedyk et al., 2014) have generally been related to increased risk for victimization, although these associations were not found in all studies (Shtayermman, 2007). Furthermore, comorbid disorders such as ADHD (Zablotsky, Bradshaw, Anderson, & Law, 2013; Sterzing et al., 2012), depression (Zablotsky et al., 2013), or multiple conditions (Zablotsky et al., 2014) have also been related to increased risk for victimization, as well as impairments in executive functioning (Kloosterman et al., 2013) and emotion regulation (Rieffe et al., 2012). These studies provide further evidence that (additional) emotional or behavioral difficulties are risk factors of victimization among youth with ASD, which is consistent with what is found among typically developing youth.

The previously mentioned factors have often been considered individual factors: that is, cognitive, behavioral, and psychological features of the child. However, contextual factors – features of the child's environment such as peers, school, and family – can act as risk and protective factors as well. Many studies have shown that peer difficulties are associated with increased risk for victimization among youth with ASD. Specifically, difficulties with making friends (Zablotsky et al., 2014), having fewer friends (Cappadocia et al., 2012), conflict in friendships (Zeedyk et al., 2014), social exclusion, rejection, and unpopularity among peers (Rowley et al., 2012; Schrooten et al., in press), and peer problems in general (Begeer et al., 2016) have all been found to be risk factors for victimization, while having positive social relationships has been found to be associated with less victimization (Hebron & Humphrey, 2014). Although peer difficulties have also been found to be a risk factor for victimization among typically developing youth, they seem to be particularly prevalent among youth with ASD because of their difficulties with social interaction and communication inherent to their condition (American Psychiatric Association, 2013; Baron-Cohen, 2000; Heerey et al., 2005).

Other contextual factors that have been associated with increased risk for victimization are school factors like educational placement, provision of special education services, and use of school transportation. Most studies indicate that educational placement in mainstream settings is related to increased risk for victimization (Hebron & Humphrey, 2014; Reid & Batten, 2006; Rowley et al., 2012; Sterzing et al., 2012; Zablotsky et al., 2014) and that attending a special school is associated with reduced exposure to bullying (Hebron & Humphrey, 2014). Furthermore, provision of special educational needs services within a mainstream school and use of school transportation were related to higher levels of victimization (Hebron & Humphrey, 2014; Sreckovic et al., 2014). These results seem to confirm that youth with less severe ASD, who are more functionally independent and who more often find themselves in situations with limited adult supervision, are more at risk for victimization.

In addition to the more well-established correlates of victimization among youth with ASD, research has indicated several other factors that have been associated with victimization among this group: sex (Cappadocia et al., 2012; Reid & Batten, 2006), age (Cappadocia et al., 2012; Hebron & Humphrey, 2014; Little, 2002), ethnicity (Sterzing et al., 2012; Zablotsky et al., 2014), socioeconomic status (Zablotsky et al., 2014), parental engagement in school (Hebron & Humphrey, 2014), and parental mental health problems (Cappadocia et al., 2012). Since research on these factors is limited, the results are difficult to interpret. These studies provide interesting preliminary evidence that demographic and family factors should be considered as potential risk or protective factors for victimization of youth with ASD. More research is definitely needed, however, to investigate if these variables are related to victimization specific to youth with ASD, to examine the differences and similarities with risk and protective factors among typically developing youth, and to establish causal directions of effects.

4.5.1 Correlates of Bullying Perpetration

Although correlates of bullying perpetration are less extensively examined than correlates of victimization, there seems to be considerable overlap in the risk and protective factors of being a perpetrator or a victim. Also in bullying perpetration, studies on the association between perpetration and autistic symptomatology have shown mixed results. Zablotsky et al. (2014) found that children with high levels of autistic traits were more likely to be perpetrators of bullying than children with low levels of autistic traits. Rowley et al. (2012), in contrast, found that children whose lack of social and communication skills were smaller reported higher levels of bullying. There are several explanations for these opposing findings. Some researchers have suggested that youth with more severe ASD are more likely to bully because they generally are more aggressive than typically developing peers (Carr, 2006), because they misinterpret social communication as hostile (Whitney, Smith, & Thompson, 1994), or as a response to previous experiences of being victimized themselves (Rose et al., 2011). Others, however, pose that more socially capable youth with ASD are likely to be more socially involved with peers, and consequently face an increased likelihood of negative social experiences including bullying perpetration (Rowley et al., 2012). Furthermore, among typically developing youth, perpetrators have been found to strategically pick victims that they have an advantage over (Salmivalli, 2010). Youth with ASD with more developed social understanding, might similarly use these skills to bully peers. Given these opposing results and explanations, investigating which aspects of autistic symptomatology are related to bullying perpetration is a fruitful area of further research.

Other aspects related to the condition of ASD, such as comorbid disorders and difficulties with emotions have also been shown to be associated with bullying perpetration. For instance, externalizing comorbid disorders such as conduct disorder, oppositional defiant disorder (Zablotsky et al., 2013) or ADHD (Montes & Halterman, 2007; Sterzing et al., 2012) have been related to increased risk of perpetration. Furthermore, bullying perpetration has been related to fewer feelings of guilt, more feelings of anger (Rieffe et al., 2012), more anxiety (Kowalski & Fedina, 2011), higher depressive symptomatology (Didden et al., 2009; Kowalski & Fedina, 2011), higher rates of emotional regulation difficulties in general (Zablotsky et al., 2013), and lower self-esteem (Didden et al., 2009). These studies provide evidence that, while internalizing problems have also been related to bullying perpetration, externalizing problems and emotion regulation difficulties seem to be particularly important correlates of bullying perpetration, which is consistent with what is found among typically developing youth.

In addition to individual factors, contextual factors have been associated with bullying perpetration as well. Specifically, fewer peer difficulties (Begeer et al., 2016) and more frequent involvement with peers (Sterzing et al., 2012) – often seen as positive for youth with ASD – have been related to increased risk of bullying perpetration. This may be due to the fact that youth with ASD who are more involved with peers, also have increased social opportunity to experience bullying involvement (Sterzing et al., 2012). However, other studies have shown associations between perpetration and more negative peer experiences, such as having difficulties in making friends (Zablotsky et al., 2014) and peer rejection (Schrooten et al., 2016). These mixed results are difficult to interpret and indicate that more insight into peer processes is needed to qualify how social experiences of youth with ASD with their peers might influence their risk of bullying perpetration.

4.5.2 Conclusion

In sum, the majority of the studies examining correlates of bullying and victimization have focused on victimization of youth with ASD. This is understandable, given that youth with ASD are particularly vulnerable to become victimized (e.g., Maïano et al., 2015; Sreckovic et al., 2014), while the risk of being involved in bullying as a bully or a bully-victim appears to be similar to typically developing peers (e.g., Maïano et al., 2015; Rose et al., 2015; Sterzing et al., 2012; Zablotsky et al., 2014). The existing literature seems to show that vulnerability for victimization is primarily related to autistic symptomatology and related internalizing problems (with externalizing emotional outbursts resulting from difficulties related to their condition), and clear difficulties in establishing and maintaining social relationships with peers. The educational context (e.g., available peer group, provision of additional support, and extent of adult supervision) seems to play a major role as well in victimization among youth with ASD. Vulnerability for bullying perpetration, in contrast, seems to be primarily related to externalizing problems, while associations with autistic symptomatology and peer difficulties are less consistent.

Research regarding the risk and protective factors of bullying and victimization among youth with ASD is still in its infancy. Research with larger samples is needed to address the problems with generalizability often found in existing studies. Furthermore, as recommended in the general bullying field (e.g., Swearer, Espelage, Vaillancourt, & Hymel, 2010), a multi-informant approach should be adopted to yield more valid results than single-informant measures (Maïano et al., 2015; Monks et al., 2003; Zablotsky et al., 2013). Moreover, various educational contexts should be considered when examining bullying and victimization among youth with ASD, as research has shown that their experiences vary across mainstream and special education settings, and across various locations in and surrounding school (e.g., school transport, playground, and classroom). Lastly, but maybe most importantly, future research would benefit from collecting longitudinal data on potential risk and protective factors to examine causes and consequences of both bullying and victimization among youth with ASD.

4.6 Prevention and Intervention

Very limited information currently exists on best practices to reduce rates of victimization among youth with ASD. Research that has made recommendations for prevention and intervention often builds upon what is known about bullying prevention among typically developing youth (Hebron & Humphrey, 2014). Systematic reviews and meta-analyses of research among the general population have shown that, although some interventions only resulted in modest positive outcomes (Merrell, Guelder, Ross, & Isava, 2008; Smith, Schneider, Smith, & Ananiadou, 2004), school-based antibullying programs generally showed a reduction in bullying and victimization by 20–23% and 17–20%, respectively (Farrington & Ttofi, 2009; Ttofi & Farrington, 2011).

Effective prevention and intervention programs involve a comprehensive strategy that approaches bullying at multiple levels. That is, not only all members of the school community, including students, teachers, and support staff but also parents should be aware of what bullying is and how to respond to it. The entire school environment should be engaged in preventing bullying and intervening when it occurs (Smith et al., 2004). In order to effectively reduce perpetration and victimization among youth, these prevention and intervention programs need to be long-lasting and intensive, probably because a considerable time period is needed to build up a strong antibullying school climate, which is endorsed by all school community members (Ttofi & Farrington, 2011). Effective elements of whole-school prevention and intervention programs contain: encouragement of positive and healthy relationships among children by adults; clear and consistent antibullying policies involving nonphysical disciplinary methods (e.g., restorative justice approaches) to address perpetration behaviors; classroom management focused on detecting and addressing bullying, and promoting the development of prosocial, communication, and conflict-resolution skills among students; active supervision of student behavior in all school locations (i.e., also in the playground and hallways); encouragement of youth to report incidences of bullying to a trusted adult; collaborations among professionals within schools to address bullying; individualized interventions for the children directly involved in bullying as victims and/or bullies; and parental involvement (Farrington & Ttofi, 2009; Smith et al., 2004; Ttofi & Farrington, 2011).

Effective prevention and intervention programs for typically developing youth have been suggested to be effective to reduce bullying and victimization among youth with ASD as well. However, several elements on each level are recommended to be intensified or added to address the needs of youth with ASD (Bitsika & Sharpley, 2014; Cappadocia et al., 2012; Fisher & Lounds Taylor, 2016; Humphrey & Hebron, 2014; Reid & Batten, 2006; Sterzing et al., 2012). First, on the individual level, the core deficits of ASD (e.g., social understanding, conversational ability, and social skills) and comorbid difficulties (e.g., behavior problems and emotion regulation difficulties) need to be targeted (Sterzing et al., 2012) in order for these students to be less likely to stand out among their peers (Sreckovic et al., 2014). To this end, youth with ASD might be trained to develop social skills (Humphrey & Hebron, 2014) and learn alternative behaviors that they can use to positively engage with peers and to replace awkward social behaviors (Bitsika & Sharpley, 2014; Sreckovic et al., 2014). In addition, interventions might want to focus part of their efforts on youth's perceptions and understanding of positive and negative social behavior (Adams et al., 2014; Sreckovic et al., 2014), since students with ASD may misperceive bullying situations (van Roekel et al., 2010) and friendships (Bitsika & Sharpley, 2014).

Second, on the level of the peer group, awareness of ASD should be raised and inclusiveness should be promoted (Cappadocia et al., 2012; Humphrey & Hebron, 2014; Reid & Batten, 2006; Sterzing et al., 2012). Awareness-raising can help typically developing peers understand why someone may act differently to them (Reid & Batten, 2006) and may increase the empathy and social skills of typically developing peers towards youth with ASD (Sterzing et al., 2012). Promoting inclusiveness may result in youth with ASD to be more integrated into protective peer groups (Sterzing et al., 2012). While some researchers also recommend specific peer engagement approaches such as peer mentoring, befriending, and buddying schemes (Reid & Batten, 2006), others discourage these due to conflicting findings for peer engagement among typically developing youth (Farrington & Ttofi, 2009; Ttofi & Farrington, 2011).

Third, on the level of teacher and support staff, teachers can actively discuss exceptionalities and difficulties among children along with modeling empathy, respect, and liking for students with ASD and other disabilities (Cappadocia et al., 2012; Humphrey & Hebron, 2014). By actively teaching peers not to avoid students who are different and serving as positive role models for (typically developing) students, teachers promote inclusiveness (Cappadocia et al., 2012; Fisher & Lounds Taylor, 2016). In line with this atmosphere of encouraging differences and individuality, teachers and support staff need to flexibly use and adjust pedagogical approaches, since "standard" pedagogic approaches often do not work for students with ASD (Humphrey & Hebron, 2014). Furthermore, in situations in which a student is victimized – especially in case of a student with ASD – more intensive adult support is needed. That is, students with ASD might need help with regulating their emotions and behavior, to cope with the negative situation, to communicate assertively, to constructively solve the problem, and/or to engage with supportive peers (Cappadocia et al., 2012). Mixed results have been found, however, for the provision of additional assistance by support staff like teaching assistants. On the one hand, support staff can enhance the academic engagement of adolescents with ASD, but their presence could also increase social distance from peers (Humphrey & Hebron, 2014), which could increase the risk of victimization.

Lastly, on the level of the entire school environment, all school community members should endorse respect for diversity and differences in all its forms (Humphrey & Hebron, 2014). In addition to that, several structural adjustments could be made to provide youth with ASD with opportunities to positively engage with peers (e.g., structured play activities during breaks; Reid & Batten, 2006) or to withdraw from social interactions when needed (e.g., provide safe havens in school; Bitsika & Sharpley, 2014). Furthermore, it is recommended to form strong school-home systems to monitor youth with ASD's bullying experiences, especially considering the fact that youth with ASD are suggested to underreport bullying and victimization to both parents and teachers (e.g., Nowell et al., 2014).

While several of the suggested prevention and intervention efforts have already been implemented with students with ASD (Sreckovic et al., 2014), their effectiveness in terms of reducing bullying and victimization has yet to be explored. Furthermore, it has to be examined to what extent the effects of current evidence-based programs among typically youth are also suitable for populations in special education (i.e., special education classrooms and/or segregated schools for special education). Initiatives to adjust whole-school approaches to such contexts have been undertaken; however, their effects on bullying and victimization have yet to be explored as well.

References

Adams, R. E., Fredstrom, B. K., Duncan, A. W., Holleb, L. J., & Bishop, S. L. (2014). Using self- and parent-reports to test the association between peer victimization and internalizing symptoms in verbally fluent adolescents with ASD. *Journal of Autism and Developmental Disorders, 44*, 861–872.

American Psychiatric Association. (2013). *Diagnostic and statistical manual of mental disorders* (5th edition). Arlington, VA: American Psychiatric Association.

Arseneault, L., Bowes, L., & Shakoor, S. (2010). Bullying victimization in youths and mental health problems: 'much ado about nothing'? *Psychological Medicine, 40*, 717–729.

Atlas, R. S., & Pepler, D. J. (1998). Observations of bullying in the classroom. *Journal of Educational Research, 92*, 86–99.

Bannon, S., McGlynn, T., McKenzie, K., & Quayle, E. (2015). The internet and young people with additional support needs (ASN): Risk and safety. *Computers in Human Behavior, 53*, 495–503.

Baron-Cohen, S. (2000). Theory of mind and autism: A fifteen-year review. In S. Baron-Cohen, H. Tager-Flusberg, & D. J. Cohen (Eds.), *Understanding other minds: Perspectives from developmental cognitive neuroscience* (pp. 3–20). New York, NY: Oxford University Press.

Bauminger, N., Shulman, C., & Agam, G. (2003). Peer interaction and loneliness in high-functioning children with autism. *Journal of Autism and Developmental Disorders, 33*, 489–507.

Bear, G. G., Mantz, L. S., Glutting, J. J., Yang, C., & Boyer, D. E. (2015). Differences in bullying victimization between students with and without disabilities. *School Psychology Review, 44*, 98–116.

Begeer, S., Fink, E., Van der Meijden, S., Goossens, F., & Olthof, T. (2016). Bullying-related behaviour in a mainstream high school for autism: Self-report and peer-report. *Autism, 20*, 562–571.

Bitsika, V., & Sharpley, C. F. (2014). Understanding, experiences, and reactions to bullying experiences in boys with an autism Spectrum disorder. *Journal of Developmental and Physical Disabilities, 26*, 747–761.

Bradshaw, C. P., Sawyer, A. L., & O'Brennan, L. M. (2007). Bullying and peer victimization at school: Perceptual differences between students and school staff. *School Psychology Review, 36*, 361–382.

Cappadocia, M. C., Weiss, J. A., & Pepler, D. (2012). Bullying experiences among children and youth with autism Spectrum disorders. *Journal of Autism and Developmental Disorders, 42*, 266–277.

Carr, A. (2006). Autism and pervasive developmental disorders. In A. Carr (Ed.), *Handbook of child and Adolescent clinical Psychology* (pp. 288–331). London: Routledge.

Carter, S. (2009). Bullying of students with Asperger's syndrome. *Issues in Comprehensive Pediatric Nursing, 32*, 145–154.

Chen, P.-Y., & Schwartz, I. S. (2012). Bullying and victimization experiences of students with autism Spectrum disorders in elementary schools. *Focus on Autism and Other Developmental Disabilities, 27*, 200–212.

Craig, W. M., Henderson, K., & Murphy, J. B. (2000). Prospective teachers' attitudes toward bullying and victimization. *School Psychology International, 21*, 5–21.

Cross, E., Piggin, R., Douglas, T., & Vonkaenel-Flatt, J. (2012). *Virtual violence II: Progress and challenges in the fight against cyberbullying*. London: Beat Bullying.

Didden, R., Scholte, R., Korzilius, H., De Moor, J., Vermeulen, A., O'Reilley, M., et al. (2009). Cyberbullying among students with intellectual and developmental disability in special education settings. *Developmental Neurorehabilitation, 12*, 146–151.

Due, P., Holstein, B. E., Lynch, J., Diderichsen, F., Nic Gabhein, S., Scheidt, P.,..., & The Health Behaviour in School-Aged Children Bullying Working Group. (2005). Bullying and symptoms among school-aged children: International comparative cross sectional study in 28 countries. *European Journal of Public Health, 15*, 128–132.

Farrington, D. P., & Ttofi, M. M. (2009). School-based programs to reduce bullying and victimization. *Campbell Systematic Reviews 2009, 6*, 1–149.

Fisher, M. H., & Lounds Taylor, J. (2016). Let's talk about it: Peer victimization experiences as reported by adolescents with autism spectrum disorder. *Autism, 20*, 402–411.

Fombonne, E. (2005). Epidemiological studies of pervasive developmental disorders. In F. R. Volkmar, R. Paul, A. Klin, & D. Cohen (Eds.), *Handbook of autism and pervasive developmental disorders* (pp. 42–69). Hoboken, NJ: Wiley.

Goossens, F. A., Olthof, T., & Dekker, P. H. (2006). New participant role scales: Comparison between various criteria for assigning roles and indications for their validity. *Aggressive Behavior, 32*, 343–357.

Hawkins, L. D., Pepler, D. J., & Craig, W. M. (2001). Naturalistic observations of peer interventions in bullying. *Social Development, 10*, 512–527.

Hebron, J., & Humphrey, N. (2014). Exposure to bullying among students with autism spectrum conditions: A multi-informant analysis of risk and protective factors. *Autism, 18*, 618–630.

Heerey, E. A., Capps, L. M., Keltner, D., & Kring, A. M. (2005). Understanding teasing: Lessons from children with autism. *Journal of Abnormal Child Psychology, 33*, 55–68.

Humphrey, N., & Hebron, J. (2014). Bullying of children and adolescents with autism spectrum conditions: A 'state of the field' review. *International Journal of Inclusive Education, 19*, 845–862.

Humphrey, N., & Symes, W. (2010a). Perceptions of social support and experience of bullying among pupils with autistic spectrum disorders in mainstream secondary schools. *European Journal of Special Needs Education, 25*, 77–91.

Humphrey, N., & Symes, W. (2010b). Responses to bullying and use of social support among pupils with autism spectrum disorders (ASDs) in mainstream schools: A qualitative study. *Journal of Research in Special Educational Needs, 10*, 82–90.

Humphrey, N., & Symes, W. (2011). Peer interaction patterns among adolescents with autistic spectrum disorders (ASDs) in mainstream school settings. *Autism, 15*, 397–419.

Juvonen, J., Nishina, A., & Graham, S. (2001). Self-views versus peer perceptions of victim status among early adolescents. In J. Juvonen & S. Graham (Eds.), *Peer harassment in school: The plight of the vulnerable and victimized* (pp. 105–124). New York: The Guilford Press.

Kasari, C., Locke, J., Gulsrud, A., & Rotheram-Fuller, E. (2011). Social networks and friendships at school: Comparing children with and without ASD. *Journal of Autism and Developmental Disorders, 41*, 533–544.

Kloosterman, P. H., Kelley, E. A., Craig, W. M., Parker, J. D. A., & Javier, C. (2013). Types and experiences of bullying in adolescents with an autism spectrum disorder. *Research in Autism Spectrum Disorders, 7*, 824–832.

Kloosterman, P. H., Kelley, E. A., Parker, J. D. A., & Craig, W. M. (2014). Executive functioning as a predictor of peer victimization in adolescents with and without an autism Spectrum disorder. *Research in Autism Spectrum Disorders, 8*, 244–254.

Kowalski, R. M., & Fedina, C. (2011). Cyber bullying in ADHD and Asperger syndrome populations. *Research in Autism Spectrum Disorders, 5*, 1201–1208.

Little, L. (2002). Middle-class mothers' perceptions of peer and sibling victimization among children with Asperger's syndrome and non-verbal learning disorders. *Issues in Comprehensive Pediatric Nursing, 25*, 43–57.

Maïano, C., Norman, C. L., Salvas, M.-C., Moullec, G., & Aimé, A. (2015). Prevalence of school bullying among youth with autism Spectrum disorders: A systematic review and meta-analysis. *Autism Research, 9*, 601–615.
Merrell, K. W., Guelder, B. A., Ross, S. W., & Isava, D. M. (2008). How effective are school bullying intervention programs? A meta-analysis of intervention research. *School Psychology Quarterly, 23*, 26–42.
Monks, C. P., Smith, P. K., & Swettenham, J. (2003). Aggressors, victims, and defenders in preschool: Peer, self-, and teacher reports. *Merrill-Palmer Quarterly, 49*, 453–469.
Montes, G., & Halterman, J. S. (2007). Bullying among children with autism and the influence of comorbidity with ADHD: A population-based study. *Ambulatory Pediatrics, 7*, 253–257.
Nowell, K. P., Brewton, C. M., & Goin-Kochel, R. P. (2014). A multi-rater study on being teased among children/adolescents with autism Spectrum disorder (ASD) and their typically developing siblings: Associations with ASD symptoms. *Focus on Autism and Other Developmental Disabilities, 29*, 195–205.
Reid, B., & Batten, A. (2006). *B is for bullied: The experiences of children with autism and their families*. London: National Autistic Society.
Rieffe, C., Camodeca, M., Pouw, L. B. C., Lange, A. M. C., & Stockmann, L. (2012). Don't anger me! Bullying, victimization, and emotion dysregulation in young adolescents with ASD. *The European Journal of Developmental Psychology, 9*, 351–370.
Rodkin, P. C., Farmer, T. W., Van Acker, R., Pearl, R., Thompson, J. H., & Fedora, P. (2006). Who do students with mild disabilities nominate as cool in inclusive general education classrooms? *Journal of School Psychology, 44*, 67–84.
Rose, C. A., Monda-Amaya, L. E., & Espelage, D. L. (2011). Bullying perpetration and victimization in special education: A review of the literature. *Remedial and Special Education, 32*, 114–130.
Rose, C. A., Simpson, C. G., & Moss, A. (2015). The bullying dynamic: Prevalence of involvement among a large-scale sample of middle and high school youth with and without disabilities. *Psychology in the Schools, 52*, 515–531.
Rowley, E., Chandler, S., Baird, G., Simonoff, E., Pickles, A., Loucas, T., et al. (2012). The experience of friendship, victimization, and bullying in children with an autism spectrum disorder: Associations with child characteristics and school placement. *Research in Autism Spectrum Disorders, 6*, 1126–1134.
Salmivalli, C. (1999). Participant role approach to school bullying: Implications for interventions. *Journal of Adolescence, 22*, 453–459.
Salmivalli, C. (2010). Bullying and the peer group: A review. *Aggression and Violent Behavior, 15*, 112–120.
Salmivalli, C., Lagerspetz, K. M. J., Björkqvist, K., Österman, K., & Kaukiainen, A. (1996). Bullying as a group process: Participant roles and their relations to social status within the group. *Aggressive Behavior, 22*, 1–15.
Salmivalli, C., Lappalainen, M., & Lagerspetz, K. M. J. (1998). Stability and change of behavior in connection with bullying in schools: A two-year follow-up. *Aggressive Behavior, 24*, 205–218.
Schroeder, J. H., Cappadocia, M. C., Bebko, J. M., Pepler, D. J., & Weiss, J. A. (2014). Shedding light on a pervasive problem: A review of research on bullying experiences among children with autism spectrum disorders. *Journal of Autism and Developmental Disorders, 44*, 1520–1534.
Schrooten, I., Scholte, R. H. J., Cillessen, A. H. N., & Hymel, S. (2016). Participant roles in bullying among Dutch adolescents with Autism Spectrum Disorders. *Journal of Clinical Child & Adolescent Psychology*. 1–14.
Schumann, L., Craig, W., & Rosu, A. (2013). Minority in the majority: Community ethnicity as a context for racial bullying and victimization. *Journal of Community Psychology, 41*, 959–972.
Shtayermman, O. (2007). Peer victimization in adolescents and young adults diagnosed with Asperger's syndrome: A link to depressive symptomatology, anxiety symptomatology and suicidal ideation. *Issues in Comprehensive Pediatric Nursing, 30*, 87–107.
Smith, P. K., Cowie, H., Olafsson, R. F., & Liefooghe, A. P. D. (2002). Definitions of bullying: A comparison of terms used, and age and gender differences, in a fourteen-country international comparison. *Child Development, 73*, 1119–1133.
Smith, D. J., Schneider, B. H., Smith, P. K., & Ananiadou, K. (2004). The effectiveness of whole-school antibullying programs: A synthesis of evaluation research. *School Psychology Review, 33*, 547–560.
Sofronoff, K., Dark, E., & Stone, V. (2011). Social vulnerability and bullying in children with Asperger syndrome. *Autism, 15*, 355–372.
Sreckovic, M. A., Brunsting, N. C., & Able, H. (2014). Victimization of students with autism spectrum disorder: A review of prevalence and risk factors. *Research in Autism Spectrum Disorders, 8*, 1155–1172.
Stassen Berger, K. (2007). Update on bullying at school: Science forgotten? *Developmental Review, 27*, 90–126.
Sterzing, P. R., Shattuck, P. T., Narendorf, S. C., Wagner, M., & Cooper, B. P. (2012). Bullying involvement and autism Spectrum disorder. *Archives of Pediatrics and Adolescent Medicine, 166*, 1058–1064.
Sutton, J., & Smith, P. K. (1999). Bullying as a group process: An adaptation of the participant role approach. *Aggressive Behavior, 25*, 97–111.
Swearer, S. M., Espelage, D. L., Vaillancourt, T., & Hymel, S. (2010). What can be done about school bullying? Linking research to educational practice. *Educational Researcher, 39*, 38–47.
Ttofi, M. M., & Farrington, D. P. (2011). Effectiveness of school-based programs to reduce bullying: A systematic and meta-analytic review. *Journal of Experimental Criminology, 7*, 27–56.
Twyman, K. A., Saylor, C. F., Saia, D., Macias, M. M., Taylor, L. A., et al. (2010). Bullying and ostracism experiences in children with special health care needs.

Journal of Developmental and Behavioral Pediatrics, 31, 1–8.

Van Roekel, E., Scholte, R., & Didden, R. (2010). Bullying among adolescents with autism Spectrum disorders: Prevalence and perception. *Journal of Autism and Developmental Disorders, 40*, 63–73.

Wainscot, J. J., Naylor, P., Sutcliffe, P., Tantam, D., & Williams, J. V. (2008). Relationships with peers and use of the school environment of mainstream secondary school pupils with Asperger syndrome (high-functioning autism): A case-control study. *International Journal of Psychology and Psychological Therapy, 8*, 25–38.

Wang, J., Ianotti, R. J., & Nansel, T. R. (2009). School bullying among adolescents in the United States: Physical, verbal, relational, and cyber. *Journal of Adolescent Health, 45*, 368–375.

Whitney, I., & Smith, P. K. (1993). A survey of the nature and extent of bullying in junior/middle and secondary schools. *Educational Research, 35*, 3–25.

Whitney, I., Smith, P. K., & Thompson, D. (1994). Bullying and children with special educational needs. In P. K. Smith & S. Sharp (Eds.), *School bullying: Insights and perspectives* (pp. 213–240). London, UK: Routledge.

Zablotsky, B., Bradshaw, C. P., Anderson, C., & Law, P. A. (2013). The association between bullying and the psychological functioning of children with autism Spectrum disorders. *Journal of Developmental & Behavioral Pediatrics, 34*, 1–8.

Zablotsky, B., Bradshaw, C. P., Anderson, C. M., & Law, P. (2014). Risk factors for bullying among children with autism spectrum disorders. *Autism, 18*, 419–427.

Zeedyk, S. M., Rodriguez, G., Tipton, L. A., Baker, B. L., & Blacher, J. (2014). Bullying of youth with autism spectrum disorder, intellectual disability, or typical development: Victim and parent perspectives. *Research in Autism Spectrum Disorders, 8*, 1173–1183.

Zych, I., Ortega-Ruiz, R., & Del Rey, R. (2015). Systematic review of theoretical studies on bullying and cyberbullying: Facts, knowledge, prevention, and intervention. *Aggression and Violent Behavior, 23*, 1–21.

5 Friendship in Autism Spectrum Disorder

Nirit Bauminger-Zviely and Yael Kimhi

Having friends is crucial to children's well-being and the development of adequate cognitive, linguistic, and social skills in typical development (Howes, 2009; Vitaro, Boivin, & Bukowski, 2009). Although the majority of individuals with autism spectrum disorder (ASD; 60–75%) have significant difficulties in friendship formation, this remains an overlooked topic. Thus, in-depth research on friendship processes in ASD is greatly needed. In this chapter, we provide descriptions of the nature, quality, and importance of friendship in ASD across development, from preschool through adulthood. We also provide a description of the children who form friendships with children with ASD as well as pointing out individual, familial, and environmental components that may contribute to friendship formation in ASD. Finally, we suggest future topics for friendship studies. Novel data will be presented based on quantitative and qualitative multidimensional assessment procedures, including semi-structured and spontaneous observations of friendship as well as self-reports and others' reports, combining current and longitudinal evaluations of friendship.

5.1 The Beginning of Friendship—Friendship in Preschoolers with ASD

Stable friendships that are based on mutual affection and that provide emotional support have been well documented for typically developing preschoolers (Howes, 1996). Interactions with friends reveal greater social complexity and intersubjectivity as affective and close interchanges than with interactions with acquaintances (Newcomb & Bagwell, 1996). Recently, studies have begun to specifically examine friendship during preschool with regard to ASD (e.g., Bauminger-Zviely, & Agam-Ben-Artzi, 2014; Bauminger-Zviely, Karin, Kimhi, & Agam-Ben-Artzi, 2014; Chang, Shih & Kasari, 2016; Freeman, Gulsrud, & Kasari, 2015; Kimhi, & Bauminger-Zviely, 2012) in contrast to previous studies, which reported on friendship among children with special needs (including but not specific to ASD; e.g., Buysee, Goldman, & Skinner, 2002; Guralnick, Neville, Hammond & Connor, 2007; Odom et al., 2006). Thus, we know very little about friendship among young children with ASD. Recent knowledge on friendship among preschoolers with ASD will be

N. Bauminger-Zviely (✉)
School of Education, Bar-Ilan University, Ramat Gan, Israel
e-mail: Nirit.Bauminger@biu.ac.il

Y. Kimhi
School of Education , Bar-Ilan University, Ramat Gan, Israel

Levinsky College of Education, Tel Aviv-Yafo, Israel

J.B. Leaf (ed.), *Handbook of Social Skills and Autism Spectrum Disorder*, Autism and Child Psychopathology Series, DOI 10.1007/978-3-319-62995-7_5

reviewed with regard to the number of identified friends, the nature and quality of friendship, characteristics of the friend, and predictions on the variables of friendship.

5.1.1 Number of Friends

Information about the number of identified friends for ASD children is provided only by Chang et al. (2016). The number of friends reported by parents (42%, n = 13) and teachers (54%, n = 17) exceeded the number of children who were identified as having friends according to observational data (20%, n = 7), following an adaptation of Howes' (1983) criteria (e.g., at least 50% of social initiation attempts with responses; at least one unit of joint engagement or games; and one positive affective exchange during the interaction). Nine (29%) sets of parents and teachers identified the same friends; however, parents reported friends from other settings in addition to school, such as family friends (n = 13), outside activities (n = 6), and the neighborhood (n = 6). Further examination of the number of friends for ASD children in preschool is still needed to clarify the gap between parents/teachers and observational reports.

5.1.2 Friendship Characteristics and Quality

Bauminger-Zviely and Agam-Ben-Artzi (2014) found same-age, same-sex, durable (mean, 13.00; range, 4–60 months) and stable friendships according to maternal reports for preschoolers with high functioning autism spectrum disorder (HFASD), with no differences from typical friendship. However, friendship duration differed between HFASD and typically developing preschool-aged children (TYP) according to teachers' reports (9.29 months; range, 4–19 HFASD; 18.60, range, TYP). Furthermore, the majority of children with HFASD had an identified friend with HFASD (62%, n = 18, nonmixed friendship), whereas none of the typically developing children did. According to maternal reports, the meeting place was similar between HFASD and TYP (69% home and preschool, HFASD, 76.7% TYP); according to teachers, however, 65.4% of friends met only at the preschool.

The quality of preschoolers' friendships was examined in a series of studies in Bauminger-Zviley's lab (i.e., Bauminger-Zviely & Agam-Ben-Artzi 2014, Bauminger-Zviely et al., 2014; Kimhi and Bauminger-Zviely 2012). These studies compared the quality of friendship between HFASD and typical development, between interactions with a friend and interactions with acquaintances (in HFASD and TYP), and, for the ASD group, the quality of friendships between mixed and nonmixed interactions (typical friends and friends with a disability, respectively). Each target child (HFSD, TYP) was videotaped at his or her preschool interacting with a friend partner and with a nonfriend partner (i.e., a child from the same preschool who was not identified as a friend) during three social situations (i.e., a construction game, drawing, and free-time snack). Using the friendship observation scale – young (FOS-Y; Bauminger-Zviely & Agam-Ben-Artzi 2014), minute-by-minute categories for each individual target child's positive social interactions and play behaviors were analyzed in addition to a global evaluation of each dyad on the dimensions of closeness, shared fun, and coengagement. Group differences emerged for sharing, social conversation, positive affect, and collaborative pretend play, with typically developing target children outperforming children with HFASD. Typical dyads also showed better dyadic friendship quality than children with HFASD on all three global dyadic categories of closeness, shared fun, and reciprocity. It is important to note that the groups did not differ significantly on several important positive social interactive behaviors, such as cooperative, prosocial, and nonverbal behaviors; parallel, social and collaborative play; and solitary pretend play. Thus, although typically developing target children showed better friendship quality with their peers, some positive social interactive behaviors were also present for the HFASD target children (Bauminger-Zviely & Agam-Ben-Artzi, 2014).

The comparison between interactions with friends and interactions with nonfriends yielded very informative results with regard to friendship quality among children with HFASD. While interacting with friends, both target children with HFASD and those with typical development showed higher levels of positive affect, more social coordinated play, and a higher frequency of the most complex form of peer-play, collaborative pretend play. Furthermore, the three dyadic friendship qualities (i.e., shared fun, closeness, and reciprocity) were higher in the friend dyads than in the nonfriend dyads for both groups. Thus, friendship for children with HFASD is related to complex interactive and play capabilities, as well as a high level of intersubjectivity and closeness.

These results were replicated in another study using the same sample, but with a different social collaborative task. In Kimhi and Bauminger-Zviely's (2012) study, dyads of children with HFASD and typical development solved a collaborative problem together with their peers (i.e., a friend and a nonfriend) in which they placed a pair of blocks, varying in color and weight, to balance a scale. Group differences emerged in favor of the typically developing group in their performance on the collaborative problem solving task with HFASD preschoolers being slower, using more irrelevant behaviors, sharing less, and using fewer coordinative gestures than the typically developing group. However, when the HFASD group interacted with friends rather than with nonfriends, they were more responsive, had more fun, and showed a higher level of reciprocity, as was assessed by the "General Dyadic Quality Evaluation" (Bauminger et al., 2008a), a global evaluation that assessed the quality of the interaction between the children throughout the problem-solving scenario,.

Another study (i.e., Bauminger-Zviely et al. 2014) based on a similar sample, in which an in-depth examination of pragmatic capabilities was conducted, yielded similar findings showing again the advantages of the interaction with friends over nonfriend. This study suggested that although typical dyads showed better pragmatic capabilities than dyads with HFASD, with regard to group differences, interactions with friends outperformed interactions with nonfriends for pivotal pragmatic skills such as reciprocal conversation, responsiveness to the interlocutor, coregulation of the conversation, appropriate reference to the other's emotions, appropriate use of facial expressions and eye contact, and a lower use of stereotypic speech. Furthermore, greater conversational adequacy, more initiations of conversational exchanges, and more responsiveness to information evoked by the partner during interactions with friends versus nonfriends were noted in both HFASD and typical friend dyads. Thus, HFASD friend dyads show more pragmatically intact and coregulated interactional behaviors than nonfriend dyads.

A more nuanced in-depth study of pragmatics and friendship with a similar sample compared children's use of speech acts (SAs; the primary illocutionary values conventionally conveyed by utterances as acts), which are crucial components of children's conversational capabilities, between groups (HFASD, TYP) and with regard to the partner (i.e., friends versus nonfriends; Bauminger-Zviely, Itshaky, & Tubul-Lavy, 2017). The main results resembled the previous results for this sample, with typically developing children showing a higher amount and diversity of SAs than the children with HFASD group. However, in both groups, interaction with a friend outperformed interaction with a nonfriend. Specifically, the HFASD group demonstrated specific difficulties with assertive acts and declarations, organizational devices, object dubbing, and pretend play as well as higher use of stereotypical speech. However, those categories showed better performance with friends than with nonfriends. Thus, the data suggest that HFASD friend dyads show more pragmatically intact and coregulated interactional behaviors than nonfriend dyads. It is important to note that pragmatics is considered a major deficit in ASD (American Psychiatric Association [APA], 2013). Thus, friendship may be an important protective factor and a beneficial social environment to enhance linguistic skills for children with HFASD. The close relationship between peer relations and language is a good fit with regard to the new Diagnostic and Statistical Manual of Mental Disorders-5 (DSM-5; 2013) definition of ASD, which combines social and communication abilities into one dimension that identifies the disorder.

An issue regarding the type of friendship emerged between mixed friends (i.e., a typically developing friend) and nonmixed friends (i.e., a friend with a disability) as one source of variability in friendship quality in ASD. Interestingly, this comparison was less informative with regard to the understanding of friendship quality in ASD. Although mixed interactions with typical friends tend to show higher social complexity than nonmixed interactions (i.e., peers with ASD), significant differences emerged for only a few positive interactive social and play behaviors. For example, in Bauminger-Zviely and Agam-Ben-Artzi (2014), higher cooperative behavior, reciprocity, and collaborative pretend play were found in mixed friendships in comparison to nonmixed friendships. Bauminger-Zviely et al.'s (2017) study on SAs presented only one significant finding, with mixed dyads exhibiting a greater variety of SAs in contrast to nonmixed dyads. Therefore, preschoolers' conversations appear more fruitful and rich when they converse in mixed dyads.

Given these findings, it seems that early friendships provide feasible and meaningful experiences for children with ASD, which may make an important contribution to children's growth in sociolinguistic skills. However, friendship is also a significant challenge for children with ASD, and not all children are able to form friendships. In the next section, we will discuss what we know about preschoolers with ASD who have friends.

5.2 Characteristics of Children Who Make Friends

Only one recent study (i.e., Chang et al., 2016) has examined spontaneous peer interactions and play when comparing preschoolers with friends to preschoolers who do not have friends. Children with friends were more likely than children without friends to be jointly engaged with their peers during free play and used higher joint attention skills. In line with these findings, Freeman et al. (2015) examined the influence of joint attention and play on the quality of friendship among 40 children as measured 5 years later via parent and child reports. The authors found that children who had better joint attention skills at the age of three reported having more closeness and less conflict in their friendships at the age of eight. Children who had better play abilities in general and specifically greater variability and flexibility in symbolic play conveyed higher levels of helpfulness in their friendships. These findings underscore the importance of early intervention in areas that include joint attention and the development of symbolic play, thus increasing children's social interest and motivation, and facilitating friendship at a later age. These are important results that link core deficits to later friendship development in ASD.

Other findings have linked developmental variables such as chronological age, intelligence, and verbal intelligence (CA, IQ, and VIQ) to better friendship qualities (e.g., Bauminger-Zviely & Agam-Ben-Artzi, 2014; Bauminger-Zviely et al., 2014), but these findings are not conclusive and do not always differentiate between children who make friends and those who do not. Furthermore, it is important to note that all studies that have examined friendship during preschool have included high-functioning children; thus, these findings may have masked IQ influences on the development of friendship. In fact, we know very little so far about friendships among less able children on the spectrum.

5.3 Characteristics of Their Partners

No direct data have examined the type of partner in preschool. In our preschool friendship project at Bauminger-Zviely's lab, we asked mothers and teachers about the factors that contributed to the development of friendship during preschool. Mothers of children with HFASD perceived close proximity to be the most important factor (e.g., "being in the same preschool"), followed by parental mediation and the child's characteristics. Children's mutual preferences and staff mediation were seen by mothers as the least important factors. The teachers agreed with the mothers with regard to the importance of being in the same preschool but evaluated the children's mutual preference and staff mediation more highly than the mothers. Teachers also thought that parental mediation was the least important influencing factor. These are preliminary data and should be regarded with caution. However, it should be noted that at the preschool age, children are dependent on the parents to arrange meetings, so partner types may be influenced by parental preferences to be acquainted with the partner's parents.

5.4 Schoolchildren with ASD

During the school-age period (usually until the age of 12), boys' friendships usually include physical rough-and-tumble group activities, or "surface-level activities" that lead to reciprocity of friendship, which includes both behavioral and affective reciprocity. Affective exchange is a significant factor in reciprocal school-age male friendships. In a meta-analytic study that examined the friendships of school-aged boys with ASD, Mendelson, Gates, and Lerner (2016) found that boys with ASD do form reciprocal friendships in which they engage in affective sharing, although it is of lower quality.

Number of Friends Information regarding the number of identified friends has been provided in various studies of school-aged children. The largest study was conducted by Mazurek and Kanne (2010), who examined a sample that included 1202 children between the ages of 4 and 17 (mean age, 9.1 years; SD, 3.5). Dyadic friendship was reported by parents according to the ADI-R item (#65) assessing friendship status. For example, (a) one or more relationships with a same-aged peer that includes sharing personal activities and seeing the individual outside of prearranged groups (this relationship has clear reciprocity); (b) one or more relationships that have some shared activities outside a prearranged group and that include some initiation, but may be limited in interests or reciprocity; (c) personal relationships with others that include seeking contact, but only in groups, school, or work; and (d) no peer relationships that involve reciprocity. The results showed that 15.2% of the children had clear, reciprocal friendships.

Another large study (i.e., Petrina, Carter, Sephenson & Sweller, 2015) that assessed school-age friendships with regard to reciprocity and mutuality included 37 boys and eight girls between the ages of 6.4 and 10.4 years (mean, 8.5; SD, 0.9). Forty-nine percent ($n = 22$) of the ASD group were in a nonmixed friendship dyad, and 51% (n = 23) were in a mixed friendship dyad. The level of friendship quality was assessed by the Friendship Quality Questionnaire (FQQ; Parker & Asher, 1993), and both friends from each dyad answered the questionnaire using a three-point response scale. According to the answers, the friendships were classified as best, regular, or nonfriendship. The results showed that 89% of the friendships (i.e., 42 out of 47) across both mixed and nonmixed dyads were reciprocated. The reciprocation rate was 19% for best friends, 15% in the mixed dyads and 24% in the nonmixed, and 55% for regular friendship, 54% in the mixed dyad and 62% in the nonmixed dyad.

5.5 Characteristics of Friendships

One of the first studies (i.e., Bauminger & Kasari, 2000) that examined the friendships of children with HFASD also examined the relationship between loneliness and friendship and whether friendship ameliorated the feeling of loneliness for these children. Loneliness and friendship were examined in a study of 22 children with HFASD (mean age, 10.74; SD, 2.14) who reported having at least one close friend, in comparison with children with typical development who were matched on IQ, CA, mother's education, gender, and ethnicity. The findings showed that although the children with HFASD felt lonely and showed a social desire to be involved with others, having a best friend did not reduce their feelings of loneliness. Despite rating their friendships as lower in quality in terms of companionship, security, and helpfulness in comparison with their typically developing peers, they rated their friendships as equal in terms of closeness. According to the authors, high levels of closeness should compensate for feelings of loneliness, as was found among the children in the control group. However, this did not occur among the children in the study group.

The friendship characteristics of 44 children and preadolescents with HFASD (ages 8–12) were examined in a binational (i.e., Israel and the USA), multidimensional study (i.e., Bauminger et al., 2008a) and were compared with 38 matched typically developing children. Most of the friendships were of the same gender (77%), and the majority of the friendships were same-age friendships. Two pairs from the ASD sample had friendships with a relative. Sixteen pairs reported having friendships with a partner with a disability. The characteristics of the friendships were examined with two scales: the Friendship Observation Scale (Bauminger, Rogers, Aviezer & Solomon, 2005), which is an interactional coding system designed to assess both minute-by-minute and global evaluations of friendship manifestations of the target child, including behaviors, verbalizations, and affect; and the Dyadic Relationships Q-Set (Park & Waters, 1989), which evaluates dyadic behavioral dimensions. The children participated in two play activities (i.e., a building and a drawing activity) that could be performed individually in a parallel manner or interactively in a shared manner. The qualities of the friendship reported by the child were assessed using The Friendship Qualities Scale (Bukowski, Hoza, & Boivin, 1994). In general, the friends showed fewer friendship-related behaviors, such as goal directedness and positive affect, in comparison with their typically developing peers. They also had less conversational flow and social conversation in both scenarios. Furthermore, the children with HFASD used fewer expressions of positive affect, had lower levels of shared fun, and presented fewer self-reports of intimacy and closeness. The children perceived their relations as limited with regard to the friendships' closeness and helpfulness. Nonetheless, some important characteristics similar to those of children with typical development were also reported by the authors. The children with HFASD reported lengthy durations of friendships with their partners (mean, 40.00 months; SD, 28.32; TYP mean, 49.11 months; SD, 36.78), a report that was verified both by the children's mothers and their friends. Another characteristic that emerged was an egalitarian relationship in which the partners maintained a balanced leader-follower relationship, with a low rate of controlling behaviors. This occurred even though the majority of the HFASD dyads (n = 28 pairs; 63.36%) involved a friend with typical development. This finding led the authors to conclude that autism influences the nature of the friendship interactions within the dyad. When examining each social situation separately, the children with HFASD showed similar nonverbal behaviors, such as shared eye contact and smiles (in the shared construction scenario), as well as sharing of experiences, attention and emotions (in the shared drawing scenario).

An in-depth examination of the same sample was conducted to identify the differences between the mixed-autism and typical development (n = 26) friendship dyads, and the nonmixed (n = 16) dyads (Bauminger et al., 2008b) in comparison to typical development. Many aspects of friendship were found to be significantly different, as was found for the preschool age. The results showed that the mixed dyads were more in accord with typical friendships in comparison to the nonmixed dyads. Their friendships were more durable and stable, and the children showed more positive affect toward each other. They were more responsive to one another and showed greater positive social orientation and cohesion. They also demonstrated more complex coordinated play than the nonmixed dyads. In sum, the mixed dyads showed more complex and responsive interaction within the friendship itself.

An essential and much neglected issue when examining the characteristics of friendships in

ASD is gender. Dean et al. (2014) examined the social relationships of 50 elementary school children with HFASD (25 male, mean age 7.7; and 25 female, mean age 7.5) in comparison to typical development via peer nomination data and focused on how gender relates to social preferences, acceptance, social connections, reciprocal friendships, and rejection. The children with ASD, both male and female, tended to be on the periphery of the various social groups and had fewer playmates with typical development. One harsh finding regarding girls with ASD was that they tended to be overlooked in social contexts. The authors found that many girls were neither accepted nor rejected but rather were off the social grid – a disturbing finding with social and emotional consequences. In contrast to girls, boys with ASD were often actively rejected, enabling their social exclusion to be easily perceived. According to the authors, the social demands of each gender are different; therefore, intervention should be planned accordingly. Female relationships and friendships incorporate the understanding of nuances such as intimacy and group conformity, whereas male relationships and friendships demand the understanding of competitive play in addition to lesser language skills. Verbal interactions are more prominent in female exchanges; thus, the core deficits of ASD may indeed be more detrimental to girls.

5.6 Characteristics of Children Who Make Friends

One of the important suppositions concerning the characteristics of children with ASD who make friends is that there is apparently no obvious or direct relationship between behavioral expressions of mentalizing and the ability to make friends (Bauminger, Solomon & Rogers, 2010; Calder, Hill & Pelicano, 2013). However, many studies have attempted to pinpoint the factors and characteristics that seem to encourage and facilitate friendships. In a study that examined what friendship means to children with ASD in inclusive settings (Calder et al., 2013), motivation for interpersonal engagement emerged as a key factor in parents' and teachers' perceptions of the children's characteristics, describing their strong desire to develop friendships.

Bauminger et al. (2010) conducted an in-depth study that examined the role played by major social-emotional variables (e.g., attachment security and mother–child relationship qualities), social-cognitive capacities (e.g., Theory of Mind, [ToM]), and developmental factors (e.g., CA, VIQ) in observed and perceived friendships of children with HFASD and typical development (i.e., 44 children with HFASD and 38 age-matched children with typical development). Overall, the authors found similar friendship predictors and developmental patterns in typical and HFASD development, such as chronological age, verbal IQ, security of attachment, mother–child relationship quality and ToM. Specifically, higher verbal capabilities appeared to be most important to the observed friendship qualities of coordinated play and responsiveness. Moreover, all observed friendship qualities appeared to improve with age, and a higher quality of mother–child relationships seemed to contribute directly to the sense of closeness, intimacy, and companionship in friendships. Thus, developmental and relationship characteristics had the strongest effect on observed behavior between friends. The interrelations between the predictors suggest that ToM and security of attachment provide compensatory and amplification mechanisms for friendship qualities. Additionally, security of attachment seems to serve as a compensatory mechanism for intimacy and companionship in friendship, especially with regard to ASD and intimacy, thus stressing the importance of a high-quality relationship with the mother for children with ASD to develop intimate friendships. Additionally, there was a similarity between the study groups in measures of attachment security as well as in the relationships that emerged between measures of attachment security and parent-child relationship qualities with friendship formation. According to the authors, these findings indicate that the construct of attachment security and internal working models can be applied to ASD and that attachment security may even contribute to social development in more comprehensive ways than friendship.

5.7 Characteristics of Their Partners

Teachers reported that when friendships are established, peers often play an important role in maintaining these friendships (Calder et al., 2013) and are often described as "warm," "kind," and "socially mature" (Bauminger & Shulman, 2003; Chamberlain, Kasari, & Rotheram-Fuller, 2007). Conn (2015) found that friends of children with ASD were often described as children on the same "wavelength" who were attuned to the children with autism and were often particularly inventive, creative, and exceptionally supportive.

5.8 Friendship in Adolescents and Adults with ASD

During adolescence, the social problems of people with ASD usually become more severe (Locke, Ishijima, Kasari, & London, 2010). According to Rossetti (2015), these individuals and adolescents with intellectual and developmental disabilities (IDD) are among those who are least likely to develop friendships, in comparison with adolescents with other disabilities. Their social networks are of lower quality, and they are often left out and marginalized (Locke et al., 2010). Nevertheless, although their friendships have been shown to have a lower quality in terms of companionship, security, and helpfulness (Bauminger & Kasari, 2000; Locke et al., 2010), the friendships themselves are often depicted as meaningful and reciprocal. With regard to friendships in adolescence, one must consider same- and other-gender factors. Therefore, we will elaborate on this issue in this section.

Friendships in adulthood are difficult to evaluate due to the paucity of research in this field, as demonstrated by the small number and low quality of adult intervention studies in general, including studies of friendship and social intervention (Howlin et al., 2015). This problem is amplified due to the social isolation that is prominent among most young adults with ASD in comparison with other groups (Shattuck, Orsmond, Wagner, & Cooper, 2011). Mehling and Tasse (2015) assessed social outcomes via a structured means analysis of 443 adults with ASD in comparison with adults with other developmental disabilities (DD). The authors found that the adults with ASD had fewer friendships although they participated in the community at similar rates as the group with DD. These results reaffirm findings concerning individuals with ASD at all ages, emphasizing that immersion or inclusion without specific intervention is less effective, and, for the most part, does not transform into friendships.

5.8.1 Number of Friends

The number of identified friends has been provided in various studies of adolescence. In a study that examined the friendship reports of 91 adolescents with ASD and their parents (i.e., Kuo, Orsmond, Cohn & Costner, 2011), 96% of the adolescents reported that they had at least one friend, and 86% of parents reported that the adolescents had at least one friend. The adolescents identified a significantly greater number of friends than their parents did; agreement between the adolescents and their parents was 60% with regard to the adolescent's best friend and 24% regarding the adolescent's three closest friends. It is interesting to note that the adolescents who reported different friends had more severe autism symptoms than those who reported at least one similar friend to their parents' report. In a study that examined the quality of reciprocated friendships of students with special educational needs (i.e., Bossaert, Colpin, Pijl & Petry, 2015), 65 adolescents reported having at least one typically developing reciprocal friend based on sociometric data. The adolescents were asked to nominate their best friends in class, and friendship was defined as a reciprocated nomination.

Locke et al. (2010) examined the friendships of seven adolescents with HFASD, all of whom identified another adolescent with ASD as a best friend (nonmixed friendship dyads). Another study examining friendship via semi-structured interviews (i.e., Sedgewick, Hill, Yates, Pickering & Pellicano, 2016), found that 10 male and 13 female adolescents in special education needs-segregated schools reported having at least one close friend in school. One of the few studies to date that has examined friendship in a sample of 108 adults with ASD (aged 18–92 years) found that 60.2% of the participants reported having a best friend (Mazurek, 2014), indicating improvement in comparison with an earlier study examining the friendships of 235 adolescents and adults with autism and found that only 8.1% of the sample had at least one close reciprocal friendship (Orsmond, Krauss & Seltzer, 2004).

5.8.2 Friendship Characteristics and Quality

Although friendships in ASD are considered to be of lower quality (Bauminger & Kasari, 2000; Locke et al., 2010) and are characterized by shorter duration and less frequent meetings (Bauminger & Shulman, 2003), some encouraging characteristics emerged regarding reciprocal friendships in ASD. In Kuo et al. (2011), 57% of the adolescents (52 adolescents) reported that they met with their friends on weekdays and on weekends for an average of 3.1 h on any given day. In a qualitative study, Rossetti (2015) examined the friendships of adolescents with ASD and found the friendships were reciprocal, meaningful, and fun. The participants showed internal motivation and attempted to maximize their interactions. They showed emotional responses and found joint ways to incorporate humor in their shared experiences. In a different study that focused on companionship, intimacy, and support in reciprocated friendships among adolescents with ASD (i.e., Bossaert et al., 2015), the authors found that these adolescents did not differ in their perception of companionship, intimacy, and support in their shared friendship in comparison with typically developing adolescents. Furthermore, although adolescents with ASD showed significantly poorer friendship qualities in terms of companionship and helpfulness, they did not differ in their reports of security, conflict, and closeness with their best friends when compared with their typically developing peers (Locke et al., 2010).

In a study that examined the social participation of 108 young adults (M = 32.4 years; SD = 12.5 years) with ASD with the ability to complete measures independently, the principal finding was exceptionally high levels of social seclusion (Mazurek, 2014). Nevertheless, 60% (n = 64) of the respondents reported having a close or best friend. More than 50% reported that they met their friend at a low-frequency rate (between every few weeks and less than once per month); the same rate was reported regarding phone contact. However, 50% reported having electronic contact with their friend from several times per day to at least once a day. In a different study (i.e., Mazurek, 2013) using the same sample, the author conducted an in-depth examination of the reasons (social connections, entertainment/information, business, family, and other) for using social network sites. The results showed that 79.2% of the participants with friends explained their use in terms of social purposes (i.e., social connections and family). As stated by the author, this finding suggests a potentially positive role of social media for adults with ASD. Furthermore, adult friendship characteristics were associated with decreased loneliness. Aspects of friendship such as having a close friend and the size of the friendship social network were significantly related to loneliness in adults with ASD, leading the author to conclude that friendship plays an important role in emotional functioning (Mazurek, 2014).

A limited number of studies have examined gender differences in adolescent friendships. One of the few studies that addressed this issue examined gender differences in social motivation and friendship experiences of adolescent girls and boys with and without ASD (Sedgewick et al., 2016). All participants attended special schools, and all were in receipt of a Statement of Special Education Needs (SEN). The adolescents completed the Friendship Qualities Scale (FQS; Bukowski et al., 1994), which assessed their perceptions of the nature of their relationship with an identified best friend. Interestingly, the results showed that the friendship quality of the girls with ASD was similar in nature to that of the nonautistic girls in terms of companionship, help, closeness, and security, with the exception of lower levels of conflict in their relationships. In contrast, the quality of the autistic boys' friendship differed; they rated their friendships as less close, less secure, and having less conflict and lower levels of helping behaviors than their typically developing peers did. The boys with ASD also reported less intimacy and more action in their relationships.

Kuo and associates (2011) found that most adolescents reported having same-gender friends but few opposite-gender friends. Male adolescents most frequently played video games or watched television with friends, which involve less direct social interactions than other activities, whereas female adolescents most frequently engaged in conversation with friends. Following video games for males and conversations for females, performing physical activities was the category in which both male and female adolescents most frequently engaged with friends. Regarding opposite-gender friends, the respondents mostly reported engaging in physical activity, such as playing ball games or swimming, which usually involves clear rules and a coach or instructor. Both boys and girls less frequently "hung out" with friends, engaged in artistic activities, listened to music, visited, or read in comparison with existing findings on typical development. Similar to typically developing adolescents, both male and female adolescents with ASD perceived more closeness and help from their female friends than from their male friends in both same- and opposite-gender friendships. In accordance with the findings of Sedgewick et al. (2016), adolescents with ASD perceived less conflict in their friendships.

5.8.3 Characteristics of Adolescents and Adults Who Make Friends

To facilitate friendships, it is important to identify the characteristics of children who make friends. Conn (2015) studied the experiences of friendship in autobiographies written by individuals with ASD and found that the individuals described their desire to have only one friend at a time and a preference for older or younger friends because younger children are easier to follow, whereas older ones can participate in serious conversations. In a large sample of children and adolescents with ASD (1202 individuals), the rates of friendships did not differ significantly based on gender; however, children and adolescents with lower IQ scores had poorer peer relationships. Furthermore, friendship was significantly related to ASD symptom severity: the more severe the ASD symptomatology, the less likely an individual was to have friends (Mazurek & Kanne, 2010). As Bauminger et al. (2008a, 2008b) stated, it may be that individuals with ASD who develop friendships have relatively higher overall social-emotional capabilities in contrast to individuals with ASD who do not have reciprocal friendships. Awareness of their social status and a desire for reciprocal high-quality friendships characterize some adolescents with higher-functioning ASD (Locke et al., 2010); however, many are also aware of their social limitations and global social deficits (Mazurek & Kanne, 2010). Contrary to typical development, in which friendship usually increases the well-being of the friends, Mazurek and Kanne (2010) found that friendships among individuals with ASD were associated with higher degrees of anxiety and depression. Adolescents with ASD who reported having one or more friends experienced the greatest levels of anxiety and depression. Surprisingly, better-quality friendships were associated with greater anxiety and depression, leading to the conclusion that having a friend does not alleviate anxiety. This finding echoes Bauminger, Shulman and Agam's findings (2003), in which children with ASD reported higher levels of loneliness than their typically developing peers as well as a lower association between social interaction and loneliness, indicating their poorer understanding of the relations between loneliness and social interaction. Regarding gender, adolescent girls with ASD have better social skills and higher social motivation than boys (Sedgewick et al., 2016), participate in "girl talk," and are able to establish friendships that are more intimate than those of boys with ASD.

5.9 Characteristics of Partners

Identifying the characteristics of adolescent partners is critical to enhance the friendships of adolescents with ASD. Adolescents entering high school are usually less understanding and less accepting in comparison to younger individuals, and their interests vary. Most importantly, the most salient feature of friendship is intimacy (Howard, Cohn & Orsmond, 2006), which is one of the more pronounced difficulties for individuals with ASD. Therefore, adolescents with ASD often find themselves sidelined socially (Locke et al., 2010). In line with Conn's findings (2015), when examining adolescent ASD friendships in general and their partners specifically, Kuo et al. (2011) found that many of the partners were younger than the adolescents with ASD. Furthermore, most were of the same gender, although adolescence is distinguished by cross-gender friendships in typical development. Moreover, half of the friends had a disability, with ASD as the leading disability. Nevertheless, according to Rossetti (2015), when friendships in adolescence do occur, the partners are usually mature, independent of cliques, and supportive of their friends with ASD. This support is, for the most part, provided with ease and confidence that is usually observed in family members rather than peers. Female friends are more likely to provide support in both same-gender and mixed-gender friendships (Kuo et al., 2011).

5.10 Environmental Support and Practical Implications

To discuss the environmental support needed to facilitate friendships in ASD, it is important to stress that in order for an individual to form and maintain friendships, interpersonal skills are necessary (Asher, Parker & Walker, 1996) to enable an inherently dyadic relationship. Therefore, when discussing interventions that can advance friendship, it is necessary to determine whether the proposed intervention aims to advance social skills or whether it is focused on advancing and maintaining friendships. Many interventions do not differentiate between promoting social skills and peer acceptance and promoting friendship. Asher et al. (1996) stated that the most important components of interventions aimed at facilitating and developing friendships are (a) instruction in specific concepts related to social interaction, (b) rehearsal and practice of these concepts while interacting with peers, and (c) reflection of the concepts taught based on individual experience. It is clear that these guidelines are in accordance with social skills intervention and are not specific enough for friendship. Developing coordinated friendships with peers is challenging and mandates interventions that include aspects specific to friendship maintenance and facilitation. A multidimensional, developmentally, and ecologically oriented curriculum can advance friendship interventions, but the content of the curriculum itself remains somewhat ambiguous. Furthermore, the location of the intervention (e.g., school, home, clinic) and the persons involved (e.g., parents, practitioners, teachers, peers) have yet to be considered. The Program for the Education and Enrichment of Relational Skills (PEERS; Laugeson & Frankel, 2010) was originally developed as a manualized, evidence-based social skills program for high-functioning adolescents with ASD (Laugeson & Frankel, 2010) that focused on making and keeping friends and managing peer conflict and rejection. The efficacy and effectiveness of parent/caregiver-assisted versions of the PEERS intervention have been established in multiple clinical trials from childhood to young adulthood (Bauminger-Zvielly, 2013). In a randomized control study of parent-assisted children's friendship training, Frankel et al. (2010) concluded that a key for the development of best friends among children with ASD may be training in the skills necessary for successful one-on-one play dates. Parents are crucial for this intervention because they can actively promote play dates. Additional crucial elements that should be considered in friendship interventions are the ability to manage conflict during a lengthy and meaningful relationship, the ability to differentiate the individual's needs from the other's needs, and increased proficiency in developing emotion-based relations.

For years, it has been clear that placing a student with ASD in an inclusive environment is not sufficient to facilitate or enable friendship. There must be an emphasis on specific interventions that focus on supporting friendship opportunities throughout the lifespan, whether in preschool or adulthood (Carter, Asmus, & Moss, 2013; Rossetti, 2015). Chang and associates (2016) examined the strategies that preschool teachers implemented during the day to encourage friendship and found that the main strategy was that of behavior regulation when the child with ASD was behaving inappropriately in the classroom. The authors found that the teacher rarely intervened to promote social skills. Nevertheless, when the teacher did encourage the children to interact and play together, the children became more aware of each other, an important first step in developing meaningful relationships. Furthermore, based on data for preschool-age children with ASD, researchers recommend early interventions that specifically target core deficits such as joint attention and communication skills to help promote meaningful friendships (Chang et al., 2016; Lawton & Kasari, 2012).

In a study that examined what friendship means to school-age children with ASD in inclusive settings, it was found that the children benefited from direct support to develop their friendship skills (Calder et al., 2013), whether the support was provided by parents or teachers. The parents facilitated friendship formation and maintenance by inviting peers home, initiated contact with others and participated in social interactions. The teachers described their role as encouraging the children to play together on the playground, encouraging peers to be supportive, and stressing inclusive messages in the classroom. The teachers also stressed that in cases where friendships had been formed, the peers saw their role as caring for the child with ASD and including him in their games. Nevertheless, both teachers and parents stressed the low priority given to supporting friendships at school in comparison to academic and behavioral issues. The same findings are apparent in preschool, where efforts are directed toward the enhancement of social skills but not necessarily the development of relationships such as friendship. This is true despite the noticeable and important contribution of friendship to the development of complex social-communicative and play capabilities during preschool.

Support at school is not the only way to assist friendships. At-home "play dates" facilitate children's social skills (Frankel, Gorospe, Chang & Sugar, 2011). Children with ASD who had more play dates engaged more successfully with peers in the school playground and engaged in higher levels of social interaction. Furthermore, better communication between teachers and parents can advance friendship formation between children with ASD and their peers. When a teacher notices a potential friendship forming in the classroom (whether in preschool, elementary, or high school), the teacher can relay this information to the parents so that they can arrange play dates outside the school setting (Chang et al., 2016).

Rossetti (2015) found that natural, inclusive settings facilitate social interaction and friendships if they provide multiple opportunities for friends to interact over time. According to the themes that emerged from the adolescent dyads in their study, it is important to enable and encourage reciprocal and meaningful interactions in natural, inclusive settings. Furthermore, encouraging interactions in multiple settings, including structured activities in after-school programs, emerged as an important means of support that can advance friendships and aid in their maintenance. Kuo and associates (2011) found that watching television and playing with a computer were the most frequent activities that adolescents with ASD engaged in with friends and that video games often served as a social bridge for adolescents with ASD and assisted them in attempting to fit in with their typically developing peers; thus, creating a context in which adolescents with ASD can socialize and expand their friendships.

A key factor in establishing and bolstering friendships among adolescents with ASD is to understand how they define friends and what characteristics of friendship they value (Kuo et al., 2011). Therefore, it would be advantageous for adolescents with ASD to discuss with their parents, therapists, and educators what social supports are needed and how the adolescents could benefit from them. It is important to stress that researchers have cautioned adult proximity as a possible barrier to friendship formation, especially by paraprofessionals (Giangreco, 2010; Giangreco & Broer, 2005), and the tendency for students to interact with individually assigned adults rather than peers. Therefore, when assessing the various social supports that are needed, it is important to use caution when providing adult assistance in school settings.

Another important and sometimes neglected aspect is individuals with typical development. The majority of studies concerning interventions to facilitate friendship are based on inclusive environments and are grounded, among other assumptions, on the understanding that the inclusion of students with special needs in regular classrooms can enrich the social climate of the classroom. The origin of this assumption is the knowledge that students can increase their insight and acceptance of diversity when a student with special needs is integrated into the classroom (Clark & Smith, 1999). To date, peer-mediated interventions are considered to be the best practice to enhance the social skills of individuals with ASD. However, the role of a peer model may at times become burdensome on children with typical development, leading to burn out in adolescence (Locke, Rotheram-Fuller & Kasari, 2012). Chang and Locke (2016) performed a systematic review of the literature concerning the benefits of peer-mediated interventions for children and adolescents with HFASD. The studies the authors reviewed included children from preschool to high school age (n = 260). In all the studies, the peers were selected via teacher nomination for various reasons, such as high levels of social skills, attendance, and social status. Furthermore, all studies reported structured peer training models to teach specific social strategies. The typically developing peers served as social role models, thereby improving the social initiations, responses, and interactions of the individuals with HFASD in all of the reported studies. These interventions can provide the basis for future friendships if, in addition to interventions for students with ASD, discussions with educators and parents are provided for students without disabilities concerning ways to provide social support and to balance this support with their social life (Rossetti, 2015).

5.11 Conclusion and Future Directions

In this chapter, friendship for individuals with ASD was reviewed by adopting developmental perspectives. Despite the difficulties children with ASD face in developing friendships, the collected data in different development periods suggest the importance of friendship. Individuals with higher IQ and verbal abilities who have better social abilities have greater chances of making friends, and some succeed more than others (Bauminger-Zviely, 2013). A sizeable amount of individuals form feasible, meaningful, and durable friendships with their peers, whether the peer is a child with typical development or with ASD. Some advantages have been reported for mixed friendships over nonmixed friendships in terms of the development of higher and more complex social and play behaviors. However, nonmixed friendships are also important to provide children with a sense of belonging and self-worth. They also make more room for equal contributions from both partners.

An important aspect of friendship is its potential role to mitigate bullying. Studies have shown that bullying has become a worldwide public health issue, and children with ASD have a particularly high incidence rate of becoming potential bullying victims (Hong, Neely & Lund, 2015; Sreckovic, Brunsting & Able, 2014) in comparison to typically developing children and children with other disabilities (Rowley et al., 2012). Rowley et al. (2012) examined the experiences of friendship and victimization (being bullied) in a sample of 100 children with ASD. They found that children with higher social abilities reported more friendships but experienced higher levels of victimization in mainstream schools. Developing interventions to promote friendships is crucial in the context of bullying. Research shows that having even one reciprocal friendship can contribute to preventing children from becoming victims of bullying (Bollmer, Milich, Harris & Maras, 2005).

Interventions should focus on the child's ability to develop relationships rather than merely sporadic interactions with peers. The developing relationships should be durable and have the qualities of closeness and togetherness between the two partners. It is also important to support these developing relationships over time. Friendships are not likely to evolve without environmental scaffolding (i.e., including parents, school staff, peers) among children with ASD, in contrast to children with typical development. It is also likely that the quality of friendships with children with ASD differ from the quality of typical friendships. However, as evident in the current review, there are many areas in which friendship with children with ASD resembles that of typical friendship. Furthermore, it is clear that friendship has an important role in providing a natural-supportive social environment for children with ASD to develop more complex social-play, pragmatic and communicative skills, as well as intersubjective capabilities.

In sum, despite the accumulated knowledge concerning friendship with children with ASD, there are still many gaps that require in-depth research. First and foremost, to our knowledge, there are no studies of friendship in other subgroups of individuals with ASD, such as minimally verbal individuals and those with lower cognitive abilities (e.g., IQ <75). Second, few studies have examined gender, including mixed-gender and nonmixed gender friendships across development. Third, we do not know enough about the friends of children with ASD. Specifically, we know little about the typically developing children who develop friendships with children on the spectrum, such as, who are they, what motivates them, and how we can encourage children with typical development to have friends with ASD. Fourth, and most importantly, there is a dire need for research concerning intervention programs that aim to develop, maintain, and expand friendships across the lifespan. Fifth, we are in a very preliminary stage in the understanding of the variables that predict or facilitate friendship in ASD.

We are in a more optimistic position today in comparison with the traditional perception of Kanner (1943), who conceptualized children with ASD as unable to develop affective ties. The data show that children with ASD develop affective-durable and meaningful friendships with their peers, but there is still much that can be done to help children on the spectrum become involved in these relationships and maintain evolving, ongoing relationships. The child's social environment and significant others within this environment seem to play pivotal roles in helping children on the spectrum to have fruitful friendships. Future studies should expend efforts to find ways to help these children make and maintain friends.

References

American Psychiatric Association. (2013). *Diagnostic and statistical manual of mental disorders: Text revision* (5th ed.). Washington, DC: Author.

Asher, S. R., Parker, J. G., & Walker, D. L. (1996). Distinguishing friendship from acceptance: Implications for intervention and assessment. In W. M. Bukowski, A. F. Newcomb, & W. W. Hartup (Eds.), *The company they keep: Friendship during childhood and adolescence* (pp. 366–405). New York, NY: Cambridge University Press.

Bauminger, N., & Kasari, C. (2000). Loneliness and friendship in high-functioning children with autism. *Child Development, 71*, 447–456.

Bauminger, N., Rogers, S. J., Aviezer, A., & Solomon, M. (2005). *The friendship observation scale (FOS)*. Davis, CA: Unpublished manual, Bar Ilan University, Israel and University of California.

Bauminger, N., & Shulman, C. (2003). The development and maintenance of friendship in high functioning children with autism, maternal perceptions. *Autism, 7*, 81–97.

Bauminger, N., Shulman, C., & Agam, G. (2003). Peer interaction and loneliness in high functioning children with autism. *Journal of Autism and Developmental Disorders, 33*, 489–507.

Bauminger, N., Solomon, N., Aviezer, A., Heung, K., Brown, J., & Rogers, S. J. (2008a). Friendship in high-functioning children with autism spectrum disorder: Mixed and non-mixed dyads. *Journal of Autism and Developmental Disorders, 38*, 1211–1229.

Bauminger, N., Solomon, N., Aviezer, A., Heung, K., Gazit, L., Brown, J., et al. (2008b). Children with autism and their friends: A multidimensional study of friendship in high-functioning autism spectrum disorder. *Journal of Abnormal Child Psychology, 36*, 135–150.

Bauminger, N., Solomon, N., & Rogers, S. J. (2010). Predicting friendship quality in autism spectrum disorders and typical development. *Journal of Autism and Developmental Disorders, 40*, 751–761.

Bauminger-Zviely, N. (2013). *Social and academic abilities in high-functioning children with autism spectrum disorders*. New York, NY: Guilford Press.

Bauminger-Zviely, N., & Agam-Ben-Artzi, G. (2014). Young friendship in HFASD and typical development: Friend versus non-friend comparisons. *Journal of Autism and Developmental Disorders, 44*, 1733–1748.

Bauminger-Zviely, N., Golan-Itshaky, A., & Tubul-Lavy, G. (2017). Speech acts during spontaneous peer conversation in preschoolers with highfunctioning autism spectrum disorder versus typical development. *Journal of Autism and Developmental Disorders, 47*, 1380–1390.

Bauminger-Zviely, N., Karin, E., Kimhi, Y., & Agam Ben Artzi, G. (2014). Spontaneous peer conversation in preschoolers with high-functioning autism spectrum disorder versus typical development. *Journal of Child Psychology and Psychiatry, 55*, 363–373.

Bollmer, J. M., Milich, R., Harris, M. J., & Maras, M. A. (2005). A friend in need: The role of friendship quality as a protective factor in peer victimization and bullying. *The Journal of Interpersonal Violence, 20*, 701–712.

Bossaert, G., Colpin, H., Pijl, S. J., & Petry, K. (2015). Quality of reciprocated friendships of students with special educational needs in mainstream seventh grade. *Exceptionality, 23*(1), 54–72. Retrieved from http://search.proquest.com/docview/1697493279?accountid=12067

Bukowski, W. M., Hoza, B., & Boivin, M. (1994). Measuring friendship quality during pre- and early adolescence: The development and psychometric properties of the friendship qualities scale. *Journal of Social and Personal Relationships, 11*, 471–484.

Buysse, V., Goldman, B. D., & Skinner, M. L. (2002). Setting events of friendship formation among young children with and without disabilities. *Exceptional Children, 68*, 503–517.

Calder, L., Hill, V., & Pellicano, E. (2013). "Sometimes I want to play by myself": Understanding what friendship means to children with autism in mainstream primary schools. *Autism, 17*, 296–316.

Carter, E. W., Asmus, J., & Moss, C. K. (2013). Fostering friendships: Supporting relationships among youth with and without developmental disabilities. *Prevention Researcher., 20*(2), 14–17.

Chamberlain, B., Kasari, C., & Rotheram-Fuller, E. (2007). Involvement or isolation? The social networks of children with autism in regular classrooms. *Journal of Autism and Developmental Disorders, 37*(2), 230–242. doi:10.1007/s10803-006-0164-4

Chang, Y. C., & Locke, J. (2016). A systematic review of peer-mediated interventions for children with autism spectrum disorder. *Research in Autism Spectrum Disorders, 27*, 1–10.

Clark, D. M., & Smith, S. W. (1999). Facilitating friendships: Including students with autism in the early elementary classroom. *Intervention in School and Clinic, 34*, 248-250.

Chang, Y. C., Shih, W., & Kasari, C. (2016). Friendships in preschool children with autism spectrum disorder: What holds them back, child characteristics or teacher behavior? *Autism: The international journal of research and practice, 20*(1), 65–74.

Conn, C. (2015). 'Sensory highs', 'vivid rememberings' and 'interactive stimming': Children's play cultures and experiences of friendship in autistic autobiographies. *Disability and Society, 30*(8), 1192–1206. doi:10.1080/09687599.2015.1081094

Dean, M., Kasari, C., Shih, W., Frankel, F., Whitney, R., Landa, R., …… & Harwood, R. (2014). The peer relationships of girls with ASD at school: Comparison to boys and girls with and without ASD. *Journal of Child Psychology and Psychiatry 55*(11), 1218–1225.

Frankel, F. D., Gorospe, C. M., Chang, Y. C., & Sugar, C. A. (2011). Mothers' reports of play dates and observation of school playground behavior of children having high-functioning autism spectrum disorders. *Journal of Child Psychology and Psychiatry, 52*(5), 571–579.

Frankel, F., Myatt, R., Sugar, C., Whitham, C., Gorospe, C., & Laugeson, E. (2010). A randomized controlled study of parent-assisted Children's Friendship Training with children having autism spectrum disorders. *Journal of Autism and Developmental Disorders, 40*(7), 827–842.

Freeman, S. F., Gulsrud, A., & Kasari, C. (2015). Brief report: Linking early joint attention and play abilities to later reports of friendships for children with ASD. *Journal of Autism and Developmental Disorders., 45*(7), 2259–2266.

Giangreco, M. F. (2010). One-to-one paraprofessionals for students with disabilities in inclusive classrooms: Is conventional wisdom wrong? *Intellectual & Developmental Disabilities, 48*(1), 1–13. doi:10.1352/1934-9556-48.1.1

Giangreco, M. F., & Broer, S. M. (2005). Questionable utilization of paraprofessionals in inclusive schools: Are we addressing symptoms or causes? *Focus on Autism and Other Developmental Disabilities, 20*(1), 10–26.

Guralnick, M. J., Neville, B., Hammond, M. A., & Connor, R. T. (2007). The friendships of young children with developmental delays: A longitudinal analysis. *Journal of Applied Developmental Psychology, 28*, 64–79.

Hong, E. R., Neely, L., & Lund, E. M. (2015). Addressing bullying of students with autism: Suggestions for families and educators. *Intervention in School and Clinic, 50*(3), 157–162.

Howard, B., Cohn, E., & Orsmond, G. I. (2006). Understanding and negotiating friendships. *Autism, 10*, 619–627.
Howes, C. (1983). Patterns of friendship. *Child Development, 54*, 1041–1053.
Howes, C. (1996). The earliest friendships. In W. M. Bukowski, A. F. Newcomb, & W. W. Hartup (Eds.), *The company they keep: Friendship in childhood and adolescence* (pp. 66–86). Cambridge, UK: Cambridge University Press.
Howes, C. (2009). Friendship in early childhood. In K. H. Rubin, W. M. Bukowski, & B. Laursen (Eds.), *Handbook of peer interactions, relationships, and groups* (pp. 180–194). New York, NY: The Guilford Press.
Howlin, P., et al. (2015). Research on adults with autism spectrum disorder: Roundtable report. *Journal of Intellectual and Developmental Disability, 40*(4), 388–393. doi:10.3109/13668250.2015.1064343
Kanner, L. (1943). Autistic disturbances of affective contact. *Nervous Child, 2*, 217–250.
Kimhi, Y., & Bauminger-Zviely, N. (2012). Collaborative problem solving in preschoolers with HFASD and with typical development. *Journal of Autism and Developmental Disorders, 42*, 1984–1997.
Kuo, M. H., Orsmond, G. I., Cohn, E. S., & Costner, W. J. (2011). Friendship characteristics and activity patterns of adolescents with an autism spectrum disorder. *Autism, 17*(4), 481–500.
Laugeson, E. A., & Frankel, F. (2010). *Social skills for teenagers with developmental and autism spectrum disorders: The PEERS treatment manual*. New York, NY: Routledge.
Lawton, K., & Kasari, C. (2012). Brief report: Longitudinal improvements in the quality of joint attention in preschool children with autism. *Journal of Autism and Developmental Disorders, 42*, 307–312.
Locke, J., Ishijima, E., Kasari, C., & London, N. (2010). Loneliness, friendship quality, and the social networks of adolescents with high-functioning autism in an inclusive school setting. *Journal of Research in Special Educational Needs, 10*, 74–81.
Locke, J., Rotheram-Fuller, E., & Kasari, C. (2012). Exploring the social impact of being a typical peer model for included children with autism spectrum disorder. *Journal of Autism and Developmental Disorders, 42*(9), 1895–1905. doi:http://dx.doi.org/10.1007/s10803-011-1437-0
Mazurek, M. O. (2013). Social media use among adults with autism spectrum disorders. *Computers in Human Behavior, 29*(4), 1709–1714.
Mazurek, M. O. (2014). Loneliness, friendship and well-being in adults with autism spectrum disorders. *Autism, 18*(3), 223–232.
Mazurek, M. O., & Kanne, S. M. (2010). Friendship and internalizing symptoms among children and adolescents with ASD. *Journal of Autism and Developmental Disorders, 40*(12), 1512–1520. doi:10.1007/s10803-010-1014-y
Mehling, M. H., & Tasse, M. J. (2015). Impact of choice on social outcomes of adults with ASD. *Journal of Autism and Developmental Disorders, 45*, 1588–1602.
Mendelson, J. L., Gates, J. A., & Lerner, M. D. (2016). Friendship in school-age boys with autism spectrum disorders: A meta-analytic summary and developmental, process-based model. *Psychological Bulletin, 142*(6), 601–622. doi:10.1037/bul0000041
Newcomb, A. F., & Bagwell, C. L. (1996). The developmental significance of children's friendship relations. In W. M. Bukowski, A. F. Newcomb, & W. W. Hartup (Eds.), *The company they keep: Friendship during childhood and adolescence* (pp. 289–321). New York, NY: Cambridge University Press.
Odom, S. L., Zercher, C., Li, S., Marquart, J. M., Sandall, S., & Brown, W. H. (2006). Social acceptance and rejection of preschool children with disabilities: A mixed-method analysis. *Journal of Educational Psychology, 98*, 807–823.
Orsmond, G. I., Krauss, M. W., & Seltzer, M. M. (2004). Peer relationships and social and recreational activities among adolescents and adults with autism. *Journal of Autism and Developmental Disorders, 34*, 245–256. doi:10.1023/B:JADD.0000029547.96610.df
Park, K. A., & Waters, E. (1989). Security of attachment and preschool friendships. *Child Development, 60*, 1076–1081.
Parker, J. G., & Asher, S. R. (1993). Friendship and friendship quality in middle childhood: Links with peer group acceptance and feelings of loneliness and social dissatisfaction. *Developmental Psychology, 29*, 611–621.
Petrina, N., Carter, M., & Stephenson, J. (2015). Parental perception of the importance of friendship and other outcome priorities in children with autism spectrum disorder. *European Journal of Special Needs Education, 30*(1), 61–74. Retrieved from http://search.proquest.com/docview/1651865799?accountid=12067
Rossetti, Z. (2015). Descriptors of friendship between secondary students with and without autism or intellectual and developmental disability. *Remedial and Special Education, 36*(3), 181–192. Retrieved from http://search.proquest.com/docview/1720060656?accountid=12067
Rowley, E., Chandler, S., Baird, G., Simonoff, E., Pickles, A., Loucas, T., & Charman, T. (2012). The experience of friendship, victimization and bullying in children with an autism spectrum disorder: Associations with child characteristics and school placement. *Research in Autism Spectrum Disorders, 6*, 1126–1134. doi:10.1016/j.rasd.2012.03.004
Sedgewick, F., Hill, V., Yates, R., Pickering, L., & Pellicano, E. (2016). Gender differences in the social motivation and friendship experiences of autistic and non-autistic adolescents. *Journal of Autism*

and Developmental Disorders, *46*(4), 1297–1306. doi:10.1007/s10803-015-2669-1

Shattuck, P. T., Orsmond, G. I., Wagner, M., & Cooper, B. P. (2011). Participation in social activities among adolescents with an autism spectrum disorder. *PloS One*, *6*(11), e27176. doi:10.1371/journal.pone.0027176

Sreckovic, M. A., Brunsting, N. C., & Able, H. (2014). Victimization of students with spectrum disorder: A review of prevalence and risk factors. *Research in Autism Spectrum Disorders*, *40*, 1067–1079.

Vitaro, F., Boivin, M., & Bukowski, W. M. (2009). The role of friendship in child and adolescent psychosocial development. In K. H. Rubin, W. M. Bukowski, & B. Laursen (Eds.), *Handbook of peer interactions, relationships, and groups* (pp. 568–588). New York, NY: Guilford Press.

Part II

Assessment

Standardized Assessment of Social Skills in Autism Spectrum Disorder

6

B.J. Freeman and Pegeen Cronin

Social skills are innate across species. As mammals, we are social creatures and our survival depends on our abilities to socially navigate the many facets of our immediate surroundings and the world at large. Kanner (1943) contrasted this marked innate predisposition of typical individuals to engage in reciprocal interactions to that of a group of 11 individuals whom he said innately lacked social interest (autism). In his original description of autism, he proposed that autism was a congenital disorder characterized by profound social deficits.

Over the past six decades, there has been an increased interest in describing, defining, and measuring how this innate lack of social interest affects development in individuals now said to have autism spectrum disorders (ASD). ASD is currently considered to be a set of heterogeneous neurodevelopmental disorders which result in significant social-communication deficits and a restricted range of interests. Persons with ASD are frequently said to have social-cognitive deficits which result in a failure to respond to social stimuli appropriately and an inability to develop meaningful social relationships (American Psychiatric Association [APA], 2013).

It is now well recognized that deficits in reciprocal social interactions are the hallmark of ASD and represent abnormalities in brain development. Soto-Icaza, Aboitiz, and Billeke (2015) in a recent review proposed a model for the development of social skills at three levels (i.e., neuronal, cognitive, and behavioral). They delineate behavioral events related to social development and the specific appearance of neuronal and cerebral events. This provides a general framework for the elaboration of cognitive models to explain social development. They conclude that cognition and social development are innately related in typical human development. However, this may not be the case with respect to ASD.

There are currently a number of measures which assess specific cognitive aspects of social skills. It is assumed that these underlying cognitive issues, either alone or in combination, can explain the social deficits associated with ASD. These include such deficits in specific social behaviors as joint attention (Mundy, 2016), theory of mind (Sorenson, 2009), empathy (Auyeung et al., 2009), and executive functioning (Pellicano, 2012) among others.

It is well documented in the literature that many individuals with ASD are able to master these skills in structured settings, but are unable to use the skills day to day. It is clear while these

B.J. Freeman, PhD (✉)
Medical Psychology, UCLA School of Medicine, Los Angeles, CA, USA
e-mail: bjf007ca@aol.com

P. Cronin, PhD
Clinical Psychologist, Cronin Assessment, Los Angeles, CA, USA

J.B. Leaf (ed.), *Handbook of Social Skills and Autism Spectrum Disorder*, Autism and Child Psychopathology Series, DOI 10.1007/978-3-319-62995-7_6

skills may be measurable, they alone cannot explain the social deficits seen in ASD. Klin, Jones, Schultz, and Volkmar (2005) addressed in detail this unique problem of how social skills are manifested with individuals with ASD. The authors point out that the discrepancy between what persons with ASD can do in a very structured task of social reasoning and how they function day to day represents one of the most "intriguing puzzles" in the field. The dilemma (e.g., the ability to verbally identify, but inability to spontaneously apply these skills in the natural environment) has created a major issue in the development of standardized measurements of social skills. Some research has been conducted defining the magnitude of this discrepancy between how individuals score on structured cognitive tests in the laboratory and how they apply these skills in the natural environment (Klin et al., 2007). While there is obviously a relationship between cognition and social skills in ASD, cognitive deficits alone cannot explain the profound social communication deficits that are the core issue in ASD.

6.1 Issues in Standardized Assessment of Social Skills

As in any area of psychometric assessment, the purpose of the assessment is of particular interest and importance. In general clinical settings, purposes of assessment include screening and diagnosis, classification and placement, selection of treatment targets, and treatment evaluations. Sigafoos, Schlosser, Green, O'Reilly, and Lanconi (2008) provide an excellent review of the purposes of communication and social skills assessments. The authors point out in some types of assessments only one evaluation is necessary, while in others ongoing and multiple evaluations will be required. It is clear in the case of measurement of social skills that ongoing behavioral observations over time in multiple environments will be required to adequately assess social competencies and deficits. Any assessment must be *flexible* and address the dynamic nature and variability of social skills among individuals and across settings.

While there is a large literature on measuring social skill competency with typical individuals, few exist in the field of ASD. Two types of social skills measures are usually performed: norm-referenced and environmentally based assessments. In norm-referenced approaches, the aim is to compare the skills of individuals with ASD with that of peers who are socially competent in order to determine how individuals with ASD compare. In environmentally based assessments, the goal is to identify discrepancies between what is required in a particular social situation and the behavior displayed by the individual with ASD (Brown, Snell & Lehr, 2006).

Wetherby and Woods (2006) reviewed the psychometric issues in measurement of social communication skills. These issues include: how the information is gathered, what social behaviors will be measured, are the items on the scale homogeneous, is the individual's behavior judged similarly by different raters in the same situation, is the measure stable from test to test, does the measure capture growth and change in the particular construct, does that measure have an empirical association with some criterion measures, does the measure differentiate ASD from other disorders, and does the measure actually measure the construct it purports to measure.

6.2 Specific Issues Unique to Standard Measurement of Social Skills in ASD

ASD represents a unique category of issues in terms of measuring social skills. If one looks at the cognitive model of social skills, it is clear that some individuals on the autism spectrum can develop specific social cognitive skills (e.g., attention to social skills, theory of mind, joint attention, and executive functioning skills) in a structured setting. However, they are uniquely unable to apply these skills in the real world. Thus, within ASD there is frequently a disconnect between the ability to learn a specific cognitive skill and the ability to apply the skill in a novel social interaction (Klin, 2000). This disconnect must be addressed in any useful measure of social skills.

Mayville (2013) discusses the importance of measuring not only social deficits, but also social competences. The large majority of standardized assessments utilized for measuring social skills in ASD are diagnostic and screening measures that focus on the individual's deficits indicative of ASD, not on their competencies. As a result, there are no specific assessments that yield the type of information needed to design an appropriate treatment program for a specific individual and adequately measure changes over time.

Other issues have hindered the development of standardized social skills measurements for individuals with ASD. One of the most important has been the definition of social skills. (See earlier chapters in this volume for a specific description of social skills as manifested in individuals with ASD.) Definitions of social skills vary from person to person and situation to situation. Until publication of the DSM-5, social and communication skills were considered to be separate entities and resulted in unsuccessful attempts to measure each independently (APA, 2013). It is now well recognized that it is not possible to separate social and communication skills because they are intimately intertwined. There is a large literature on language and communication assessments and standardized psychometric tests have been developed to measure language skills. However, the problem with the measurement of communication skills is similar to the measurement of social skills for individuals with ASD; that is, they are unable to utilize the skills that they are able to demonstrate in structured settings (Freeman, 2011).

Emphasis in social skills research has been on treatment rather than assessment. Reichow and Volkmar (2010) reviewed the scientific literature on social skills treatment. The authors reported one of the major problems in assessing treatment effectiveness is the lack of assessment tools that allow for the measurement of meaningful changes in behavior as the result of an intervention. Typically, in studies of social skills treatment effectiveness, idiosyncratic measures are developed by the examiners for the particular study and focus on only one or two aspects of social skills. This makes it particularly difficult to compare treatment outcome studies.

Another complicating factor in measuring social skills in ASD has been recently identified. Rankin, Weber, Kang, and Lerner (2016) reported that the specific social deficits associated with ASD were positively correlated with parent reported importance. However, they were negatively correlated to importance when rated by individuals with ASD. These results were consistent with previous results reported by Johnson, Filliter, and Murphy (2009), who found significant discrepancies between parent and self-ratings of autistic traits and empathy. Individuals with ASD reported fewer autistic traits and more empathy than parents. Thus, the individuals with ASD saw themselves as less impaired than others perceived them.

Still another consideration in the development of standardized assessments has been the developmental nature of ASD. Cunningham (2012) reviewed the measurement of social interaction with very young children. Cunningham concluded that one of the barriers to drawing conclusions about optimal treatments is the absence of a "gold standard" to measure social interaction with very young children (Cunningham, 2012). Cunningham points out that there are currently no psychometrically sound outcome measures that adequately describe the complex social skill profiles of individuals with ASD, which are also sensitive to change.

The purpose of this chapter is to review the scales that are currently in use for measuring social skills in individuals with ASD. A variety of diagnostic screening scales which involve some measurement of social skill deficits are available. These include general behavior rating measures with an added autism rating scale, autism specific screening scales for early diagnosis and general screening, diagnostic evaluation scales, and adaptive behavior measures. There are only two standardized measures of social skills, the Social Skills Improvement System (SSiS; Gresham & Elliot, 2008) and the Social Responsiveness Scale, Second Edition (SRS-2; Constantino & Gruber, 2012), which attempt to identify social competencies and deficits, which may lead to evaluation and treatment planning.

6.3 Screening Instruments

Screening instruments by definition do not provide diagnosis. Their purpose is to identify behaviors that may reflect a diagnosis of ASD and require further evaluation (Sigafoos et al., 2008). They provide some information regarding the social skill deficits that define ASD. These measures can be divided into three categories: general behavior measures with an autism scale, screening instruments for early diagnosis, and autism specific screening instruments.

Several commonly utilized standardized measures designed to identify emotional and behavioral disorders in the general population have recently been applied with children with ASD. One of the most commonly used scales is the Child Behavior Checklist (CBCL; Achenbach & Rescorla, 2000, 2001; Bérubé and Achenbach 2006. Rescorla, Kim, and Oh (2015) reported that a group with ASD scored higher on the Withdrawn and DSM-Pervasive Developmental Problems scales than individuals with other psychiatric and developmental problems. So, Greaves-Lord et al. (2013) reported that the teacher form of the CBCL was reliable in screening of children for ASD. In an earlier preliminary study, Biederman et al. (2010) reported that the CBCL could be used to distinguish children with ASD from those with other types of psychiatric problems. Volker et al. (2010) also compared the profiles of 62 children with high functioning ASD to 62 typically developing children using the BASC-2. Their results indicated that, with the exception of the Somatization, Conduct Problems and Aggression scales, the ASD group scored higher than the typical individuals on all the scales. The Conners Comprehensive Behavior Rating Scales (Conners, 2014) has also been recently updated to include a separate scale for ASD, but there is little research regarding its use as a screening tool for ASD. Both of these measures are, in fact, merely screening instruments. While they may be helpful in identifying comorbid psychiatric diagnoses, they do not yield specific profiles of social deficits and competencies and are not useful in designing specific treatment interventions.

Gamliel and Yirmiya (2009) provide an excellent review of the most commonly used screening instruments for very young children and their theoretical basis. The majority of these are research instruments not in widespread use. They include: the Autism Observation Scale for Infants (AOSI; Bryson, Zwaigenbaum, McDermott, Rombough & Brian, Bryson et al. 2007); the First Year Inventory (FYI; Reznick, Baranek, Reavis, Watson & Crais, 2007); the Communication and Symbolic Behavior Scales (CSBS; Wetherby & Prizant, 1993); the Early Social Communication Scale (ESCS; Mundy, Hogan & Doehring, 1996); the Screening Tool for Autism in Two-Year-Olds (STAT; Stone, Coonrod, Turner & Pozdol, 2004); and the Modified Checklist for Autism in Toddlers (CHAT and M-CHAT; Baron-Cohen, Allen & Gilberg, 1992). Gamliel and Yirmiya conclude that all of these measures reflect some aspect of social skills in ASD, but are focused on identifying deficits. Thus, the screening instruments do not provide adequate information to design treatment programs or measure change over time.

While none of these instruments are in widespread use outside of research, the M-CHAT has been the most studied. The M-CHAT (Robbins, Fein & Barton, 1999; Robbins, Fein, Barton & Green, 2001; Robbins & Dumont-Mathieu, 2006) is a 23-item yes or no checklist completed by parents. The M-CHAT does not provide a specific measure of social skills; rather it provides information on early social development in general. Kleinman et al. (2008), in a detailed review, concluded that the measure shows promise for early detection of ASD, but more research is needed for it to become a general screening instrument. This is an extremely important area of research as the American Academy of Pediatrics (AAP, 2006) recently endorsed screening of all children at 18 months for ASD. This recommendation has not been implemented due to the lack of a reliable standardized screening instrument.

There are a number of additional screening instruments for ASD that are in widespread use. While the majority of these scales have been found to be reliable and valid for use as screeners for ASD in general, they rarely provide a detailed description of an individual's social skills and do not assess competencies. Commonly used instruments in this category include: the Childhood Autism Rating Scale, Second Edition (CARS2; Schopler, Van Bourgondien, Wellman & Love, 2010); the Autism Screening Instrument for Educational Planning – Third Edition (ASIEP-3; Krug, Arick & Almond, 2008); the PDD Behavior Inventory (PDDBI; Cohen & Sudhalter, 2005); the Gillian Autism Rating Scales – Second Edition (GARS-2; Gilliam, 1995, 2006); the Autism Spectrum Rating Scales (ASRS; Goldstein & Naglieri, 2008); and the Social Communication Questionnaire (SCQ; Rutter, Baily & Lord, 2003a).

In addition, prior to the DSM-5 diagnostic criteria, there were a number of scales purporting to screen for Asperger's Syndrome. These scales may remain useful in order to gather specific information regarding specific social skill deficits of individuals with ASD. Examples of these scales include Gilliam Asperger's Disorder Scale (GADS; Gilliam, 2001); Asperger's Syndrome Diagnostic Scale (ASD; Myles, Jones-Bock & Simpson, 2000); Krugs Asperger's Disorder Index (KADI; Klin et al., 2007); Childhood Asperger's Syndrome Test (CAST; Scott, Baron-Cohen, Bolton, & Brayne, 2002; and Asperger's Syndrome Questions (ASSQ; Ehlers, Gillberg & Wing, 1999).

In summary, all of these screening instruments measure aspects of social deficits associated with ASD and may be useful in identifying individuals that may require further evaluation. However, no screening instruments provide enough information for program development, they do not adequately describe social competencies, and do not measure outcome or change over time.

6.4 Diagnostic Measures Specific to ASD

The Autism Diagnostic Interview – Revised (ADI-R; Rutter, Le Couteur, and Lord 2003) and the Autism Diagnostic Observation Schedule (ADOS; Lord, Rutter, DiLavore & Risi, 2001) are based on the DSM-IV criteria for Autistic Disorder (American Psychiatric Association [APA], 1994; ICD-10, World Health Organization [WHO], 1992) and represent the gold standards for diagnosis.

The ADI-R is a semi-structured interview that contains five sections: opening questions, communication, social development and play, repetitive and restricted behavior, and general behavior problems. Behaviors are rated on a 0–3 scale and are coded as to whether they occurred before or after 5 years of age. The Reciprocal Social Interaction items map directly onto the DSM-IV as well as DSM-5 criteria (e.g., peer relationships, sharing enjoyment, and social-emotional reciprocity). Because of its length, the ADI-R is primarily used as a diagnostic research instrument.

The ADOS is a highly structured behavioral observation instrument for assessment of social interactions, communication, play, and imaginative use of toys. Each skill is rated on a scale from 0 to 3. The ADOS consists of five modules that are administered based on the individual's age and level of language development. The Reciprocal Social Interaction items include such behaviors as use of eye contact, nonverbal communication, directing facial expressions to others, shared enjoyment in interaction, communication, affect, and understanding emotions, as well as insight into one's own behavior. The ADOS may be helpful in identifying basic social deficits in a highly structured situation. However, it does not provide information on the presence/absence of these behaviors in the natural environment. Recently, algorithms on the ADOS were updated (Autism Diagnostic Observation Schedule, Second Edition (ADOS-2; Lord, Rutter et al., 2012) to reflect changes in the diagnostic criteria in the DSM-5 (APA, 2013).

Both the ADI-R and ADOS are the gold standards for diagnosis and can provide useful information on specific deficits; thus, they can be helpful in designing treatment programs for a specific individual. Research is underway to study if the ADOS can be utilized to measure change in social skills.

6.5 Adaptive Behavior Measurements

There are standardized measures of social adaptive behavior and behavior problems in the general population, which are frequently used to obtain information regarding social skills functioning in individuals with ASD. These types of measures are potentially useful since they reflect actual behavior and not potential. In addition, these scales generally have several forms (i.e., parent, teacher, and self-report) and provide multiple sources of information about how the behaviors of individuals with ASD differ from the norm and, more importantly, how the individual actually functions in the natural environment. This information is important for differential diagnosis. While overall scores may have limited usefulness in designing treatment programs and identifying social competencies, they do provide useful information. Volkmar et al. (1987) reported that individuals with ASD typically score lower on measures of adaptive behavior than on cognitive tests. Freeman, Del'Homme, Guthrie and Zhang (1999) and more recently Kenworthy, Case, Harms, Martin and Wallace (2010) reported that while adaptive changes in communication skills are positively related to IQ scores, changes in social skills were not. These results confirm the use of adaptive functioning measures in assessing changes in adaptive deficits even in higher functioning individuals with ASD. Furthermore, the relationship between social abilities and ASD exists independent of intelligence. These results support the theory that social skills are at least, in part, independent of cognitive skills.

The Vineland Adaptive Behavior Scales, Second Edition (Vineland-II; Sparrow, Cicchetti and Balla, 2005) has recently been reviewed and updated. In addition to separate norms for children with ASD, it can be used to measure the severity of ASD. The Vineland-II (2005) and Vineland-3 (Sparrow, Cicchetti and Saulnier, 2016) tools assess skills in four domains: communication, daily living skills, socialization, and motor skills. The scale also includes a maladaptive behavior index. Each domain is further divided into three subdomains. For example, the Socialization domain is subdivided to assess interpersonal relationships, play and leisure time skills, and coping skills in the home and community. The Vineland II and Vineland-3 scales and other measures of adaptive behavior ask whether an individual exhibits the skill and if that behavior occurs independently and consistently. The scales measure actual behaviors, not potential behaviors.

The updated Adaptive Behavior Assessment System, Third Edition (ABAS-3; Harrison & Oakland, 2015) measures adaptive behavior skills from birth to 89 years. It is divided into three age groupings: 0–5 years, 5–21 years, and 16–89 years. As with the Vineland scales, separate forms are available for parents and teachers. The ABAS-3 divides skills into three primary domains that cover 10 skill areas: Conceptual (communication, functional academics, self-direction); Social (leisure, social); and Practical (community, home living/school living, health and safety, self-care, work). While individuals with ASD are included in the norms, separate norms for this population are not available. To date, little research has focused on the use of the ABAS in ASD and no specific profile for ASD has been identified.

The Scales of Independent Behavior – Revised (SIB-R; Bruininks, Woodcock, Weatherman & Hill, 1996) is designed to measure adaptive behavior from infancy to mature adults. Measured skill areas include: Motor skills (gross motor and fine motor), Social and Communication Skills (social interaction, language comprehension, language expression), Personal Living Skills (eating and meal preparation, toileting, dressing, personal self-care, domestic skills), Community Living Skills (time and punctuality, money and value, home/community, and orientation), and Maladaptive Behaviors (internalized, asocial, and externalized). As with the ABAS, little, if any, research into how individuals with ASD score on this assessment has been conducted.

In general, measures of adaptive behavior provide normative assessment data to assess social deficits for individuals with ASD. They can be utilized to identify gross strengths and weaknesses, and to measure changes over time. Unfortunately, such instruments tend to measure social skills globally and do not provide enough information to design individual treatment programs. For a complete review of adaptive behavior assessments, see Chapter Seven in this handbook.

6.6 Social Skills Improvement System (SSiS) and Social Responsiveness Scale (SRS-2)

There are currently only two measures, the Social Skills Improvement System Rating Scales (SSiS; Gresham & Elliott, 2008); and the Social Responsiveness Scale – Second Edition (SRS-2; å & Gruber, 2012), that can measure social competencies and deficits. Both of these instruments have good reliability, validity, and involve multiple raters including the individual with ASD. They also provide at least some information on social competencies as well as deficits. In addition, both scales are directly tied to treatment.

6.6.1 Social Skills Improvement System (SSiS)

According to Gresham and Elliott (2008), in a review of the earlier Social Skills Rating Scales (SSRS; Gresham & Elliott, 1990), the Social Skills Improvement System (SSiS) provides an evidence-based, multitiered assessment and intervention to help identify students who have social issues. This group of measures (SSiS Performance Screening Guide, SSiS Classroom Intervention Program, SSiS Rating Scales, and SSiS Intervention Guide) can be utilized for both individual and universal screenings of students at risk for academic and social behavioral difficulties, to help plan interventions, and to evaluate progress on targeted skills.

The SSiS Rating Scale (Gresham & Elliott, 2008) is designed to assess individuals and small groups in order to evaluate social skills, problem behaviors, and academic competence. It utilizes multiple forms (parent, teacher, and student) to provide a comprehensive picture across home, school, and community settings. Designed to replace earlier versions of the SSRS, this substantially revised tool incudes updated norms, improved psychometric properties, and new subscales. The multirater SSiS Rating Scales help measure: social skill competencies (i.e., communication, cooperation, assertion, responsibility, empathy, engagement, and self-control); problem behaviors (i.e., externalizing, bullying, hyperactivity/inattention, internalizing, and autism spectrum); and academic competence (i.e., reading achievement, math achievement, and motivation to learn).

The SSiS rates frequency (never, seldom, often, and almost always) and importance of behaviors on a 0–4 scale. By adding importance to the rating scale, the SSiS provides a systematic look at how the rater and the person being rated actually perceive the importance of the behaviors. As noted, this has been a common problem in measures of social behavior in ASD. Since this is a multirater assessment, behaviors across environments can be compared. In addition to measuring social competencies and behavioral deficits, the SSiS also has an academic competency scale, which is aimed at examining how a student's social behaviors affect his or her academic functioning in the classroom. As noted above, the SSiS is linked to a general education classroom intervention plan as well as a specific individualized plan.

According to the authors (Gresham and Elliott, 2008) the mean score differences between individuals with ASD and typical individuals were elevated on all of the scales and were statistically significant. They report that these results are consistent with expectations that individuals with ASD exhibit major deficits in social skills and academic skills, and tend to show more problem behaviors than typical children and adolescents. The greatest mean difference on all of the subscales was on the autism spectrum scale, as would be expected.

Consistent with best practice guidelines the SSiS incorporates multiple sources of information across multiple environments including home, school/academic, and community settings.

Measuring social skills competencies in these areas clearly helps to both identify information about an individual's social adaptation challenges and contrast behaviors across settings, such as the general education classroom and the home setting. Alternatively, direct comparisons identify social deficits respective to the environment, and as such the SSiS is a good first step, as it remains a screening instrument for social skill deficits and competencies and should not be used alone to assess social skills for individuals with ASD. There is no adult form for the SSiS.

6.6.2 Social Responsiveness Scale (SRS-2)

The recently revised Social Responsiveness Scale (SRS-2; Constantino & Gruber, 2005, 2012) is a 65-item objective measure of symptoms associated with ASD. The scale has been widely used not only as a diagnostic screening tool, but also as a measure of severity in ASD. There are four forms of the instrument allowing ratings to be collected on individuals from ages 2.5 years through adulthood. Ratings can be obtained from both caregivers and teachers, and the adult form can be used to collect self-information. Behaviors on this scale are rated on a four-point scale from 0 (never) to 4 (almost always). Items focus on the individual's ability to engage in appropriate reciprocal social interaction and communication. One of its strengths is its ability to identify social communication problems in a wide variety of individuals, some of whom do not meet criteria for ASD. An additional strength is its ability to identify and measure autism symptom severity in the natural environment. The SRS-2 scales measure social awareness, social cognition, social communication, social motivation, autistic mannerisms, and also generate an overall score. Constantino and Gruber (2012) reviewed in detail the peer-reviewed literature regarding use of the SRS. (These studies are discussed in detail on pages 65–69 of the manual.) The Social Responsiveness Scale has been correlated with a number of other measures of ASD.

While the authors report that the SRS might be useful in measuring change over time, Wang, Sandall, Davis and Thomas (2011), in a study comparing the SSRS and the Preschool and Kindergarten Behavior Scales – Second Edition (PKBS-2; Merrell, 2002), reported that both scales were helpful in assessing young children with ASD in the natural setting. However, their usefulness in detecting how social skills progress over time or as a result of intervention outcomes for young children with ASD may not be satisfactory.

Bölte, Westerwald, Holtmann, Freitag, and Poustka (2010) reported that the SRS appeared to be a better screening measure than the Social and Communication Disorders Checklist (SCDC; Skuse, Mandy, & Scourfield, 2005). The SRS was found to have higher correlations with the ADI-R, ADOS, and SCQ. These authors support the use of the SRS in screening individuals in the natural environment for an ASD. Schanding, Nowell, and Goin-Kochel (2012) also reported the SRS to be a better screener than the SCQ when teacher ratings were taken into account, confirming the need for multiple raters when attempting to measure social skills in the natural environment. Duku et al. (2013) examined the measurement properties of the SRS and concluded that this measure showed enhanced psychometric properties in measuring social responsiveness in individuals with ASD.

A more recent study (Reszka, Boyd, McBee, Hume & Odom, 2014) examined the use of the SRS as a measure of autism symptom severity as described in the DSM-5. While the ADOS, CARS, ADI-R, and SRS were found to be reliable and valid measures, there was some disagreement among the measures with regard to classification of the individual in the categorization of autism symptom severity (Cholemkery, Medda, Lempp & Freitag, 2016), indicating that much more research is needed at this point before the SRS can be utilized alone as a measure of severity of autism.

Duvekot, van der Endr, Verhulst, and Greaves-Lord (2015) compared the screening accuracy of the parent and teacher reported SRS scores and compared this with an ASD classification according to several other measures. These included the Developmental Dimensional and Diagnostic Interview (3Di; Skuse et al., 2004) and the ADOS in individuals referred to a mental health clinic. Their findings indicated that the SRS was a useful screening tool among clinically referred individuals. Duvekot et al. further stress that the different observers may give different results and have different insights into an individual's social functioning across environments, as individuals function differently in different environments.

In another study of the usefulness of the SRS-2 teacher evaluation, Nelson et al. (2016) examined the factor structure and internal consistency of special education teaching staff ratings on the SRS-2. They reported that there was a four-factor solution that included: social awareness and competence, restricted and repetitive behaviors and interests, atypical social communication, and social avoidance. The subjects in the study tended to be individuals who were more impaired in language and social skills. Thus, they concluded that the SRS for this population did have a four-factor structure, but the four factors were different than that reported by the authors. Again, more research is needed to ascertain if these are valid factors for looking at social skills on the SRS.

Thus, the SRS has adequate psychometric properties as a screening tool for ASD. In addition, it provides some information regarding social competencies in four areas. At this point, much more research is needed to identify the competencies and deficits identified on the SRS before it can be used as a measure of severity and change over time. As with the SSiS, the SRS cannot be used in isolation to define social skills, diagnose, or design treatment programs for individuals with ASD.

6.7 Environmental-Based Assessments

Typically, there have been two types of environmentally based assessments. The first type involves attempts to measure generalization of treatment interventions in the natural environment. Very few studies have addressed how social skills treatment generalizes to the natural environment (Owens, Granader, Humphrey & Baron-Cohen, 2008). The primary reasons for the lack of research center on the intensity required of direct observation, its limited feasibility, and difficulty deriving reliable information across multiple occasions and environments (White, Keonig & Scahill, 2007; McMahon, Vismara & Solomon, 2013).

Dekker, Nanta, Muldur, Sytema, and Bildt (2016) reviewed the methodological issues encountered when attempts are made to measure behaviors in the natural environment as a result of a specific social skills training program. These typically involve short observation in only one environment and look at only one or two behaviors (Frankel, Gorospe, Chang & Sugar, 2011; Humphrey & Symes, 2011).

Dekker et al. (2016) describe the development of a new blind direct observation measure, the Social skills Observation Measure (SOM). They investigated the psychometric properties of the measure and proposed adding a quality measure in addition to the frequency measure of behaviors examined. Each observation consisted of two separate observation periods consisting of 15 1-minute intervals, one in an unstructured setting and one in the classroom. The children did not know they were being observed. Researchers focused on very specific behaviors including: solitary play, cooperative play, aggression, social initiations, and quality of behavior. Results indicated that the SOM had good reliability, but poor convergent validity between parent and teacher reports on standardized measures. This study continues to support one of the major issues in social skills assessment, that is, that standardized measures may not actually reflect accurately the individual's behavior.

The second type of environmentally based assessment is direct behavior assessment. Taubman, Leaf and McEachin (2011) describe in detail the analysis of social skills and present programs for addressing social skill deficits for individuals with ASD. It is clear from the literature that each child needs to be observed individually to determine exactly what social competencies and deficits are present. Thus, individuals need to be observed in natural, and sometimes contrived, social circumstances. Information indicating presence or absence of the behavior, frequency, duration, and quality of behaviors needs to be specified. Behavior assessments should also frequently include reports of significant parties (i.e., parents and teachers, and sometimes peers) and should document progress over time. Questionnaires are designed specifically for a particular child and specifically for his or her social skills assessment. In addition, standardized assessments discussed in this chapter may also be utilized as a starting point to a behavioral assessment.

When a social behavior assessment is completed, multiple sources of information are obtained through objective measurement on the behavioral functioning of an individual's skills and deficits. This specific and individualized information can be readily used to inform a specific treatment or education plan as well as measure change over time. This is the component lacking in most standardized measurement instruments described in this chapter. However, the information obtained through behavior assessment cannot accurately be compared to information for typically developing peers. Further, because individualized information is pinpointed, idiosyncratic measurement may occur, that is, only measurement of unique or even minimally pertinent segments of social competency may be involved. Taubman et al. (2011) describe a particular social skills assessment protocol to guide and assist not only the assessment of skill deficits and competencies, but also the development of necessary instructional programming.

6.8 Future Areas for Research

As reviewed here there are many checklists that screen for social communication strengths and weaknesses and frequency of behaviors across settings and people. Measures rely on the reporter's perception of behaviors and frequency. Future research considerations must keep in mind that there is an overreliance on checklists to identify specific weaknesses or areas of treatment in lieu of a complete evaluation. Therefore, with increased efforts for brevity the risk grows for missing individuals who require a complete evaluation and intervention. Thus, future research and implementation of checklists must take into account that the community at large is eager for efficient, easy-to-read, and quickly scored checklists. Developers must continue to evaluate the efficacy and appropriate implementation of measures intended to screen rather than diagnose and the importance of multiple sources of information that possibly includes measures sold by other publishers.

Ultimately, results identify symptoms or factors characteristic of autism spectrum disorder that may or may not require evaluation and intervention. In light of the inconsistency of ASD social deficits across people and settings, future research might identify measures, possibly in electronic format, that require reporters to complete the same measure at different intervals. This might alleviate response bias of "never" or "always" observing a given behavior. Further, this provides the opportunity to administer a checklist that takes less time to complete in one sitting, yet measures factors or symptoms across specific intervals of time, providing more information about an individual. Similarly, future research must focus on extrapolating the factors and symptoms to track improvement.

As noted here, checklists are utilized to identify symptoms and factors associated with psychiatric diagnoses, including ASD. Therefore, because checklists are screening information for the presence or absence of symptoms and frequency, they are not specific to developmental expectations. This is necessary, and not surprising, as the intent is to identify abnormalities that are not associated with age expectations. Yet, checklists that screen for more than ASD may cloud or distract from screening further for ASD as symptoms or factors reported are scored under other categories such as depression or anxiety. As Volker et al. (2010) reported, all BASC-2 scales were elevated for individuals with ASD. This warrants that each screening measure provides normative data for sample populations of individuals with ASD.

6.9 Conclusions

Attempt to develop standardized measures of social skills for individuals with ASD have been exploding over the past few years. New tools are being developed that are designed for a variety of purposes and focus on various aspects in the social skill arena. While some instruments may be useful in gathering general information and are psychometrically sound, no single instrument yields the information needed to develop a specific social skills program for a specific child and measure change over time. Standardized assessments are useful guides, but only tell us how children with ASD differ from typical children.

Standardized assessment instruments may eventually be designed to measure social skill deficits and competencies in general for individuals with ASD. These tools will aid in diagnosis and provide a measure of response to treatment. However, standardized measures will never provide the comprehensive information required to design and implement appropriate social skills programs for a specific individual and adequately measure behavior change over time. Rather, individualized behavior assessment of social skills in the natural environment utilizing multiple sources of information, multiple modes of assessment, multiple observations, across multiple observers and environments, should become the standard of practice and should be included in every assessment of individuals with ASD.

References

Achenbach, T.M., & Rescorla, L.A. (2000, 2001). *Manual for the ASEBA school-age forms & profiles*. Burlington, VT: University of Vermont, Research Center for Children, Youth, & Families. (online) (www.ASEBA.org).

American Academy of Pediatrics, & Council on Children with Disabilities, Section on Developmental Behavioral Pediatrics, Bright Futures Steering Committee, Medical Home Initiatives for Children with Special Needs Project Advisory Committee. (2006). Identifying infants and young children with developmental disorders in the medical home: An algorithm for developmental surveillance and screening. *Pediatrics, 118*(1), 405–420.

American Psychiatric Association. (1994). *Diagnostic and statistical manual of mental disorders* (4th ed.). Arlington, VA: Author.

American Psychiatric Association. (2013). *Diagnostic and statistical manual of mental disorders* (5th ed.). Arlington, VA: Author.

Auyeung, B., Wheelwright, S., Allison, C., Atkinson, M., Samarawickrema, N., & Baron-Cohen, S. (2009). The children's empathy quotient and systemizing quotient: Sex differences in typical development and in autism spectrum conditions. *Journal of Autism and Developmental Disorders, 39*, 1509–1521.

Baron-Cohen, S., Allen, J., & Gillberg, C. (1992). Can autism be detected at 18 months?: The needle in the haystack and the CHAT. *British Journal of Psychiatry, 161*, 839–843.

Bérubé, R. L., & Achenbach, T. M. (2006). *Bibliography of published studies using the Achenbach system of empirically based assessment*. Burlington, VT: University of Vermont, Research Center for Children, Youth & Families. (online, www.ASEBA.org)

Biederman, J., Petty, C. R., Fried, R., Wozniak, J., et al. (2010). Child behavior checklist clinical scales discriminate referred youth with autism spectrum disorder: A preliminary study. *Journal of Developmental and Behavioral Pediatrics, 31*, 485–490.

Bölte, S., Westerwald, E., Holtmann, M., Freitag, C., & Poustka, F. (2010). Autistic traits and autism spectrum disorders: The clinical validity of two measures presuming a continuum of social communication skills. *Journal of Autism and Developmental Disorders, 41*, 66–72.

Brown, F., Snell, M. E., & Lehr, D. (2006). Meaningful assessment. In M. E. Snell & F. Brown (Eds.), *Instruction for students with severe disabilities* (6th ed.pp. 67–110). Upper Saddle River, NJ: Pearson.

Bruininks, R. H., Woodcock, R. W., Weatherman, R. F., & Hill, B. K. (1996). *Scales of independent behavior – Revised (SIB-R)*. Itasca, IL: Riverside Publishing Company.

Bryson, S. E., Zwaigenbaum, L., McDermott, C., Rombough, V., & Brian, J. (2007). The autism observation scale for infants: Scale development and reliability data. *Journal of Autism and Developmental Disorders, 38*, 731–738.

Cholemkery, H., Medda, J., Lempp, T., & Freitag, C. M. (2016). Classifying autism Spectrum disorders by ADI-R: Subtypes or severity gradient? *Journal of Autism and Developmental Disorders, 46*, 2327–2339.

Cohen, I. L., & Sudhalter, V. (2005). *The PDD behavior inventory*. Lutz, FL: Psychological Assessment Resources.

Conners, K. (2014). *Conners comprehensive behavior rating scales (Conners CBRS)*. New York, NY: Multi-Health Systems.

Constantino, J. N., & Gruber, C. P. (2005). *Social responsiveness scale*. Torrance, CA: Western Psychological Services.

Constantino, J. N., & Gruber, C. P. (2012). *Social responsiveness scale – second edition (SRS-2)*. Torrance, CA: Western Psychological Services.

Cunningham, A. B. (2012). Measuring change in social interaction skills of young children with autism. *Journal of Autism and Developmental Disorders, 42*, 593–605.

Dekker, V., Nauta, M. H., Mulder, E., Sytema, S., & de Bildt, A. (2016). A fresh pair of eyes: A blind observation method for evaluating social skills of children with ASD in a naturalistic peer situation in school. *Journal of Autism and Developmental Disorders, 46*, 2890–2904.

Duku, E., Vaillancourt, T., Szatmari, P., Pathways in ASD Study Team, et al. (2013). Investigating the measurement of the social responsiveness scale in preschool children with autism spectrum disorders. *Journal of Autism and Developmental Disorders, 43*, 860–868.

Duvekot, J., van der Ende, J., Verhulst, F. C., & Greaves-Lord, K. (2015). The screening accuracy of the parent and teacher-reported social responsiveness scale (SRS): Comparison with the 3Di and ADOS. *Journal of Autism and Developmental Disorders, 45*, 1658–1672.

Ehlers, S., Gillberg, C., & Wing, L. (1999). A screening questionnaire for Asperger syndrome and other high-functioning autism spectrum disorders in school age children. *Journal of Autism and Developmental Disorders, 29*, 129–141.

Frankel, F., Gorospe, C. M., Chang, Y. C., & Sugar, C. A. (2011). Mothers' reports of play dates and observation of school playground behavior of children having high-functioning autism spectrum disorders. *Journal of Child Psychology and Psychiatry, 52*, 571–579.

Freeman, B. J. (2011). Assessment of social skills in ASD: A User's guide. In M. Taubman, R. Leaf, & J. McEachin (Eds.), *Crafting connections*. New York, NY: DRL Books.

Freeman, B. J., Del'Homme, M., Guthrie, D., & Zhang, F. (1999). Vineland adaptive behavior scale scores as a function of age and initial IQ in 210 autistic children. *Journal of Autism and Developmental Disorders, 29*, 379–384.

Gamliel, I., & Yirmiya, N. (2009). Assessment of social behavior in autism spectrum disorder. In S. Goldstein, J. A. Naglieri, & S. Ozonoff (Eds.), *Assessment of autism spectrum disorders* (pp. 138–170). New York, NY: The Guilford Press.

Gilliam, J. E., (1995; 2006). *Gilliam autism rating scale*. Austin, TX: Pro-Ed.

Gilliam, J. E. (2001). *Gilliam asperger's disorder scale*. Austin, TX: Pro-Ed.

Goldstein, S., & Naglieri, J. A. (2008). *Autism Spectrum rating scales (ASRS)*. New York, NY: Multi-Health Systems.

Gresham, F. M., & Elliott, S. N. (1990). *Social skills rating system (SSRS). Circle*. Pines, MN: American Guidance Service.

Gresham, F., & Elliott, S. N. (2008). *Social skills improvement system (SSiS)*. Minneapolis, MN: Pearson Assessments.

Harrison, P. L., & Oakland, T. (2015). *Adaptive behavior assessment system* (3rd ed.). Torrance, CA: Western Psychological Services.

Humphrey, N., & Symes, W. (2011). Peer interaction patterns among adolescents with autistic spectrum disorders (ASD) in mainstream school settings. *Autism, 15*, 397–419.

Johnson, S. A., Filliter, J. H., & Murphy, R. R. (2009). Discrepancies between self- and parent-perceptions of autistic traits and empathy in high functioning children and adolescents on the autism spectrum. *Journal of Autism and Developmental Disorders, 39*, 1706–1714.

Kanner, L. (1943). Autistic disturbances of affective contact. *Nervous Child: Journal of Psychopathology, Psychotherapy, Mental Hygiene, and Guidance of the Child, 2*, 217–250.

Kenworthy, L., Case, L., Harms, M. B., Martin, A., & Wallace, G. L. (2010). Adaptive behavior ratings correlate with symptomatology and IQ among individuals with high-functioning autism spectrum disorders. *Journal of Autism and Developmental Disorders, 40*, 416–423.

Kleinman, J. M., Robins, D. L., Ventols, P. E., et al. (2008). The modified checklist for autism in toddlers: A follow-up study investigating the early detection of autism Spectrum disorders. *Journal of Autism and Developmental Disorders, 38*, 827–839.

Klin, A. (2000). Attributing social meaning to ambiguous visual stimuli in higher functioning autism and Asperger syndrome: The social attribution task. *Journal of Child Psychology and Psychiatry, 41*, 831–846.

Klin, A., Saulnier, C. A., Sparrow, S. S., Cicchetti, D. V., Volkmar, F. R., & Lord, C. (2007). Social and communication abilities and disabilities in higher functioning individuals with autism spectrum disorders: The Vineland and the ADOS. *Journal of Autism and Developmental Disorders, 37*, 748–759.

Klin, A., Jones, W., Schultz, R., & Volkmar, F. (2005). The enactive mind, or from actions to cognition: Lessons from autism. In F. R. Volkmar, R. Paul, A. Klin, & D. Cohen (Eds.), *Handbook of autism and pervasive developmental disorders* (pp. 682–703). New York, NY: Wiley.

Krug, D. A., Arick, J. R., & Almond, P. J. (2008). *Autism screening instrument for educational planning, Third edition (ASIEP-3)*. Austin, TX: Pro-Ed.

Lord, C., Rutter, M., DiLavore, P. C., & Risi, S. (2001). *Autism diagnostic observation schedule (ADOS)*. Los Angeles, CA: Western Psychological Services.

Lord, C., Rutter, M., DiLavore, P. C., Risi, S., Gotham, K., & Bishop, S. (2012). *Autism diagnostic observation schedule, second edition (ADOS-2)*. Torrance, CA: Western Psychological Services.

Mayville, E. (2013). The assessment of social skills. In P. F. Gerhardt & D. Crimmins (Eds.), *Social skills and*

adaptive behavior in learners with autism spectrum disorders (pp. 17–32). Baltimore, MD: Brookes.
McMahon, C. M., Vismara, L. A., & Solomon, M. (2013). Measuring changes in social behavior during a social skills intervention for higher-functioning children and adolescents with autism spectrum disorder. *Journal of Autism and Developmental Disorders, 43*, 1843–1856.
Merrell, K. W. (2002). *Preschool and kindergarten behavior scales, second edition (PKBS-2): Examiner's manual*. Austin, TX: PRO-ED.
Mundy, P. (2016). *Autism and joint attention: Development, neuroscience and clinical fundamentals*. New York, NY: Guilford Press.
Mundy, P., Hogan, A., & Doehring, P. (1996). *A preliminary manual for the abridged Early social-communication scales*. Coral Gables, FL: University of Miami.
Myles, B. S., Jones-Bock, S. J., & Simpson, R. L. (2000). *Asperger syndrome diagnostic scale*. Wood Dale, IL: Stoelting.
Nelson, A. T., Lopata, C., Volker, M. A., Thomeer, M. L., Toomey, J. A., & Dua, E. (2016). Exploratory factor analysis of SRS-2 teacher ratings for youth with ASD. *Journal of Autism and Developmental Disorders, 46*, 2905–2915.
Owens, G., Granader, Y., Humphrey, A., & Baron-Cohen, S. (2008). LEGO therapy and the social use of language programme: An evaluation of two social skills interventions for children with high functioning autism and Asperger syndrome. *Journal of Autism and Developmental Disorders, 38*, 1944–1957.
Pellicano, E. (2012). The development of executive function in autism. *Autism Research and Treatment, 2012*, 146132.
Rankin, J. A., Weber, R. J., Kang, E., & Lerner, M. D. (2016). Parent- and self-reported social skills importance in autism Spectrum disorder. *Journal of Autism and Developmental Disorders, 46*, 273–286.
Reichow, B., & Volkmar, F. R. (2010). Social skills intervention for individuals with autism: Evaluation for evidence-based practices with a best evidence synthesis framework. *Journal of Autism and Developmental Disorders, 40*, 149–166.
Rescorla, L., Kim, Y. A., & Oh, K. J. (2015). Screening for ASD with the Korean CBCL/1½–5. *Journal of Autism and Developmental Disorders, 45*, 4039.
Reszka, S. S., Boyd, B. A., McBee, M., Hume, K. A., & Odom, S. L. (2014). Brief report: Concurrent validity of autism symptom severity measures. *Journal of Autism and Developmental Disorders, 44*, 466–470.
Reznick, J. S., Baranek, G. T., Reavis, S., Watson, L. R., & Crais, E. R. (2007). A parent-report instrument for identifying one-year-olds at risk for an eventual diagnosis of autism: The first year Inventory. *Journal of Autism and Developmental Disorders, 37*, 1691–1710.
Robbins, D. L., & Dumont-Mathieu, T. M. (2006). Early screening for autism spectrum disorders: Update on the modified checklist for autism in toddlers and other measures. *Journal of Developmental & Behavioral Pediatrics, 27*(Supplement 2), S111–S119.
Robbins, D. L., Fein, D., & Barton, M. L. (1999). *The modified checklist for autism in toddlers* (M-CHAT). Storrs, CT: Self-published.
Robbins, D. L., Fein, D., Barton, M. L., & Green, J. A. (2001). The modified checklist for autism in toddlers: An initial study investigating the early detection of autism and pervasive developmental disorders. *Journal of Autism and Developmental Disorders, 31*, 131–144.
Rutter, M., Bailey, A., & Lord, C. (2003). *Social communication questionnaire*. Los Angeles, CA: Western Psychological Services.
Rutter, M., Le Couteur, A., & Lord, C. (2003). *Autism diagnostic interview – Revised* (ADI-R). Los Angeles, CA: Western Psychological Services.
Schanding, G. T., Jr., Nowell, K. P., & Goin-Kochel, R. P. (2012). Utility of the *social communication questionnaire – current* and *social responsiveness scale* as teacher-report screening tools for autism spectrum disorders. *Journal of Autism and Developmental Disorders, 42*, 1705–1716.
Schopler, E., Van Bourgondien, M. E., Wellman, G. J., & Love, S. R. (2010). *Childhood autism rating scale, second edition* (CARS-2). Los Angeles, CA: Western Psychological Services.
Scott, F., Baron-Cohen, S., Bolton, P., & Brayne, C. (2002). The CAST (Childhood Asperger Syndrome Test): Preliminary development of a UK screen for mainstream primary-school aged children. *Autism, 6*, 9–31.
Sigafoos, J., Schlosser, R. W., Green, V. A., O'Reilly, M., & Lancioni, G. E. (2008). Communication and social skills assessment. In J. Matson (Ed.), *Clinical assessment and intervention for autism Spectrum disorders* (pp. 165–188). London, UK: Elsevier.
Skuse, D. H., Mandy, W. P. L., & Scourfield, J. (2005). Measuring autistic traits: Heritability, reliability, and validity of the social and communication disorders checklist. *British Journal of Psychiatry, 187*, 568–572.
Skuse, D., Warrington, R., Bishop, D., Chowdhury, U., Lau, J., Mandy, W., & Place, M. (2004). The developmental, dimensional and diagnostic interview (3di): A novel computerized assessment for autism spectrum disorders. *Journal of the American Academy of Child and Adolescent Psychiatry, 43*, 548–558.
So, P., Greaves-Lord, K., van der Ende, J., Verhulst, F. C., Rescorla, L., & de Nijs, P. F. A. (2013). Using the child behavior checklist and the Teacher's report form for identification of children with autism spectrum disorders. *Autism, 2013*(17), 595–607.
Sorenson, L. (2009). Autism, asperger's and theory of mind: A literature review. Cognitive and Children's Thinking Seminar: 295–590.
Soto-Icaza, P., Aboitiz, F., & Billeke, P. (2015). Development of social skills in children: Neural and behavioral evidence for the elaboration of cognitive models. *Frontiers in Neuroscience, 9*, 333.

Sparrow, S., Cicchetti, D., & Balla, D. (2005). *Vineland adaptive behavior scales – second Edition*. Circle Pines, MI: AGS Publishing.

Sparrow, S., Cicchetti, D., & Saulnier, C. A. (2016). *Vineland adaptive behavior scales – third edition*. Bloomington, MN: Pearson.

Stone, W. L., Coonrod, E. E., Turner, L. M., & Pozdol, S. L. (2004). Psychometric properties of the STAT for early autism screening. *Journal of Autism and Developmental Disorders, 34*, 691–701.

Taubman, M., Leaf, R., & McEachin, J. (2011). *Crafting connections*. New York, NY: DRL Publications.

Volker, M. A., Lopata, C., Smerbeck, A. M., Knoll, V. A., Thomeer, M.,. L., Toomey, J. A., & Rodgers, J. D. (2010). BASC-2 PRS profiles for students with high-functioning autism spectrum disorders. *Journal of Autism and Developmental Disorders, 40*, 188–199.

Volkmar, F. R., Sparrow, S. S., Goudreau, D., Cicchetti, D. V., Paul, R., & Cohen, D. J. (1987). Social deficits in autism: An operational approach using the Vineland adaptive behavior scales. *Journal of the American Academy of Child and Adolescent Psychiatry, 26*, 156–161.

Wang, H., Sandall, S. R., Davis, C. A., et al. (2011). Social skills assessment in young children with autism: A comparison evaluation of the SSRS and PKBS. *Journal of Autism and Developmental Disorders, 41*, 1487.

Wetherby, A. M., & Prizant, B. (1993). *Communication and symbolic behavior scales – normed edition*. Baltimore, MD: Brookes.

Wetherby, A., & Woods, J. (2006). Effectiveness of early intervention for children with autism spectrum disorders in the second year of life. *Journal of Autism and Developmental Disorders, 37*, 960–975.

White, S., Keonig, K., & Scahill, L. (2007). Social skills development in children with autism spectrum disorders: A review of the intervention research. *Journal of Autism and Developmental Disorders, 37*, 1858–1868.

World Health Organization (1992). *International classification of diseases,* 10th Revision (ICD-10). Geneva, Switzerland: Author.

Assessment of Adaptive Behavior and Autism Spectrum Disorder

7

Pegeen Cronin and B.J. Freeman

7.1 Assessment of Adaptive Behavior and Autism Spectrum Disorder

Measurement of adaptive behavior has its roots in the identification of what we now know as intellectual disabilities (ID; formerly mental retardation). Scheerenberger (1983) in his book, *A History of Mental Retardation*, traces attempts to define ID and adaptive behavior back to as early as the seventeenth century. By the nineteenth century, intellectual disability was principally identified and defined as awareness and understanding of surroundings, ability to engage in regular economic and social life, dependence on others, the ability to attain one's basic health and safety, and individual responsibility (Brockley, 1999). Thus, initial definitions of ID focused on a person's ability to navigate their world. However, with the development of intelligence quotient (IQ) tests, the focus of defining ID turned to cognitive tests scores that were considered to be fixed in time, easier to measure, and believed to be representative of an individual's overall functioning. As a result, many checklists, IQ tests, and inventories evolved to measure specific cognitive abilities and aspects of personality. By shifting this focus, evaluation and measurement of independent adaptive functioning progressed much more slowly. We have now come full circle with the *Diagnostic and Statistical Manual of mental Disorders* (DSM-5; American Psychiatric Association, 2013), which emphasizes adaptive behavior as the primary focus when defining intellectual disability.

As early as the 1920s, Edgar Doll, a psychologist at the Vineland School, identified test construction and reliability issues with intelligence testing measures. Furthermore, he recognized the inconsistency among individuals over time that could result in an inaccurate and inconsistent picture of a disability when test scores alone were utilized. In the early 1920s, Doll identified a "*scorecard*" of functional adaptive skills to track an individual's progress prior, during, and following treatment at the Vineland school. In 1936 (revised in 1965), the Vineland Social Maturity Scale, a 117-item scale, was published and became the first measure of adaptive behavior for the next several decades. It was derived from a concerted effort to study behavior and learning characteristics of the most severely intellectually disabled. In spite of Doll's work, there remained an over reliance on IQ to determine how a person functions throughout the twentieth century.

P. Cronin, PhD
Clinical Psychologist, Cronin Assessment,
Los Angeles, CA, USA
e-mail: askdrcronin@gmail.com

B.J. Freeman, PhD (✉)
Medical Psychology, UCLA School of Medicine,
Los Angeles, CA, USA
e-mail: bjf007ca@aol.com

J.B. Leaf (ed.), *Handbook of Social Skills and Autism Spectrum Disorder*, Autism and Child Psychopathology Series, DOI 10.1007/978-3-319-62995-7_7

However, over time and with repeat iterations of the gold standard diagnostic manuals for ID, the American Psychiatric Association (APA) DSM-5 and the American Association on Intellectual and Developmental Disabilities (AAIDD, 2010), adaptive behavior has become increasingly important in differential diagnosis of not only intellectual disabilities but autism spectrum disorders (ASD) as well. Currently, adaptive behaviors are viewed as multidimensional and include social, practical, and conceptual skills as they occur in the natural environment. Practical skills include areas of daily living, self-care including health maintenance, occupational independence, community adaptation including safety awareness, transportation, and following routines and schedules. Social skills include social perception, avoiding victimization, social responsibility, self-esteem, gullibility, and social problem solving. Conceptual skills pertain to language, including reading and writing, money, temporal concepts, and number concepts. Currently, concerns remain that measures of adaptive behavior do not measure all these dimensions of independent functioning (Greenspan, 2008). In spite of the fact that the DSM-5 (American Psychiatric Association, 2013) goes so far as to stress that development of adaptive skills better defines intellectual disabilities than IQ, the instruments used continue to suffer from several methodological issues that hinder interpretation, and no one instrument alone can define an individual's adaptive functioning overall.

7.2 Methodological Issues in Measuring Adaptive Behavior

Edgar Doll (1935) was the first to propose that no clinical diagnosis is complete without an estimate of social competence. Similarly, he pointed out that the most important principles inherent in adaptive behavior are that it is age-related, increases and becomes more complex with age, and there are different priorities relative to age. Adaptive functioning begins at birth and becomes more complex with age, is defined by cultural norms, and is not only affected by changes in age and development but also by changes in environment, intervention, and personal experiences (Sparrow, Balla, & Cicchetti, 1984; Sparrow, Cicchetti, &Balla, 2005; and Sparrow, Cicchetti, &Saulnier, 2016). Of particular importance is that adaptive behavior is defined by *typical performance*, not ability. *Typical performance* fluctuates over time based on a variety of circumstances including illness, trauma, or environment including environmental expectations. It is important to distinguish *typical performance* from ability. Further, adaptive behavior measurements are best made by report of a "third party." Thus, the individual being evaluated is not the individual primarily interviewed with regard to current functioning. There can be difficulty if the third party does not have direct experiences, or has biased perceptions or faulty memories. All of these variables must be taken in account when measuring adaptive behavior.

Any instrument must measure abilities reliably across all ages. Since adaptive behavior is defined by typical performance in the natural environment, it is dynamic. Thus, any instrument that purports to measure adaptive behavior must measure multiple dimensions of behavior and must take a developmental approach to identify expectations based on age and cultural norms. Measurement of adaptive behavior is thus complex and requires obtaining qualitative and quantitative information as part of the evaluation process. Results should highlight areas of need for intervention necessary to promote personal independence across environments for an individual. The examiner must be experienced in the selected measure and its scoring system. The reporter must have a current working knowledge and familiarity with the individual undergoing evaluation. Items to be measured on adaptive behavior scales are rated on a scale or dimension necessitating knowledge of developmental and normative expectations to determine the individual's *typical* performance or functioning level, not capabilities. It is important not to let functioning in other areas, such as cognitive functioning, influence ratings of adaptive behavior (Sparrow et al., 1984).

There are several ways to measure adaptive functioning: surveys or checklists completed by individuals familiar with the client's typical performance, structured/unstructured interview with an individual most familiar with the individual's functioning, direct observation, and self-report from the individual undergoing evaluation. Each of these formats has methodological strengths and weaknesses. The direct interview method with a standardized measure is preferred and has the most validity, while self-report has the least. It has been well documented that individuals' perceptions in self-report overestimate and possibly exaggerate their typical abilities (American Association on Intellectual and Developmental Disabilities, 2010; Edgerton, 1993). Different from other psychological measures, there is little evidence that measures of adaptive functioning are significantly affected by ethnic or racial bias (Reschly, 2002). Yet, as measuring adaptive functioning relies in part on cultural expectations and norms; the examiner must have the experience to recognize whether differences in an examinee's culture might be affecting adaptive functioning expectations.

One of the most common pitfalls in measurement of adaptive information is making assumptions not only based on cognitive abilities or IQ but also based on symptom severity, family status, socioeconomic status, education level, or age. While most standardized measures address the core areas of adaptive functioning, a comprehensive review is also necessary across multiple sources of information, including psychological, educational and medical records, and direct evaluation to assess adaptive functioning (American Association on Intellectual and Developmental Disabilities, 2010). The Individuals with Disabilities Education Act (2004) also promotes the importance of measuring adaptive functioning as part of an evaluation.

While a structured interview with a trained clinician is the preferred method, checklists or screening instruments may provide the opportunity to efficiently collect information from a number of reporters to compare the individual's typical performance across settings and people. However, checklists may pose an issue with reading level and language processing skills. Most checklists require at least fifth grade or higher reading level. Reading and comprehension abilities might further thwart someone unfamiliar with specific expectations or assumptions in responding about the person's *typical* behaviors rather than the individual's capabilities. Often there is confusion in perceptions with regard to what an individual *will* or *can* do. Emphasis in the measurement of adaptive functioning should be on what an individual *will* do independently on a consistent basis relative to age and cultural expectations. In attempts to address some of these issues, checklists are best completed in the clinic setting to insure focus and comprehension. When completed elsewhere, at home or at work, there are risks including but not limited to distraction, including those unrelated to the individual, and completing the checklist. Furthermore, checklists also must be carefully analyzed as respondents might have to guess, or if they are unfamiliar with an area of an individual's functioning, this affects scoring. Thus, the interview format by a skilled clinician continues to demonstrate the best validity albeit the disadvantage is that relative to checklists, it takes longer. However, interviews alone are not sufficient. Structured interviews and direct observation in the natural environment combined provide the most information regarding an individual's adaptive behavior.

7.3 Commonly Utilized Measures of Adaptive Functioning

7.3.1 Vineland Adaptive Behavior Scales: Third Edition (Sparrow et al., 2016)

The Vineland Social Maturity Scale (Doll, 1936, 1965) was revised in 1984 by Sara Sparrow and her colleagues at Yale University. The Vineland Adaptive Behavior Scale (VABS) is now in its third edition (Sparrow et al., 2016) and is one of the most frequently used measures of adaptive behavior particularly in the field of ASD research. The VABS-3 assesses an individual's daily independent functioning necessary for everyday living in three primary domains of adaptive functioning: communication, daily living skills (e.g., self-help skills) and socialization, and in the optional area of motor skills. Additional information is gathered relative to maladaptive or problem behaviors that cause difficulty with daily and overall functioning. This information can be helpful in diagnosis or intervention planning and may also be used as a screener to determine if a more in-depth assessment of problematic behavior is warranted.

Results are reported as standard scores, v-scale scores, percentile rank, and age equivalent scores, as well as qualitative status in the three domains. Standard scores for the VABS-3 have a mean of 100 and a standard deviation of 15 points. *V*-Scale scores range from 1 to 24 and have a mean of 15 and a standard deviation of 3. This allows one to compare the relative functioning of individuals to those in the normative population. Each behavior is scored on a 3-point scale (i.e., 2 = always, 1 = sometimes, 0 = never). A basal or sequence of consistent scores is expected below an individual's chronological age, and a ceiling or sequence of "no score" items is expected relative to how an individual's functioning measures at or above chronological age. Results are presented as a quantitative average of adaptive functioning. The quantitative scores should be used as a baseline to guide appropriate intervention and to facilitate adaptive functioning. The VABS is a measure of current functioning, not capabilities. Some scores may not reflect an individual's behavior in all situations; they simply represent how the parent or teacher sees the child.

There have been several changes in the VABS-3. First, the motor skills scale has been removed from the overall adaptive behavior score. However, it can still be used to gather the information in younger children. Sparrow et al. (2016) report all forms of the VABS-3 have adequate validity and reliability and can provide useful information if used properly. Each form's normative sample is based on a large-scale national study that provided the information on validity and reliability and information in special groups (e.g., individuals with intellectual disabilities and ASD). Like its predecessor, the VABS-3 has both parent and teacher forms. Data can be gathered by thorough interview (e.g., parent/caregiver and teacher comprehensive interview forms) or by parent or teacher report (e.g., parent/caregiver and teacher comprehensive forms). In addition, there are shortened domain-level screening forms that can be completed by parent and teacher. As discussed, there are major cautions about the use of the parent or caregiver screening questionnaires. It is recommended that these be administered in the clinic setting. The examiner must ensure that the parent or caregiver has the abilities to adequately comprehend the item content; unintentionally, there could be distortions including possible inadvertent exaggeration of the child's competencies or other emotionally driven responses. Therefore, it is necessary to review the parent or caregiver report with the respondent after it is completed.

7.3.2 Adaptive Behavior Assessment System: Third Edition (Harrison & Oakland, 2005)

The Adaptive Behavior Assessment System (ABAS; Harrison & Oakland, 2000, 2003, 2005), like the VABS, is designed to assess adaptive behavior and related skills in multiple areas in comparison to chronological age. These skill areas encompass the practical, everyday skills required to function and meet environmental demands, including those needed to effectively and independently care for oneself and to interact with others. Five distinct forms are designed for the purpose of gaining critical insight into adaptive functioning from parents, teachers, and adults alike. These include a preschool form (ages 0–5), school age form (ages 5–21), and adult rating form (ages 16–89). The ABAS-3 is utilized for evaluating levels of adaptive skills and specifying treatment goals for individuals with learning disabilities or other types of learning, behavioral, medical, or psychological problems. Specific behaviors and activities are rated based on how often the child/individual engages in the behavior or performs the activity without help.

The ABAS-3 measures behaviors grouped into three categories—conceptual, social, and practical—that each yields a domain standard score as well as a composite score. Standard scores in the three domains have a mean of 100 and a standard deviation of 15 points. Subtest scores are reported as T-scores with a mean of 10 and a standard deviation of 3. Qualitative levels are also reported. Each behavior is rated on a 4-point scale. A *0* score indicates that the individual is not able to perform the behavior. If the individual is able to perform the behavior, the respondent then rates how often he or she performs the behavior without reminders and without help: 1 = never (or almost never) when needed, 2 = sometimes when needed, and 3 = always (or almost always) when needed.

The conceptual domain encompasses three skill areas: *communication*, which assesses an individual's speech, vocabulary, listening, conversation, and nonverbal communication skills; *functional academics*, which assesses the ability to perform basic academic skills such as reading, writing, and mathematics, as well as functional skills such as measurement, telling time, and money skills (e.g., making change); and *self-direction*, which assesses the ability to make independent choices, exhibit self-control, and take responsibility when appropriate.

The social domain is made up of two subtests: *leisure* and *social skills*. The *leisure* subtest measures skills needed for engaging in and planning individual leisure and recreational activities. The *social* subtest measures skills needed to interact socially and to get along with others. Therefore, the social domain might inadvertently overestimate the social abilities of an individual with ASD because it includes a substantial number of questions about solitary activities in the *leisure* area.

The practical domain assesses skills in four areas: *community use*, *home/school living, health and safety,* and *self-care*. The area of *community use* measures the ability to function appropriately in the community. *Home living* assesses skills needed to function on a daily basis in the household, and *school living* assesses the child's ability to function appropriately in the school environment. The area of *health and safety* looks at the ability to protect one's own physical well-being, and *self-care* represents the ability of the individual to care for their own needs.

Harrison and Oakland (2005) address the difficulty of measuring adaptive behavior reliably since the behavior itself may not be consistent. They report adequate reliability across diagnostic categories for the ABAS-3 and adequate validity across all ABAS measures. They point out, however, that the use of any test is influenced by assessor's theory as well as the empirical data. Furthermore, professional users of tests have an ongoing responsibility to "acquire, share and examine evidence that informs the users as to ways in which the instrument can and should be used" (p. 113). A word of caution, the ABAS-3 is typically completed outside of a clinical setting and not by interviews. Therefore, results should be viewed in light of the previous discussion regarding use of checklists.

7.3.3 Scales of Independent Behavior-Revised (Bruininks, Woodcock, Weatherman & Hill, 1996)

The Scales of Independent Behavior-Revised (SIB-R, Bruininks et al., 1996) is an older measure that is not frequently utilized in clinical settings for diagnosis or program planning. The SIB-R provides a comprehensive norm-referenced assessment of 14 areas of adaptive behavior across four adaptive domains (i.e., motor skills, social interaction and communication, personal living, and community living) and eight areas of maladaptive behavior across three maladaptive domains (i.e., internalized, asocial, and externalized). The SIB-R is primarily designed to measure functional independence and adaptive functioning in home, school, employment, and community settings. SIB-R response forms include full-scale, short, and early development. Behavior is rated on a 4-point scale: 0 = never; 1 = does, but not well; 2 = does fairly well 75% of the time; and 3 = does very well or almost always. Maladaptive behavior is rated on a 6-point scale, from not serious (0) to extremely serious (5). Results are reported as standard and age-equivalent scores, percentile rank, broad independence score, relative mastery index, and a support score. The support score predicts the level of support the individual will require based on maladaptive behavior and functional limitations.

The SIB-R *can* be administered using a structured interview procedure or as a checklist. In spite of issues discussed above, the manual suggests the checklist administration procedure is often preferred when a face-to-face interview is not practical. According to the authors, these options give examiners maximum flexibility when using the SIB-R. The manual reports adequate reliability and validity. Unlike the VABS and ABAS, there is little data to support use of the SIB-R in evaluation of ASD.

7.3.4 Behavior Assessment System for Children, Third Edition (Reynolds & Kamphaus, 2015)

The Behavior Assessment System for Children (BASC-3; Reynolds & Kamphaus, 2015), currently in its third revision, is frequently used in educational settings. While not a comprehensive measure of adaptive behavior, it includes an adaptive subscale. The BASC-3 uses a multimethod, multidimensional approach to evaluating behavior and self-perception of children ages 2 years 6 months to 18 years. It was designed to facilitate differential diagnosis and educational classification of a variety of emotional and behavioral difficulties and aid in the design of treatment programs. The BASC-3 includes parent and teacher rating scales, a self-report of personality, a structured developmental history, and a student observation system. Items are rated on a 4-point scale (i.e., 0 = never, 1 = sometimes, 2 = often, and 3 = almost always). Raw scores are summed to yield T-scores. The adaptive skills composite consists of: adaptability, social skills, leadership, activities of daily living, and functional communication. The BASC-3 is reported to be a clinically sound approach to assessing multiple domains of personality (Swart, 2005). However, it does not provide a comprehensive measure of adaptive behavior and primarily relies on checklist ratings of behavior.

7.3.5 Adaptive Behavior and ASD

ASD represents a group of heterogeneous neurodevelopmental disorders resulting in social communication deficits and a restricted range of interests (American Psychiatric Association, 2013). There is a general consensus among clinicians and researchers alike that impairments in adaptive behavior particularly in the social area are the hallmark of ASD. Thus, measurement of adaptive behavior becomes an essential component of any evaluation. Focus has been on using adaptive behavior measures to define the discrepancy shown between cognitive skills and the ability to use skills in the natural environment. Klin, Jones, Schultz, and Volkmar (2005) have described this unique problem as one of the most intriguing puzzles in the field.

The first step in understanding this issue is to examine how data are generated. Cognitive test results are gathered in an artificial environment, and conditions are created to optimize performance (Sattler, 2008). Adaptive behavior measures are designed to reflect an individual's typical performance in the natural environment. In addition to defining the actual discrepancy between the two areas, research has also attempted to examine how adaptive behavior changes over time. While a number of studies have examined the role of adaptive behavior in ASD, many of the results are idiosyncratic to a particular study. Results are highly dependent on how ASD is defined, sample studied, and measures of adaptive functioning actually utilized.

7.3.5.1 Adaptive Behavior and Evaluation

As noted, assessment of adaptive behavior is a required component of a comprehensive developmental evaluation. There is a direct relationship between IQ and adaptive behavior in typical development and in intellectual disability (Lee &

Park, 2007; Liss et al., 2001). While individuals with ASD and individuals with ID are more likely to show delays on measures of adaptive functioning, individuals with ASD are more likely to show variability across subdomains. Generally, with ASD, the higher the cognitive functioning, the greater the difference between adaptive functioning and cognitive abilities. Individuals with ID usually present with a consistent scoring profile across areas, while individuals on the autism spectrum demonstrate an inconsistent scoring profile along with the variability within domain scores. Adaptive functioning in individuals with ASD is evident for progress in some areas and not others, and deficits are often more evident with age (Sweizy, Stuart, Korzekwa, & Pozdol, 2008). Specifically, the gap between standard scores or age equivalencies and cognitive/intellectual abilities increases as individuals age. There is also some evidence that individuals with ASD may acquire adaptive skills at a slower rate than cognitive skills.

There have been a number of studies that have attempted to understand the role of adaptive behavior in both diagnosis and long-term outcome in ASD. In an early study, Dominick, Davis, Lainhart, Tager-Flusberg, and Folstein (2007) reported that use of a measure of adaptive behavior as part of a comprehensive diagnostic evaluation for autism, specifically the use of the Autism Diagnostic Interview-Revised (ADI-R; Rutter, LeCouter, & Lord, 1994) and the Autism Diagnostic Observation Schedule (ADOS; Lord, Rutter, DiLavore, & Risi, 2003), was improved with the use of a measure of adaptive functioning. As would be expected, individuals with ASD exhibited their greatest deficits in terms of social skills including intrinsic motivation that is the underlying core drive to initiate and pursue the ability to independently function and assimilate in one's culture (Bolte & Poustka, 2002; Kenworthy, Case, Harms, Martin, & Wallace, 2010; Liss et al., 2001). Understanding these profiles is essential in developing treatment programs and outcome measures.

The following is a review of studies to date. An attempt was made to group studies by factors measured to examine their relationship to each other. However, this was not always possible as most studies examined multiple aspects of the role of adaptive behavior in ASD.

7.3.5.2 Adaptive Functioning in Early Childhood

There have been a number of studies examining adaptive behavior and how it develops in very young children. Perry, Flanagan, Dunn Geier, and Freeman (2009) identified an *autism profile* with 290 young children diagnosed with autism. With higher functioning children, IQ was higher than adaptive functioning measured by the VABS-II, while the opposite profile occurred with the lower functioning children. Significant differences were found between age equivalents but not standard scores, with the autism group showing lower scores in the areas of socialization and communication. Correlational analyses between age, cognitive level, and adaptive levels were also reported and indicated severity of autism accounted for only a modest amount of the variance in socialization and daily living skills.

Ray-Subramanian, Huai, and Weismer (2011) reported that these profiles were evident by age two. They compared cognitive functioning as measured on the Bayley-II to adaptive functioning as measured on the VABS-II, and social communication disability as measured by the ADOS, a semistructured measure of social communication. Social communication scores were predicted by age and Bayley-II scores, while overall ADOS scores were not. Daily living skills were significantly correlated with nonverbal ability and overall ADOS algorithms. Only VABS-II receptive language correlated with ADOS scores. Again, as in Perry et al., severity of autism on the ADOS did not predict social communication on the VABS-II. However, in this sample, daily living skills were correlated with severity.

Using the ABAS-II, Milne, McDonald, and Comino (2013) examined the relationship between adaptive behavior and developmental ability in 152 preschoolers with and without autism, and with and without developmental delay. They found that overall adaptive function was closely correlated with developmental ability. The authors reported that the autism group without developmental delay had lower adaptive skills than predicted from developmental level. The practical and social domains discriminated the children with autism, with this group scoring lower in both domains. In a similar study, Paul, Loomis, and Chaworska (2014) examined adaptive behavior in children younger than 2 years with ASD. Their results confirmed those of Ray-Subramanian et al., (2011) who had reported that VABS daily living skills were significantly correlated with nonverbal ability and overall ADOS algorithms, while VABS receptive language correlated only with the ADOS.

Malhi and Singh (2015) also examined the relationship among intellectual functioning, symptom severity, and adaptive behavior in children (mean age = 4.79 years) referred to a pediatric tracking hospital in India utilizing the Indian version of the Vineland Social Maturity Scale and Children's Autism Rating Scale (CARS). Even using outdated measures, results were consistent with other studies showing adaptive behavior scores in the lower functioning children with ASD were significantly higher than their IQ scores, while the opposite was true in higher functioning children.

Flanagan et al. (2015) also examined the stability of cognitive and adaptive function in preschoolers between initial diagnosis and school entry at 6 years of age. IQ increased 18 points in 2-year-olds, 12 points in 3-year-olds, and 9 points in 4-year-olds. Adaptive behavior scores increased only 4 points across age groups. At school entry, 24% of children met criteria for intellectual disability (cognitive and adaptive behavior scores less than 70). No children with both scores greater than or equal to 70 at diagnosis later met criteria for intellectual disability. Outcomes were more variable for children with initial delays in both areas (i.e., in 57%, both scores remained less than 70). Thus, change in IQ was directly related to age at diagnosis, while changes in adaptive behavior were not. Findings are particularly relevant to clinicians who may inaccurately diagnose young children with ASD as also ID. In addition, it appears that IQ alone could not account for adaptive behavior deficits. While IQ showed a consistent increase, changes in adaptive behavior scores were minimal. These results once again point to the importance of focusing on adaptive skills in treatment programs.

Yang, Paynter, and Gilmore (2016) examined the adaptive functioning profiles of 77 young children with ASD using the VABS-II. They analyzed factors associated with adaptive function. Consistent with previous *research* and with the original VABS, a VABS profile for children with ASD was identified—highest scores were in motor skills, and lowest scores were in socialization. These scores were correlated with age and nonverbal ability, but not ADOS scores, further supporting that each of these measures is intended to evaluate different aspects of an individual.

Balboni, Tasso, Muratori, and Cubelli (2016) utilized item content analysis on the VABS-II to further examine the autism profile in preschool children with autism. They noted that frequently reported socialization delays in ASD were primarily the result of playing and imitating skills, not in other social skills. They suggest that item content categories on theVABS-II may yield a better clinical description than overall scores and may better identify behaviors that should be the focus of treatment.

Green and Carter (2014) examined the course of daily living skills (DLS) development in toddlers with ASD. Using the VABS -II, they assessed 162 children at three annual time points. Hierarchical linear models showed that age, development quotient (DQ), and autism symptom severity predicted the initial DLS and DLS growth. They found that improvement in DLS greatly reduced parenting stress and is important to focus on during treatment. Thus, it seems that while severity of autism does not predict social skills on the VABS in toddlers, it does predict daily living skills, which has a direct impact on family function.

7.3.5.3 Adaptive Behavior and Stress

Hall and Graff (2011) further examined the relationship between adaptive behavior and family stress. They conducted a descriptive study with 75 parents or primary caregivers of children with

ASD. Adaptive behaviors of children with ASD, family support networks, parenting stress, and parent coping were measured. Confirming the results reported in Toddlers, an association between low adaptive functioning in children with autism and increased parenting stress creates a need for additional family support. The authors point out that professionals should have up-to-date knowledge of the supports available to families and refer families to appropriate resources to avoid overwhelming them with unnecessary and inappropriate referrals.

7.3.5.4 Adaptive Behavior and Development

Mazefsky, Williams, and Minshew (2008) examined the role of family history and variability in adaptive functioning in 77 autistic individuals (mean age = 18 years) with average intellectual development. Adaptive behavior was measured with the VABS-II. Family history of depression and shyness accounted for the most variance in VABS scores, particularly in the social domain. The authors conclude that family history variables may affect prognosis and are important to consider in both diagnosis and treatment.

Kenworthy et al. (2010) utilized caregiver reports on the ABAS-II to compare the profiles of 40 high-functioning individuals (12–21 years of age) with ASD and 30 typically developing individuals matched on age, IQ, and sex. Similar to previous studies utilizing the VABS in younger children, the ASD group showed particular deficits on the Social scale. Within the ASD group, adaptive communication skills were positively related with IQ. Autistic behavior ratings correlated negatively to ABAS scores in the typically developing but not the ASD group. Thus, results were consistent with the previous studies that found IQ is related to communication scores but not severity of ASD on adaptive behavior measures. This study provides additional support for the idea that adaptive behavior is an independent construct of IQ and must be examined separately.

Baghdadli et al. (2012) examined change in trajectories of adaptive behavior from early childhood to adolescence. Utilizing the VABS–II, this study examined changes in scores in 152 children over an almost 10-year period [Time 1: 4.9(±1.3) years; Time 2: 8.1(±1.3) years; Time 3: 15(±1.6) years]. Important deficits remained at adolescence in the adaptive abilities of children with ASD, but changes in adaptive skills showed two distinct growth rates. Analyses revealed that low growth trajectories for both social and communication outcomes were associated with the following characteristics at 5 years of age: low cognitive and language skills, presence of epilepsy, and severity of autism. Thus, risk factors at this age were low language and severity of autism for both social and communication outcomes 10 years later. They also reported that hours of early intervention were a protective factor for communication. Thus, it appears that while severity of autism is not predictive in very young children, it becomes increasingly important to consider as children with ASD age and more importantly is sensitive to intervention.

7.3.5.5 Adaptive Functioning and Daily Living Skills

Daily living skills have become an important predictor of independence and quality of life. Smith, Greenberg, and Mailick (2012) indicated that as individuals with ASD continued into adulthood in their late twenties, there was a plateau in daily living skills in the ASD group. Other studies have noted that higher cognitive functioning is predictive of better daily living skills in adulthood. Living in an advantaged area was also positively correlated with DLS. However, living with a single parent was associated with lower levels of daily living skills (Smith et al., 2012) and increased family stress. Gray et al. (2014) reported that community skills rather than self-help skills predicted independent living; thus, it is clear that independence in the community should play a significant role in treatment programs.

Matthews et al. (2015) examined adaptive functioning during the transition to adulthood in individuals diagnosed with ASD. Profiles on the VABS-II were examined by age and intellectual ability for 75 participants with ASD (ages 16–58 years). Results confirmed the gap between cognitive and adaptive functioning in an older group of individuals. DLS were a relative strength compared to communication and socialization in adults, but not adolescents. In general, highest subdomain scores were observed for writing skills and lowest scores were observed in interpersonal skills. Regardless of cognitive ability, all standard scores were well below average, indicating there may be a need for lifelong intervention that targets adaptive functioning independent of cognitive functioning.

Hus Bal, Kim, Cheong, and Lord (2015) in a longitudinal study examined individuals with ASD from ages 2 to 21 years. They report that early childhood nonverbal mental age was shown to be the strongest predictor of DLS attainment for both diagnostic groups, one with individuals on the autism spectrum and the other a sample of nonspectrum individuals. Specifically, the predictive variables were nonverbal mental age, receptive language, and social communication impairment at 2 years old, and these delineated high versus low daily living skills. Further, 20 hours a week of intervention before the age of 3 years was also associated with a positive daily living skills trajectory. For those who were in the group identified as highest daily living skills, they still were approximately 7 years below age level at 21 years of age, and the low daily living skills group had an even greater deficit of approximately 16 years. While the sample size was small, there was a slight decline from 18 to 21 years of age in daily living skills that has also been evident in prior research. It was notable that individuals on the autism spectrum show slower development of daily living skills, even though daily living skills were positively correlated with cognitive skills and early language abilities. Thus, intervention for individuals with ASD of all ages must include an emphasis on daily living skills.

Duncan and Bishop (2013) examined the gap between cognitive abilities and daily living skills in adolescents with ASD and average intelligence. DLS standard scores on the VABS-II were examined with 417 adolescents. All participants had at least average intelligence and a diagnosis of ASD. Descriptive statistics and regression analysis were used to examine the prevalence and predictors of a DLS deficit, defined as below average DLS in the context of average intelligence quotient. Approximately half of the adolescents were identified as having a DLS deficit. Autism symptomatology, intelligence quotient, maternal education, age, and sex accounted for only 10% of the variance in predicting a DLS deficit. Identifying factors associated with better or worse DLS may help shed light on the variability in adult outcome in individuals with ASD with average intelligence. This study also is consistent with earlier studies showing the importance of remediation in DLS from an early age.

7.3.5.6 Adaptive Functioning, IQ, and Severity of ASD

While studies reviewed to date have provided some information of the role of IQ and/or developmental level in adaptive behavior, several other studies have examined this relationship directly. Black, Wallace, and Kenworthy (2009) investigated the relationship of discrepancies between verbal IQ (VIQ) and nonverbal IQ (NVIQ), known as an IQ split, and autism symptoms and adaptive behavior in a sample of high-functioning (mean full scale [FSIQ] = 98.5) school-age children with ASD divided into three groups: high VIQ (n = 18); high NVIQ (n = 24); and equivalent VIQ and NVIQ (n = 36). Discrepancy between high VIQ and NVIQ was associated with autism social symptoms, but not communication symptoms or repetitive behaviors. On the other hand, high VIQ and NVIQ scores alone were associated with better adaptive communication, but not socialization or daily living skills. Thus, IQ discrepancy may result in a better description than IQ alone. Better verbal abilities have typically been associated with better functional outcomes in autism. However, discrepantly high VIQs in high-functioning children may also be associated with more social difficulties. Thus, as previously reported, the relationship between IQ and adaptive behavior is extremely complex and varies with age.

Kanne et al. (2011) examined the relationship between VABS subscales and IQ. The VABS composite was negatively correlated with age.

Negligible associations were found between autism symptomatology and adaptive behavior. Results indicated that the gap between IQ and adaptive impairments decreases in lower functioning individuals with ASD, while higher functioning and older individuals have a greater gap between IQ and adaptive skills. These results are consistent with other studies that examined how the gap between cognitive and adaptive behavior changes with development.

Oliveras-Rentas, Kenworthy, Roberson, Martin, and Wallace (2012) examined changes in Wechsler Intelligence Scales for Children (WISC-IV) profiles and its relation to symptomatology and adaptive functioning. This study reported WISC-IV profiles on 56 high-functioning (IQ > 70) children with ASD and correlated the profiles with ASD, ADHD symptomatology, and adaptive functioning. The ASD WISC-IV profile included strengths in matrix reasoning and similarities, weaknesses on comprehension, and the subtests comprising the processing speed index (i.e., coding, symbol search). The comprehension subtest correlated negatively with social symptoms. Processing speed task performance correlated negatively with communication symptoms and positively with communication abilities, indicating its importance to functional outcomes in ASD. These results confirm those of Black et al. (2009) and are consistent with profile analyses in toddlers. This study also points out the differences between communication ability and performance.

Chang, Lung, Yen, and Yang (2013) investigated the relationship among cognitive level, autistic severity, and adaptive functioning in 94 high-functioning children with ASD. Parents and teachers both completed the ABAS-II and the Social Responsiveness Scale (SRS; Constantino & Gruber, 2005, 2012). Results revealed that average general adaptive composites scores (home: 74.0; school: 74.6) were below average FSIQ (84.8). Profile analysis revealed that social domain was the weakest among the adaptive abilities assessed both at school and home. Cognitive abilities had a positive relationship with adaptive function, while autistic severity had a weak negative relationship with adaptive function. Also, the younger the age the child was diagnosed, the less severe the current symptoms of autism. This study confirms earlier studies that emphasize early intervention and that autism severity shows a weak relationship to adaptive behavior and further confirms importance of treatment.

Utilizing the ABAS-II, Hill, Gray, Kamps, and Varela (2015) examined the moderating effects of intellectual functioning and ASD symptom severity on the relation between age and adaptive functioning for 220 youth with ASD. Results indicate that there was a three-way interaction among age (4–16 years), intellectual functioning (NVIQ), and autism severity (ADOS score). The association between ASD symptom severity and adaptive functioning was weak for younger children with higher intellectual functioning and older children with lower intellectual functioning, again confirming the complex and dynamic interaction of cognitive abilities, age, and adaptive functioning.

7.3.5.7 Adaptive Behavior in ASD on the BASC-2

The VABS-3 and ABAS-3 are the most commonly utilized measures in both clinical and research settings. However, in educational settings, the BASC-2 is frequently administered. It is important to note that the BASC-2 is a checklist and has a subscale entitled adaptive behavior. Unlike the VABS-3 and ABAS-3, it is not a comprehensive measure of adaptive functioning.

Volker et al. (2010) compared the BASC-2 Parent Rating Scale (PRS) profiles of 62 children with high-functioning autism spectrum disorder (HFASD) with those of 62 typically developing children matched by age, gender, and ethnicity. Results indicated that except for the somatization, conduct problems, and aggression scales, significant differences were found between the HFASD and typically developing groups on all PRS scores. Mean HFASD scores were in the clinically significant range on the behavioral symptoms index, atypicality, withdrawal, and developmental social disorders scales. At-risk range HFASD means were obtained on the adaptive skills composite, all adaptive scales, remaining content scales (except bullying), and hyperactivity, attention problems, and depression clinical scales. Screening indices suggested that the developmental social disorders scale was highly effective in differentiating between the two groups. While providing a profile of how HFASD children function on the BASC-2, differentiating them from typical development does not yield the information needed to adequately measure adaptive behavior and design appropriate treatment programs.

Lopata et al. (2013) examined the relationship among three measures of adaptive behavior to (a) document the parent-rated VABS-II, BASC-2, and ABAS-II adaptive behavior profiles of 6- to 11-year-olds with HFASD (including relative strengths and weaknesses); (b) examine the extent to which these measures yielded similar scores on comparable scales; and (c) assess potential discrepancies between cognitive ability and adaptive behavior across the measures. All three adaptive measures revealed significant deficits overall for the sample, with the VABS-II and ABAS-II indicating relative weaknesses in social skills and strengths in academic-related skills. Cross-measure comparisons indicated significant differences in the absolute magnitude of scores. In general, the VABS-II yielded significantly higher scores than the BASC-2 and ABAS-II. However, the VABS-II and ABAS-II yielded scores that did not significantly differ for adaptive social skills, which are a critical area to assess for children with HFASD. Results also indicated significant discrepancies between the children's average IQ scores and their scores on the adaptive domains and composites of the three adaptive measures. This study confirms previous results regarding the gap between cognitive and adaptive behavior.

Doobay, Foley-Nicpon, Ali, and Assouline (2014) also examined cognitive, adaptive, and psychosocial differences in high-functioning individuals with ASD using both the BASC and the VABS. The purpose of the study was to provide an empirical account of the intellectual, adaptive, and psychosocial functioning of individuals with superior scores on IQ tests and with ASD. Forty youth with high cognitive ability and ASD and a control group of 41 youth with high cognitive ability without ASD were compared. In comparison to the control group, the ASD group showed poorer functioning on measures of processing speed on cognitive tests. In addition, individuals in the ASD group, while scoring in the average ranges overall, showed a 28-point discrepancy between their Full Scale IQ and Processing Speed IQ on the WISC-IV. Within the area of adaptive functioning, there was a highly significant group difference in all three domains on the VABS. The greatest difference between groups was, as would be expected, in the social domain. Furthermore, the social domain in the ASD group was the only score below average. However, while the scores on DLS were adequate, they were one standard deviation below mean adaptive behavior composite scores. Psychosocial functioning was measured on the BASC-2, and a number of subscales were elevated to the at-risk or clinically significant range for the ASD group. These results must be interpreted with caution because individual items will be scored on multiple scales. For example, an item might ask about repetitive speech or conversation difficulties and might be scored on each of the scales for social skills, anxiety, atypical behavior, and adaptive functioning. On the parent forms, 75% reported concerns on the atypical behavior, social withdrawal, and adaptability subscales. Teachers reported concerns in only 50% of the ASD group. On the self-report measure, no differences were reported between groups. These results have significant implications for diagnosis and intervention for high ability individuals with ASD.

Lopata et al. (2016) compared teacher and parent ratings of ASD-related symptoms in 120 high-functioning 6- to 12-year-old children with ASD on the Developmental Social Disorder (DSD) scale of the BASC-2. Both parent and teacher ratings were higher than reported in the normative estimates. In addition, there was a significant difference in parent and teacher ratings with parents reporting more symptoms in the at-risk range. This study is consistent with Doobay et al. (2014) and is clinically very important as it confirms the often observed discrepancy between parent and teacher reports. The BASC-2 may be useful in identifying comorbid conditions in ASD and their relationship to adaptive functioning, but has limited value in describing adaptive behavior overall.

7.3.5.8 Adaptive Behavior: Executive Functioning and Other Comorbidities

As our understanding has increased of the importance of the role adaptive behavior has in prognosis in ASD, so has interest in how other variables such as executive functioning may relate to it. Williams, Mazofsky, Walker, Minshew, and Goldstein (2014) examined abstract reasoning and problem solving abilities in relation to adaptive functioning. Measures of conceptual reasoning, a laboratory measure of problem-solving, and a measure of adaptive functioning in the natural environment were administered to children and adults with and without autism. The individuals with autism had weaker conceptual reasoning ability than individuals with typical development of similar age and cognitive ability. For the autism group, their flexible thinking scores were significantly correlated with laboratory measures of strategy formation and rule shifting and with reported overall adaptive behavior but not socialization scores. Therefore, in autism, flexibility of thought is potentially more important for adaptive functioning in the natural environment than conceptual reasoning or problem-solving. This study clearly points out one of the major problems in ASD, that is, the inability of cognitive tasks to predict behavior in the natural environment.

Pugliese et al. (2016) examined longitudinal change in adaptive behavior in 64 children and adolescents with ASD without ID. These individuals were evaluated on multiple occasions, and the effect of prior estimates of executive function problems on future adaptive behavior scores was examined. Compared to standardized estimates for their developmental stage, adaptive behavior in most participants was impaired and did not improve over time. Prior executive function predicted later adaptive behavior in daily living skills and socialization domains after controlling for age and IQ. Self-monitoring behaviors robustly predicted later adaptive behavior in all domains. Results support targeting treatment of adaptive skills in ASD, as well as the importance of assessing for executive function problems that may contribute to adaptive behavior difficulties.

Wallace et al. (2016) further examined real-world executive function and adaptive behavior profiles, using the ABAS, in individuals with ASD with comorbid anxiety and depression. Little is known about real-world measures of executive function among adults with ASD. This study examined parent-reported real-world executive function problems among 35 adults with ASD without ID and their correlations with adaptive functioning and comorbid anxiety and depression symptomatology. A variable executive function profile was found with prominent deficits occurring in flexibility and metacognition. Flexibility problems were associated with anxiety-related symptoms, while metacognition difficulties were associated with depression symptoms and impaired adaptive functioning (metacognition-adaptive functioning relationship was moderated by ADHD symptoms). These persistent executive function problems are predictors of broader functioning and therefore remain an important treatment target among adults with ASD.

7.3.5.9 Adaptive Behavior Measure Comparison

In addition to the study comparing BASC-2 to VABS (i.e., Doobay et al., 2014), Wells, Condillac, Perry, and Factor (2011) examined the utility and construct validity of three widely used measures of adaptive behavior, as rated by staff: the Vineland Adaptive Behavior Scales-Classroom Edition (VABS-Classroom; Sparrow et al., 1985), the Scales of Independent Behavior-Revised (SIB-R; Bruininks et al., 1996), and the Adaptive Behavior Scale-School, Second Edition (ABS-S: 2; Nihira, Leland, & Lambert, 1993). The authors found a strong positive relationship between mental age and adaptive skills on all three measures. Thus, as mental age increased so did overall adaptive skills. There were only moderate negative correlation between severity of autism and adaptive behavior among the measures. Results do not suggest any one measure is superior to another. Rather, selecting a measure of adaptive behavior depends on several factors such as age, purpose of assessment, and time required to complete the measure.

7.3.6 Conclusion and Future Directions

Adaptive behavior is vital to the understanding of individuals with developmental disabilities, especially those with ASD. Knowledge regarding the relationship of ASD and adaptive behavior is critical to research, treatment, and defining quality of life. While a review of current research has yielded some conflicting results at times, several general statements can be made. First, individuals with ASD even with normal intelligence show significant deficits in adaptive behavior, particularly in the area of socialization. However, cognitive skills alone cannot predict adaptive functioning. There is generally a gap between cognitive skills and performance—the intriguing puzzle described by Klin et al. (2005). This gap appears to be differentially affected by cognitive skills and age. In lower functioning individuals (those with both ASD and ID), adaptive skills may become higher than cognitive skills as they transition into adolescence and adulthood. On the other hand, the gap increases in higher functioning individuals.

In addition, severity of autism does not predict adaptive behavior generally but is correlated with daily living skills and increased stress in families. Thus, measurement of adaptive behavior is very complex. Research indicates that age, cognitive skills, and severity of autism all interact in affecting adaptive behavior particularly daily living skills. Other variables such as family stress, comorbid psychiatric conditions, and level of executive functioning also affect adaptive skills in the natural environment. It is important for the clinician to be aware of all of these variables as well as the strengths and weaknesses of measures used prior to undertaking an evaluation.

Measures selected should be a function of the purpose of the evaluation and becomes one of the most important decisions a clinician has to make. There is no one measure that has been found to be superior and that captures all aspects of adaptive functioning. Measures available yield some important information, but alone cannot provide a complete picture of how an individual functions across environments. Thus, in addition to a structured interview using current available standardized measures, an ongoing behavioral assessment is necessary to develop an appropriate treatment program.

Much more research is needed to inform how adaptive behavior is related to outcome and quality of life in ASD. In addition, how to identify strengths not just weaknesses should be a focus so that individuals with ASD can learn to function independently in the natural environment. This should become a priority for research and all clinicians.

References

American Association on Intellectual and Developmental Disabilities (AAIDD). (2010). *Intellectual disability: Definition, classification, and systems of supports* (11th ed.). Washington, DC: Author.

American Psychiatric Association. (2013). *Diagnostic and statistical manual of mental disorders* (5th ed.). Arlington, VA: American Psychiatric Publishing.

Baghdadli, A., Assouline, B., Sonie, S., Pernon, E., Darrou, C., Michelon, C., & Pry, R. (2012). Developmental trajectories of adaptive behaviors from early childhood to adolescence in a cohort of 152 children with autism spectrum disorders. *Journal of Autism and Developmental Disorders, 42*(7), 1314–1325.

Balboni, G., Tasso, A., Muratori, F., & Cubelli, R. (2016). The Vineland-II in preschool children with autism spectrum disorders: An item content category analysis. *Journal of Autism and Developmental Disorders, 46*(1), 42–52.

Black, D. O., Wallace, G. L., Sokoloff, J. L., & Kenworthy, L. (2009). Brief report: IQ split predicts social symptoms and communication abilities in high-functioning children with autism spectrum disorders. *Journal of Autism and Developmental Disorders, 39*(11), 1613–1619.

Bolte, S., & Poustka, F. (2002). The relation between general cognitive level andadaptive behaviordomains in individuals with autism with and without co-morbid mental retardation. *Child Psychiatry & Human Development, 33*(2), 165–172.

Brockley, J. A. (1999). History of mental retardation: An essay review. *History of Psychology*, *2*(1), 25–36.

Bruininks, R. H., Woodcock, R. W., Weatherman, R. F., & Hill, B. K. (1996). *Scales of Independent Behavior – Revised (SIB-R)*. Itasca, IL: Riverside Publishing Company.

Chang, C. L., Lung, F. W., Yen, C. F., & Yang, P. (2013). Adaptive behaviors in high-functioning Taiwanese children with autism spectrum disorders: An investigation of the mediating roles of symptom severity and cognitive ability. *Journal of Autism and Developmental Disorders*, *43*(6), 1347–1355.

Constantino, J. N., & Gruber, C. P. (2005). *Social responsiveness scale*. Los Angeles, CA: Western Psychological Services.

Constantino, J. N., & Gruber, C. P. (2012). *Social responsiveness scale* (2nd ed.). Los Angeles, CA: Western Psychological Services.

Doll, E. A. (1935). A genetic scale of social maturity. *The Journal of Orthopsychiatry*, *5*(2), 180–188.

Doll, E. A. (1936). *The vineland social maturity scale, Publication of the Training School at Vineland. Departmental Research Series* (vol. 3). New Jersey/ Circle Pines, MI: American Guidance Service.

Doll, E. A. (1965). *The vineland social maturity scale*. Circle Pines, MI: American Guidance Service,Inc..

Dominick, K. C., Davis, N. O., Lainhart, J., Tager-Flusberg, H., & Folstein, S. (2007). Atypical behaviors in children with autism and children with a history of language impairment. *Research in Developmental Disabilities: A Multidisciplinary Journal*, *28*(2), 145–162.

Doobay, A. F., Foley-Nicpon, M., Ali, S. R., et al. (2014). Cognitive, adaptive and psychosocial differences between high ability youth with and without autism spectrum disorder. *Journal of Autism and Developmental Disorders*, *44*(8), 2026–2040.

Duncan, A. W., & Bishop, S. L. (2013). Understanding the gap between cognitive abilities and daily living skills in adolescents with autism spectrum disorders with average intelligence. *Autism*, *19*(1), 64–72.

Edgerton, R. B. (1993). *The cloak of competence*. Berkeley/Los Angeles, CA: University of California Press.

Flanagan, H. E., Smith, I. M., Vaillancourt, T., Duku, E., Szatmari, P., Bryson, S., … Georgiades, S. (2015). Stability and change in the cognitive and adaptive behaviour scores of preschoolers with autism spectrum disorder. *Journal of Autism and Developmental Disorders*, *45*(9), 2691–2703.

Gray, K. M., Keating, C. M., Taffe, J. R., Brereton, A. V., Einfeld, S. L., Reardon, T. C., & Tonge, B. J. (2014). Adult outcomes in autism: Community inclusion and living skills. *Journal of Autism and Developmental Disorders*, *44*(12), 3006–3015.

Green, S. A., & Carter, A. S. (2014). Predictors and course of daily living skills development in toddlers with autism spectrum disorders. *Journal of Autism and Developmental Disorders*, *44*(2), 256–263.

Greenspan, S. (2008). *Annals of gullibility: Why we get duped and how to avoid it*. Westport, CT: Praeger Publishers.

Hall, H. R., & Graff, J. C. (2011). The relationships among adaptive behaviors of children with autism, family support, parenting stress and coping. *Issues in Comprehensive Pediatric Nursing*, *34*(1), 4–25.

Harrison, P. L., & Oakland, T. (2000). *Adaptive behavior assessment system*. San Antonio, TX: The Psychological Corporation.

Harrison, P. L., & Oakland, T. (2003). *Adaptive behavior assessment system* (2nd ed.). San Antonio, TX: The Psychological Corporation.

Harrison, P. L., & Oakland, T. (2005). *Adaptive behavior assessment system* (3rd ed.). Torrance, CA: WPS Publishing.

Hill, T. L., Gray, S. A. O., Kamps, J. L., & Varela, E. R. (2015). Age and adaptive functioning in children and adolescents with ASD: The effects of intellectual functioning and ASD symptom severity. *Journal of Autism and Developmental Disorders*, *45*(12), 4074–4083.

Hus Bal, V., Kim, S.-H., Cheong, D., & Lord, C. (2015). Daily living skills in individuals with autism spectrum disorder from 2 to 21 years of age. *Autism*, *19*(7), 774–784.

Individuals with Disabilities Education Act, 20 U.S.C. § 1400 (2004).

Kanne, S. M., Gerber, A. J., Quirmbach, L. M., Sparrow, S. S., Cicchetti, D. V., & Saulnier, C. A. (2011). The role of adaptive behavior in autism spectrum disorders: Implications for functional outcome. *Journal of Autism and Developmental Disorders*, *41*(8), 1007–1018.

Kenworthy, L., Case, L., Harms, M. B., Martin, A., & Wallace, G. L. (2010). Adaptive behavior ratings correlate with symptomatology and IQ among individuals with high-functioning autism spectrum disorders. *Journal of Autism and Developmental Disorders*, *40*(4), 416–423.

Klin, A., Jones, W., Schultz, R. T., & Volkmar, F. R. (2005). The enactive mind, or from actions to cognition: Lessons from autism. In F. R. Volkmar, R. Paul, A. Klin, & D. Cohen (Eds.), *Handbook of autism and pervasive developmental disabilities* (pp. 682–703). New York: Wiley.

Lee, H. J., & Park, H. R. (2007). An integrated literature review on the adaptive behavior of individuals with Asperger syndrome. *Remedial and Special Education*, *28*(3), 132–139.

Liss, M., Harel, B., Fein, D., Allen, D., Dunn, M., Feinstein, C., & Rapin, I. (2001). Predictors and correlates of adaptive functioning in children with developmental disorders. *Journal of Autism and Developmental Disorders*, *31*(2), 219–230.

Lopata, C., Donnelly, J. P., Jordan, A. K., Thomeer, M. L., McDonald, C. A., & Rodgers, J. D. (2016). Brief report: Parent-teacher discrepancies on the developmental social disorders scale (BASC-2) in the assessment of high-functioning children with ASD. *Journal of Autism and Developmental Disorders*, *46*(9), 3183–3189.

Lopata, C., Smith, R. A., Volker, M. A., Thomeer, M. L., Lee, G. K., & McDonald, C. A. (2013). Comparison of adaptive behavior measures for children with HFASDs. *Autism Research and Treatment, 2013*, 1–10. doi:10.1155/2013/415989

Lord, C., Rutter, M., DiLavore, P., & Risi, S. (2003). *Autism diagnostic observation schedule*. Los Angeles, CA: Western Psychological Services.

Malhi, P., & Singh, P. (2015). Adaptive behavior functioning in children with autism. *Indian Journal of Pediatrics, 82*(8), 677–681.

Matthews, N. L., Smith, C. J., Pollard, E., Ober-Reynolds, S., Kirwan, J., & Malligo, A. (2015). Adaptive functioning in autism spectrum disorder during the transition to adulthood. *Journal of Autism and Developmental Disorders, 45*(8), 2349–2360.

Mazefsky, C. A., Williams, D. L., & Minshew, N. J. (2008). Variability in adaptive behavior in autism: Evidence for the importance of family history. *Journal of Abnormal Child Psychology, 36*(4), 591–599.

Milne, S. L., McDonald, J. L., & Comino, E. J. (2013). Adaptive function in preschoolers in relation to developmental delay and diagnosis of autism spectrum disorders: Insights from a clinical sample. *Autism, 17*(6), 743–753.

Nihira, K., Leland, H., & Lambert, N. (1993). *Adaptive behavior scale – Residential and community: Examiner's manual* (2nd ed.). Austin, TX: Pro-Ed.

Oliveras-Rentas, R. E., Kenworthy, L., Roberson, R. B., Martin, R., & Wallace, G. L. (2012). WISC-IV profile in high-functioning autism spectrum disorders: Impaired processing speed is associated with increased autism communication symptoms and decreased adaptive communication abilities. *Journal of Autism and Developmental Disorders, 42*(5), 655–664.

Paul, R., Loomis, R., & Chaworska, K. (2014). Adaptive behavior in toddlers under two with autism spectrum disorders. *Journal of Autism and Developmental Disorders, 44*(2), 264–270.

Perry, A., Flanagan, H. E., Dunn Geier, J., & Freeman, N. L. (2009). Brief report: The vineland adaptive behavior scales in young children with autism spectrum disorders at different cognitive levels. *Journal of Autism and Developmental Disorders, 39*(7), 1066–1078.

Pugliese, C. E., Anthony, L., Strang, J. F., Dudley, K., Wallace, G. L., Naiman, D. Q., & Kenworthy, L. (2016). Longitudinal examination of adaptive behavior in autism spectrum disorders: Influence of executive function. *Journal of Autism and Developmental Disorders, 46*(2), 467–477.

Ray-Subramanian, C. E., Huai, N., & Weismer, S. (2011). Brief report: Adaptive behavior and cognitive skills for toddlers on the autism spectrum. *Journal of Autism and Developmental Disorders, 41*(5), 679–684.

Reschly, D. J. (2002). Minority overrepresentation: The silent contributor to LD prevalence and diagnostic confusion. In R. Bradley, L. Danielson, & D. P. Hallahan (Eds.), *Identification of learning disabilities: Research to practice* (pp. 361–368). Mahwah, NJ: Lawrence Erlbaum.

Reynolds, C. R., & Kamphaus, R. W. (2015). *Behavior assessment system for children* (3rd ed.). San Antonio, TX: The Psychological Corporation.

Rutter, M., LeCouteur, A., & Lord, C. (1994). *Autism diagnostic interview – Revised*. Los Angeles, CA: Western Psychological Services.

Sattler, J. M. (2008). *Assessment of children: Cognitive foundations* (5th ed.). San Diego, CA: Author.

Scheerenberger, R. C. (1983). *A history of mental retardation*. Baltimore: P.H. Brookes.

Smith, L. E., Greenberg, J. S., & Mailick, M. R. (2012). Adults with autism: Outcomes, family effects, and the multi-family group psychoeducation model. *Current Psychiatry Reports, 14*(6), 732–738.

Sparrow, S. S., Balla, D. A., & Cicchetti, D. V. (1984). *Vineland adaptive behavior scales*. Circle Pines, MN: American Guidance Service.

Sparrow, S. S., Balla, D. A., & Cicchetti, D. V. (1985). *Vineland adaptive behavior scales: Classroom edition*. Circle Pines, MN: American Guidance Service.

Sparrow, S. S., Cicchetti, D. V., & Balla, A. D. (2005). *Vineland adaptive behavior scales* (2nd ed.). Circle Pines, MN: American Guidance Service.

Sparrow, S. S., Cicchetti, D. V., & Saulnier, C. A. (2016). *Vineland adaptive behavior scales* (3rd ed.). Bloomington, MN: NCS Pearson, Inc..

Swart, G. T. (2005). The clinician's guide to the Behavior Assessment System for Children (BASC). *The Canadian Child and Adolescent Psychiatry Review, 14*(3), 90.

Sweizy, N. B., Stuart, M., Korzekwa, P., & Pozdol, S. (2008). Assessment of independent living/adaptive skills. In J. L. Matson (Ed.), *Clinical assessment and intervention for autism spectrum disorders* (pp. 193–219). Amsterdam: Elsevier.

Volker, M. A., Lopata, C., Smerneck, A. M., Knoll, V. A., Thomeer, M. L., Toomey, J. A., & Rodgers, J. D. (2010). BASC-2 PRS profiles for students with high-functioning autism spectrum disorders. *Journal of Autism and Developmental Disorders, 40*(2), 188–199.

Wallace, G. L., Kenworthy, L., Pugliese, C. E., Popal, H. S., White, E. I., Brodsky, E., & Martin, A. (2016). Real-world executive functions in adults with autism spectrum disorder: Profiles of impairment and associations with adaptive functioning and co-morbid anxiety and depression. *Journal of Autism and Developmental Disorders, 46*(3), 1071–1083.

Wells, K., Condillac, R., Perry, A., & Factor, D. (2011). A comparison of three adaptive behaviour measures in relation to cognitive level and severity of autism. *Journal of Developmental Disabilities, 15*(3), 55–63.

Williams, D. L., Mazefsky, C. A., Walker, J. D., Minshew, N. J., & Goldstein, G. (2014). Associations between conceptual reasoning, problem solving, and adaptive ability in high-functioning autism. *Journal of Autism and Developmental Disorders, 44*(11), 2908–2920.

Yang, S., Paynter, J. M., & Gilmore, L. (2016). Vineland adaptive behavior scales: II profile of young children with autism spectrum disorder. *Journal of Autism and Developmental Disorders, 46*(1), 64–73.

Curriculum-Based Assessment of Social Development: Goal Selection and Sequencing

8

Raymond G. Romanczyk, Kaylie Wiseman, and Hannah Morton

Impaired and unusual social development is the central characteristic of individuals diagnosed with autism spectrum disorder (ASD). Leo Kanner first identified a syndrome he termed early infantile autism and stated, "The outstanding pathognomonic fundamental disorder is the children's inability to relate themselves in the ordinary way to people and situations from the beginning of life" (Kanner, 1943, p. 242). As part of his description he also emphasized that individuals presented as aloof, rather than as withdrawn. This is a key concept as aloof implies having a lack of value for social interaction, while withdrawn implies that social interaction has aversive qualities.

Over time with the evolution of the diagnostic criteria for ASD, a broader population is defined wherein there are subgroups (Eagle, Romanczyk, & Lenzenweger, 2010) that encompass the aloof description and the avoidance description. Currently, the fifth edition of the *Diagnostic and Statistical Manual of Mental Disorders* (DSM-5) of the American Psychiatric Association (2013) presents two primary categories of symptomatology:

A. Persistent deficits in social communication and social interaction
B. Restricted, repetitive patterns of behavior, interests, or activities

These two categories can interact in a negative manner with respect to social development. For example, restricted interests can limit the quality and frequency of discussion among social partners having a conversation.

There are numerous social development deficits observed in the population of individuals diagnosed with ASD. Some important deficits are:

- Decreased attention to the voices of others
- Using another person as a tool (e.g., grabbing someone's hand to get a desired item)
- Little or no interest in other children
- Failure to initiate social interactions with peers
- Poor understanding of gestures
- Limited use of gestures to communicate
- Lack sharing enjoyment with others
- Poor eye gaze
- Poor gaze following
- Poor joint attention
- Poor isolate and cooperative play
- Responding inappropriately to facial expressions

R.G. Romanczyk (✉) • K. Wiseman • H. Morton
Institute for Child Development, Binghamton University, Binghamton, NY, USA
e-mail: rromanc@binghamton.edu; kwisema1@binghamton.edu; hmorton2@binghamton.edu

J.B. Leaf (ed.), *Handbook of Social Skills and Autism Spectrum Disorder*, Autism and Child Psychopathology Series, DOI 10.1007/978-3-319-62995-7_8

Within this context of deficits in social development, remediation/treatment is often referred to as teaching social skills. Within the broad literature in child development is the construct of social competence, often referred to as interpersonal skills, interpersonal competence, social skills, and communication competence (Segrin, 2000). All of these terms refer to a similar construct, which can be defined as the ability to appropriately and effectively interact with other people (Baron, 2000). This phrase "appropriately and effectively" is an understandable colloquial phrase but is imprecise and incomplete. Romanczyk, White, and Gillis (2005) presented a model that differentiates social skills from skilled social behavior. Social skills can be viewed as components, or building blocks, that are necessary for skilled social behavior. However, having specific individual social skills does not necessarily result in skilled social behavior. The complex repertoire of skilled social behavior requires not only the individual skills but also complex monitoring and analysis of social situations and interactions to constantly moderate the content, combination, and timing of the use of individual skills. They presented a conceptual process diagram to illustrate the complexity of this dynamic (see Fig. 8.1).

As the authors stated in their article, this diagram, as with any diagram of a complex process, is not exhaustive and underscores the complexity of the clinical task of establishing complex skilled repertoires for individuals who present with significant deficits. This figure is intended to represent in part the complex process of skilled social behavior and is not a goal selection or priority tool and is not intended as a behavior analytic analysis of common colloquial terms such as motivation, paralinguistic, attention, awareness, etc. Rather, it illustrates a midpoint in consumer-provider discussions of the complex skilled social behavior repertoire and highlights the difficulty of addressing social repertoire deficits in individuals diagnosed with ASD.

This difficulty is further compounded by our relative lack of clear knowledge of the causal mechanism(s) for the social development deficits. For example, much has been written concerning the motivation for social interaction. Simply put, individuals diagnosed with ASD do not experience reward aspects of social interaction. Ferster (1961) hypothesized that the social environment did not produce reinforcing effects. In the broader autism literature, researchers such as Argyle and Kendon (1967), McFall (1982), Dodge and Murphy (1984), Chevallier, Kohls, Troiani, Brodkin, and Schultz (2012), and others have hypothesized such a deficit but comprehensive research has been lacking. Likewise, hypotheses concerning "mindblindness," have received much attention, (e.g., Barron-Cohen, 1995). Other hypotheses such as aversion to eye gaze, which has support in specific research for children diagnosed with Fragile X syndrome (Bruno, Garrett, Quintin, Mazaika, & Reiss, 2014; Cohen et al., 1988), add further complexity to this area. A recent review of the literature on social reward processing in ASD concludes that "…nearly half of the studies reviewed here either find contradictory evidence or support a broader range of deficits in reward processing" (Bottini, 2016, p. 24). Thus, one can reasonably conclude that attention to social motivation is important from a clinical perspective but may not provide a complete picture of the multiple possible mechanisms contributing to the performance deficit.

8.1 Curriculum-Based Assessment

A curriculum is broadly defined as the content and sequence of instruction. Wolery and Winterling (1997) provide a more comprehensive definition of a curriculum: "an organized description of a body of content, assessment procedures, and methods for teaching selected skills," (p. 88) which is based on a conceptual foundation. The description and use of curriculum-based assessment (CBA) and the related concept of curriculum-based measurement (CBM) have increased substantially over the last four decades (Deno & Mirkin, 1977). It was developed in the field of education for typical learners and extended into special education (Deno, 1985; Deno & Fuchs, 1987; Fuchs & Dino, 1991; Jones, Southern, &

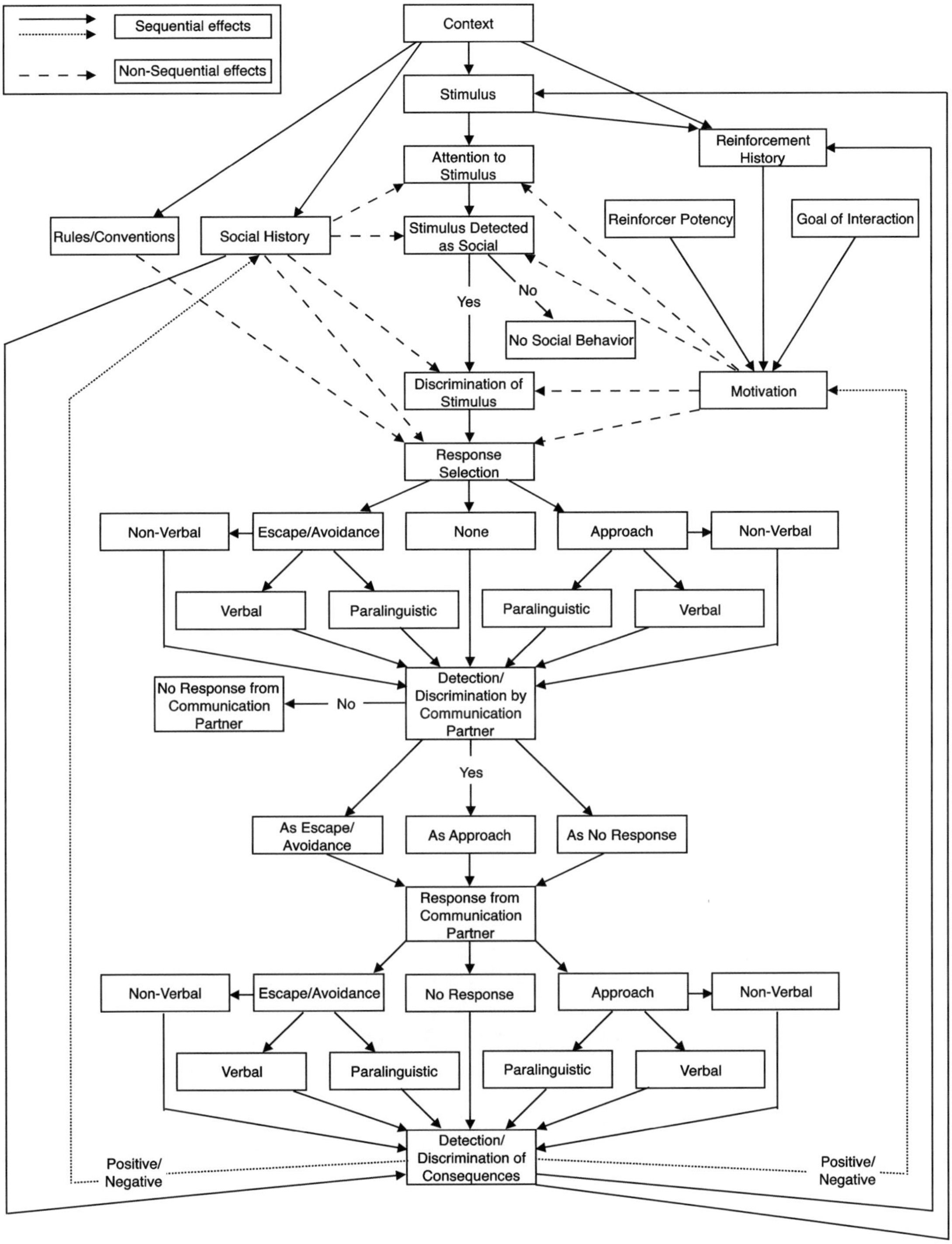

Fig. 8.1 Romanczyk et al. (2005) schematic representation of social competence

Brigham, 1998; Shinn, 2008). Although there are many definitions, a straightforward description for the current context by Deno (1987) seems appropriate: "Curriculum-based assessment (CBA) can be defined as any set of measurement activities that uses direct observation and recording of a student's performance in the local curriculum as a basis for gathering information to make instructional decisions" (p. 41). With the emphasis on direct measurement, it is not surprising that CBA has strong roots in applied behavior analysis (Shinn, 2013).

Most curriculum-based assessments are criterion based and thus focus on determining a child's individual profile of strengths and weaknesses (Rubin & Laurent, 2004). It is argued that this approach provides information regarding skills that are currently in the child's repertoire, skills that are emerging, and skills that are not yet displayed by the child. Additionally, many curriculum-based assessments are designed to examine the child's skills in relation to skills outlined in the curriculum, thereby explicitly linking assessment to intervention. By conceptualizing a child's abilities in this way, an individualized curriculum, used as a goal selection process, is intended to best meet the child's functional needs (Najdowski, Gould, Lanagan, & Bishop, 2014). Ongoing instructional decisions can thus be made based on direct observations of a child's ability to complete curricular objectives.

Although the area of CBA has a wealth of research and debate, this chapter will focus on evaluating the utility and validity of the CBA approach with extant curricula that address social development deficits in individuals diagnosed with ASD. For this purpose, curricula were defined as a codified set of developmentally arranged specific behaviors/skills intended to guide intervention implementation.

8.2 Curriculum-Based Assessment for Autism Spectrum Disorder

A multitude of curricula exist for educating children diagnosed with ASD; however, not all include a CBA component. We have selected for review CBAs that are tied to a curriculum for young children (defined as birth through 10 years of age) diagnosed with ASD, as this is a crucial developmental period for skill acquisition. Although we are highlighting CBAs that examine social skills, many of the models reviewed focus on multiple domains for a more comprehensive intervention approach. Additionally, although many curricula are designed for children diagnosed with ASD or other special needs, some can also be used for children with more global delays. Many of the models reviewed are based on the principles of applied behavior analysis (ABA) or were developed from a developmental and/or relationship focused framework. Available curricula and accompanying CBAs are described below. Summary information to assist in evaluating the CBAs is presented in Tables 8.1 and 8.2. Table 8.3 provides operational definitions for the information available in the preceding tables.

8.2.1 The Assessment of Basic Language and Learning Skills: Revised (ABLLS-R; Partington, 2006)

The *Assessment of Basic Language and Learning Skills-Revised* (ABLLS-R; Partington, 2006) is a criterion-referenced assessment tool and intervention guide designed for children diagnosed with developmental or language delays. Based on the principles of behavior analysis, it encompasses 522 skills across 25 skill sets, which each correspond to a letter of the alphabet. Areas include receptive language, labeling, self-help, social interaction, classroom routines, gross motor, and fine motor; the skills within each area progress in developmental sequence. The assessment protocol is conducted by observing the child's behavior and abilities along each skill area, and parents can also provide input for their child's abilities. The assessment can take 10–14 h and should be readministered every 6–12 months for progress monitoring. The ABLLS-R guide supports the identification of intervention goals as well as writing Individualized Education Program (IEP) goals for learning and progress tracking. However, the curriculum does not itself

Table 8.1 Summary information for social skills specific curriculum-based assessments

CBA	Ages	ASD specific	Developmental progression	Setting	Family involvement	Reliability/validity research	Outcome research	Other available research
DO-WATCH-LISTEN-SAY	Young children	Y	N	School or home	N	N	N	N
POWER	K-12 grades	N	N	Any	Y	N	N	N
Socially Savvy	Preschool+	N	N	Any	Y	N	N	N

Table 8.2 Summary information for curriculum-based assessments covering broad developmental domains

CBA	Ages	ASD specific	Developmental progression	Setting	Family involvement	Reliability/validity research	Outcome research	Other available research
ABLLS-R	Birth to 12 years	N	N	School or community	Y	N	Y	Y
ACE	3–22 years	Y	Y	School	Y	Y	N	N
AEPS	Birth to 6 years	N	Y	Any	Y	N	N	Y
BCP	1–14 years	N	Y	School or community	Y	N	N	Y
Brigance IED III*	Birth to 7 years	N	Y	Any	Y	N	N	Y
Carolina	Birth to 5 years	N	Y	School or home	Y	N	N	Y
Eden	Pre-K-12 grades	Y	Y	Any	Y	N	N	N
ESDM	1–5 years	Y	Y	Any	Y	N	Y	Y
HELP	Birth to 6 years	N	Y	Any	Y	Y	N	Y
PEP-3	6 months–7 years	Y	N	Any	Y	Y	N	Y
PIRK	Preschool age	N	N	School	N	N	Y	N
SCERTS	Birth to 10 years	Y	Y	Any	Y	N	N	N
SKILLS	Infant to adolescent	Y	Y	Any	Y	Y	N	Y
STAR	Birth to 8 years	Y	Y	School	N	N	Y	Y
VB-MAPP	Birth to 4 years	Y	Y	School or community	N	Y	Y	Y

See note. Summary information for the Brigance IED III refers to the criterion-referenced version

Table 8.3 Definitions for summary information

Summary information	Definition
ASD specific	Intended for use solely for individuals diagnosed with ASD
Developmental progression	Includes a hierarchical sequencing of skills based on progression in typical development
Family involvement	Family members provide input in the assessment process (i.e., comment on child abilities, help inform goal selection)
Reliability/validity research	At least one peer-reviewed, empirical study examines the reliability and/or validity of the assessment measure
Other domains	Covers developmental domains in additional to social skills that are typically covered by comprehensive treatment models for ASD (i.e., motor, language, adaptive, play, executive function, cognition, academic skills)
Outcome research	At least one peer-reviewed, empirical study examines the efficacy or effectiveness of the model with children with ASD (can include assessment or intervention components)
Other available research	At least one peer-reviewed, empirical study examines components of the model or the model's utility for a purpose other than examining outcomes for children with ASD as described above or strictly for the purposes of reliability or validity

contain specific activities or lessons that directly map on to the skills identified in the assessment. It is available in several additional languages including Spanish, Italian, French, Japanese, Arabic, Hebrew, and Norwegian. Uniquely, there is also a web-based version of the assessment, WebABLLS, which supports multidisciplinary coordination in assessment and skills tracking for an individual child.

The ABLLS-R has been used to measure progress in a behavioral educational model (Lambert-Lee et al., 2015) and Intensive Behavior Intervention (IBI; Sharma, Heywood, & Rajkumar, 2010) for children diagnosed with ASD. Additionally, Lin and Kubina (2004) describe integrating the ABLLS with learning channels for optimally descriptive behavioral definitions. Portions of the ABLLS have also been used to evaluate transfer of stimulus control in tacting instruction methods within a single-case design (Bloh, 2008). There are currently no peer-reviewed studies evaluating the validity or reliability of this measure.

8.2.2 Assessment, Evaluation, and Programming Systems, Second Edition (AEPS; Bricker, Capt, & Pretti-Frontczak, 2002)

The Assessment, Evaluation, and Programming Systems, Second Edition (AEPS; Bricker et al., 2002) is a CBA that aims to link assessment, goal development, intervention, and evaluation. It is appropriate for children ages birth through 6 years with disabilities or those at risk for developmental delays. It may be used with children up to 9 years of age if developmentally appropriate. Skills from six major developmental areas are assessed including, social, social communication, cognitive, adaptive, fine motor, and gross motor skills. These are further subdivided into a developmental progression of skills (referred to as strands) and smaller units of goals and objectives that build toward broader skill domains. Children are assessed in a naturalistic environment while engaging in developmentally appropriate activities. The AEPS includes assessment activities that consist of scripts and directions for the examiner to create engaging testing activities incorporating test items. Caregiver report of child skills and input from any professionals working with the child are also included. Assessment items are scored as 0 (the child cannot perform the skill), 1 (the child inconsistently performs the skill), or 2 (the child consistently performs the skills). Rating criteria are provided for each test item. This permits examination of skills present in the child's repertoire and items that require intervention and provides the basis for the development of specific intervention goals. The model also includes information on developing IEP and Individual Family Service Plan (IFSP) goals. Notably, with this model, it is possible to observe and collect data for multiple children across domains at one time, thus improving the efficiency of the assessment for those working in center or school-based programs.

The curriculum volume of the AEPS maps onto the assessment with a similar sequencing of items, thus allowing one to match the skills identified during assessment with goals for intervention. This linking of items from assessment to intervention also permits evaluation of child progress in reaching intervention goals. Research conducted using the AEPS has demonstrated its utility for generating appropriate IEP goals (Notari & Bricker, 1990; Pretti-Frontczak & Bricker, 2000). It has also been utilized to assist in determining eligibility for accessing state and federal early intervention and early childhood special education services under the Disabilities Education Improvement Act (Bricker et al., 2008; Bricker, Yovanoff, Capt, & Allen, 2003). No peer-reviewed research is available examining outcomes of this model for children diagnosed with ASD.

8.2.3 Behavioral Characteristics Progression (BCP): Birth to 14 Years (http://www.vort.com/BCP-Birth-14-years-Behavioral-Characteristics-Progression/)

The behavioral characteristics progression (BCP; VORT Corporation, 2015–2016) is a criterion-referenced curriculum-based assessment with instructional activities. The BCP includes 2,300 skills or "behavioral characteristics" that comprise 56 domains or "strands." The strands are grouped into seven goal areas: cognition, language, gross motor, fine motor, social, self-help, and vocational. Each strand progresses in a continuous developmental sequence that terminates with appropriate abilities. The BCP assessment record screens for "identifying behaviors" to reveal strands for intervention and to support writing IEP goals. Many (1,900) of the skills also map onto activities for intervention. The program should be implemented by a teacher or professional; however, high priority is placed on including the parent for generalization to the home setting. Progress is tracked on each child's individual assessment record, which provides space for noting skill mastery. There are currently no peer-reviewed studies documenting the validity or reliability of the BCP.

8.2.4 Brigance Inventory of Early Development (IED) III (French, 2013)

The Brigance IED III (French, 2013) is a curriculum-based assessment tool designed specifically for special education with standardized (norm-referenced) and non-standardized (criterion-referenced) inventories. Both provide a comprehensive skill assessment that aligns with state and Common Core standards, albeit with somewhat different purposes.

8.2.4.1 Brigance IED III Standardized

The IED III Standardized includes 55 norm-referenced assessments, which involve a standardized assessment with kit materials and a stimulus book. The IED III Standardized evaluates a child's abilities in five domains: physical development, language development, academic skills/cognitive development, adaptive behavior, and social and emotional development. These domains allow for comparison of the child's standardized scores and percentile ranks to same-age peers through the chronological age of 7 years and 11 months. In this way, the IED III Standardized results can also be used to inform referral recommendations. This assessment administration requires up to 1 h per child and should be administered by a trained professional.

8.2.4.2 Brigance IED III

The IED III is criterion referenced for the identification of strengths and weaknesses within individual students. It assesses skills in physical development, language development, literacy, mathematics and science, daily living, and social and emotional development. Assessment may occur through child observation and input from parent/caregiver interview. Results can be used to inform the development of IEP goals and lesson planning for children below the developmental age of eight as well as to monitor progress.

8.2.4.3 Brigance Readiness Activities Inventory

The readiness activities are a separate manual that links with the skills listed in the IED III. It includes 300 activities, each of which lists the objective (skill being taught), domain of the skill, rationale for teaching it, related skills, developmental sequence, recommendations for teaching, and examples of difficulties the child may experience when learning the new skill. It includes student activity pages and letters to be sent to the family with at-home activities; the latter are also available in Spanish.

Although reliability and validity statistics are included in the Standardization and Validation Manual for the IED III, these data have not been published in any peer-reviewed sources.

8.2.5 The Carolina Curriculum (Johnson-Martin, Attermeier, & Hacker, 2004; Johnson-Martin, Hacker, & Attermeier, 2004)

The Carolina Curriculum (Johnson-Martin, Attermeier, & Hacker, 2004; Johnson-Martin, Hacker, & Attermeier, 2004) is an assessment and intervention curriculum for young children (birth to 5 years) with mild to severe disabilities. There are separate volumes for infants and toddlers from birth through 3 years (the Carolina Curriculum for Infants and Toddlers with Special Needs; CCITSN) and preschoolers ages 2–5 years (The Carolina Curriculum for Preschoolers with Special Needs; CCPSN). The curriculum is intended for use by professionals in the child's home or school environment. Assessment is conducted in the child's natural environment either with or without caregivers present. The curriculum is sequenced in a developmental progression including 22 teaching sequences in an assessment log covering five developmental areas: personal-social, cognition, communication, fine motor, and gross motor. Assessment consists of a brief observation of the child engaging in skills or activities included in the sequence. If skills do not occur naturally, the examiner or caregiver attempts to engage the child in specified activities to help elicit the skill. The assessment is used to determine a child's strengths and weaknesses and select items in need of the most attention. Each assessment item is linked directly to a curriculum item that describes the instructional methods for teaching the skill.

Castro, Pinto, and Maia (2011) examined the association between the content of *the Carolina Curriculum for Preschoolers with Special Needs* (CCPSN) and the International Classification of Functionality, Disability, and Health for Children and Youth (ICF-CY; World Health Organization, 2007), an international classification system of child functioning. This was conducted due to the lack of measures available to assess functioning that maps onto the ICF-CY. Results revealed high overlap between the CCPSN and two domains on the ICF-CY: body functions and activities and participation. These two domains encompass a large variety of functional skills including the ability to carry out actions needed to develop interpersonal relationships and complete daily tasks of living, as well as the lower-order bodily functions required to complete such tasks (World Health Organization, 2007). Two other domains of the ICF-CY, body structures and environmental factors, are not covered by the CCPSN. Notably, these two domains are not focused on functional abilities of the child but rather include structural factors that may be considered prerequisites for the ability to display functional skills. Additionally, Del Giudice et al. (2006) demonstrated the efficacy of *The Carolina Curriculum for Infants and Toddlers with Special Needs* implemented by parents of children with Down syndrome. No information is available on the efficacy of this model for children with ASD, which is a limitation of the model.

8.2.6 DO-WATCH-LISTEN-SAY Social and Communication Intervention for Children with Autism (Quill, 2000)

DO-WATCH-LISTEN-SAY (Quill, 2000) exclusively addresses the social and communication needs of children through both assessment and manualized intervention components. The *Assessment of Social and Communication Skills for Children with Autism* contains questionnaires and checklists to better understand a child's abilities and objectives for intervention in more than 100 subskill areas. Subskills identified through the assessment correspond to activities for intervention. Although intervention is outlined through the curriculum guidelines, it can also be integrated with other treatment strategies and models (Cohen, 2001). DO-WATCH-LISTEN-SAY encompasses skills in social reciprocity, imitation, solitary play, social play, group skills, and social communication. The curriculum is designed to be implemented in the home or school setting and includes considerations for children with various communication abilities, including those who use augmentative or alternative communication. Child progress can also be tracked via data collection forms and charts. There is currently no published validity or reliability data for this assessment.

8.2.7 Eden Autism Assessment and Curriculum Series (EDEN; edenautism.org)

The Eden Autism Assessment and Curriculum Series (EDEN; Eden Faculty, 2010) includes a series of manuals designed for use by professionals, teachers, and parents to facilitate ABA-based interventions for individuals diagnosed with ASD. It is appropriate for individuals across the lifespan, from infancy to adulthood. The Eden School Series, applicable for children and adolescents from Pre-K to grade 12, focuses on cognitive skills, speech and language, vocational education, self and domestic care, physical education, recreation, and leisure. Additional volumes include an infant and toddler curriculum, adult employment curriculum, and adult residential curriculum. The Eden Autism Assessment provides a mechanism to identify student strengths and weaknesses, which informs goal selection. The assessment measure also links directly to lesson plans and is used to track child progress across domains as intervention progresses within the Eden Autism Curriculum. A subscription-based software program is also available (Eden's Learning Management System), which links assessment and intervention. The Eden Autism Assessment and Curriculum Series was developed and updated based on the experience and clinical expertise of Eden faculty. Field tests have been utilized to examine the implementation and effectiveness of teaching programs focusing on curricular objectives. No published outcome data or empirical work evaluating the model is available.

8.2.8 Early Start Denver Model (ESDM; Rogers & Dawson, 2010)

The ESDM (Rogers & Dawson, 2010) is a comprehensive early intervention approach for children diagnosed with ASD ages 12–36 months and can extend up to 60 months of age. The model is an adaptation of the original Denver model (Rogers, Herbison, Lewis, Pantone, & Reis, 1986) for preschool-age children. ESDM incorporates knowledge of typical development and the effects of ASD on a child's developmental trajectory. It was developed from several complementary approaches and emphasizes increasing social motivation and utilizing naturalistic and child-directed instruction for both assessment and intervention purposes. The ESDM curriculum includes a developmentally sequenced curriculum checklist with corresponding item descriptions of specific skills across ten domains: receptive communication, expressive communication, joint attention, imitation, social skills, play skills, cognitive skills, fine motor, gross motor, and self-care. The checklist is utilized prior to intervention to generate learning objectives, which are designed to be accomplished within a 12-week period. The checklist is readministered following the 12-week period to develop new objectives based on the child's progress since the initial assessment. If a child does not demonstrate progress in a certain area following a 12-week period, a decision tree is included in the model to help determine why this might be the case and how to proceed. Caregiver and/or teacher report is included within the checklist to determine whether the child can perform skills that may not have been observed during assessment sessions.

In comparison to other curriculum models for ASD, empirical support for the ESDM is demonstrated by a randomized controlled trial and several other empirical studies investigating outcomes of ESDM for children with ASD, such as cognitive functioning, adaptive behavior, social communication, receptive language, normalized patterns of brain activity in response to faces, and ASD diagnosis (Dawson et al., 2012; Dawson et al., 2010; Vivanti et al., 2014). The effectiveness of a training workshop to help disseminate the model to community early intervention programs has also been examined, demonstrating high levels of fidelity (80% or better) post-training for all professionals attending the workshop (Vismara, Young, & Rogers, 2013). Finally, parent delivery of ESDM has been investigated, which has not been demonstrated to be more effective than treatment as usual (Rogers et al., 2012).

8.2.9 Hawaii Early Learning Profile (HELP; http://www.vort.com)

The Hawaii Early Learning Profile (HELP; VORT Corporation, 2005–2016) is a curriculum-based assessment tool that was initially developed through the Enrichment Project for Handicapped Infants, a federal grant program, from 1971 to 1979. Although the HELP assessment and curriculum are designed to be used together, either can be used on its own. It is split into two separate curricula based on the age of the child (0–3 years and 3–6 years), with each program outlined separately below:

8.2.9.1 HELP: 0–3 years

This product assesses 685 skills across six domains: cognitive, language, gross motor, fine motor, social-emotional, and self-help (Warshaw, 2006). These skills and behaviors were identified based on growth charts, standardized tests, and literature at the time of the curriculum development. The skills are grouped into 59 concepts or "strands," which progress in developmental sequence and are linked to curriculum materials for intervention efforts. The administration manual also provides suggestions for adaptations for children with disabilities, as well as cultural considerations for interacting with families. A separate at-home product ("*Help… At Home*") provides handouts for families that introduce skills and provide instructions and activities for parent involvement.

8.2.9.2 HELP: 3–6 Years (Second Edition; Previously "HELP for Preschoolers"; Wheat & Baker, 2010)

This product is designed to extend the use of HELP 0–3 for older children and assesses 585 skills across the same six domains, which are grouped into 47 developmentally sequenced strands (Wheat & Baker, 2010). Notably, three new strands in HELP 3–6 are specifically designed for children with special needs: sign language, speechreading, and wheelchair skills. HELP 3–6 also includes considerations for individual- or group-level assessment.

Similarly, both products provide charts for visually tracking skill level and progress in development. Additionally, the skills in HELP 3–6 are sequenced with the same ID numbers as HELP 0–3 for ease of transition from the latter to the former. Uniquely, underlying deficits in mental processes are hypothesized for children who persist with difficulty in certain assessment areas. HELP also emphasizes the importance of the family's involvement and includes parent questions for assisting the parents with informing their child's assessment. In this way, the assessment portion begins with a parent interview and is not solely based on professional observation. Parents are also encouraged to facilitate play and interactions with their child during assessment observation. An additional book focuses on considerations for curriculum implementation with parents with disabilities. HELP also suggests involvement of a multidisciplinary team, when applicable. Select HELP curriculum products are also available in Spanish.

Components of HELP have been used in published research, including to measure development of motor skills before and after a pediatric strength intervention (Sayers, Cowden, Newton, Warren, & Eason, 1996), to estimate children's developmental abilities in retrospective chart review (Coplan & Jawad, 2005), and to inform professional training (Belcher et al., 2005).

When compared with other CBAs and standardized assessments, HELP assessment results align well with the norm-referenced Gesell Developmental Schedules-Revised-Adaptive Domain (GDS-R; Knobloch, Stevens, & Malone, 1980) and provide the least variable and most representative results (Bagnato & Murphy, 1989). Furthermore, Bagnato and Murphy (1989) conclude that the HELP "may be one of the best curriculum-imbedded assessment choices" (p. 58); however, many of the CBAs in this chapter were not included in their comparison.

8.2.10 The New England Center for Children Autism Curriculum Encyclopedia; New England Center for Children: Core Skills Assessment (NECC-CSA; acenecc.org)

The Autism Curriculum Encyclopedia (ACE) is an educational web-based software system developed by the New England Center for Children (NECC; The New England Center for Children: Autism Education and Research, 2017). It is designed for use by teachers and professionals to create programs, based on the principles of ABA, for children, adolescents, and young adults (ages 3–22 years) diagnosed with ASD spanning various levels of functioning. The curriculum covers a broad array of skills including social, communication, self-help, discrimination, recreation and physical education, health and safety, community, academic, and vocational. Within ACE, assessment is conducted with the New England Center for Children-Core Skills Assessment (NECC-CSA). The CSA measures 52 foundational skills across the domains covered by the ACE. These skills are considered prerequisites for higher-level learning and independent functioning (e.g., ability to respond to one's name when called, requesting wants and needs). The CSA delineates specific skills needed to achieve broader objectives. Skills are rated as yes (i.e., present), no (i.e., not present), or emerging based either on direct observation or informant report. Skills are evaluated annually to assess child progress. The ACE skills assessment is also available as a next step following the CSA for a more comprehensive assessment of a child's level of functioning across domains. This assessment evaluates all skills within the ACE curriculum, beyond the foundational skills. Both the CSA and ACE skills assessments are linked directly to lesson plans providing instructional methods for teaching skills identified as an area of need via the assessments. Since the assessment is tied to a software program, raw data from the assessment can be entered into a computer application, which provides a performance score indexing the child's skill level. The NECC-CSA was designed by senior professionals at NECC based on clinical expertise and empirical work examining skill selection, and curricula for individuals with ASD (Dickson et al., 2014). Dickson et al., (2014) also demonstrated the social validity of the foundational skills comprising the CSA across professionals and parents of NECC and the wider community.

8.2.11 POWER-Solving Social Skills Curriculum (http://power-solving.com)

POWER-Solving (POWER-Solving, LLC, 2016) is a curriculum for the development of social skills in elementary through high school-age students who have deficits in this area (e.g., ASD, social communication disorder, attention deficit hyperactivity disorder, oppositional defiant disorder, nonverbal learning disabilities, or subclinical presentations). The program is based on the social information processing model (Crick & Dodge, 1994), which outlines six stages that individuals work through in a social situation.

The POWER-Solving Rating Scale is an assessment tool for identifying areas of strength and intervention goals. Specific aspects of social situations are split into four modules: introduction, social conversation, developing friendships, and anger management. The curriculum teaches a "toolbox" – the five steps of the POWER-Solving approach. Rather than teaching discrete skills, students are taught to apply the POWER-Solving steps when they encounter a problem in a social situation; this approach is intended to encourage generalization of social skills and problem-solving beyond a structured or clinical setting. The assessment and curriculum can be used as a primary tool or can be integrated within other programs.

Although the primary facilitator of the POWER-Solving curriculum is usually the teacher or other professional in a school setting, other mental health professionals can conduct the assessment and program implementation in clinical settings, and parents can be trained for home use. The POWER-Solving program has not been validated in any peer-reviewed sources.

8.2.12 Preschool Inventory of Repertoires for Kindergarten (PIRK; Greer & McCorkle, 2003)

The Preschool Inventory of Repertoires for Kindergarten (PIRK; Greer & McCorkle, 2003) was developed as a criterion-referenced assessment tool and an inventory of curricular objectives to help prepare children for typical school settings. It is based on research in ABA. PIRK is categorized into six domains: academic literacy and problem-solving, communication abilities, community of reinforcers, self-management skills, social self-management, and physical and motor skills. The social self-management domain focuses on teaching social skills necessary for appropriate interaction with others across settings. This domain also provides support in reducing stereotypic, self-injurious, and aggressive behaviors, as they may interfere with successful social interaction with others. Within these six domains, 266 long-term objectives are specified each with a number of sub-objectives. PIRK can be used to assess a child's current skill level in each domain and apparent deficits, which is then used to select appropriate objectives for intervention.

Two recent studies have investigated the use of PIRK for children diagnosed with ASD attending special education schools (McGarrell, Healy, Leader, O'Connor, & Kenny, 2009; Waddington & Reed, 2009). Both studies reported that children assessed and instructed with the PIRK curriculum demonstrated improvements in areas important for transitioning to typical schools including behavior management, social skills, intellectual functioning, adaptive behavior, and communication skills. Although empirical support is available demonstrating the effectiveness of the PIRK model, there are no randomized controlled trials available to document the efficacy of the PIRK curriculum.

8.2.13 Psychoeducational Profile Revised-Third Edition (PEP-3; Schopler, Lansing, Reichler, & Marcus, 2005)

The PEP-3 (Schopler, Lansing, Reichler, & Marcus, 2005) is a standardized, norm-referenced scale that assesses the development of communication skills, motor skills, and maladaptive behaviors in children diagnosed with ASD ages 2–7 years old. These three composite scales are divided into ten subtests: cognitive, expressive language, receptive language, fine motor, gross motor, visual motor imitation, affective expression, social reciprocity, characteristic motor behaviors, and characteristic verbal behaviors. The PEP-3 consists of 172 items in total, and administration time is 45–90 min. Internal consistency of the measure is 0.90, test-retest reliability is 0.94, and the measure is significantly correlated with other standardized measures covering similar domains (e.g., Vineland Adaptive Behavior Scales, Childhood Autism Rating Scale-2). The PEP-3 is used as an assessment tool to inform the design of individualized curriculums and includes both direct observation and caregiver report. It can be utilized across school and home-based intervention programs for young children with ASD. For example, the TEACCH model, a clinical service and professional training program developed at the University of North Carolina Chapel Hill, utilizes the PEP-3 to determine curricular objectives. However, since the skills assessed by the PEP-3 do not directly map onto curriculum items, this assessment is not as efficient at linking assessment to intervention. It would thus be most useful for curriculums without a corresponding curriculum-based assessment and one that maps closely to the domains and items assessed by the PEP-3. Strengths of the PEP-3 are its inclusion of nonverbal, untimed, easy items, concrete testing materials, and flexible testing processes that make the measure suitable for children with differing levels of ASD severity and functioning (Lee et al., 2016). There is a Chinese version (The Chinese Psychoeducational Profile-Third Edition, CPEP-3), and a short form with 73 items also exists (SF-PEP3) and is recommended as a more efficient tool for the purposes of progress monitoring (Lee et al., 2016).

8.2.14 Social Communication Emotional Regulation and Transactional Support Model (SCERTS; Prizant, Wetherby, Rubin, Laurent, & Rydell, 2006)

In comparison to many other models of assessment and intervention for ASD, the SCERTS model (Prizant, Wetherby, Rubin, Laurent, & Rydell, 2006) is specifically focused on developing social communication skills for children diagnosed with ASD. It is intended for use with children from early intervention to the early school years (birth to 10 years). The SCERTS model was designed based on empirical work on the typical course of development as well as the effect of ASD on development. The curriculum may be used with children with and without cognitive and language delays and concentrates on social communication, emotion regulation, and transactional support. The curriculum-based assessment accompanying the model, referred to as the SCERTS Assessment Process (SAP) was designed for use by clinicians and educators for the purposes of educational planning and determining necessary environmental supports (Rubin & Laurent, 2004). Skills within the assessment are organized based on a developmental sequence. The SAP should be used with children who are already identified as having a delay and are thus in need of an IEP or an IFSP.

The assessment process includes a range of possible strategies in order to obtain the most representative sample of a child's abilities across individuals and settings and determine any variability in skills. Assessment strategies are listed from least to most intrusive and outlined below.

8.2.14.1 Interviewing Significant Others and/or Having Familiar People Complete Assessment Questionnaires

Used as an initial method of gathering information, interviews and developmental questionnaires, referred to collectively as SAP-R, are conducted with individuals familiar with the child (e.g., parents, other family members, teachers). This is used to create an initial picture of the child's strengths, areas of need, and available supports.

8.2.14.2 Observation of Daily Activities That Occur in Natural Environments

In the SAP-O component, the child is directly observed in familiar naturalistic settings (e.g., school, home, community sites) with social partners that are typically encountered. This provides information about a child's typical functioning. A scoring system is utilized, and operational definitions are provided to determine if the child is using the skill independently and consistently (scored as 2), the child is practicing the skill and using it inconsistently (scored as 1), or the child is learning the skill and is not able to demonstrate it without support (scored as 0).

8.2.14.3 Behavior Sampling and Elicited Responses

Also utilized as part of the SAP-O, this strategy is used as needed to obtain more specific information about a child's skills. It involves setting up specific activities and challenges to observe how the child responds. This can be particularly useful for eliciting low-frequency behaviors. For example, a snack activity may be conducted to observe requests, protests, and the child's ability to make choices.

Information gleaned from the SAP-R and SAP-O is summarized on the SAP summary form as a method of compiling and integrating all information; strengths and needs are documented. Before proceeding, parents are asked to validate results from the SAP-O to ensure it is a representative of the child's behavior, and the child's strengths, needs, and concerns of the family are discussed. Objectives for intervention are determined based on skills that are most functional, address family priorities, and map onto areas of need. The assessment process is described as ongoing, wherein an initial assessment process guides development of goals and is used throughout intervention to document progress and make adjustments to a child's program as necessary. Daily and weekly logs are used for ongoing progress monitoring, and program modification is considered every 3 months. The emphasis on ecologically valid assessment and the corresponding large degree of family involvement across assessment, goal selection, and intervention can be considered strengths of this model. The SCERTS model was derived from several decades of empirical and clinical work; however, the model itself has not been systematically evaluated.

8.2.15 Shaping Knowledge Through Individual Life Learning Systems (SKILLS): The Online Autism Solution (https://www.skillsforautism.com)

SKILLS: The Online Autism Solution (Skills Global LLC, 2016) is a web-based assessment and curriculum for children with ASD from infancy through adolescence. The SKILLS program is based on the principles of ABA, is aligned with the Common Core standards, and contains assessment, curriculum, and progress tracking components. Assessment is provided across eight learning areas: social, motor, language, adaptive, play, executive functions, cognition, and academic. Completion of the assessment provides activities and lessons for individualized intervention from a selection of nearly 4,000 options in three areas: executive function, social cognition, and language. Each assessment question and intervention activity has an age assigned to it for developmental mapping and lists prerequisite skills needed. SKILLS can also be used to create IEP goals and to form a behavioral intervention plan (BIP) for challenging behavior, if warranted. As a digital program, SKILLS also contains the logbook application for data collection on mobile devices and tablets. These data can be used to create charts and reports for progress tracking. Although SKILLS was initially designed for use by professionals, its user-friendly interface can also be used by families in the home setting, although professional consultation may be necessary. Parents can also report on their child's skills to complete assessment questions; indirect assessment can reduce time demand for the professional (Persicke et al., 2014). The program also allows for online collaboration among team members for the same child.

The SKILLS Assessment has been found to have excellent concurrent validity, as evidenced by moderate to high correlations between assessment results and a child's abilities as noted by direct observation (Persicke et al., 2014). The SKILLS Language Index has also been shown to have good internal consistency and excellent test-retest and inter-rater reliabilities (Dixon, Tarbox, Najdowski, Wilke, & Granpeesheh, 2011). Finally, an individual review by Pritchard (2013) highlights the accessibility of the curriculum as well as the opportunity for ongoing development of the program due to its online nature. These findings preliminarily suggest that the SKILLS Assessment is recommended as a comprehensive indirect assessment tool for children diagnosed with ASD (Persicke et al., 2014); however, additional data are still needed on the psychometric properties of this tool (Dixon et al., 2011).

8.2.16 Socially Savvy: An Assessment and Curriculum Guide for Young Children (Ellis & Almeida, 2015a)

Socially Savvy is designed to decompose the complexity of social interaction into skills that can be pursued for intervention (Ellis & Almeida, 2015a). It includes an assessment checklist, which is completed via direct observation in a social setting over a 2-week period to evaluate a young child's skills and deficits. The checklist outlines social development in seven areas: joint attending, social play, self-regulation, social/emotional, social language, classroom/group behavior, and nonverbal. The manual also provides 50 play-based teaching activities for intervention that specifically address skills in several different areas simultaneously. Finally, the curriculum includes sample IEP goals and ideas for data collection and tracking progress. Although it is geared toward preschool children, the content could be adapted for other ages. This program can be implemented by professionals or parents and was the topic of a training workshop at the 42nd annual convention of the Association for Behavior Analysis International (ABAI; Ellis & Almeida, 2015b, May). Neither validity nor reliability data have been published for this CBA in any peer-reviewed sources.

8.2.17 Strategies for Teaching Based on Autism Research (STAR) Program; Arick, Loos, Falco, & Krug, 2004; STAR Autism Support, 2013–2016)

The STAR program (Arick et al., 2004; STAR Autism Support, 2013–2016) is an ABA-based program for teaching skills to children up to 8 years old diagnosed with ASD. The STAR program has three levels of the curriculum, each of which progress in sequential difficulty according to a child's developmental and verbal abilities. The program includes a comprehensive curriculum-based assessment, which informs individualized goal selection from 169 detailed lesson plans and teaching materials for six skill areas: receptive language, expressive language, spontaneous language, functional routines, academics, and play and social skills. The assessment and curriculum align with the Common Core standards, and implementation of the STAR program also includes data collection for progress tracking. Finally, the STAR Media Center is an additional online resource to support implementing curriculum materials, which includes training videos, visual aids, printable worksheets, and staff schedule templates.

The STAR program is based on evidence-based practices outlined by The National Professional Development Center and National Standards Project (National Autism Center, 2009, 2015), including discrete trial training, pivotal response training, and teaching within functional routines. The STAR program has been shown to significantly improve the skill acquisition of children diagnosed with ASD (Bacon et al., 2014) and to produce significant improvement in cognitive abilities when teachers demonstrate high fidelity to program implementation (Pellecchia et al., 2015). The STAR program was also implemented in Kindergarten through second grade autism support public school classrooms in Philadelphia, PA, as part of the Autism Instructional Methods Study (AIMS). This study demonstrated mixed results in cognitive outcomes when compared to a structured teaching environment, although both conditions demonstrated gains (Mandell et al., 2013). Due to the importance of implementation fidelity, rigorous staff training is an essential consideration for conducting this program. The practices of the STAR program have also been used in staff training for the Autism Outcome Study, an effort by the Oregon Department of Education to evaluate progress and outcomes in children diagnosed with ASD (Arick et al., 2003).

8.2.18 The Verbal Behavior Milestones Assessment and Placement Program (VB-MAPP; Sundberg, 2008)

The VB-MAPP (Verbal Behavior Milestones Assessment and Placement Program (VB-MAPP; Sundberg, 2008) is perhaps the most widely used CBA for children diagnosed with ASD and/or language delays. It is a criterion-referenced tool informed by the principles of ABA, as well as Skinner's (1957) analysis of verbal behavior with five different components.

8.2.18.1 Milestones Assessment

This assessment evaluates 170 learning and language milestones split into three levels based on developmental age: 0–18 months (Level 1), 18–30 months (Level 2), and 30–48 months (Level 3). Between 9 and 13 separate measurements of skills are included, depending on the level. The child's overall skill development can also be determined to fall in one of these three levels. This assessment should be conducted by a trained professional and takes between 2 and 10 h per child, with longer administration times occurring at the higher levels. It can be conducted with standard classroom materials, and a kit with materials is also available. Within this assessment, the Early Echoic Skills Assessment (EESA) is an additional subtest created by Barbara E. Esch, Ph.D., CCC-SLP, BCBA. Although the VB-MAPP does address social skills, it is conceptualized as a language-based assessment used to categorize verbal operants by their function (e.g., tact, mand, intraverbal).

8.2.18.2 Barriers Assessment

This assessment evaluates 24 potential barriers to learning and language development that may hinder a child's progress. The identification of barriers is useful for individualized intervention strategies. A high score (the presence of barriers) can be related to a low score on the Milestones Assessment (the absence of skills).

8.2.18.3 Transition Assessment

This assessment evaluates the student's progress in 18 assessment areas for success in moving to a less restrictive environment. These data can be useful to inform prioritization of IEP goals and decisions about educational placement.

8.2.18.4 Task Analysis and Skills Tracking

This fourth component breaks down the skills in the milestones assessment even further to facilitate progress tracking and nuanced conceptualization of a child's abilities. Approximately 900 specific skills are included and can also inform specific activities for growth.

8.2.18.5 Placement and IEP Goals

This final component informs the writing of IEP goals and intervention needs based on the results of the other four assessment components to ensure a balanced intervention curriculum.

The VB-MAPP is available in several other languages, including Chinese, French, Italian, Polish, Russian, and Spanish. Additionally, a protocol and scoring form is provided for each of the assessments. A digital application is also available for mobile devices.

Sundberg and Sundberg (2011) identified a positive correlation between child age and correct responses on the intraverbal subtest of the VB-MAPP, reflecting the sequential nature of the items on this subtest and its construct validity in measuring a child's intraverbal abilities. Although chronological age was the best predictor of intraverbal skill abilities in typically developing children, correct responses on previous subtest items were a better predictor for children with ASD in this study. Thus, the language-learning sequence of children diagnosed with ASD may differ from typically developing children and is likely not tied as strongly to chronological age. Accordingly, children diagnosed with ASD may have difficulty mastering skills of which they are otherwise able if corequisite language skills are expected in task instruction or completion.

Additionally, the VB-MAPP has good external validity with another CBA, Promoting the Emergence of Advanced Knowledge Relational Training System (PEAK; Dixon et al., 2015). However, Dixon et al. (2015) also note a ceiling effect of the VB-MAPP scores in comparison to PEAK total scores. Thus, the VB-MAPP may be more useful for children with nuanced skill abilities, or those who are more delayed. The extended age range of the PEAK assessments also likely contributes to this ceiling effect. PEAK is not discussed separately in this chapter because it does not explicitly include a social domain.

8.3 Summary and Conclusions

Upon review of the utility of 18 publicly available CBAs for use with young children diagnosed with ASD, we offer conclusions and recommendations for researchers and practitioners. CBAs are tools that can provide information beyond what is typically derived from standardized measures of social skills used with children diagnosed with ASD. Specifically, CBAs produce information regarding a child's strength and weaknesses in a particular developmental domain. A profile documenting a child's current strengths or skill repertoire and deficits is more informative for intervention purposes than standardized assessments, which determine where a child falls on specific skills relative to same-age peers. Criterion-referenced assessment may be particularly relevant in the domain of social skills, as children diagnosed with ASD have a core deficit in this area and are likely to fall significantly below same-age peers on standardized social skills measures. CBAs are also more sensitive to short-term improvements across time than standardized assessments, as skills are delineated into a progression toward obtaining broader objectives. Additionally, many CBAs allow for the direct linking of skill deficits, as identified by the assessment, to intervention goals and specific instructional methods that can be utilized to help a child acquire the skill. Thus, CBAs offer distinct advantages over other commonly used forms of social skills assessment. Further, assessment of social skills and instruction within a child's educational curriculum is particularly useful as acquisition of age appropriate social skills is crucial for successful integration into typical educational settings.

The CBAs for social skills with children diagnosed with ASD reviewed here have been evaluated based on the inclusion or absence of a variety of criteria notable across assessments (see Tables 8.1 and 8.2). Although the presented CBAs are linked to intervention goals, not all are linked directly to specific instructional methods for teaching identified goals. Those that more seamlessly incorporate assessment and intervention, such as the Assessment, Evaluation, and Programming Systems, as well as SKILLS, the STAR program, and the HELP may provide advantages to practitioners in terms of time and ease with which goals can be implemented. They also allow for more direct evaluation of whether the intervention is producing its intended effect and child progress over time. Additionally, those that are linked to a developmental progression, including many of the CBAs reviewed here, provide guidance in determining where a child's skills fall in relation to expectations for their chronological age, as well as whether prerequisite developmental skills must be achieved prior to acquisition of age-appropriate skills. Additionally, models that focus on short-term acquisition of goals and more frequent reevaluation permit more delimited and efficient instruction, prevent the continuation of goals when minimal progress is made, and are essential to understand a child's learning patterns (Gould et al., 2011). The ESDM and the SCERTS model emphasize reevaluation of skills after a 3-month period.

Another consideration in the selection of a CBA is the domain(s) that each covers. All of the tools reviewed here include a social component; however, there are a wide variety of other domains covered. Some curricula take a more comprehensive approach, covering a breadth of developmental areas and can be used to conceptualize a child's strengths and weaknesses in social and other areas simultaneously (e.g., ABLLS-R, HELP, SKILLS). This approach can be advantageous for children with more global delays and for use by teachers and clinicians who are not exclusively focused on social skill development in their intervention efforts. According to Gould, Dixon, Najdowski, Smith, and Tarbox (2011), eight domains comprise a comprehensive assessment: social, motor, language, adaptive, play, executive functions, cognition, and academic skills. Of the CBAs evaluated in this chapter, SKILLS exclusively covers all of these areas. Comprehensive skill assessment and intervention may be useful to maximize a child's learning potential as she/he is encouraged to make developmental strides equitably across multiple domains (Najdowski et al., 2014). Alternatively, other curricula focus more specifically on the assessment of social skills (e.g., POWER-Solving, SCERTS, Socially Savvy). These programs excel in providing focused intervention by breaking down social development even further into specific skill areas. When a specialized CBA is selected, it should be supplemented by other programs for increased scope of intervention (Najdowski et al., 2014). Of note, the POWER-Solving program is the only assessment reviewed here that does not include specific goals. Rather, a generalization approach is taken by teaching a problem-solving skill set with the goal of applying this skill to a variety of situations.

Although most of the curriculum models reviewed were established from empirical work on typical development, development in ASD, and behavioral principles for instruction of children diagnosed with ASD, most of these curricula have not been empirically evaluated. Several exceptions to this are the Early Start Denver Model, HELP, and SKILLS. In comparison to other curriculums for young children diagnosed with ASD, the efficacy of these models has been investigated. A number of empirical studies have documented the validity and reliability of these models; most notably, ESDM has also been used in a randomized controlled trial. These and other curricula have also been utilized in peer-reviewed studies investigating the models as implemented with children diagnosed with ASD (i.e., PIRK, the STAR Program, VB-MAPP).

For clinicians or researchers working with children from a wider age range, several of the curricula reviewed here span developmental levels (i.e., ACE, BCP, EDEN, POWER-Solving, Skills). These CBAs may be beneficial for use with a wider age demographic of children, or for longitudinal use as a child ages. Additionally, due to the developmental nature of these criterion-based assessments, they may still be appropriate for individuals with skill impairments who have a chronological age beyond that prescribed in the curriculum. However, age-appropriate adaptations may be necessary for intervention activities in chronologically older individuals.

Finally, the CBAs available for children diagnosed with ASD differ with respect to the extent to which caregivers are incorporated in assessment and treatment planning. The involvement of caregivers into several of the models presented is crucial as it helps practitioners obtain a more complete picture of child functioning; lack of information can be a concern when relying exclusively on direct observation, or on report from an otherwise singular source. Caregiver involvement also promotes generalization of skills across settings, as parents are given a voice in contributing to their child's skill assessment and development. The SCERTS and HELP models in particular are noted for their large caregiver component. These models emphasize involvement of caregivers in the assessment process, goal selection, and in determining additional supports that may be required to assist the child in developing and maintaining skills.

Recommendations

1. Although some models do have documented empirical support, many of the CBAs and corresponding curricula reviewed in this chapter have not been systematically evaluated. Therefore, there is a need for more research examining outcomes for the model as a whole as well as whether the CBAs employed within the models are effective and efficient in determining goals for intervention. Reliability and validity data would also provide further support for the use of these models. Finally, social validation studies are useful for ensuring that selected domains and goals are considered meaningful to children, families, and professionals.
2. Relatedly, it will be important for researchers to evaluate the effects of various curriculum models against other available models that teach social skills. This would be useful for determining the relative ease of use, efficiency, and effectiveness of each model, as well as whether certain domains of functioning (e.g., communication, motor, social, adaptive) might be best served by certain models. An examination of potential moderating factors (e.g., IQ, verbal ability) would also be productive for determining which models might be best suited to any given child and family.

3. As discussed above, not all available CBAs are linked directly with specific instructional objectives and methods of teaching. Those that are most closely linked to intervention include NECC-CSA, Eden, and *the Carolina Curriculum*. These models might be particularly useful for center or school-based programs that require higher levels of standardization.

To best meet the individualized needs of the child, the selection of a CBA should include consideration of the domains addressed in this chapter. Although most CBAs do involve a learning curve or training process, the ability to tailor interventions to specific child weaknesses is highly valued. The importance of skill assessment and goal selection cannot be overemphasized, especially in the social domain for children diagnosed with ASD. The integration of CBA and intervention into existing educational programming can also be considered for children already receiving services. Due to the widespread interspersal of social demands throughout daily interactions, the involvement of a team of professionals and caregivers across multiple settings should be prioritized to facilitate optimal learning and generalizability of a child's social skills.

8.3.1 Admonition

While the use of a CBA approach can be very beneficial, particularly with respect to facilitating communication between consumers and service provides, (i.e., having a common reference and vocabulary), effective intervention is an idiographic process. There does not exist, and there may never exist, a codified system such as a curriculum that will have sufficient detail and supporting research to adequately match goal sequence and priority with a given individual's characteristics and prior learning history, in the context of current need and priorities. There will always be a need for specific and precise assessment of the individual and the development of an iterative, ongoing assessment of goal selection, progress, and teaching methods, as well as sensitivity to collateral issues that can arise. Increased social interaction, for instance, can lead to not only positive interactions but also negative ones, such as hostility or bullying. Thus, clinicians must always be planning "a few steps ahead" for both planned and unplanned impact of the ongoing development of simple to complex social interaction repertoires.

References

American Psychiatric Association. (2013). *Diagnostic and statistical manual of mental disorders* (5th ed.). Arlington, VA: American Psychiatric Publishing.

Arick, J., Loos, L., Falco, R., & Krug, D. (2004). *Star program: Strategies for teaching based on autism research*. Austin, Texas: Pro-Ed.

Arick, J. R., Young, H. E., Falco, R. A., Loos, L. M., Krug, D. A., Gense, M. H., & Johnson, S. B. (2003). Designing an outcome study to monitor the progress of students with autism spectrum disorders. *Focus on Autism and other Developmental Disabilities, 18*(2), 75–87.

Argyle, M., & Kendon, A. (1967). The experimental analysis of social performance. In L. Berkowitz (Ed.), *Advances in experimental social psychology*. New York, NY: Academic Press.

Bacon, E. C., Dufek, S., Schreibman, L., Stahmer, A. C., Pierce, K., & Courchesne, E. (2014). Measuring outcome in an early intervention program for toddlers with autism spectrum disorder: Use of a curriculum-based assessment. *Autism Research and Treatment, 2014*, 964704. doi:10.1155/2014/964704

Bagnato, S. J., & Murphy, J. P. (1989). Validity of curriculum-based scales with young neurodevelopmentally disabled children: Implicates for team assessment. *Early Education and Development, 1*(1), 50–63.

Baron, R. A. (2000). Psychological perspectives on entrepreneurship: Cognitive and social factors in entrepreneurs success. *Current Directions in Psychological Science, 9*, 15–18.

Baron-Cohen, S. (1995). *Mindblindness: An essay on autism and theory of mind*. Cambridge, MA. London: The MIT Press.

Bottini, S. (2016). *A systematic review of the experimental analysis of social reward processing in individuals with autism spectrum disorder (unpublished manuscript)*. Binghamton, New York: Binghamton University.

Belcher, H. M. E., Butz, A. M., Wallace, P., Hoon, A. H., Reinhardt, E., Reeves, S. A., & Pulsifer, M. B. (2005). Spectrum of early intervention services for children with intrauterine drug exposure. *Infants & Young Children, 18*(1), 2–15.

Bloh, C. (2008). Assessing transfer of stimulus control procedures across learners with autism. *The Analysis of Verbal Behavior, 24*, 87–101.

Bricker, D., Capt, B., & Pretti-Frontczak, K. (2002). AEPS assessment, evaluation, and programming system for infants and children. In *Volume 2 test birth to three years and three to six years* (2nd ed.). Baltimore, MD: Brookes Publishing.

Bricker, D., Clifford, J., Yovanoff, P., Pretti-Frontczak, K., Waddell, M., Allen, D., & Hoselton, R. (2008). Eligibility determination using a curriculum-based assessment: A further examination. *Journal of Early Intervention, 31*(1), 3–21. doi:10.1177/1053815108324422

Bricker, D., Yovanoff, P., Capt, B., & Allen, D. (2003). Use of a curriculum-based measure to corroborate eligibility decisions. *Journal of Early Intervention, 26*(1), 20–30. doi:10.1177/105381510302600102

Bruno, J. L., Garrett, A. S., Quintin, E. M., Mazaika, P. K., & Reiss, A. L. (2014). Aberrant face and gaze habituation in fragile x syndrome. *American Journal of Psychiatry, 171*(10), 1099–1106.

Castro, S., Pinto, A. I., & Maia, M. (2011). Linking the Carolina curriculum for preschoolers with special needs to the ICF-CY. *The British Journal of Developmental Disabilities, 57*(113), 133–146. doi:10.1179/096979511798967043

Chevallier, C., Kohls, G., Troiani, V., Brodkin, E. S., & Schultz, R. T. (2012). The social motivation theory of autism. *Trends in Cognitive Sciences, 16*(4), 231–239.

Cohen, S. (2001). Do-watch-listen-say: Social and communication intervention for children with autism. *Journal of the Association for Persons with Severe Handicaps, 26*(2), 127–131.

Cohen, I. L., Fisch, G. S., Sudhalter, V., Wolf-Schein, E. G., Hanson, D., Hagerman, R., … Brown WT. (1988). Social gaze, social avoidance, and repetitive behavior in fragile X males: A controlled study. *American Journal of Mental Retardation, 92*(5), 436–446.

Coplan, J., & Jawad, A. F. (2005). Modeling clinical outcome of children with autistic spectrum disorders. *Pediatrics, 116*(1), 117–122.

Crick, N. R., & Dodge, K. A. (1994). A review and reformulation of social information-processing mechanisms in children's social adjustment. *Psychological Bulletin, 115*, 74–101.

Dawson, G., Jones, E. J. H., Merkle, K., Venema, K., Lowy, R., Faja, S., … Webb, S. J. (2012). Early behavioral intervention is associated with normalized brain activity in young children with autism. *Journal of the American Academy of Child and Adolescent Psychiatry, 51*(11), 1150–1159. doi:10.1016/j.jaac.2012.08.018

Dawson, G., Rogers, S., Munson, J., Smith, M., Winter, J., Greenson, J., … Varley, J. (2010). Randomized, controlled trial of an intervention for toddlers with autism: The early start denver model. *Pediatrics, 125*(1), e17–e23. doi:10.1542/peds.2009.0958

Del Giudice, E., Titomanlio, L., Brogna, G., Bonaccorso, A., Romano, A., Mansi, G … Andria, G. (2006). Early intervention for children with down syndrome in southern Italy: The role of parent-implemented developmental training. *Infants and Young Children, 19*(1), 50–58. doi:10.1097/00001163-200601000-00006

Deno, S. L. (1985). Curriculum-based measurement: The emerging alternative. *Exceptional Children, 52*, 219–232.

Deno, S. L. (1987). Curriculum-based measurement. *Teaching Exceptional Children, 20*(1), 40–42.

Deno, S. L., & Mirkin, P. K. (1977). *Data-based program modification: A manual*. Reston, VA: Council for Exceptional Children.

Deno, S. L., & Fuchs, L. S. (1987). Developing curriculum-based measurement systems for data-based special education problem solving. *Focus on Exceptional Children, 19*(8), 1–16.

Dickson, C. A., MacDonald, R. P. F., Mansfield, R., Guilhardi, P., Johnson, C., & Ahearn, W. H. (2014). Social validation of the New England center for children-core skills assessment. *Journal of Autism and Developmental Disorders, 44*, 65–74. doi:10.1007/s10803-013-1852-5

Dixon, M. R., Belisle, J., Stanley, C., Rowsey, K., Daar, J. H., & Szekely, S. (2015). Toward a behavior analysis of complex language for children with autism: Evaluating the relationship between PEAK and the VB-MAPP. *Journal of Developmental and Physical Disabilities, 27*, 223–233.

Dixon, D. R., Tarbox, J., Najdowski, A. C., Wilke, A. E., & Granpeesheh, D. (2011). A comprehensive evaluation of language for early behavioral intervention programs: The reliability of the SKILLS language index. *Research in Autism Spectrum Disorders, 5*, 506–511. doi:10.1016/j.rasd.2010.06.016

Dodge, K. A., & Murphy, R. R. (1984). The assessment of social competence in adolescents. *Advances in Child Behavior Analysis and Therapy, 3*, 61–96.

Eagle, R., Romanczyk, R. G., & Lenzenweger, M. (2010). Classification of children with autism Spectrum disorders: A finite mixture modeling approach to heterogeneity. *Research in Autism Spectrum Disorders, 4*(4), 772–781. doi:10.1016/j.rasd.2010.02.001

Eden Faculty. (2010). *Eden Autism Assessment and Curriculum Series*. Retrieved from http://edenautism.org/for-educators/services/%20eden-autism-assessment-and-curriculum-series/

Ellis, J. T., & Almeida, C. (2015a). *Socially savvy: An assessment and curriculum guide for young children*. New York, NY: DRL Books.

Ellis, J. T. & Almeida, C. (2015b, May). *Socially savvy: An assessment and curriculum guide for young children*. Workshop offered at the 41st annual meeting of the Association for Behavioral Analysis International.

Ferster, C. B. (1961). Positive reinforcement and behavioral deficits of autistic children. *Child Development, 32*, 437–456.

French, B. F. (2013). *Brigance Inventory of Early Development (IED III)*. North Billerica, MA: Curriculum Associates LLC.

Fuchs, L. S., & Deno, S. L. (1991). Paradigmatic distinctions between instructionally useful measurement. *Exceptional Children, 57*, 488–501.

Gould, E., Dixon, D. R., Najdowski, A. C., Smith, M. N., & Tarbox, J. (2011). A review of assessments for determining the content of early intensive behavioral intervention programs for autism spectrum disorders. *Research in Autism Spectrum Disorders, 5*, 990–1002. doi:10.1016/j.rasd.2011.01.012

Greer, R. D., & McKorkle, N. (2003). *Preschool Inventory of Repertoire for Kindergarten (PIRK)* (vol. Yonkers, NY). CABAS and the Fred S Keller School.

Johnson-Martin, N. M., Attermeier, S. M., & Hacker, B. J. (2004). *The Carolina curriculum for infants and toddlers with special needs (CCITSN)* (3rd ed.). Baltimore, MD: Brookes Publishing.

Johnson-Martin, N. M., Hacker, B. J., & Attermeier, S. M. (2004). *The Carolina curriculum for preschoolers with special needs (CCPSN)* (2nd ed.). Baltimore, MD: Brookes Publishing.

Jones, E. D., Southern, W. T., & Brigham, F. J. (1998). Curriculum-based assessment: Testing what is taught and teaching what is tested. *Intervention in School and Clinic, 33*(4), 239–249.

Kanner, L. (1943). Autistic disturbances of affective contact. *The Nervous Child, 2*, 217–250.

Knobloch, H., Stevens, F., & Malone, A. F. (1980). *The Gesell developmental schedules-revised, manual of developmental diagnosis*. New York, NY: Harper and Row.

Lambert-Lee, K. A., Jones, R., O'Sullivan, J., Hastings, R. P., Douglas-Cobane, E., Thomas, J. E., … Griffith, G. (2015). Translating evidence-based practice into a comprehensive educational model within an autism-specific special school. *British Journal of Special Education, 42*(1), 69–86. doi:10.1111/1467-8578.12090

Lee, C., Su, C., Chiang, F., Chen, Y., Hsieh, C., & Fu, C. (2016). Developing a short form of the psychoeducational profile-third edition for children with autism spectrum disorder. *Research in Autism Spectrum Disorders, 21*, 37–50. doi:10.1016/j.rasd.2015.09.008

Lin, F.-Y., & Kubina, R. M., Jr. (2004). Learning channels and verbal behavior. *The Behavior Analyst Today, 5*(1), 1–14.

Mandell, D. S., Stahmer, A. C., Shin, S., Xie, M., Reisinger, E., & Marcus, S. C. (2013). The role of treatment fidelity on outcomes during a randomized field trial of an autism intervention. *Autism, 17*(3), 281–295. doi:10.1177/1362361312473666

McGarrell, M., Healy, O., Leader, G., O'Connor, J., & Kenny, N. (2009). Six reports of children with autism spectrum disorder following intensive behavioral intervention using the preschool inventory of repertoires for kindergarten (PIRK). *Research in Autism Spectrum Disorders, 3*, 767–782. doi:10.1016/j.rasd.2009.02.006

McFall, R. M. (1982). A review and reformulation of the concept of social skills. *Behavioral Assessment, 4*, 1–33.

Najdowski, A. C., Gould, E. R., Lanagan, T. M., & Bishop, M. R. (2014). Designing curriculum programs for children with autism. In J. Tarbox, D. R. Dixon, P. Sturmey, & J. L. Matson (Eds.), *Handbook of early intervention for autism spectrum disorders: Research, policy, and practice* (pp. 227–259). New York, NY: Springer.

National Autism Center. (2009). *Findings and conclusions: National standards project, phase 1*. Randolph, MA: Author.

National Autism Center. (2015). *Findings and conclusions: National standards project, phase 2*. Randolph, MA: Author.

Notari, A. R., & Bricker, D. D. (1990). The utility of using a curriculum-based assessment instrument in the development of individualized education plans for infants and young children. *Journal of Early Intervention, 14*, 117–132.

Partington, J. W. (2006). *Assessment of Basic Language and Learning Skills-Revised (The ABLLS-R): An assessment, curriculum guide, and skills tracking system for children with autism or other developmental disabilities*. Pleasant Hill, CA: Behavior Analysts Inc..

Pellecchia, M., Connell, J. E., Beidas, R. S., Xie, M., Marcus, S. C., & Mandell, D. S. (2015). Dismantling the active ingredients of an intervention for children with autism. *Journal of Autism and Developmental Disorders, 45*, 2917–2927. doi:10.1007/s10803-015-2455-0

Persicke, A., Bishop, M. R., Coffman, C. M., Najdowski, A. C., Tarbox, J., Chi, K., … Deering, A. (2014). Evaluation of the concurrent validity of a skills assessment for autism treatment. *Research in Autism Spectrum Disorders, 8*, 281–285. doi:10.1016/j.rasd.2013.12.011

POWER-Solving, LLC (2016). *POWER-solving: Stepping stones to solving life's everyday social problems*. Retrieved from http://power-solving.com

Pretti-Frontczak, K., & Bricker, D. (2000). Enhancing the quality of individualized education plan (IEP) goals and objectives. *Journal of Early Intervention, 23*, 92–105.

Pritchard, J. K. (2013). Skills™. *Behavior Analysis in Practice, 6*(1), 1–6.

Prizant, B. M., Wetherby, A. M., Rubin, E., Laurent, A. C., & Rydell, P. J. (2006). *The SCERTS model: A comprehensive educational approach for children with autism spectrum disorders* (Vol. 1). Baltimore, MD: Brookes Publishing.

Quill, K. A. (2000). *DO-WATCH-LISTEN-SAY: Social and communication intervention for children with autism*. Baltimore, MD: Paul H. Brookes Publishing Company.

Rogers, S. J., & Dawson, G. (2010). *Early start Denver model for young children with ASD: Promoting language, learning, and engagement*. New York, NY: Guilford Press.

Rogers, S. J., Herbison, J., Lewis, H., Pantone, J., & Reis, K. (1986). An approach for enhancing the symbolic, communicative, and interpersonal functioning of young children with autism and severe emotional handicaps. *Journal of the Division of Early Childhood, 10*, 135–148.

Rogers, S. J., Estes, A., Lord, C., Vismara, L., Winter, J., Fitzpatrick, A … & Dawson, G. (2012). Effects of a brief early start Denver model (ESDM)-based parent intervention on toddlers at risk for autism spectrum disorders: A randomized controlled trial. *Journal of the American Academy of Child & Adolescent Psychiatry, 51*(10), 1052–1065. doi:10.1016/j.jaac.2012.08.003.

Romanczyk, R. G., White, S., & Gillis, J. M. (2005). Social skills vs skilled social behavior: A problematic distinction in autism spectrum disorders. *Journal of Early and Intensive Behavioral Intervention, 2*(3), 177–193.

Rubin, E., & Laurent, A. C. (2004). Implementing a curriculum-based assessment to prioritize learning objectives in asperger syndrome and high-functioning autism. *Topics in Language Disorders, 24*(4), 298–315.

Sayers, L. K., Cowden, J. E., Newton, M., Warren, B., & Eason, B. (1996). Qualitative analysis of a pediatric strength intervention on the developmental stepping movements of infants with down syndrome. *Adapted Physical Activity Quarterly, 13*, 247–268.

Schopler, E., Lansing, M. D., Reichler, R. J., & Marcus, L. M. (2005). *Psychoeducational profile: TEACCH individualized psychoeducational assessment for children with autism spectrum disorders* (3rd ed.). Austin, TX: Pro-Ed.

Segrin, C. (2000). Social skill deficits associated with depression. *Clinical Psychology Review, 20*, 379–403.

Sharma, P., Heywood, A., & Rajkumar, D. (2010). Brief report: IBI training: Social and play skills upon entry as predictors of outcome in children with autism spectrum disorder. *Journal on Developmental Disabilities, 16*(3), 76–77.

Shinn, M. (2008). Best practices for using curriculum based measurement in a problem solving model. In B. Irby, G. Brown, R. Lara-Alecio, & S. Jackson (Eds.), *The handbook of educational theories* (pp. 783–792). Charlotee, NC: Information Age Publishing.

Shinn, M. (2013). Curriculum-based measurement. In A. Thomas & J. Grimes (Eds.), *Best practices in school psychology IV* (pp. 243–262). Bethesda, MD: National Association of School Psychologists.

Skills Global LLC (2016). *Skills solutions for behavioral health.* Retrieved from https://www.skillsforautism.com

Skinner, B. F. (1957). *Verbal behavior.* New York, NY: Appleton-Century-Crofts.

Sundberg, M. L. (2008). *Verbal behavior milestones assessment and placement program-guide.* Concord, CA: AVB Press.

Sundberg, M. L., & Sundberg, C. A. (2011). Intraverbal behavior and verbal conditional discriminations in typically developing children and children with autism. *The Analysis of Verbal Behavior, 27*, 23–43.

STAR Autism Support (2013–2016). *STAR autism support.* Retrieved from http://starautismsupport.com

The New England Center for Children: Autism Education and Research (2017). About the ACE: Customizable curriculum. Retrieved from http://www.acenecc.org/about-the-ace/

Vismara, L. A., Young, G. S., & Rogers, S. J. (2013). Community dissemination of the early start Denver model: Implications for science and practice. *Topics in Early Childhood Special Education, 32*(4), 223–233. doi:10.1177/0271121411409250

Vivani, G., Paynter, J., Duncan, E., Fothergill, H., Dissanayake, C., & Rogers, S. J. (2014). Effectiveness and feasibility of the early start Denver model implemented in a group-based community childcare setting. *Journal of Autism and Developmental Disorders, 44*(12), 3140–3153. doi:10.1007/s10803-014-2168-9

VORT Corporation (2005–2016). Hawaii early learning profile. Retrieved from: http://www.vort.com/

VORT Corporation (2015–2016). BCP: Birth-14 years (behavioral characteristics progression). Retrieved from: http://www.vort.com/BCP-Birth-14-years-Behavioral-Characteristics-Progression/

Waddington, E. M., & Reed, P. (2009). The impact of using the "preschool inventory of repertoires for kindergarten" (PIRK) on school outcomes of children with autism spectrum disorders. *Research in Autism Spectrum Disorders, 3*, 809–827. doi:10.1016/j.rasd.2009.03.002

Warshaw, S. P. (2006). *Inside HELP: Administrative and reference manual for HELP (the Hawaii early learning profile) birth - 3 years.* Retrieved from http://www.vort.com/Inside-HELP.html

Wheat, J., & Baker, T. (2010). *HELP 3-6 Assessment Manual (2nd Ed.).* Teaford, P. (Ed.). Retrieved from http://www.vort.com/HELP-3-6-Assessment-Manual-2nd-Ed.html

Wolery, M., & Winterling, V. (1997). Curricular approaches to controlling severe behavior problems. In N. N. Singh (Ed.), *Prevention and treatment of severe behavior problems: Models and methods in developmental disabilities* (pp. 87–120). Pacific Grove, CA: Brooks/Cole.

World Health Organization (2007). *International Classification of Functioning, Disability, and Health-Version for Children and Youth: ICF-CY.* WHO Workgroup for Development of Version of ICF for Children and Youth.

Part III

Social Skills Interventions

Evidence-Based Interventions

9

Florence D. DiGennaro Reed, Matthew D. Novak, Amy J. Henley, Denys Brand, and Mary E. McDonald

Our everyday lives contain numerous examples of the pursuit of quick fixes and fad treatments lacking objective research to support their use. Recently, the 2016 summer Olympics featured athletes who practice cupping, an inexpensive treatment that promotes blood flow by pulling the skin away from the body using suction cups. The bodies of swimmers, gymnasts, and other athletes contained circular bruising, which sparked dozens of hours of media coverage and Internet stories promoting this "healing" practice (e.g., Axon, 2016). Athletes are not the only victims of these types of unsubstantiated practices. Readers of this book have likely fallen prey to clever marketing schemes and anecdotes promulgating a particular intervention.

We suspect many readers have attempted a new weight-loss strategy or wellness fad promising improved health and well-being without carefully examining the evidence supporting claims of its effectiveness. For example, in 2013 the cotton ball diet gained popularity on the Internet and attracted the attention of adolescent and teen girls (Neporent, 2013). The goal of the diet is to curb hunger and subsequently reduce food intake by consuming several cotton balls soaked in juice before eating. Unfortunately, the diet is associated with life-threatening health risks, such as choking, malnutrition, intestinal blockages and obstruction, and toxicity resulting from processing chemicals including bleach (Schaefer, 2015). Despite limited evidence of effectiveness and the possibility of great harm, females across the country pursued this weight-loss strategy.

Examples of unsubstantiated weight-loss products, exercise regimens, medical treatments, and other interventions abound. The Internet is saturated with anecdotal stories of effectiveness and other false claims, which make it challenging to separate legitimate treatment options from offerings by "snake oil salesmen." Humans are not immune to their effects. This phenomenon is often found in resources for autism treatment as well. In fact, Romanczyk, Gillis, White, and DiGennaro (2008) identified 414 interventions listed on 16 frequently visited websites that share information about autism. The interventions were varied, including biological, educational, psychological, experiential, and combinational approaches. Despite this variety, only a small number met criteria to be rated as having strong ($n = 2$) or moderate ($n = 7$; 5 of which were center-based programs and not interventions per se) support and many popular treatments continue to lack evidence of effectiveness or show evidence of harming treatment recipients.

F.D. DiGennaro Reed (✉) • M.D. Novak • A.J. Henley • D. Brand
Department of Applied Behavioral Science, University of Kansas, Lawrence, KS, USA
e-mail: fdreed@ku.edu

M.E. McDonald
Department of Specialized Programs in Education, Hofstra University, Hempstead, NY, USA

J.B. Leaf (ed.), *Handbook of Social Skills and Autism Spectrum Disorder*, Autism and Child Psychopathology Series, DOI 10.1007/978-3-319-62995-7_9

Table 9.1 Red flags checklist for identifying pseudoscience

Red Flags	Applicable?
High "success" rates are claimed.	
Rapid effects are promised.	
The intervention is said to be effective for many symptoms or disorders.	
The "theory" behind the intervention contradicts objective knowledge (and sometimes common sense).	
An overuse of ad hoc hypotheses designed to immunize claims from falsification.	
The intervention is said to be easy to administer, requiring little training or expertise.	
Other proven treatments are said to be unnecessary, inferior, or harmful.	
Promoters of the intervention are working outside of their area of expertise.	
Promoters benefit financially or otherwise from adoption of the treatment.	
Testimonials, anecdotes, or personal accounts are offered in support of claims about the intervention's effectiveness, but little or no objective evidence is provided.	
Obscurist language is used and prevents consumers from understanding.	
Catchy, emotionally appealing slogans are used in marketing the treatment.	
Belief and faith are said to be necessary for the intervention to "work."	
Skepticism and critical evaluation are said to make the intervention's effects evaporate.	
Promoters resist objective evaluation or scrutiny of the treatment by others.	
Negative findings from scientific studies are ignored or dismissed.	
There is a reversed burden of proof required.	
There is evasion of peer review.	
There is an absence of self-correction.	
Critics and scientific investigators are often met with hostility, and are accused of persecuting the promoters, being "close-minded," or having some ulterior motive for "debunking" the treatment.	

Note. Content adapted from Lilienfeld, Lynn, and Lohr (2003) and Association for Science in Autism Treatment (1999).

Why are some parents of individuals with autism and their service providers attracted to unsubstantiated interventions? Romanczyk and Gillis (2004) describe seven strategies parents often use to assist them in their decision making, which may also apply to practitioners:

- *They know what's best*: Place trust in a service provider and defer to his or her judgment.
- *Hedge your bets:* Seek several options simultaneously in the hopes a treatment package will be effective.
- *Fanatical focus:* Pursue a single course with overwhelming intensity and focus.
- *Hope for the best:* Forgo formal treatment and participate in typical activities that are available.
- *Cure du jour:* Pursue new treatments as they appear and drop the current program.
- *A friend told me:* Implement treatments that appeared to work for the child of someone they know or about whom they have read.
- *Guru selection:* Follow and believe in a single, specific "expert."

Recognizing that these potentially flawed decision-making strategies may be adopted, both parents and professionals must be aware of the warning signs of interventions promulgated by service providers or treatment agents. The use of a checklist may be helpful when faced with the myriad of interventions that exist for individuals with autism to help parents identify warning signs of pseudoscience. As such, Table 9.1 summarizes a number of red flags that should be contemplated when considering a new intervention.

9.1 Different Approaches to Understanding Phenomena

Approaches to understanding phenomena can be broadly classified as science, pseudoscience, and antiscience (Green & Perry, 1999). *Science* is a systematic approach by which we come to understand the causes underlying various phenomena (Cooper, Heron, & Heward, 2007) and operates on the assumption of determinism. Determinism is a philosophical position that holds that the universe is orderly and events do not occur at random, but are related in a lawful and systematic way to other events. Science allows us to uncover and understand the lawful and orderly relations between events through the process of observation and experimentation (Spata, 2003).

From a scientific perspective, knowledge about how the natural world works is gained through the application of the scientific method (Singleton, Straits, & Straits, 1993). Generally, the scientific method begins by proposing a hypothesis about the relationship between two or more events. To test the hypothesis, one or more experiments are conducted to produce data that either support or contradict the hypothesis (Cozby, 1997). To provide a believable demonstration of a lawful relation between events, experiments must consist of clearly defined dependent and independent variables that are measured objectively, accurately, and reliably (Green & Perry, 1999). Moreover, experiments must be conducted with a high degree of control, which is achieved through strong research designs that ensure study procedures rule out the effects of extraneous variables, thereby demonstrating a functional relation. The independent replication of results is also an important feature of the scientific method (Johnston & Pennypacker, 2009). Thus, scientific understanding of phenomena is based on an *accumulated* body of evidence produced using the scientific method. We advocate that science should be the foundation on which treatments for people with autism are based (Green & Perry, 1999).

In contrast to a scientific understanding of phenomena, *pseudoscience* attempts to make claims, beliefs, speculations, and untested assumptions *appear* scientific despite a lack of evidence to support them (Green & Perry, 1999; Shermer, 2002). Commonly used methods of promoting pseudoscience include making grandiose claims without empirical support, a reliance on anecdotes and testimonials as the main sources of evidence, avoiding the peer-review process that accompanies publishing in scientific journals, using scientific jargon, and a tendency to promote relevant materials in newsletters, books, and on the Internet (Normand, 2008; Travers, Ayers, Simpson, & Crutchfield, 2016). Pseudoscience is further characterized by errors in critical thinking and invalid logic (Travers, Tincani, & Lang, 2014). Promoters of pseudoscience rely on several errors in thinking and reasoning to communicate their message. For example, the straw man fallacy consists of misrepresenting the arguments of people who do not support the pseudoscientific claim and using the misrepresentations to attack opponents (Travers et al., 2016). Another error, shifting the burden of proof, requires individuals who doubt a claim to provide the proof of their doubt (Travers et al., 2016). Additionally, promoters may engage in confirmation bias (i.e., only paying attention to information that supports their own arguments and beliefs) and the ad hoc fallacy (i.e., a rationale for a particular claim is changed in the face of evidence to the contrary in an effort to maintain beliefs; McNally, 2003; Travers et al., 2016).

Unfortunately, for a variety of reasons, the field of autism is rife with treatment procedures that amount to little more than pseudoscience. Applying pseudoscientific interventions and procedures must be avoided because it diverts valuable time and resources from scientifically validated treatments (Horner et al., 2005; Lerman et al., 2008). In extreme cases, the application of interventions and procedures based on pseudoscience has been associated with significant harm, including death. For example, Baxter and Krenzelok (2008) reported a case in which a 5-year-old boy with autism went into cardiac arrest and later died after being given the wrong chelating agent by a physician during chelation therapy (an unproven procedure for treating autism that involves removing lead and various other heavy metals from the bloodstream through the injection of chelating agents).

Antiscience is the outright rejection of objective scientific data in favor of subjective personal beliefs or ideologies (Green & Perry, 1999). Promotors of antiscience rely on many of the same tactics as promotors of pseudoscience. A prime example of antiscience in the field of autism is facilitated communication (Biklen, 1992). Facilitated communication involves a facilitator assisting an individual—often with limited independent communication skills—to type messages with a keyboard. A facilitator may provide hand-over-hand guidance by physically moving the hand of an individual toward or away from the keyboard so the individual can communicate his or her message. Advocates of facilitated communication believe it works by unlocking an individual's hidden and intact writing and communication abilities to enable genuine self-expression (Travers et al., 2016).

However, a large body of objective and empirically based scientific research, conducted over many years, has provided overwhelming evidence showing the *facilitator* authors the message (Jacobson, Mulick, & Schwartz, 1995; McDonald, Pace, Blue, & Schwartz, 2012; Mostert, 2001, 2010; Romanczyk, Arnstein, Soorya, & Gillis, 2003). Despite the overwhelming amount of scientific evidence documenting facilitated communication as an ineffective treatment option for individuals with autism, its usefulness as an effective treatment is still being promoted by facilitated communication advocates whose arguments are centered around anecdotal evidence and data produced from flawed research designs (Mostert, 2010). Given the lack of scientific evidence to support facilitated communication as a viable treatment, some authors have attempted to provide alternative explanations for facilitated communication, including spirituality (e.g., Bilu & Goodman, 1997) and questioning what it means to have a disability (e.g., Biklen & Kliewer, 2006). Thus, continued practice of facilitated communication, despite the overwhelming amount of scientific evidence to the contrary, can be considered an antiscientific approach to treatment. As is the case with pseudoscience, treatments based on antiscience can produce great harm to clients and their families or caregivers, and should be avoided at all cost.

9.2 Distinguishing Empirical Evidence and Evidence-Based Practice

Empirical evidence refers to the collective body of knowledge gained through the process of observation and experimentation and serves the purpose of providing support for or against hypotheses or theories (Spata, 2003). Evidence-based practice (EBP) is a term used to describe the process of using results from high-quality research to inform clinical practice, while also taking into consideration clinical experience and expertise, and the individual characteristics, culture, and preferences of a client (Lilienfeld, Ritschel, Lynn, Cautin, & Latzman, 2014; Odom, Collet-Klingenberg, Rogers, & Hatton, 2010). For practitioners to identify EBPs, they must be knowledgeable of the empirical evidence regarding efficacy and effectiveness of treatments and procedures to determine whether enough empirical evidence exists to classify them as evidence based (Rogers, 1998). Being familiar with the empirical evidence can help practitioners distinguish between treatments that are evidence based (e.g., discrete-trial teaching; Lovaas, 1987), and those that are not (e.g., facilitated communication; Biklen, 1992).

9.2.1 Why Is EBP Important?

Use of the term EBP has become increasingly popular in recent years, which may be due to a heightened emphasis among practitioners and consumers attempting to identify "what works" in clinical service delivery (DiGennaro Reed & Reed, 2008; Maffei-Almodovar & Sturmey, 2013; Nathan & Gorman, 2015; Roth & Fonagy, 2004). Moreover, professional service providers across many disciplines are often called upon to document the effectiveness of their practice by demonstrating how their practice produces desired outcomes relative to alternative treatment options, and at what cost. Evidence-based practice guidelines were developed to help practitioners and parents make informed, unbiased decisions that will lead to desired outcomes for individuals served (New York State Department of Health Early Intervention Program, 1999). These guidelines may also serve to provide a general outline of different treatments and their empirical support.

Many professional agencies (e.g., Behavior Analyst Certification Board®, Inc. [BACB®], National Association of School Psychologists) recognize the importance of EBP and dictate the use of EBP in their professional and ethical guidelines. The *Professional and Ethical Compliance Code for Behavior Analysts* states that behavior analysts should "rely on professionally derived knowledge based on science and behavior analysis" (BACB®, 2016a, Section 1.01) and "have the responsibility to recommend scientifically supported, most-effective treatment procedures" (BACB®, 2016a, Section 2.09). Similarly, the National Association of School Psychologists' *Principles for Professional Ethics* states that school psychologists should provide services that "the profession considers to be responsible, research-based practice" (NASP, 2010, Principle II.3.2). Through these regulations, professional agencies attempt to ensure their members provide the best possible treatment, which ultimately produces meaningful long-term outcomes for service recipients.

Federal and state governments use information about EBP when determining how to allocate funding, which further underscores the importance of relying on evidence to inform treatment decisions. Recent federal acts have placed an emphasis on the use of EBP in identifying and implementing educational programs (e.g., Individuals with Disabilities Education Act of 2004; Every Student Succeeds Act of 2015). Notably, the Every Student Succeeds Act of 2015 is among the first pieces of federal legislation on education to specifically use the term "evidence-based practice." Additionally, in 2012, the U.S. Office of Management and Budget issued a memorandum instructing department heads of federal agencies to consider evidence of effectiveness when evaluating programs and awarding funds (Zients, 2012).

9.2.2 Definition of EBP

Several independent groups and researchers have worked to develop a definition of EBP (e.g., American Psychological Association [APA], 2005; American Psychological Association Presidential Task Force of Evidence-Based Practice, 2006; American Speech-Language Hearing Association, 2005; Horner et al., 2005; Slocum et al., 2014) and, although no standard definition has been adopted, most definitions contain the same core components. Generally, most definitions state that a practice is evidence-based if it incorporates (a) use of the best-available research evidence, (b) clinical expertise on the part of the practitioner, and (c) client values and contextual factors of the situation.

9.2.2.1 Best-Available Research Evidence

Just as several groups have attempted to define EBP, there has been mixed discussion for what exactly comprises an empirically supported treatment (Chambless et al., 1998; Horner et al., 2005; National Autism Center, 2009; New York State Department of Health Early Intervention Program, 1999; Tweed, Connolly, & Beaulieu, 2009). One set of criteria offered by Horner et al. (2005) focused on describing methods for evaluating single-case research designs. Specifically, the criteria are: (a) the procedure is operationally defined, (b) the context for use is specifically defined, (c) the procedure is implemented with fidelity, (d) results must be functionally related to changes in the independent variable, and (e) results have been replicated by at least five studies conducted by three different research teams across three locations, with a minimum of 20 participants. These criteria provide a means by which consumers of scientific literature may evaluate a study's procedures and how the results may or may not align with previous findings from the same procedure.

9.2.2.2 Reviews of the Literature

Several organizations have reviewed various practices and evaluated their strength of evidence according to a predefined standard.

Generally, interventions are evaluated based on their quality or the quantity of research support and then categorized along a spectrum ranging from those practices with established support to practices with limited support. A report by the APA Division 12 Task Force on Psychological Interventions (Chambless et al., 1998) provided specific criteria for each category. The APA task force determined that a "well-established" treatment must contain treatment manuals, list relevant participant characteristics, be conducted by at least two different research teams, and have either two experiments conducted as between-group randomized control trials or nine experiments conducted as single-case research designs. Practices that do not meet these criteria may still be labeled as "probably efficacious" if they list participant characteristics, are conducted by two different research teams, and have either two randomized control trials or three single-case research designs. Some organizations (e.g., Maine Department of Health and Human Services, National Autism Center) have also distinguished between those practices that have insufficient evidence to form a conclusion from those that have evidence suggesting they may harm or produce no effect.

For example, a review by the Maine Department of Health and Human Services (i.e., Tweed et al., 2009) evaluated 11 studies that used the principles of applied behavior analysis (ABA) to address social skills with children with autism. The review committee found eight of the studies had strong or adequate research evidence, which met the criteria to conclude that the use of ABA for social skills is an established practice. In another review of the literature, the National Autism Center published results of its National Standards Project, which synthesized the strength of evidence supporting educational and behavioral interventions for children and adults with autism in two reports (National Autism Center, 2009, 2015). Across both reports, interventions based on the principles of ABA (e.g., comprehensive behavioral treatment, modeling) met criteria as established interventions.

The aforementioned reviews and their criteria describe what constitutes an *empirically supported treatment*; however, they do not sufficiently articulate what constitutes *EBP*. In addition to research evidence supporting a particular treatment or procedure, practitioners must also incorporate their clinical expertise and the values of a client and his or her family. That is, practitioners must make decisions on whether a treatment effectively addresses relevant treatment goals for a client.

9.2.2.3 Clinical Expertise

Practitioners must use their clinical expertise to integrate empirically supported treatments with the specific characteristics of their clients to produce services with the highest likelihood of success. Specifically, clinical expertise refers to a practitioner's level of competence and ability to evaluate and apply the scientific literature to produce effective client outcomes (Stricker & Trierweiler, 1995). This competence can take shape through several components, including: (a) assessment, diagnostic judgment, systematic case formulation, and treatment planning; (b) clinical decision making, treatment implementation, and monitoring of patient progress; (c) interpersonal expertise; (d) continual self-reflection and acquisition of skills; (e) appropriate evaluation and use of research evidence in both basic and applied science; (f) understanding the influence of individual and cultural differences on treatment; (g) seeking available resources, as needed; and (h) having a cogent rationale for clinical strategies (APA, 2005). Practitioners must use contextual information to inform decisions ranging from which treatment to implement, to whether they are adequately qualified to continue serving a client. Thus, the use of clinical expertise is a critical component of EBP because it requires that practitioners evaluate and understand aspects of providing treatment that extend beyond scientific findings alone.

9.2.2.4 Client Values and Context

The third and final component for EBP is the incorporation of any client-specific information which may influence the generality or maintenance of a treatment. Clinical interventions that are implemented without consideration of client-specific variables may be limited in the extent to which they produce meaningful long-term outcomes (Norcross, 2002). When preparing a treatment plan, practitioners should consider information about the client's preferences, goals, values, and religious or cultural practices, as well as contextual information such as age, developmental progress, academic skill level, and socioeconomic status. For example, a practitioner may be presented with a choice between two equally effective treatments for teaching a new skill. In deciding which treatment to implement, the practitioner should consider the client's current skill level while also engaging in discussion with caregivers and clients about their preferences. Furthermore, if the treatment relies on the use of positive reinforcers, then the practitioner should also conduct a stimulus preference and reinforcer assessment to ensure that functional reinforcers are being used.

9.3 Keeping Abreast of the Scientific Literature

In addition to accessing the reviews described previously, a number of other possible sources for contacting the literature are available. It is important to recognize, however, that practitioners face a number of barriers to keeping abreast of the scholarly literature. Carr and Briggs (2010) provide an excellent overview of several barriers to maintaining competence through frequent contact with the literature. More importantly, they provide suggestions for ameliorating these difficulties such that practitioners may more readily manage this important responsibility. One notable barrier involves searching the literature. Carr and Briggs recommend using a relatively more comprehensive search engine such as the ERIC database—for which the BACB® provides free access to certified individuals—rather than relying on databases that publishers frequently make available for searching within a specific journal. However, in this ever-changing world of technology and the Internet, we urge practitioners to consider several other important activities and resources, which we describe next.

9.3.1 The Search

A frequently daunting task—yet an essential prerequisite for contacting the literature—is conducting the search. Literature searches commonly yield hundreds or even thousands of results, many of which are irrelevant to the problem or question at hand. As noted by Carr and Briggs (2010), Google Scholar (https://scholar.google.com) is a powerful search engine for identifying relevant literature. Two features of Google Scholar are particularly beneficial. First, the *cited by* function returns a list of all articles that have cited a given publication. The *cited by* function may be especially helpful for practitioners who are familiar with a fundamental article on a topic of interest. For example, suppose Brian is a practitioner interested in functional analysis. Brian selects *cited by* for the seminal article on functional analysis by Iwata, Dorsey, Slifer, Bauman, and Richman (1982). His search returns 1084 articles related to functional analysis from which he may further restrict his search to include a specific publication timeframe (e.g., 2015–2016) and/or search for key terms within the results (e.g., self-injurious behavior), returning a manageable 36 results. The *cited by* feature can help reduce the required effort to search, facilitate identification of appropriate literature, and reduce the overall quantity of articles, including the number that have not been peer reviewed and irrelevant articles identified in search results. Second, Google Scholar provides a link to sources where an article can be accessed, discussed in more detail in the next section.

Numerous organizations provide access to up-to-date treatment summaries based on recent empirical research, which is an additional option for practitioners. For example, the Association for Science in Autism Treatment (www.asatonline.org) provides brief synopses of current research related to the treatment of autism. Treatment summaries may decrease the effort associated with conducting a literature search, thereby improving the efficiency with which practitioners identify articles. It is important to note, however, that treatment summaries are intended to provide a brief overview in a reader friendly format. As such, treatment summaries likely do not contain sufficient methodological detail to facilitate accurate implementation of a treatment with a service recipient; readers will likely need to consult the original article for use with a client.

Although posting to online forums (e.g., Facebook©) can provide useful information in a short timeframe, we strongly encourage readers to use caution when relying on information obtained from online forums for several reasons. First, when searching for treatment options for a client, it is difficult to strike the right balance regarding the type and quantity of client information to share. Responders without sufficient information about a client's history, environment, and target behavior may provide inappropriate or even harmful recommendations. Conversely, providing too much detail may violate ethical codes of conduct and an individual's right to privacy or confidentiality (Behavior Analyst Certification Board, 2016a; van Houten et al., 1988). Online forums can also make it difficult to evaluate the qualifications of individuals who respond to inquiries. However, we recognize that if the resources mentioned in this chapter have been exhausted, it may sometimes be necessary to consult online forums. When using online forums, we therefore recommend asking individuals for helpful resources (e.g., names of relevant experts or scholarly publications) from which you can consult as opposed to soliciting specific treatment advice.

9.3.2 Accessing Article Content

Another major barrier recognized by Carr and Briggs (2010) is the difficulty accessing content identified through a search. Many databases only provide access to article titles and abstracts, which do not provide sufficient detail to allow a practitioner to implement those procedures with a service recipient. Moreover, the costs associated with purchasing a single article or subscribing to a journal may prohibit practitioners from staying abreast of the scholarly literature. One noteworthy change since Carr and Briggs is the popularization of ResearchGate© (www.researchgate.net); a free social networking site for individuals to share their previous and ongoing research. ResearchGate© provides a platform for researchers to post publications, book chapters, conference posters, data sets, and more for members to freely access. Google Scholar search results provide a link to articles that are available on ResearchGate©; an integrated method for accessing articles identified through a literature search decreases the effort involved in contacting the literature. Nonetheless, not all of the research posted on ResearchGate© has undergone peer review and should be viewed with more skepticism than published research. Publishers may also restrict when content may be posted; thereby limiting the availability of up-to-date research.

Although they are relatively fewer in number, open access journals are another viable option for individuals who do not have access to paid journal subscriptions. Articles published in fully open access journals and journals that support open access (i.e., authors pay publication fees to provide open access for their article) are freely available to subscribers and the wider public with permitted reuse. Open access obviates financial barriers associated with accessing the literature; however, the effort required to find appropriate and sufficient behavior analytic research to keep abreast of the literature and inform practice may be high because of the relatively few behavior analytic journals supporting open access (e.g., *Research in Autism Spectrum Disorders*) or publication of behavior analytic work in open access journals. Alternatively, in November of 2016, the BACB® announced that it will be adding free subscriptions to several of the leading behavior analytic journals including: *Journal of Applied Behavior Analysis*, *Journal of the Experimental Analysis of Behavior*, and *Behavioral Interventions*, with more to come in subsequent years (Behavior Analyst Certification Board, 2016b). Lastly, authors are often willing to share their work via email if an interested reader contacts them.

9.4 Scientific Skepticism

After making contact with the literature using one or a combination of the methods previously described, it is important to evaluate an experiment's merit and the utility of identified studies for a given situation or purpose. Research is an evolving process and perfect experiments do not exist despite researchers' best efforts. Instead, researchers walk a fine line in which they must constantly balance practical and logistical constraints with experimental control. As a result, research varies widely in terms of methodological rigor. The compromises researchers make when designing an experiment may vary along a continuum with some experimental features being more critical to the validity of a study than others. In some situations, a number of relatively minor methodological weaknesses may render a study's results equally as questionable as one major methodological flaw (Herbert, 2000). Study evaluation is further complicated by the fact that experimental designs are intended to be flexible and adaptable to meet the needs of a particular research question rather than having a set of concrete rules for how to design an experiment (Johnston & Pennypacker, 2009). Therefore, demonstrating scientific skepticism and critical analysis is necessary when examining the merit of a study and attempting to discriminate methodologically rigorous studies from those with less convincing evidence. Although there are no hard-and-fast rules, we provide some considerations for evaluating a study's merit for readers (Table 9.2; for more information, see also Horner et al., 2005). Scientific skepticism is also necessary to ensure practitioners select the most effective and appropriate treatment or teaching procedure for a client. For example, practitioners should ask whether it is reasonable to generalize a study's findings to their current situation. It is important for practitioners to evaluate if a study is applicable to the setting (including the available supports to implement the plan), the function of the presenting problem, and whether the treatment or procedure is within the skillset of the interventionist, among others. Table 9.3 provides questions readers may ask when evaluating the appropriateness of published studies.

9.5 A Model for Addressing Implementation of Unsubstantiated Interventions

Even after ample consideration, parents or other service providers may decide to implement an unsubstantiated treatment. Under these circumstances, it is important to remain as objective as possible, advocate for the client, and assist the family and colleagues, all while adhering to ethical guidelines. Note that federal law requires students with disabilities to receive the support services that are necessary to allow them to benefit from their education (Heflin & Simpson, 1998). However, over the years the interventions or procedures that constitute "support services" has greatly expanded and may include pseudoscientific or antiscientific interventions, such as facilitated communication (Le Mars Community School District, 1992). These interventions are upheld in the court even when there may be no evidence to support the intervention or, in the case of facilitated communication, evidence documenting the intervention is not effective (Tostanoski, Lang, Raulston, Carnett & Davis, 2014).

Upon learning that a parent or colleague intends to implement an unsubstantiated treatment, an initial reaction may be to confront decision makers by telling them there is no evidence to support the intervention and it should not be used. However, a hasty or aggressive response that fails to consider their perspective or interests may not be the most effective way to assure the client receives appropriate treatment. Because it is recommended that professionals develop a set of guidelines to facilitate a decision-making process (Heflin & Simpson, 1998), we conclude the chapter by proposing a data-based decision-making model that can be implemented by partnering with parents and other professionals in the

Table 9.2 Questions to ask when evaluating published studies

Component	
Introduction	
Is the rationale reasonable and does it logically flow from the purpose of the study?	**Y/N**
Methods	
Were all study variables and procedures described clearly and with adequate detail for replication and/or implementation? (e.g., participants, participant selection, setting, apparatus, and/or study materials, independent and dependent variables, observation and recording procedures, procedures for measuring and quantifying reliability of the dependent *and* independent variables)	**Y/N**
Did the author(s) provide objective and specific operational definitions of all independent and dependent variables?	**Y/N**
Was the primary dependent variable observable and measurable behavior?	**Y/N**
Was only one independent variable manipulated at a time? If more than one variable was manipulated, did the author(s) recognize this and attribute behavioral change to the combinations of variables manipulated rather than one of the variables?	**Y/N**
Did the author(s) measure reliability of the dependent *and* independent variables for approximately or greater than 30% of observations in every condition?	**Y/N**
Was the level of reported reliability sufficient to allow confidence in appropriateness of definitions and procedures and a functional relation between independent and dependent variables?	**Y/N**
Was a contingent relation demonstrated between the independent and dependent variable(s)?	**Y/N**
Was experimental control demonstrated?	**Y/N**
Did the author(s) collect at least three baseline data points for each participant/behavior/setting?	**Y/N**
Were baseline data stable or trending in the direction opposite of the desired change prior to introduction of the independent variable?	**Y/N**
Was the sequence of conditions adequate to allow conclusions to be made about the effects of the independent variable(s)? Can sequential effects of conditions be eliminated as accounting for behavioral change?	**Y/N**
Were individuals responsible for data collection independent and/or blind to the experimental conditions? (i.e., did they have a vested interest in the study outcome)?	**Y/N**
Were precautions taken to minimize reactivity?	**Y/N**
Were independent variables implemented and dependent variables measured consistently across conditions?	**Y/N**
Multiple baseline: Were treatment effects replicated when reinstated or implemented across individuals, behaviors, or settings? Reversal: Did the behavior reverse to pre-intervention levels? Alternating treatments/multi-element: Is there clear differentiation in level between conditions?	**Y/N**
Results	
Were data presented graphically?	**Y/N**
Were data analysis techniques appropriate?	**Y/N**
Was the behavior of interest changed?	**Y/N**
Can plausible alternate accounts of the results be eliminated?	**Y/N**
Were idiosyncrasies in the data discussed?	**Y/N**
Were generalization data collected and reported?	**Y/N**

event an unsubstantiated intervention will be implemented. The purpose of the model is to set parameters for reasonable and informed decision making by both parents and professionals (Simpson, 1995) and should not be interpreted to mean that partnership implies agreement with intervention implementation. If the intervention is going to be implemented despite one's best efforts, this model allows for the application of data-based decision making for a client. The model includes the following components assuming consultation with parents and possibly clients or other service providers:

- *Informational meeting:* Meet with parents to learn about the intervention and expected outcomes. Often, parents may not know what the expected outcomes are and this is an opportu-

Table 9.3 Key questions for practitioners to ask regarding the appropriateness of intervention selection

Question	
Does this intervention address assessment results and the client's needs, desires, and strengths?	Y/N
Are there sufficient published research articles in peer-reviewed journals documenting the efficacy or effectiveness of the proposed intervention method?	Y/N
Does the current setting have the necessary resources to implement the intervention consistent with the procedures documented in the published studies?	Y/N
Is there any evidence of harm associated with this intervention? Have positive alternatives been exhausted? If yes, what are the risks? Is there adequate client protection?	Y/N
What position statements from respected professional organizations support or do not support the intervention?	Y/N
Are the intervention procedures consistent with professional guidelines and standards of practice in the interventionist's chosen field (e.g., Behavior Analyst Certification Board, American Psychological Association, National Association of School Psychologists, National Association for the Education of Young Children, Council for Exceptional Children)?	Y/N
What are the credentials of the interventionist? What kind of training and supervision would the interventionist need to have before implementing the intervention? Is that particular training and experience documented and substantiated?	Y/N
What types of ongoing supervision and professional support are available for the interventionist?	Y/N
Does the interventionist have sufficient time and resources to devote to implementing and monitoring the intervention?	Y/N
What is the expected outcome? Can the team measure the effects of the intervention and share data regularly to document potential changes, no changes, or worsening outcomes?	Y/N
What happens during a typical treatment session?	Y/N
How involved are parents and primary caregivers in the day-to-day delivery of a client's intervention? Do they have the time and ability to implement the intervention?	Y/N
What type of data will the interventionist collect and how often?	Y/N

Note. These questions were informed by our professional experiences and adaptations from several resources including McDonald and DiGennaro Reed (in press), Autism Special Interest Group of the Association for Behavior Analysis (2007), Association for Science in Autism Treatment (n.d.), and Autism Spectrum Therapies (n.d.), and Celiberti et al. (2004).

nity to be sure that there are expected outcomes and to clarify them. Service providers cannot measure the effect of an intervention when they do not know what to measure.

- *Research the intervention:* Before and after the meeting, conduct your own research on the intervention and its efficacy in the literature. Table 9.3 provides a detailed checklist of considerations for intervention selection and use. Be clear about what behavior parents are looking to affect with the intervention at this stage. This information will help determine which behaviors are priorities and which you may be able to address alternately with an evidence-based intervention.
- *Do no harm:* If the intervention has been shown to be harmful, initiate a discussion about the previous outcomes and communicate that the present decision-making model will not be applicable and terminate involvement consistent with ethical guidelines. For example, practitioners consulting with a parent who intends to treat their child to Miracle Mineral Solution, which has been linked to serious injury and death (Connett, 2015), should not pursue this proposed decision-making model.
- *Decision making:* Meet with parents again and discuss your findings and their plans related to the intervention. The parents will decide whether to move forward with the intervention.
- *Clarify and operationalize:* If the parents decide to move forward with the intervention, clarify and operationalize the expected outcomes. What behavior will you be recording? What are the expected changes in the behavior? What is the timeframe for the expected behavior change?

- *Data systems:* Set up your data collection systems and record baseline, as needed, for new (unlearned) behavior that you may begin recording. For behavior already being recorded, make phase change lines on existing graphs. Criterion should be set for behavior change based on the expected outcomes and timeline, which will allow for clear data-based decision making in the future.
- *Prepare for the effects of intervention:* Prepare for any side effects or direct effects of the intervention, such as an initial increase in a particular behavior. Expect temporary changes in behavior (e.g., student begins a diet and he engages in behavior when he sees other students' snacks) or quite possibly, long-term effects of intervention.
- *Ongoing evaluation:* Review data daily and meet with parents weekly to review the effects and expected outcomes. Take note of any changes in the target behavior and other behavior, or anticipated or unanticipated side effects.
- *Modification or termination:* Upon review and data analysis of the proposed expected outcomes, a decision will be made to continue, terminate, or modify the intervention. The goal of the data-based decision-making model is that if an intervention is not showing the expected outcomes or possibly even showing negative outcomes (e.g., increase in self-injurious behavior, decrease in verbal initiations), the parents will agree to stop the intervention based on pre-agreed criteria and a review of the data.

9.6 Conclusion

The purpose of this chapter is to share information about the risks of pseudoscience and antiscience and educate readers on the importance of adopting evidence-based interventions and how to do so. To accomplish this task, we synthesized resources into easy-to-use checklists and models that can be quickly adopted when needed. Table 9.1 provides a checklist to help identify red flags associated with pseudoscientific interventions. Moreover, this chapter details recommendations to guide efforts to stay abreast of the scholarly literature in affordable and resource-sensitive ways. Recognizing that readers will, at some point, be required to evaluate the scientific merit of a published study, Table 9.2 lists numerous questions to inform this crucial and necessary activity. Moreover, Table 9.3 contains a detailed checklist of considerations for intervention selection and use. The chapter also presents a decision-making model to facilitate a collaborative, data-based evaluation of unsubstantiated treatments in the event readers are part of a team that decides to pursue an unestablished treatment despite the lack of empirical support.

In a world of quick fixes and fad autism treatments, professionals must frequently avoid falling prey to clever marketing schemes and are challenged to ensure the provision of effective and ethical services. In addition to maintaining knowledge and implementation of science-based treatments and EBP, we recommend readers refer to their ethical guidelines when they encounter situations similar to those presented in this chapter. We also encourage readers to identify a colleague who may serve as an "ethics mentor" to discuss ethical dilemmas or difficult situations in a supportive manner. Finally, behavior analysts may seek guidance by contacting a hotline resource offered by the Association for Behavior Analysis International (see https://www.abainternational.org/Miscellaneous/ABAIHotLine.aspx).

References

American Psychological Association. (2005). *Policy statement of evidence-based practice in psychology.* Retrieved from http://www.apa.org/practice/resources/evidence/evidence-based-statement.pdf

American Psychological Association Presidential Task Force of Evidence-Based Practice. (2006). Evidence-based practice in psychology. *American Psychologist, 61*, 271–285.

American Speech-Language-Hearing Association. (2005). *Evidence-based practice in communication disorders.* Retrieved from http://www.asha.org/policy/PS2005-00221/

Association for Science in Autism Treatment. (1999, Spring). *Pseudoscientific therapies: Some warning signs*. Retrieved from http://www.asatonline.org/wp-content/uploads/2014/08/spring99.pdf

Association for Science in Autism Treatment. (n.d.). *Some questions to ask before writing the next story about autism treatment*. Retrieved from http://www.asatonline.org/for-media-professionals/top-10-questions-to-ask/

Autism Special Interest Group of the Association for Behavior Analysis. (2007). *Consumer guidelines for identifying, selecting, and evaluating behavior analysts working with individuals with autism spectrum disorders*. Retrieved from http://www.apbahome.net/downloads/AutGuidelines.pdf

Autism Spectrum Therapies. (n.d.). *Good questions to ask*. Retrieved from http://autismtherapies.com/journey/build-your-team.php?article=questions-to-ask

Axon, R. (2016). Cupping helps heal the USA men's Olympic gymnastics team. *USA Today*. Retrieved from http://www.usatoday.com/story/sports/olympics/rio-2016/2016/08/06/usa-mens-gymnastics-cupping-game-ready-jake-dalton-sam-mikaluk/88336190/

Baxter, A. J., & Krenzelok, E. P. (2008). Pediatric fatality secondary to EDTA chelation. *Clinical Toxicology*, *46*, 1083–1084.

Behavior Analyst Certification Board. (2016a). *BACB Professional and ethical compliance code for behavior analysts*. Retrieved from http://bacb.com/wp-content/uploads/2016/03/160321-compliance-code-english.pdf

Behavior Analyst Certification Board. (2016b, November). New journal resources for BCBAs and BCaBAs. *BACB Newsletter*. Retrieved from http://bacb.com/wp-content/uploads/2016/11/1611-newsletter.pdf

Biklen, D. (1992). Typing to talk: Facilitated communication. *American Journal of Speech-Language Pathology*, *1*, 15–17.

Biklen, D., & Kliewer, C. (2006). Constructing competence: Autism, voice, and the 'disordered' body. *International Journal of Inclusive Education*, *10*, 169–188.

Bilu, Y., & Goodman, Y. C. (1997). What does the soul say? Metaphysical uses of facilitated communication in the Jewish ultraorthodox community. *Ethos*, *25*, 375–407.

Carr, J. E., & Briggs, A. M. (2010). Strategies for making regular contact with the scholarly literature. *Behavior Analysis in Practice*, *3*, 13–18.

Celiberti, D., Buchanan, S., Bleecker, F., Kreiss, D., & Rosenfeld, D. (2004). The road less traveled: Charting a clear course for autism treatment. In *Autism: Basic information* (pp. 17–31). Robbinsville, NJ: Autism New Jersey.

Chambless, D. L., Baker, M. J., Baucom, D. H., Beutler, L. E., Calhoun, K. S., Crits-Christoph, P., …, & Johnson, S. B. (1998). Update on empirically validated therapies, II. *The Clinical Psychologist*, *51*, 3–16.

Connett, D. (2015, November). Autism: Potentially lethal bleach. Retrieved from http://www.independent.co.uk/life-style/health-and-families/health-news/autism-potentially-lethal-bleach-cure-feared-to-have-spread-to-britain-a6744291.html

Cooper, J. O., Heron, T. E., & Heward, W. L. (2007). *Applied behavior analysis* (2nd ed.). London: Pearson.

Cozby, P. C. (1997). *Methods in behavioral research* (6th ed.). London: Mayfield Publishing Company.

DiGennaro Reed, F. D., & Reed, D. D. (2008). Towards an understanding of evidence-based practice. *Journal of Early and Intensive Behavioral Intervention*, *5*, 20–29.

Every Student Succeeds Act of 2015, Pub. L. No. 114–95 §1177 (2015).

Green, G., & Perry, L. (1999). Science, pseudoscience, and antiscience. *Science in Autism Treatment*, *1*, 5–6.

Heflin, L. J., & Simpson, R. (1998). Interventions for children and youth with autism: Prudent choices in a world of exaggerated claims and empty promises. Part II: Legal/policy analysis and recommendations for selecting interventions and treatments. *Focus on Autism and other Developmental Disorders,* 13, 212–220.

Herbert, J. D. (2000). Defining empirically supported treatments: Pitfalls and possible solutions. *the Behavior Therapist, 23*, 113–121.

Horner, R. H., Carr, E. G., Halle, J., McGee, G., Odom, S., & Wolery, M. (2005). The use of single-subject research to identify evidence-based practice in special education. *Exceptional Children*, *71*, 165–179.

Individuals with Disabilities Education Act, 20 U.S.C. § 1400 (2004).

Iwata, B. A., Dorsey, M. F., Slifer, K. J., Bauman, K. E., & Richman, G. S. (1982/1994). Toward a functional analysis of self-injury. *Journal of Applied Behavior Analysis*, *27*, 197–209.

Jacobson, J. W., Mulick, J. A., & Schwartz, A. A. (1995). A history of facilitated communication: Science, pseudoscience, and antiscience. *American Psychologist*, *50*, 750–765.

Johnston, J. M., & Pennypacker, H. S. (2009). *Strategies and tactics of behavioral research* (3rd ed.). New York, NY: Routledge.

Le Mars Community School District. (1992). 19 IDELR 284.

Lerman, D. C., Sansbury, T., Hovanetz, A., Wolever, E. W., Garcia, A., O'Brien, E., & Adedipe, H. (2008). Using behavior analysis to examine the outcomes of unproven therapies: An evaluation of hyperbaric oxygen therapy for children with autism. *Behavior Analysis in Practice*, *1*, 50–58.

Lilienfeld, S. O., Lynn, S. J., & Lohr, J. M. (2003). Science and pseudoscience in clinical psychology: Initial thoughts, reflections and considerations. In S. O. Lilienfeld, S. J. Lynn, & J. M. Lohr (Eds.), *Science and pseudoscience in clinical psychology* (pp. 1–38). New York, NY: Guilford Press.

Lilienfeld, S. O., Ritschel, L. A., Lynn, S. J., Cautin, R. L., & Latzman, R. D. (2014). Why ineffective psychotherapies appear to work: A taxonomy of causes of spurious therapeutic effectiveness. *Psychological Science*, *9*, 355–387.

Lovaas, O. I. (1987). Behavioral treatment and normal education and intellectual functioning in young children. *Journal of Consulting and Clinical Psychology*, *55*, 3–9.

Maffei-Almodovar, L., & Sturmey, P. (2013). Evidence-based practice and crisis intervention. In D. D. Reed, F. D. DiGennaro Reed, & J. K. Luiselli (Eds.), *Handbook of crisis intervention and developmental disabilities* (pp. 49–69). New York, NY: Springer.

McDonald, M. E., & DiGennaro Reed, F. D. (in press). Autism spectrum disorder: Distinguishing science and pseudoscience. In J. Naglieri, S. Ozonoff, & S. Goldstein (Eds.), *Assessment of autism spectrum disorders* (2nd ed.). New York, NY: Guilford Press.

McDonald, M. E., Pace, D., Blue, E., & Schwartz, D. (2012). Critical issues in causation and treatment of autism: Why fads continue to flourish. *Child & Family Behavior Therapy, 34*, 290–304.

McNally, R. J. (2003). The demise of pseudoscience. *The Scientific Review of Mental Health Practice,* 2(2). Retrieved from http://www.srmhp.org/0202/pseudoscience.html

Mostert, M. P. (2001). Facilitated communication since 1995: A review of published studies. *Journal of Autism and Developmental Disorders, 31*, 287–313.

Mostert, M. P. (2010). Facilitated communication and its legitimacy – Twenty-first century developments. *Exceptionality, 18*, 31–41.

Nathan, P. E., & Gorman, J. M. (Eds.). (2015). *A guide to treatments that work* (4th ed.). New York, NY: Oxford University Press.

National Association of School Psychologists. (2010). *Principles for professional ethics*. Retrieved from https://www.nasponline.org/assets/Documents/StandardsandCertification/Standards/1_ Ethical Principles.pdf

National Autism Center. (2009). *National Standards Project: Findings and conclusions*. Randolph, MA: National Autism Center.

National Autism Center. (2015). *National Standards Project, phase 2: Findings and conclusions. Addressing the need for evidence-based practice guidelines for autism spectrum disorder*. Randolph, MA: National Autism Center.

Neporent, L. (2013). Dangerous diet trend: The cotton ball diet. *ABC News*. Retrieved from http://abcnews.go.com/Health/dangerous-diet-trend-cotton-ball-diet/story?id=20942888.

New York State Department of Health Early Intervention Program. (1999). *Clinical practice guideline report of the recommendations, autism/pervasive developmental disorders assessment and intervention for young children (age 0–3 years) (publication no. 4215)*. Albany, NY: NYS Department of Health.

Norcross, J. C. (Ed.). (2002). *Psychotherapy relationships that work: Therapist contributions and responsiveness to patient needs*. New York: Oxford University Press.

Normand, M. P. (2008). Science, skepticism, and applied behavior analysis. *Behavior Analysis in Practice, 1*, 42–49.

Odom, S. L., Collet-Klingenberg, L. C., Rogers, S. J., & Hatton, D. D. (2010). Evidence-based practices in interventions for children and youth with autism spectrum disorders. *Preventing School Failure: Alternative Education for Children and Youth, 54*, 275–282.

Rogers, S. J. (1998). Empirically supported comprehensive treatments for young children with autism. *Journal of Clinical Child Psychology, 27*, 168–179.

Romanczyk, R. G., Arnstein, L., Soorya, L. V., & Gillis, J. (2003). The myriad of controversial treatments for autism: A critical evaluation of efficacy. In S. O. Lilienfeld, S. J. Lynn, & J. M. Lohr (Eds.), *Science and pseudoscience in clinical psychology* (pp. 363–398). New York, NY: Guilford Press.

Romanczyk, R. G., & Gillis, J. M. (2004). Treatment approaches for autism: Evaluating options and making informed choices. In D. Zager (Ed.), *Autism: Identification, education, and treatment* (pp. 515–535). Hillsdale, NJ: Erlbaum.

Romanczyk, R. G., Gillis, J. M., White, S., & DiGennaro, F. D. (2008). Comprehensive treatment packages for ASD: Effectiveness and cost-benefit. In J. Matson (Ed.), *Autism spectrum disorder: Evidence based assessment and treatment across the lifespan* (pp. 351–381). Burlington, MA: Elsevier Science.

Roth, A., & Fonagy, P. (2004). *What works for whom? A critical review of psychotherapy research* (2nd ed.). New York, NY: Guilford Press.

Schaefer, A. (2015). 4 ways the cotton ball diet could kill you. *Healthline*. Retrieved from http://www.healthline.com/health/eating-disorders/ways-the-cotton-ball-diet-could-kill-you#1

Shermer, M. (2002). *Why people believe weird things: Pseudoscience, superstition, and other confusions of our time*. New York, NY: MJF Books.

Simpson, R. L. (1995). Children and youth with autism in an age of reform: A perspective on current issues. *Behavioral Disorders, 21*, 7–20.

Singleton, R. A., Straits, B. C., & Straits, M. M. (1993). *Approaches to social research* (2nd ed.). New York: Oxford University Press.

Slocum, T. A., Detrich, R., Wilczynski, S. M., Spencer, T. D., Lewis, T., & Wolfe, K. (2014). The evidence-based practice of applied behavior analysis. *The Behavior Analyst, 37*, 41–56.

Spata, A. V. (2003). *Research methods: Science and diversity*. New York, NY: Wiley.

Stricker, G., & Trierweiler, S. J. (1995). The local clinical scientist: A bridge between science and practice. *American Psychologist, 50*, 995–1002.

Tostanoski, A., Lang, R., Raulston, T., Carnett, A., & Davis, T. (2014). Voices from the past: Comparing the rapid prompting method and facilitated communication. *Developmental Neurorehabilitation, 17*, 210–223.

Travers, J. C., Ayers, K., Simpson, R. L., & Crutchfield, S. (2016). Fad, pseudoscientific, and controversial interventions. In R. Lang, T. Hancock, & N. Singh (Eds.), *Early intervention for young children with autism spectrum disorder* (pp. 257–293). New York, NY: Springer.

Travers, J. C., Tincani, M. J., & Lang, R. (2014). Facilitated communication denies people with disabilities their voice. *Research and Practice for Persons with Severe Disabilities, 39*, 195–202.

Tweed, L., Connolly, N., & Beaulieu, A. (2009). *Interventions for autism spectrum disorders: State of the evidence*. Augusta, ME: Muskie School of Public Service and the Maine Department of Health and Humans Services.

van Houten, R., Axelrod, S., Bailey, J. S., Favell, J. E., Foxx, R. M., Iwata, B. A., & Lovaas, O. I. (1988). The right to effective behavioral treatment. *Journal of Applied Behavior Analysis, 21*, 381–384.

Zients, J. (2012). *Use of evidence and evaluation in the 2014 budget*. Office of Management and Budget: Memorandum to the heads of executive agencies.

Discrete Trial Teaching and Social Skill Training: Don't Throw the Baby Out with the Bathwater

10

Mary Jane Weiss, Jennifer Hilton, and Samantha Russo

Discrete trial teaching (DTT) is a method of instruction that enables highly individualized instruction and the rapid presentation of targets in discrete units. Repetition is a fundamental aspect of DTT, and its formal structure lends itself to the presentation of many learning opportunities in a short period of time. Many learners with autism specturm disorder (ASD) may require repetition, and do not obtain knowledge without multiple learning trials (Smith, 2001). For this reason, DTT has been a foundational instructional technique for teaching students with autism, and has been lauded as an efficient means of imparting knowledge, especially when learner motivation is low (Smith, 2001). However, many people believe that DTT is most relevant to instruction in building compliance, imitation, and appropriate toy play (Lovaas, 1987), and consider going outside of applied behavior analysis (ABA) to address social skill deficits through methods such as cognitive-behavioral therapy (Lopata, Thomeer, Volker, & Nida, 2006), Social Stories™ (Adams, Gouvousis, VanLue, & Waldron, 2004), Relationship Development Intervention® (RDI; Gutstein, Burgess, & Montfort, 2007), Social Thinking® (Leaf et al., 2016), and other types of interventions.

It is understandable that people might not glean the relevance of DTT for social skill instruction. After all, the ultimate outcomes for social skills instruction are very divergent from the instructional context. Goals often include the spontaneous demonstration of skills in novel, untrained contexts with the hope that the learner will adapt to each context and adjust his or her response accordingly. These are lofty goals for instructors, who may be attracted to interventions that seem more aligned with these outcomes. Behavior analysts may be tempted to explore practices that are not empirically validated to be effective, which dilutes the effectiveness of intervention and erodes the public's perception of the impact potential of ABA.

However, a variety of different skills can be successfully and efficiently taught through the use of DTT, including social skills. Behavior analytic research has investigated teaching of a number of different social skills through the use of DTT. Previously published literature includes teaching affective behavior (DeQuinzio, Townsend, Sturmey, & Poulson, 2007; Gena, Couloura, & Kymissis, 2005), increasing social interactions and initiations (Garcia-Albea, Reeve, Reeve, & Brothers, 2014; Garfinkle & Schwartz, 2002; Groskreutz, Peters, Groskreutz, & Higbee, 2015), teaching children to offer help to others (Harris, Handleman, & Alessandri, 1990; Reeve, Reeve, Townsend, & Poulson, 2007), sharing (Marzullo-Kerth, Reeve, Reeve, & Townsend,

M.J. Weiss (✉) • J. Hilton • S. Russo
Endicott College, Beverly, MA, USA
e-mail: mjinnj@gmail.com

J.B. Leaf (ed.), *Handbook of Social Skills and Autism Spectrum Disorder*, Autism and Child Psychopathology Series, DOI 10.1007/978-3-319-62995-7_10

2011), teaching empathy skills (Schrandt, Townsend, & Poulson, 2009), teaching perspective taking skills (LeBlanc et al., 2003), and increasing joint attention (Jones, Carr, & Feeley, 2006; Kasari, Freeman, & Paparella, 2006; Krstovska-Guerrero & Jones, 2013). While all of these different skills have been taught using DTT, various procedures within discrete trial methodology were utilized, and at times DTT was applied in slightly nuanced and unique ways.

The literature demonstrates the use of a variety of instructional techniques under discrete trial methodology including: modeling (Schrandt et al., 2009), prompting (Pollard, Betz, & Higbee, 2012), error correction (Francisco & Hanley, 2012; Gena et al., 2005; Nientimp & Cole, 1993), multiple exemplar training (Marzullo-Kerth et al., 2011), progressive intertrial intervals (Francisco & Hanley, 2012), priming sessions (Nientimp & Cole, 1993; Zanolli, Daggett, & Adams, 1996), video modeling (Gena et al., 2005; LeBlanc et al., 2003; Marzullo-Kerth et al., 2011), observational learning (DeQuinzio et al., 2007; Garfinkle & Schwartz, 2002; MacDonald & Ahearn, 2015), behavioral skills training (Peters & Thompson, 2015), script fading (Garcia-Albea et al., 2014; Groskreutz et al., 2015; Ledbetter-Cho et al., 2015), and computer-based instruction (Simpson, Langone, & Ayres, 2004). Each of these instructional techniques is individually supported in the behavior analytic research showing positive results in the instruction of a number of different target skills, making these techniques valued components of DTT. Because of the support the literature provides for the success of these methods to teach varying social skills, the use of DTT should be considered when attempting to teach different social targets.

DTT has been applied to social skill deficits for several decades, with a long history of impressive outcomes (Smith, 2001). When social skills are taught exclusively in the natural environment, there may not be enough opportunities for the individual to practice the skill to mastery. Conversely, DTT of social skills allows for additional practice of skills, which can then be trained to generalize into the appropriate settings. For this reason, DTT was applied to these targets, just as it was applied to many learning, academic, and other skills (Smith, 2001). Social responding and social initiations were the initial targets of social skills interventions. Within DTT there are a number of different prompting hierarchies that can be used to facilitate correct responding. This facilitation of correct responding, coupled with the multiple opportunities for responding provided in DTT, can potentially be beneficial for the learning of social skills. Much of the social skills research focuses on the use of different types of prompts to teach skills. However, these prompting strategies are often applied within a DTT format. Hence, these studies are reviewed, as they do illustrate the use of DTT, though the emphasis may be on the strategic application of prompts.

10.1 Using Prompting and Modeling Within DTT

Prompting and modeling are essential components of DTT because they allow for errorless learning, which is considered to be important for learners on the autism spectrum (Delprato, 2001). There are many different types of prompts and prompt hierarchies that may be successful in the teaching of social skills. In particular, the use of progressive prompt delays may be beneficial in teaching skills that require verbal modeling (Delprato, 2001). Delaying the provision of the prompt may help reduce dependence on prompting and may facilitate independent responding. In an early demonstration of the use of DTT to address social responding, Nientimp and Cole (1993) used a constant time delay within DTT to teach three participants to vocally respond to social greetings. Schrandt et al. (2009) also used a combination of prompt delays, modeling, manual prompts, behavioral rehearsals, and reinforcement in a discrete trial format to teach empathy responses. Time delay prompts have also been shown to be beneficial in teaching intraverbal responses. For example, Ingvarsson and Hollobaugh (2010) demonstrated the acquisition of intraverbal responses using a discrete trial format and a progressive prompt delay. A different approach to prompting was utilized by Jones et al. (2006). If responding to the discriminative stimulus during joint attention training did not occur, a gaze alternation or tracing a visual path to the toy with an edible reinforcer was utilized. Both prompting procedures were then faded using a most-to-least prompting procedure paired with a time delay.

In addition to the effectiveness of the progressive prompt delay, experimenters have shown success with different sized blocks of trials when using the discrete trial format to teach social skills (Jones et al., 2006; Nientimp & Cole, 1993; Schrandt et al., 2009). Nientimp and Cole (1993) presented instruction in blocks of 10 trials across five different targeted greetings (e.g., "Hi" and "hello") with generalization probes conducted by typically developing peers following baseline (i.e., no prompting) conditions. Jones et al. (2006) also used 10 trials per session to teach joint attention skills. In contrast, Schrandt et al. (2009) presented training sessions in much larger blocks consisting of 30 trials, seven of which were training, and three of which were nontraining probe trials per response category. Each trial consisted of a discriminative stimulus (i.e., vignette using a doll or puppet), a response from the participant, and a prompt delay sequence to prevent errors from occurring. Starting at a 0-s delay, the prompts were faded to a 1-s delay and then to a 3-s delay. During these training trials reinforcement in the form of token delivery and behavior specific praise were delivered for correct unprompted responses.

Other experimenters have exposed participants to multiple shorter blocks of trials in a given day. In one study, Jones, Feeley, and Takacs (2007) exposed participants to up to six 10-trial sessions per day in which opportunities were contrived for the participants to engage in spontaneous language. Opportunities for each target response were initially presented in isolation and, following mastery, these responses were then interspersed with previously mastered targets. Other experimenters have interspersed training trials with probe trials, such as in Gena et al. (2005) who conducted a series of 14 trials, four of which were probe trials and 10 were training trials. The number of trials used in DTT is an important consideration—the instructor must strike a balance between providing adequate opportunities for practice of the skill and the tolerance threshold of the learner. Perhaps even more importantly, the behavior analyst must ensure that generalization is demonstrated, and that skills transfer to natural environments and contexts.

Behavior analysts must consider not only the amount of trials used in training sessions, but also the type of prompting hierarchy that should be employed. In using a constant time delay prompting procedure, Nientimp and Cole (1993) found that all participants showed increases in accurate responding to social greetings, two reaching 100% accuracy across trials while the third increased to 50% accuracy across trials. The acquisition of manding for information has also been demonstrated through the use of DTT and prompt delay procedures. Ingvarsson and Hollobaugh (2010) taught participants the response "I don't know, please tell me," when presented with a question for which they did not know the answer. All participants acquired the intended response, and the authors concluded that the fast-paced format of DTT may have led to the quick acquisition demonstrated by this procedure.

Other experimenters have targeted empathetic responses such as happiness or excitement, sadness or pain, and frustration. Schrandt et al. (2009) demonstrated increases in empathetic responding as treatment was introduced across response categories when using dolls and puppets to present different scenarios. Most importantly, generalization was demonstrated across training to nontraining probes and from dolls to actual people. Individuals may be required to engage in a number of different empathetic or sympathetic social responses dependent upon the situation in which they find themselves. Jones et al. (2007) demonstrated that children were able to learn a variety of different spontaneous responses including "Bless you", "What?", and "Are you ok?". The participants were able to demonstrate generalized responding in the form of responding to staff members who were not a part of the initial study in a novel setting (Jones et al., 2007).

Despite the success of DTT in training generalized responding in some studies, others have found the intended response to be acquired by all participants in the experimental setting, but found mixed results across participants during generalization probes (e.g., Ingvarsson & Hollobaugh, 2010). When teaching social skills, it is essential for the instructional methods to encourage and achieve quick acquisition of target skills and the generalization of those skills across settings, people, and time. In the absence of these outcomes, the skill is not likely to be demonstrated within the natural environment.

In addition to the social skills mentioned up to this point, DTT can also be used to teach individuals with autism to engage in spontaneous responses, which is an essential component of reciprocal responding in social situations. Tactile prompts have also been explored for their utility in helping the development of social responses, especially within the response class of social initiations. Shabani et al. (2002) were able to teach three phrases, "Look at this," "I have [object label]," and "Do you want to play?" The tactile prompt was placed in the participant's pocket, and, during training, the adult would activate the tactile prompt and immediately provide a verbal prompt of the initiation statement. If the participant successfully imitated the verbal model, an edible was provided. Across sessions, the verbal model was gradually faded using a progressive most-to-least prompting hierarchy until the participant independently initiated a social interaction following the tactile prompt. Although the tactile prompt was successful in increasing verbal initiations across all three participants, the experimenters were unable to successfully fade the prompt.

Using a multiple probe design across behaviors, Krstovska-Guerrero and Jones (2013) implemented intervention sessions in a discrete trial format with 10 opportunities to respond per session with 1–3 sessions per day. A prompting procedure with a most-to-least hierarchy combined with a time delay was used across trials. Three skills were targeted and each built off the previous (1) smile, (2) look and smile, and (3) gaze shift and smile. Generalization was evaluated with each participant's mother, a novel interventionist, and novel materials. All targeted responses increased with all participants and maintenance and generalization was effectively demonstrated. Whalen and Schreibman (2003) used a behavior modification technique with components of DTT and pivotal response training to target joint attention responding and joint attention initiations. This hybrid intervention consisted of using clear prompts, interspersing mastered tasks with unlearned tasks, allowing the child to choose the activity, taking turns with the child, contingent reinforcement of correct responses, and direct response-reinforcer relationships. This intervention proved to be effective for increasing joint attention for all five participants. In addition, social validation measures completed by naïve observers supported positive changes in each participant.

10.2 Error Correction and DTT

One of the reasons that DTT is so successful is because of the multiple opportunities for practice and reinforcement. Since individuals will be performing a skill many times in DTT, it is essential that they perform that skill correctly, rather than having multiple opportunities to practice the skill incorrectly. This is usually approached through using errorless learning. In other situations, when errorless learning is not used or is used only initially, it is vital that an error correction system be put in place. There are many different types of error correction used in DTT, but nearly all protocols involving DTT include some sort of error correction component.

Some error correction procedures simply involve providing an additional trial of the targeted skill in order to give an opportunity for extra practice following an error (e.g., Francisco & Hanley, 2012). Other error correction procedures involve the use of a model prompt for the targeted response. For example, Gena et al.

(2005) utilized a model prompt to teach children to model the facial expressions of others. When a child emitted an erroneous response, the therapist would state "Look (emotion) like me," and provide a model prompt of the targeted response. In another study various facial expressions were taught to learners with ASD (i.e., DeQuinzio et al., 2007), participants were provided with a verbal prompt, "Do this," and a model prompt. Reinforcement was withheld when an error occurred. If still unsuccessful, the verbal prompt, "Do this," was provided, the model prompt was provided, and two facial motor movements were repeatedly provided (i.e., the model would open and close her eyes). Finally, a manual prompt in which the model physically prompted the action was utilized. During error correction procedures, if the motor imitation sequence was unsuccessful, a manual prompt was used to ensure a successful response.

In some cases, if an error or an echolalic response occurs, an error correction procedure consisting of "No, you should say (correct response)" has been implemented (e.g., Nientimp & Cole, 1993). In addition to traditional error correction procedures, some studies in the area of social skills have used video modeling as an error correction procedure. For instance, LeBlanc et al. (2003) intended to teach perspective taking; correct answers were reinforced, while incorrect responses resulted in replaying a video model and additional prompting. The participants were shown a video, the video was paused, and perspective taking questions were asked. Correct answers were reinforced, while incorrect responses resulted in replaying the video and a prompt to pay attention until the correct answer was achieved.

As mentioned above, error correction is an important component of DTT. There are a number of different error correction procedures that may be selected and can be successful, but it is essential for behavior analysts to be aware of the benefits of errorless learning for learners on the autism spectrum. This can be particularly important in the social domain where children with autism may be stigmatized for social interactions that do not meet social norms.

10.3 Multiple Exemplar Training and DTT

One of the concerns with DTT is that it will promote rote responding that only occurs in the specific instructional setting associated with DTT which can be intensified by teaching with limited materials or in restricted contexts (Miranda-Linne & Melin, 1992). When teaching social skills, it is particularly important that the skills the individual learned generalize to the natural environment so that s/he can engage socially with others. One way to promote generalized responding is the use of multiple exemplar training. When multiple exemplars are used to teach social skills, individuals will not respond to the specific stimulus presented in DTT; but, rather, to a class of stimuli intended to occasion a particular response (Miranda-Linne & Melin, 1992). Thus, it is particularly important to ensure that multiple exemplars are used when teaching social skills to individuals with ASD.

Marzullo-Kerth et al. (2011) used multiple exemplar training to teach children with autism to share. Participants in this study were taught to share across multiple classes of materials (e.g., art, snack, toys) and generalization of skills was assessed. The procedure in the study followed a DTT approach by using a cue, prompting (if required), a response, a consequence, and an intertrial interval. An error correction procedure was used in which the materials were removed, a video model was presented, and then if the appropriate response was still not emitted a physical prompt was used to complete the response. Following intervention, all four participants learned to share and generalized sharing across novel stimuli, novel adults, novel settings, and novel peers. Multiple exemplars were also used by Charlop-Christy and Daneshvar (2003) to teach a perspective taking task using video modeling. This procedure involved using variations of the "Sally-Ann Task," in which participants view a scenario and are asked questions regarding the perspective of the different characters in the scenario. The multiple exemplars used in this study included different characters taking part in different scenarios with similar perspective taking questions being asked to participants. Finally, multiple peers have been utilized within multiple exemplar training to encourage stimulus generalization when training social skills to learners with autism (Gaylord-Ross, Haring, Breen, & Pitts-Conway, 1984). When using DTT, it is important to program for generalization to avoid rote responding. One of the ways in which this can be completed is through multiple exemplar training (Miranda-Linne & Melin, 1992). This should be an important consideration for behavior analysts who are attempting to train social skills that will easily generalize into the natural environment. Preparing learners for the myriad responses they are likely to encounter in the natural environment is more easily accomplished with the use of multiple exemplars.

10.4 Progressive Intertrial Intervals in DTT

One important component of DTT is the intertrial interval (ITI). Research has shown that short ITIs lead to favorable acquisition of target skills. Francisco and Hanley (2012) compared the effects of the lengths of different ITIs on the acquisition of social skills with two preschool aged children. Using a concurrent multiple baseline design, the use of distributed and progressive ITIs was assessed. In the distributed ITI condition, participants were provided with five trials during the morning session of preschool and five trials during the afternoon session of preschool for each targeted social skill. These trials took place roughly every 30 min during each session. The conditions were identical for the progressive ITIs, with the exception of progressively increasing ITIs following the initial response opportunity. Thus, following the first trial, opportunities were presented 3 s, 10 s, 30 s, 2 min, 4 min, and 16 min after one another. The results of this study indicated no improvement following the distributed ITI condition, but immediate improvement following the implementation of the progressive ITI condition. These results indicate that initially short ITIs can be useful when teaching social skills in a trial-based format.

10.5 Using Priming Sessions Within DTT

Priming is a well-known procedure in which a stimulus is presented prior to the start of sessions to increase the establishing operation and/or the reinforcing effects of the stimulus (Roantree & Kennedy, 2006). Zanolli et al. (1996) used DTT in priming sessions to compare rates of spontaneous initiations of children with autism to their typically developing peers. Priming sessions were conducted prior to the activity with the same materials, in a low demand situation with easy to complete activities and reinforcement delivered on a rich schedule. Target responses included, "Give me that," "Look at me," "Show me yours," "Smile," "Touch," and "Look," in a random order. Two of the participants were exposed to 14 trials per session, while the third participant was exposed to 10 trials per session. Priming sessions had successful outcomes in the subsequent treatment sessions. Moreover, the priming sessions successfully increased spontaneous initiations, produced salient initiations, increased successful responding to initiations, and increased rate of initiation above average rates of typically developing peer's initiations. As previously discussed, Nientimp and Cole (1993) used a constant time delay within DTT to teach three participants to verbally respond to social greetings. To start each training session, participants were provided with two warm up trials for each of the five target greetings (i.e., hi, what's up, hello, yo, and hey). During this priming procedure, the teacher presented the greetings and then immediately prompted the correct response. The results showed that independent accurate social interactions increased while at the same time echolalic responding decreased. This research supports the use of priming as a tool that can be used to promote the success of DTT for social skills targets (Nientimp & Cole, 1993; Zanolli et al., 1996).

Kasari et al. (2006) implemented a slightly different approach to priming. The teaching procedure included 5 to 8 min of DTT to prime the goal of treatment. The least-to-most prompting hierarchy consisted of a verbal, model, then a physical prompt. This prompting hierarchy was used to achieve a social interaction or a communicative attempt which was then maintained through positive reinforcement. This same skill was then taught in a semistructured session away from the table in a more natural setting. This occurred on the floor, with a child driven, rather than a teacher-directed approach. Imitation of the child's behavior with toys, and incorporating child's activity interests into play routines were two different strategies commonly used on the floor. The target skill was taught using systematic prompting and reinforcement. Results indicated that both the formal and less structured interventions were effective in increasing joint attention among participants.

10.6 Using Video Modeling Within DTT

Video modeling is a powerful tool that can be used to teach individuals with ASD to engage in a variety of different social skills, such as utilizing appropriate affect (Gena et al., 2005), sharing (Marzullo-Kerth et al., 2011), helping (Reeve et al., 2007), and perspective taking (LeBlanc et al., 2003). There are many potential benefits to the use of video modeling to teach social skills, including the heightened interest that the learner may have in the use of technology. Additionally, when filming video models, behavior analysts are able to focus explicitly on the target of instruction, making it more salient for the learner. There are a number of different types of presentations used in video modeling including showing peers, adults, or even the participant engaging in the target skill. This is generally referred to as first person point-of-view or third person point-of-view. In addition, some video models include voice overs that explain the scenario, while other video models simply include the dialogue relevant to the social skill being taught. Overall, video modeling serves as an effective tool for teaching social skills to individuals on the autism spectrum (Bellini & Akullian, 2007).

One effective strategy for the use of video modeling is the use of a trial-based format which, as previously mentioned, allows for fast-paced instruction and multiple opportunities for responding and reinforcement. Gena et al. (2005) utilized video modeling, in vivo modeling, reinforcement, and error correction procedures to increase the affective behaviors of sympathy, appreciation, and disapproval. All participants demonstrated contextually appropriate affective responding following both the in vivo and video modeling treatments. Additionally, this skill generalized to novel scenarios, and novel therapists. These results maintained at follow up sessions, 1 month and 3 months following the conclusion of treatment. Reeve et al. (2007) used a multiple baseline design across participants to teach a generalized helping repertoire across tasks. In addition, a multicomponent treatment package consisting of a discriminative stimulus, training, consequences, and generalization was implemented across participants. Helping behavior in this study was defined as cleaning, replacing broken materials, picking up objects, sorting materials, locating objects, carrying objects, putting items away, and setting up an activity. In the presence of the discriminative stimuli used in training, all four participants engaged in appropriate helping responses. Novel stimuli were used to assess generalization of helping responses in probe conditions. Generalization trials showed an increase of the target helping response across novel stimuli, novel settings, and novel therapists.

In addition to the absence of the social awareness required to help others when they need it, a lack of empathy displayed by children with autism has been well documented in the literature. Video modeling has also been used in conjunction with reinforcement to teach children with autism the skill of perspective taking, which is a component of empathy. LeBlanc et al. (2003) taught perspective taking to three children with autism using video modeling and reinforcement. The authors evaluated these procedures through the use of a multiple baseline design. The participants were shown a video, the video was paused, and perspective taking questions (about how others might perceive situations or feel about them) were asked. The training sessions were completed after three consecutive correct trials. All of the participants failed the primary tasks during baseline, and then went on to master the tasks following intervention. Generalization was also demonstrated across novel vocal or motor responses, which all participants also demonstrated. Another important social skill that is sometimes required to be directly taught to individuals with autism, is sharing. Marzullo-Kerth et al. (2011) used multiple exemplar training to teach children with autism to share. Participants in this study were taught to share across multiple classes of materials (e.g., art, snack, toys) and generalization of skills was assessed.

The effects of video modeling have been found to generalize from training conditions to the natural environment for a variety of skills. LeBlanc et al. (2003) found video modeling to be an effective procedure to increase perspective taking skills and generalization was demonstrated with two out of the three participants by successfully answering questions regarding an untrained exemplar. Marzullo-Kerth et al. (2011) were also able to demonstrate generalization with sharing by conducting probes for sharing in novel settings, with novel people, and with novel stimuli. The effects of the treatment package were evaluated using a multiple baseline design, which demonstrated that the treatment package was effective in increasing sharing behavior across all three participants with evidence of skill maintenance and generalization. Gena et al. (2005) were able to demonstrate similar effects in increasing the affective behavior of three participants using video modeling and in vivo modeling. During the in vivo modeling condition, the appropriate response was modeled, and verbal and gestural prompts were used to guide the participant to imitate the model. Reinforcement was delivered following an appropriate display of affective responses. If an error occurred during the in vivo modeling condition, the therapist modeled the appropriate facial expression and provided a full verbal model, that is, "Say 'I am so sorry for you.'" During the video modeling condition the same procedures were utilized; however, the error correction procedure was different. The error correction procedure in this condition consisted of playing a video of a peer modeling the behavior and a verbal prompt from the therapist, that is, "you do it too." All participants demonstrated contextually appropriate affective responding following both the in vivo and video modeling treatments. Additionally, this skill generalized to novel scenarios and novel therapists. These results maintained at follow up sessions, 1 month and 3 months following the conclusion of treatment. It is essential that social skills taught through procedures such as video modeling are able to generalize to a variety of settings and people so that individuals with autism can be taught to be competent in these areas.

Video modeling can be an important tool that can be very successful in the teaching of social skills when combined with the DTT format. When using video modeling in this way, the learner not only gets multiple opportunities to practice the targeted social skill, but s/he also gets multiple opportunities to observe the correct performance of the skill. These components tied together with the traditional parts of discrete trial instruction. Using cues and prompts, either delivered by a person or by a video, is a necessary component of DTT (Smith, 2001). These multiple opportunities for observation and practice may contribute to the learning of skills. Additionally, if a learner is interested in technology, there may be an increased level of attention to the instruction because of the format in which it is presented. Thus, video modeling should be considered when attempting to teach social skills to some learners with ASD.

10.7 Observational Learning Within DTT

Social skills involve many complex conversational exchanges that may serve a wide variety of functions. Observational learning is an important component of social skills training because individuals must be able to observe the behavior of others and adjust their own behavior to the social situation. Observational learning occurs when an individual is able to observe the response of another individual and then engage in responding based on this observation. While this is a skill that develops without explicit training within the typically developing population, individuals on the autism spectrum may need to be explicitly taught this skill (Varni, Lovaas, Koegel, & Everett, 1979). Observational learning can be extended into many areas, and becomes increasingly relevant as children age. Many children use it informationally and can use the skill to ascertain what to do in class, to learn new skills, or to solve novel problems.

Despite the importance of observational learning as a skill for learners on the autism spectrum, there are a number of prerequisite skills that are necessary before observational learning can take place. In particular, an individual must attend to the relevant stimuli within the environment in order to appropriately adjust his behavior to the situation. Additionally, the individual must be able to accurately imitate the behavior of others in order for observational learning to take place. Once these prerequisite skills have been taught, individuals with ASD can benefit from observational learning as it pertains to the acquisition of social skills (MacDonald & Ahearn, 2015).

Observational learning can be beneficial for teaching a variety of different skills, including the imitation of facial expressions (DeQuinzio et al., 2007), play skills (MacDonald & Ahearn, 2015), and social interactions (Garfinkle & Schwartz, 2002). In order to establish observational learning, the prerequisite skills must be established, which can be done through the use of DTT. Individuals should be taught to attend, engage in delayed imitation, and discriminate among consequences (MacDonald & Ahearn, 2015). Once these skills have been taught, individuals are prepared to take part in observational learning. Taking the time to adequately train the prerequisite skills will allow the learner to access associated reinforcers more quickly and may reduce the prompting required during observational learning sessions.

MacDonald and Ahearn (2015) taught individuals with autism to engage in observational learning using a trial-based format for a variety of different tasks including a hidden item task, a computer task, an academic task, a construction toy task, and a building toy task. For each of these tasks, skills were taught in blocks of nine trials and least-to-most physical prompting was used to facilitate correct responding. During preassessment, none of the participants performed the observational learning tasks independently. Following training on a specific task, appropriate responses were demonstrated on an untrained task for five of the six participants. Another study targeting the teaching of observational learning, or imitation, Garfinkle and Schwartz (2002) utilized a multiple baseline design across four male participants aged 3 years, 7 months to 5 years, 5 months to teach imitation of a peer's social interactions. Teaching sessions were referred to as small group peer imitation training. Specifically, the training procedure consisted of four steps and was repeated until every child went through the training procedure two times. The training procedure consisted of (1) the teacher provided instructions to the small group, (2) the leader was selected, (3) a prompt was provided to promote initiation, and (4) praise was given for imitative acts. Following intervention participants demonstrated increased social behavior in both the proximity to peers and the amount of peer interactions. Peer imitation behavior also increased in both small group and free play settings.

DeQuinzio et al. (2007) used DTT with modeling, prompting, and the delivery of reinforcement in order to improve children with autism's imitation skills of various facial expressions presented on a model. The authors utilized a least-to-most prompting hierarchy along with an error correction procedure in order to have participants imitate the facial expression on the model. All three participants responded to facial models during 80–90% of training trials. Additionally, through the pattern of responding, it was concluded that facial expression was an effective discriminative stimulus. Reinforcement only occurred following a correct imitative response of the facial model and never following error correction procedures. Harris et al. (1990) taught three adolescent males to offer assistance using prompting and confederate reinforcement. Similarly, Reeve et al. (2007) taught a generalized repertoire of helping skills in children with autism. Harris et al. (1990) used a confederate peer by having the peer state their inability to accomplish a task (e.g., “I can’t button this jacket”) and then verbally prompting the participant to ask, “Can I help you?” After the participant helped, the confederate peer would provide thanks to the participant. The intervention was evaluated in two ways; a multiple baseline design across participants on the first trained task and a multiple baseline across tasks for each participant. Training time varied from a minimum of 5 days to a maximum of 15 days. All three participants showed increases in rate of learning as training progressed, evident by acquisition of tasks two to three in less time than acquisition to task one.

The variety of skills targeted demonstrates the utility of DTT for teaching observational learning and/or the prerequisites in different settings ranging from academics to toy play. Some treatment packages have been found to be effective in teaching observational learning of motor responses (MacDonald & Ahearn, 2015), while other studies have shown effectiveness in the teaching of facial expressions (DeQuinzio et al., 2007) and social interactions (Garfinkle & Schwartz, 2002). Overall, observational learning is an essential component of social interactions because individuals must be able to attend to the actions of others, as well as imitate the behavior of others, if they are going to be socially effective. By directly teaching the skills related to observational learning, behavior analysts are teaching pivotal behaviors that will allow for the performance of a variety of different social skills.

10.8 Behavioral Skills Training Within DTT

Behavioral skills training (BST) is centered around the principles of clear instruction, with multiple exposures of someone practicing the skill who already displays competence (e.g., modeling). The learner who is acquiring the skills then gets to practice the skill with the competent person, while receiving positive and corrective feedback. This procedure has been demonstrated to be an effective teaching procedure for a variety of skills including social skills (Stewart, Carr, & LeBlanc, 2007). A brief overview of BST will be discussed here, and more specific information regarding BST and DTT can be found in the chapter on BST.

BST has been used in a trial based format and was used to teach accurate tacting of listener behavior. Peters and Thompson (2015) taught four children between the ages of 5 and 9 years old to tact listener behavior as an initial component of their experiment. However, the skill of tacting nonvocal listener behavior failed to improve the target response of regaining listener interest. Participants were then taught to ask a question of an uninterested listener in order to regain the interest of a conversation partner. Again, BST was used to teach the skill and a trial-based format was used to determine mastery of the skill. Following this intervention, all participants acquired the skill of asking a question of an uninterested listener in order to regain the interest of the listener within 36 teaching trials. Three out of four participants demonstrated generalization of learned skills at follow up, while the fourth participant required additional training. The experimenters included two subsequent experiments testing the utility of BST which was evaluated in a trial-based format. Specifically, the experimenters examined the teaching of a variety of skills related to responding to the interest of a conversation partner, and all experiments demonstrated positive results.

Conversational exchanges pose many different challenges for individuals on the autism spectrum. Children with autism often demonstrate difficulty with appropriately responding to the interests of their conversation partners, which contributes to the difficulty that these individuals experience in making and maintaining friendships with peers (Peters & Thompson, 2015). Furthermore, it may serve to stigmatize them as they engage in off-task conversation or fail to respond in ways that build natural banter. Teaching the identification of interest and disinterest could make individuals with autism more sensitive to cues emitted from others, and might reduce conversational difficulty and awkwardness (Peters & Thompson, 2015).

10.9 Script Fading Within DTT

Scripts and script fading procedures have been used in a trial-based format to teach individuals on the autism spectrum to engage in language surrounding social interactions required for play (Garcia-Albea et al., 2014). Trial-based script training procedures have also been used to teach individuals with autism to share toys, which is an essential social skill with which individuals with autism often experience difficulty (Ledbetter-Cho et al., 2015). Social scripts have also been found to be effective in teaching social commenting and other social skills for individuals on the autism spectrum (Groskreutz et al., 2015). Script fading procedures involve providing individuals with a prompt for the language required for a social situation. This may come in the form of a written script or an auditory script, and prompting procedures are used to encourage the learner to imitate the script appropriately. As the learner is successful with the use of a script, the script is gradually faded until the learner independently emits the appropriate response. Script fading procedures have been found to be effective in increasing scripted and unscripted interactions for individuals on the autism spectrum.

Script fading procedures have been modified and used in a variety of ways. Some interactions may occur in the presence of naturally occurring stimuli while others are controlled by a teacher. By varying procedures, a technology has been developed in which script fading has contributed to increases in appropriate meaningful social exchanges. Garcia-Albea et al. (2014) placed a series of toys on shelves in a treatment room and participants could access each toy once per session, allowing for one trial with each toy. Audio buttons containing recorded social scripts were attached to each toy and participants were required to approach the toy they wanted to play with, press the audio button, and accurately repeat the social script to gain access to each toy. Prior to the start of intervention there were no observed responses across any participants. Following intervention all participants demonstrated increases in scripted, unscripted and novel responses. Generalization was demonstrated during multiple exemplar training across untaught stimuli. This intervention was able to successfully demonstrate that control over the response by the participant was maintained by the appropriate environmental stimuli. Groskreutz et al. (2015) taught participants to use multiple exemplars of different script frames to appropriately comment on toys. The script frames were attached to various aspects of each toy and a total of 15 trials of script training took place per session. If participants did not independently engage with the scripts, least-to-most physical prompting was used to guide participants to use the script. The participants met mastery criteria for the script frames in two to seven sessions. Groskreutz et al. (2015) extended the current literature on extended script frame procedures by including a novel script-frame procedure. This novel script-frame procedure may have contributed to stimulus generalization which occurred with untrained play activities, and untrained comments.

Ledbetter-Cho et al. (2015) used script training to teach three boys, diagnosed with ASD, between the ages of 4 and 6 years to initiate peer interactions related to sharing toys. The procedure involved having all three boys sit together at a table in a therapy room. Each boy was provided with a set of toys in a random order and instructed to share the toys with his friends. During the script training phase of the experiment, the child was expected to read the script associated with the toys provided. Each of the participants demonstrated improved communication skills with their peers following the introduction of the script. An area that all participants continued to struggle with throughout the intervention was responding to peer initiations. This could be explained by the fact that responses to a peer were not scripted. Pollard et al. (2012) combined the use of a trial-based format and script fading to teach individuals with autism to make bids for joint attention. Three children between the ages of 4 and 7 years were taught to make bids for joint attention using this procedure. Scripts stating "Look, it's a _____," were attached to different toys in the experimental setting. Physical prompting was used to orient the child to the script and a 2 s prompt delay was used to prompt the participants to engage in the intended verbal response. All participants independently initiated bids for joint attention following treatment. For two of the three participants an increase in unscripted language was also observed. These results support the hypothesis that scripts are effective for teaching joint attention, and extended the previous literature by assessing generalization in natural environments.

Once the intended response is acquired using a social script, the script must be faded so that the individual engages in the response independently. While all script procedures involve some form of fading, how the script is faded occurs in different ways. When a written script is used, words can be removed from the end of the script as the mastery criterion is met for each phase. Some learners may require a gradual fading of the script, while other learners may be able to learn scripts more quickly. In some cases, an entire script may not be used, but, rather, a script frame (e.g., Groskreutz et al., 2015). Groskreutz et al. (2015) taught children to use different script frames, such as "Look, it's a _____," when engaging in commenting during play. Pollard et al. (2012) used a similar script-frame procedure to teach individuals with autism to engage in joint attention with toys. Participants were taught to request attention using a script frame with this procedure.

Scripts and script-fading procedures can be used to teach a variety of different verbal responses associated with several different areas of social skills such as bids for joint attention (Pollard et al., 2012) and conversation skills about toys (Garcia-Albea et al., 2014). Scripts and script-fading procedures were demonstrated in the articles referenced above to be effective in teaching participants to engage in scripted and unscripted responses and the responses often generalized to novel conversation partners.

10.10 Computer-Based Instruction Within DTT

The discrete trial format of teaching can be administered in many different ways, including by teachers or through the use of a computer program. Some benefits of the use of a computer program include more efficient and accurate delivery of instruction (Ramdoss et al., 2011). Simpson et al. (2004) utilized a computer program to improve social skills for four participants with autism. The computer program provided a video model of different social skills. The students were exposed to four different videos and had the opportunity to watch each video twice. A teacher was present to provide verbal prompts to assist the student in successfully navigating the software. Each student was exposed to three daily sessions consisting of 12 trials per day. Each session was 45 min and the sessions were dispersed throughout the participants' school day. All participants showed gains in the targeted social skills following implementation of the computer-based intervention used in this study. The combination of computer-based intervention and DTT has many advantages. For example, individuals are often very interested in teaching programs that are presented through a computer, which may increase compliance with the intervention (Simpson et al., 2004). Additionally, as previously mentioned, the use of computer-based programs can minimize some of the instructor errors as well as decrease the delay to reinforcement, and regulate the systematic fading of prompts based on student performance (Ramdoss et al., 2011). The combination of the heightened interest levels in computer-based instruction and the fast-paced nature of DTT can lead to beneficial outcomes in terms of increased performance of targeted social skills.

10.11 Conclusion

As previously mentioned, there are many potential benefits of using DTT to teach social skills, including the increased number of opportunities to practice social skills that may occur less frequently in the natural setting. Additionally, DTT can be brought into the natural setting to promote the generalization of social skills taught through this method. Generalized results remain the essential outcome for these interventions, yet some generalized effects have been documented, including in crucial yet elusive skills such as perspective taking and joint attention. It is important for clinicians to utilize DTT in appropriate contexts, including to address social skill deficits. With a primary focus on efficiency and effectiveness, behavior analysts value evidence-based interventions that lead to socially significant changes. While the field values naturalistic approaches and continues to embrace and assimilate them, we must not be too hasty to abandon effective interventions and approaches.

Within DTT, there are many considerations that can assist clinicians in making intervention as naturalistic as possible. For example, interspersing trials throughout the day in naturally occurring or carefully contrived contexts may be preferable to doing massed trials in a noncontextual manner. Furthermore, varying language used across trials can be helpful in programming for generalization. Using multicomponent packages that incorporate multiple evidence-based elements is also a useful way to target these deficits. Overall, the literature demonstrates that DTT is a useful tool that can be used to teach individuals social skills. Increasing social interactions through DTT has been taught using a multitude of teaching procedures including: peer imitation (Garfinkle & Schwartz, 2002), constant time delays (Nientimp & Cole, 1993), and modeling, prompting, and reinforcement (Shabani et al., 2002; Zanolli et al., 1996). Initiations and responses (Groskreutz et al., 2015), verbal responses to social greetings (Garcia-Albea et al., 2014), eye contact (Jones et al., 2006), in seat and on task behavior, following questions from adults, and imitation skills (DeQuinzio et al., 2007; Garfinkle & Schwartz, 2002) were all taught under the umbrella of social skills using DTT.

There are many formats which DTT can be presented in, including formal and less formal contexts and instruction that is presented by live teachers, video models, and computer programs. The use of DTT should be strongly considered when attempting to teach any of the previously mentioned social skills considering the success of this method reported in the supporting literature. Future research should focus on demonstrating the generality of the skills taught in social skills interventions, as this remains the ultimate and most socially significant outcome of instruction. In addition, more research on the variations of instructional arrangements, the use of a variety of prompts, and on the modalities of instruction (e.g., live, video, and computer models) will help to identify the most efficient approaches to teaching specific skills.

References

Adams, L., Gouvousis, A., VanLue, M., & Waldron, C. (2004). Social story intervention: Improving communication skills in a child with an autism spectrum disorder. *Focus on Autism and Other Developmental Disabilities*, *19*(2), 87–94.

Bellini, S., & Akullian, J. (2007). A meta-analysis of video modeling and video self modeling interventions for children and adolescents with autism spectrum disorders. *Exceptional Children*, *73*(3), 264–287.

Charlop-Christy, M., & Daneshvar, S. (2003). Using video modeling to teach perspective taking to children with autism. *Journal of Positive Behavior Interventions*, *5*(1), 12–21.

Delprato, D. (2001). Comparisons of discrete-trial and normalized behavioral language intervention for young children with autism. *Journal of Autism and Developmental Disorders*, *31*(3), 315–325.

DeQuinzio, J., Townsend, D., Sturmey, P., & Poulson, C. (2007). Generalized imitation of facial models by children with autism. *Journal of Applied Behavior Analysis*, *40*(4), 755–759.

Francisco, M., & Hanley, G. (2012). An evaluation of progressively increasing intertrial intervals on the acquisition and generalization of three social skills. *Journal of Applied Behavior Analysis*, *45*(1), 137–142.

Garcia-Albea, E., Reeve, S., Reeve, K., & Brothers, K. (2014). Using audio script fading and multiple-exemplar training to increase vocal interactions in children with autism. *Journal of Applied Behavior Analysis*, *47*(2), 325–343.

Garfinkle, A., & Schwartz, I. (2002). Peer imitation increasing social interactions in children with autism and other developmental disabilities in inclusive preschool classrooms. *Topics in Early Childhood Special Education*, *22*(1), 26–38.

Gaylord-Ross, R., Haring, T., Breen, C., & Pitts-Conway, V. (1984). The training and generalization of social interaction skills with autistic youth. *Journal of Applied Behavior Analysis, 17*(2), 229–247.

Gena, A., Couloura, S., & Kymissis, E. (2005). Modifying the affective behavior of preschoolers with autism using in-vivo or video modeling and reinforcement contingencies. *Joural of Autism and Developmental Disorders, 35*(5), 545–556.

Groskreutz, M., Peters, A., Groskreutz, N., & Higbee, T. (2015). Increasing play-based commenting in children with autism spectrum disorder using a novel script-frame procedure. *Journal of Applied Behavior Analysis, 48*(2), 442–447.

Gutstein, S., Burgess, A., & Montfort, K. (2007). Evaluation of the relationship development intervention program. *Autism, 11*(5), 397–411.

Harris, S., Handleman, J., & Alessandri, M. (1990). Teaching youths with autism to offer assistance. *Journal of Applied Behavior Analysis, 23*(3), 297–305.

Ingvarsson, E., & Hollobaugh, T. (2010). Acquisition of intraverbal behavior: Teaching children with autism to mand for answers to questions. *Journal of Applied Behavior Analysis, 43*(1), 1–17.

Jones, E., Carr, E., & Feeley, K. (2006). Multiple effects of joint attention intervention for children with autism. *Behavior Modification, 30*(6), 782–834.

Jones, E., Feeley, K., & Takacs, J. (2007). Teaching spontaneous responses to young children with autism. *Journal of Applied Behavior Analysis, 40*(3), 565–570.

Kasari, C., Freeman, S., & Paparella, T. (2006). Joint attention and symbolic play in young children with autism: A randomized controlled intervention study. *Journal of Child Psychology and Psychiatry, 47*(6), 611–620.

Krstovska-Guerrero, I., & Jones, E. (2013). Joint attention in autism: Teaching smiling coordinated with gaze to respond to joint attention bids. *Research in Autism Spectrum Disorders, 7*(1), 93–108.

Leaf, J., Kassardjian, A., Oppenheim-Leaf, M., Cihon, J., Taubman, M., Leaf, R., & McEachin, J. (2016). Social thinking (R): Science, pseudoscience, or antiscience? *Behavior Analysis in Practice, 9*(2), 152–157.

LeBlanc, L., Coates, A., Daneshvar, S., Charlop-Christy, M., Morris, C., & Lancaster, B. (2003). Using video modeling and reinforcement to teach perspective taking skills to children with autism. *Journal of Applied Behavior Analysis, 36*(2), 253–257.

Ledbetter-Cho, K., Lang, R., Davenport, K., Moore, M., Lee, A., Howell, A.,…, & O'Reilly, M. (2015). Effects of script training on the peer-to-peer communication of children with autism spectrum disorder. *Journal of Applied Behavior Analysis, 48*(4), 785–799.

Lopata, C., Thomeer, M., Volker, M., & Nida, R. (2006). Effectiveness of a cognitive-behavioral treatment on the social behaviors of children with asperger disorder. *Focus on Autism and Other Developmental Disabilities, 21*(4), 237–244.

Lovaas, O. I. (1987). Behavioral treatment in normal educational and intellectual functioning in young autistic children. *Journal of Consulting and Clinical Psychology, 55*(1), 3–9.

MacDonald, J., & Ahearn, W. (2015). Teaching observational learning to children with autism. *Journal of Applied Behavior Analysis, 48*(4), 800–816.

Marzullo-Kerth, D., Reeve, S., Reeve, K., & Townsend, D. (2011). Using multiple-exemplar training to teach a generalized repertoire of sharing to children with autism. *Journal of Applied Behavior Analysis, 22*(2), 279–294.

Miranda-Linne, F., & Melin, L. (1992). Acquisition, generalization, and spontaneous use of color adjectives: A comparison of incidental teaching and traditional discrete trial procedures for children with autism. *Research in Developmental Disabilities, 13*(3), 191–210.

Nientimp, E., & Cole, C. (1993). Teaching socially valid social interaction responses to students with severe disabilities in an integrated school setting. *Journal of School Psychology, 30*(4), 343–354.

Peters, L. C., & Thompson, R. H. (2015). Teaching children with autism to respond to conversation partner's interest. *Journal of Applied Behavior Analysis, 48*(3), 544–562.

Pollard, J., Betz, A., & Higbee, T. (2012). Script fading to promote unscripted bids for joint attention in children with autism. *Journal of Applied Behavior Analysis, 45*(2), 387–393.

Ramdoss, S., Lang, R., Mulloy, A., Franco, J., O'Reilly, M. O., Didden, R., & Lancioni, G. (2011). Use of computer- based interventions to teach communication skills to children with autism spectrum disorders: A systematic review. *Journal of Behavioral Education, 20*(1), 55–76.

Roantree, C. F., & Kennedy, C. H. (2006). A paradoxical effect of presession attention on sterotype: Antecednet attention as an establishing, not an abolishing operation. *Journal of Applied Behavior Analysis, 39*(3), 381–384.

Reeve, S., Reeve, K., Townsend, D., & Poulson, C. (2007). Establishing generalized repertoire of helping behavior in children with autism. *Journal of Applied Behavior Analysis, 40*(1), 123–136.

Schrandt, J., Townsend, D., & Poulson, C. (2009). Teaching empathy skills to children with autism. *Journal of Applied Behavior Analysis, 42*(1), 17–32.

Shabani, D. B., Katz, R. C., Wilder, D. A., Beauchamp, K., Taylor, C. R., & Fischer, K. J. (2002). Increasing social initiations in children with autism: Effects of tactile prompts. *Journal of Applied Behavior Analysis, 35*(1), 79–83.

Simpson, A., Langone, J., & Ayres, K. M. (2004). Embedded video and computer based instruction to improve social skills for students with autism. *Education and Training in Developmental Disabilities, 39*(3), 240–252.

Smith, T. (2001). Discrete trial training in the treatment of autism. *Focus on Autism and Other Developmental disabilities, 16*(2), 86–92.

Stewart, K. K., Carr, J. E., & LeBlanc, L. A. (2007). Evaluation of family- implemented behavioral skills training for teaching social skills to a child with Asperger's disorder. *Clinical Case Studies, 6*(3), 252–262.

Varni, J. W., Lovaas, O. I., Koegel, R. L., & Everett, N. L. (1979). An analysis of observational learning in autistic and normal children. *Journal of Abnormal Psychology, 7*, 31–43.

Whalen, C., & Schreibman, L. (2003). Joint attention training for children with autism using behavior modification procedures. *Journal of Child Psychology and Psychiatry, 44*(3), 456–468.

Zanolli, K., Daggett, J., & Adams, T. (1996). Teaching preschool age autistic children to make spontaneous initiations to peers using priming. *Journal of Autism and Developmental Disorders, 26*, 407–422.

11 Incidental Teaching: Happy Progress

Shahla Alai-Rosales, Karen A. Toussaint, and Gail G. McGee

The purpose of any teaching program is learner progress. We teach so that our students diagnosed with autism spectrum disorder (ASD) can learn under the most normalized conditions possible and continue to develop in successful ways across settings and time. Incidental teaching is a contextualized instruction that takes advantage of naturally occurring opportunities – "incidents" – to teach valued skills in the context of child preference and use (Hart & Risley, 1968; Haring, 1992).

The aim of this chapter is to present the potential benefits of incidental teaching for increasing social competence for children with autism. Competencies are comprised of groups of *behaviors* under the conditions of use that lead to particular *outcomes*. In this context, social *behavior* covers a wide expanse and can include diverse skills such as orienting, imitating, communicating, sharing, and negotiating. The social *outcomes* resulting from our teaching success also cover a wide expanse, ranging from play partnerships to situational friendships to enduring and loving companionships. Specific competency goals will vary for each child and the values and norms of their social community. Our examples and recommendations focus on social *behaviors*, with the understanding that the practitioner will place these goals in the context of meaningful competencies. The essence of incidental teaching for social skills is to make the most of motivating variables and present conditions to help the learner learn component social skills, maintain social engagement, and develop mutually beneficial relationships.

This chapter is organized within the context of evidence-based practice (Slocum et al., 2014). That is, successful clinical work is based on sound understanding of the basic mechanisms and principles, best available research evidence, and clinical experience and wisdom (Sackett, Rosenberg, Gray, Haynes, & Richardson, 1996). For that reason, we first provide a description of the theoretical framework supporting incidental teaching, illustrate incidental teaching procedures, summarize the empirical evidence base, and end the chapter with key recommendations based on the theory, research, and our clinical experience.

11.1 Theoretical Framework and Basic Procedures

We cover the theory behind the procedures because it is one of the three driving forces for successful evidence-based practice. If a practitioner

S. Alai-Rosales, Ph.D., BCBA-D (✉) • K.A. Toussaint
Department of Behavior Analysis, College of Health and Public Service, University of North Texas, 1155 Union Circle, #310919 Denton, Texas 76203
e-mail: shahla.alai-rosales@unt.edu

G.G. McGee
Department of Psychiatry and Behavioral Sciences, Emory University, Atlanta, GA, USA

J.B. Leaf (ed.), *Handbook of Social Skills and Autism Spectrum Disorder*, Autism and Child Psychopathology Series, DOI 10.1007/978-3-319-62995-7_11

understands the theory and basic mechanisms, they may be better able to implement the procedures with fidelity and generalize and extend the procedures to new situations and teaching problems (Johnston, 2014; BACB 5th Edition Task List, 2017). While there is a fair amount of research specifically addressing incidental teaching, there are many areas not studied. Yet, a child's world is full of potential incidental teaching opportunities, those we notice and those we create. This means that incidental teaching has the potential to be a pervasive teaching strategy across the child's day. To make the best of these opportunities, it is helpful to understand the basic principles that are believed to be responsible for successful behavior change. This is analogous to master chefs who understand the chemistry principles behind recipes. This knowledge allows them to successfully adopt, adapt, and create far beyond a box recipe.

Incidental teaching procedures were derived from common preschool practices that emphasize teaching within and through children's high-preference play activities. The procedures were formalized, behaviorally conceptualized, and applied to the language development of children living in poverty during the late 1960s and 1970s at the University of Kansas' Center for Research in Early Childhood Education (see Hart & Risley, 1968, 1974, 1975, 1980, 1982). The approach was then extended to other populations and domains (e.g., McGee, Jacobs, & Regnier, 1993; McGee, Krantz, Mason, & McClannahan, 1983; O'Brien, Porterfield, Herbert-Jackson, & Risley, 1979; Warren, McQuarter, & Rogers-Warren, 1984). Furthermore, the empirical research base supporting incidental teaching is noted as a powerful influence on the later development of several effective naturalistic teaching models (e.g., Kaiser, Hancock, & Nietfeld, 2000; Koegel, O'Dell, & Koegel, 1987; Laski, Charlop & Schreibman, 1988; Rogers-Warren & Warren, 1980; Sundberg & Partington, 1998) and is considered an "established practice" within evidence-based practice (see, for example, National Autism Center, 2015).

Incidental teaching is conceptualized within operant learning theory. Operant learning, one type of learning studied in behavior analysis, conceptualizes behavior by considering time and how behaviors change in relation to sequences of events in time. The theory is that behavior is viewed as amenable to change by arranging the type and timing of physical and social environmental events. These events will shift probabilities related to increases or decreases in behavior. Temporal events are broken down into units, and the process is described as a *contingency*, a dependent relation between different events in time. The theory is supported by thousands of experiments verifying the operant processes of learning involved in stimulus control (the events that come before behavior) and consequence control (the reinforcing or punishing events that come after behaviors). For examples of this research base one can refer to textbooks such as *Learning* by Charles Catania (2013).

Incidental teaching involves physical or social events in the child's natural environment with natural interaction partners and events specific to the child's interests. The dependent relations, or contingencies, are arranged around child interests and taught under the conditions of use. In the context of social behavior, incidental teaching is a way of arranging contingencies to produce improved changes in behavior between interaction partners. The basic assumption, from a behavioral standpoint, is that all social interactions are contextually dependent and interaction partners will mediate one another's behavior through a process of contingent interactions (Skinner, 1957; Haring, 1992). Haring (1992) describes this process:

> The skill has to be understood in relation to the goals that a child has for his or her social behavior, the quality of support that the social behavior receives from others, and the power of the simple presence and responsiveness of others in the child's natural settings to increase the occurrence of the behavior. In other words, a more contextualistic analysis considers the goals and functions of the behavior from the child's perspective, as well as the social responses that the child receives in interactions with others, which reinforces social behavior. (p. 309)

When considering social behavior, the contingency involves the discriminative actions and consequences of the social partners. It also involves the motivation for the child to respond under the social contingencies. A typical method of illustrating an operant contingency is presented in Fig. 11.1.

A contingency is a dependent relation in time. Each event has an effect on subsequent events. The stimulus conditions, represented in the schematic as $\mathbf{S^{D\Delta}}$, are those antecedent events that set the occasion for a response to occur (discriminative stimuli or S^D) or not occur (delta stimuli or S^Δ). This part of the process is called *stimulus control*. **R** stands for the response topography of the behavior. This is what the child does, or is to do, in response to the stimulus conditions. The response will be strengthened or weakened by what follows, the consequent stimuli (for our purposes, $\mathbf{S^{R+}}$ or $\mathbf{S^{R-}}$). The stimuli that follow the response will affect the increase or decrease of the response. This is called *reinforcer control*. Motivating operations (**MO**) are those events that alter the reinforcing value of the consequent stimuli; they increase or decrease the value of a consequence. Environmental arrangements are methods to arrange motivation and insure that preferred events and materials are accessible but regulated by the interaction partner. The MO is an essential part of the incidental teaching contingency.

Consideration of all four parts of the contingency and their relationship to one another is considered critical to the success of incidental teaching procedures. Contingencies are arranged around the child's interests, and the stimulus and reinforcement conditions are at the full or approximate criterion conditions in the natural environment. Three factors are especially important in the incidental teaching contingency: (1) child preference; (2) teacher responsiveness to child progress, initiations, and affect; and (3) response specific reinforcers.

First, the child has to indicate in some way that there is a preference for an activity or event. This creates the teaching "incident" and is commonly called a "child-initiated" learning opportunity. The child initiation indicates a preference (hopefully a reinforcing event), and especially in the case of social development, it is preferable that it is a positive reinforcement contingency (i.e., producing approach behaviors), rather than contingencies involving negative reinforcement (i.e., producing escape behaviors) or punishment contingencies (i.e., producing avoidance behaviors). In this regard, a child that is approaching the social partner and displaying indices of favorable affect (e.g., happiness) is more likely to be ready and responsive to an incidental teaching interaction and under the control of positive reinforcement contingencies. For example, a young child reaches for a blue car in a closed container that only his big brother can open. Smiles and eyebrow raises accompany the young child's reach and not grimaces or tears. The big brother can use this initiation as a signal to start an incidental teaching interaction. From a theoretical and methodological point of view, this increases the chance that there will be a reinforcing consequence for the behavior being taught and that the brother has been arranging the right balance of response requirements so his sibling is still happily initiating and approaching the social situation. There is precedent for considering affect as a component part of naturalistic teaching procedures (Koegel, Bimbela, & Schreibman, 1996).

Fig. 11.1 Schematic of a contingency

MO
motivating operation

$S^{D\Delta}$ ⟶ R ⟶ S^{R+}

Discriminative Stimulus
Delta Stimulus

Response

Positively Reinforcing Stimulus

The second point is that incidental teaching requires a responsive teacher that observes and adjusts to the learner's progress. That is, the teaching should be progressive with the learner engaging in increasingly more complex social responses under increasingly more complex conditions. For example, at first the brother may require just a simple vocalization, "blue car." But in order to be progressive, the activity and the target should become more complex and socially robust. For example, the siblings might set up a race track and additional interactions can be added, such as requesting to "crash the cars" or adding instructions to be followed, such as, "Give me the truck so I can crash into your car," or actions to imitate, such as adding pieces of the track during the play activity before getting access to the zipline to activate the car through the track. Of course, while the response requirements are made increasingly complex and diverse, the teacher maintains a balance between the response requirements and access to reinforcement. This is more likely to ensure positively reinforcing contingencies and is accomplished by relying on indicators such as child approach and initiations that are accompanied by indices of happiness and enjoyment (Green & Reid, 1996).

Third, the child's response and the consequence must be related and consistent. For example, the child asks for a blue car and gets a blue car, not a green bus, a potato chip, or a token. From a theoretical point of view, specific response-reinforcer relationships may contribute to the strengthening of a given contingency (Davison & Nevin, 1999; Koegel & Williams, 1980; Schreibman et al., 2015), and from a methodological point of view, it is more likely to be a useful and functional contingency in the child's daily life (Dyer & Peck, 1987). That is, the responses taught are ones more likely to be used in the natural environment, and the contingency will be maintained. For this reason, assessment in the natural environment plays a critical role in the incidental teaching process.

Like all educational programs, we begin with envisioning and assessing. Participation by the stakeholders in the child's life is an essential component to incidental teaching. It is especially important because the arrangement of the teaching should be tailored to the goals and the conditions of the child's natural environment. The stakeholders are the key players in this social environment, and understanding their behaviors and preferences is a critical component of the assessment process. The assessment process continues as reasonable, meaningful, and potentially generative stakeholder goals are understood. Assessment also involves analysis of current child skills and environments, in particular, the incorporation of variables of the current and subsequent least restrictive environments (Brown et al., 1979) and cues related to the criterion discriminations in the natural environment (Etzel & LeBlanc, 1979). All of this is accomplished through a series of ecological assessments, stakeholder interviews, and curriculum guides (see, e.g., Division for Early Childhood, 2014; McLean, Bailey, & Wolery, 2004; Noonan & McCormick, 2014; Odom, McConnell & McEvoy, 1992; Taubman, Leaf & McEachin, 2011; see Chaps. 6, 7, and 8).

As specific goals are agreed upon, the design of the teaching programs begins. A key feature of incidental teaching is the teacher's use of naturally occurring incidents to set the occasion for teaching desired social behavior. There are approaches to naturally occurring opportunities: 1) noticing present child preferences in an existing environment or 2) intentionally introducing regulated access to high-preference events. In most cases, children with ASD will require both approaches due to the restricted activities and interests that are part of the defining features of ASD. To some degree, a technology for arranging enticing and favorable incidental teaching environments has been developed. For example, McGee, Morrier, and Daly (2001) provide extensive descriptions for creating an incidental teaching environment in inclusive early childhood education settings. McGee and colleagues suggest arranging the overall physical structure, rotating provision of high- and neutral-preference toys and activities, and providing methods for creating specific incidental teaching opportunities. In every case, the environment is arranged so that children must respond in order to access desired social and physical events. Textbooks such as *An Activity-Based Approach to Early Intervention* by Johnson, Rahn, and Bricker (2015) and *Teaching Young Children with Disabilities in Natural Environments* by Noonan and McCormick (2014) also provide examples of specific strategies to create incidental teaching opportunities. For example, Noonan and McCormick summarize six specific ways to arrange the environment, or motivating operations (MOs), that include having interesting materials and activities, having items visible but out of reach, offering inadequate or missing portions, providing choice situations, setting up situations where assistance is needed to complete the activity, and creating unexpected or "silly" circumstances. In every case where interest is evoked, the child may initiate and that is the opportunity, the incident, that allows teaching to occur.

To illustrate the theoretical concepts and basic incidental teaching procedures, we provide two simple examples. The first is an example of social orientation with a very young child and the second an example of social bidding with an older child.

11.1.1 Social Orienting Example

Social orientation between communication partners is considered an important behavior for a variety of reasons. Orienting to your social partner can indicate interest and attention, comfort, or discomfort, can allow a person to reference to another to get information about the world, and can be a means to learn basic skills related to developing other skills, such as those related to communication and emotional competencies. These are just a few of the reasons social orienting may be considered a teaching goal.

In our example, Jamal is a 2-year-old boy with autism. Jamal does not make eye contact, looks away when others look at him, and does not call people by their names. Jamal spends most of his time running in circles around the house, opening and closing doors, and stacking books. There are two activities he seems to enjoy – rough housing and tickle games. His parents are being coached in the use of incidental teaching to expand his social skills. In this case, his enjoyment of tickling is the social consequence, and his family members are the interaction partners that set the occasion for and provide the desired social consequences. The parents begin with an interaction that has been going on for several weeks. Jamal pulls their hands, and then they tickle him until he is tired and moves away to one of his solitary activities. His parent described the current interaction with some discomfort: "it feels as if he is just interested in our hands." The goal of adding incidental teaching is to increase Jamal's orienting behavior and to foster more social relationships between Jamal and his parents. Figure 11.2 provides a schematic of the incidental teaching sequence Jamal's parents will use to increase nonvocal, social behavior. Each step is described below (see Fig. 11.2).

11.1.1.1 MO

To begin the incidental teaching, the motivating operations (**MOs**) are arranged. First, instead of waiting until *Jamal* stops the activity, the parent pauses the activity momentarily until he reaches, and then they start tickling again. This allows a brief period of deprivation (instead of waiting until he satiates, that is, gets tired and uninterested and leaves) and multiple chances to practice the

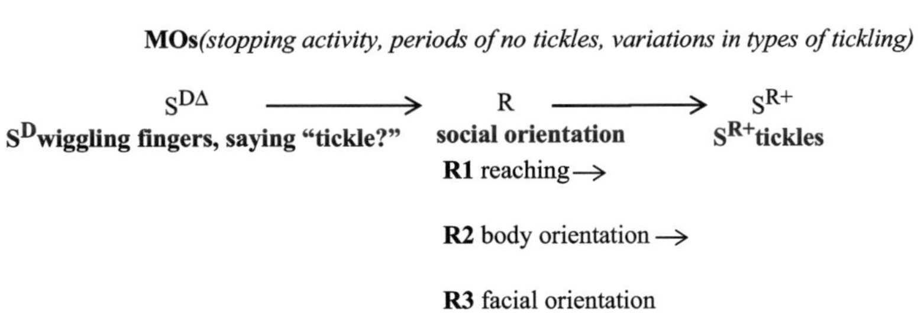

Fig. 11.2 Schematic of a contingency analysis applied to an example of Jamal's social orienting

response. Perhaps more importantly, it also teaches the back and forth nature and reciprocity of a social relationship.

11.1.1.2 S^D

Second, the parent makes a clear facial expression (e.g., eyebrows raised, smiling anticipation) and movement (e.g., fingers wiggling in the air by their faces) to signal (the $\mathbf{S^D}$) they are ready to have fun and tickle just as soon as he makes an approximation to the target response.

11.1.1.3 R

Third, parents require increasingly more complex responses. At first, the parent requires Jamal to reach (**R1**), and as Jamal does this successfully, they then require him to also turn his body toward them (**R2**) and finally to look at them (**R3**). This changing response requirement is a shaping process that is progressed through the consequences (final part of the contingency).

11.1.1.4 S^{R+}

The final part of the contingency involves the consequence stimuli. The fun tickles are the positively reinforcing consequence (S^{R+}) that immediately follows Jamal's social orientations. As his social responding consistently increases, the response requirements increase and become progressively more complex.

Finally, the parents began to introduce additional opportunities and embed other social responses into the interaction. For example, his mom began making raspberries on his belly instead of tickles. To initiate this, she made the raspberry sound when Jamal looked at her, which made Jamal laugh a lot and continue looking at his mom in anticipation. His mom recognizes the laughter, looking as a happy initiation, and waits until he looks before she makes another sound. In his parent's words, "now it feels a lot more like we are connecting and communicating."

11.1.2 Social Bid Example

Figure 11.3 provides an example of an incidental teaching interaction for social bids. Devon is 11; attends a science, math, and technology charter school; and is strong in math but requires special supports in his other subjects. He is described as socially isolated and spends most of his time alone playing video games or collecting statistics on basketball and baseball players. His favorite

MOs *("forgetting" the phone, arranging for cousins to play NBA2K®)*

$S^{D\Delta}$ ⟶ R ⟶ S^{R+}

Antecedent cues, S^D	**social bids**	**desired consequences**
games ends for players		
Cousin asks "who's next?"	**R1** "Can I play?"	S^{R+}cousin gives controller
Ball is in cousin's hands by basket	**R2** "Shoot it!"	S^{R+}cousin makes shot
(dad prompts, "Tell him to shoot it!")		(hopefully)
fades prompt using words, then gesture of shoot motion		
Ball is in cousin's hand	**R3** "Pass, I'm open"	S^{R+}cousin passes ball
(dad prompts, "Tell him to pass it!")		
fades prompt using words, then gesture of pass motion		

Fig. 11.3 Schematic of a contingency analysis applied to an example of Devon's social bids

game is NBA2K®. He plays the game either by himself or with his dad. His father has worked with him on social tolerance for the last few weeks. At first his dad just sat with him while he played, and now he plays with Devon for short periods. They play "coop," meaning they each have a controller and the screen is split so both can play. His dad has been intentionally playing coop for longer durations to increase Devon's tolerance for having someone play at the same time. His intervention team has decided that his interest in NBA2K® will be a good way to work on social activities with others and that incidental teaching would be an appropriate method. They decide to work on social bids. Social bids are a way to get the attention of others, indicate interest, and make requests. Every weekend Devon's family gets together with his maternal grandmother, aunts, uncles, and cousins. Normally he only engages with his dad's phone amidst the family cooking, eating, and socializing. On the other hand, several of the cousins congregate in the family room to play video games. Dad has recruited their help to get Devon more involved.

11.1.2.1 MO

To arrange favorable conditions for incidental teaching, the motivating operations (**MOs**) are addressed. First, Dad forgets his phone in the car. This creates an opportunity to play NBA2K® in other ways. Second, he asks the cousins to play it for a while, which they are happy to do. He also asks them to play coop style. Dad makes himself available to go into the family room with Devon.

11.1.2.2 S^D

Second, his dad chooses a couple of social bids to work on and decides on the signals and prompts for each response (the **S^Ds**). He will encourage one of the cousins to ask, "Who wants the controller?" Dad will also prompt bids to shoot and pass. The prompting will begin with verbal and then gestural cues. The prompting will be faded quickly as Devon is successful.

11.1.2.3 R

Third, as the opportunity arises, Dad and the cousins will require responses specific to Devon's initiations and interests. They provide the controller when he comes into the room and asks to play (**R1**), they shoot the ball when he says shoot (**R2**), and they pass it to him when he asks for a pass (**R3**). This example uses Dad's prompting rather than shaping. In this case, access to the reinforcing consequence is more time dependent (i.e., the opportunity to pass lasts about 2 s), and the responses are all ones that Devon has made with his dad at home. For these reasons, prompting seems to be more efficient.

11.1.2.4 S^{R+}

The final part of the contingency, the consequence stimuli, involves the events that happen after Devon's social bids (S^{R+}). Getting the controller, making points, and getting access to the ball should all increase the probability that Devon will make these responses more frequently with his cousins during family weekend time.

Finally, the family started to introduce additional opportunities and embed other social responses into interactions. For example, his cousins started asking him to bring his other versions of NBA2K®, and they asked him questions about the various stats of players. They looked for online baseball games and set up opportunities for social interactions around that interest. He started to have roles for engagement during family weekends, as opposed to isolation and forbearance until it was over.

Each of these examples illustrates the basic conceptualization of the incidental teaching interaction within the three-term contingency of operant learning theory. In our next section, we review key literature on incidental teaching applications.

11.2 Empirical Evidence

In the first clinical description of individuals with ASD, Leo Kanner noted that social isolation was the most salient characteristic of this group (Kanner, 1943). The current clinical description of ASD categorizes this social dysfunction as social-communicative deficits that are manifested across three specific areas: (a) deficits in social-emotional reciprocity, (b) deficits in nonverbal communication, and (c) deficits in maintaining/understanding relationships (American Psychiatric Association, 2013). In the following, we review the empirical base on incidental teaching of social behavior and describe the relevance of each application to the domain of social-communicative deficits in ASD.

11.2.1 Origins of Incidental Teaching

In a series of seminal studies on enriching language, Hart and Risley (1968, 1974, 1975) established an instructional framework for increasing spontaneous, elaborate speech for disadvantaged preschoolers. Hart and Risley (1968) demonstrated that traditional instruction increased children's "knowledge," or correct labeling, of colors when queried, but the children still lacked the "skill" as they were seldom observed to use color names outside of the instructional setting. To promote spontaneity, it was necessary to create learning opportunities or incidents under the control of natural, environmental cues; to promote complexity, it was necessary for teachers to prompt elaborated language and contingently deliver relevant, preferred stimuli. Accordingly, Hart and Risley (1975) outlined the basic process of incidental teaching: (1) the teacher places numerous, preferred materials in an area that is out of reach yet visible to the child, (2) the child initiates or requests an item, (3) the teacher may prompt the child to provide a more elaborated request dependent upon the quality of the initiation, and (4) the teacher provides access to the preferred item. After implementation of incidental teaching procedures, preschoolers' spontaneous use of complex language is generalized to free-play periods with peers and maintained after the discontinuation of the teaching methods.

11.2.2 Applications to Autism Spectrum Disorder

Given the advantages of enhanced generalization, incidental teaching procedures were incorporated into instructional programming for individuals with ASD to address the limited generalization yielded from analog teaching procedures, such as discrete trial teaching (McGee, Morrier, & Daly, 1999). Discrete trial teaching produced rapid skill acquisition for individuals with ASD by arranging adult-initiated learning opportunities that were under highly controlled stimulus conditions and included contingent access to highly preferred, yet often artificial, and unrelated items (e.g., receiving food for pointing to "circle"). As a result, learners quickly expanded their skill repertoire, but the skills failed to maintain over time and generalize to natural stimulus conditions (Lovaas, Koegel, Simmons, & Long, 1973). In contrast, skills taught using incidental teaching, such as reading (McGee, Krantz, & McClannahan, 1986), receptive identification (McGee et al., 1983), and preposition use (McGee, Krantz, & McClannahan, 1985), are readily generalized for individuals with ASD.

Although research on incidental teaching has demonstrated wide success with preschool populations, incidental teaching procedures can also be successfully applied to the adult population. For example, Farmer-Dougan (1994) showed increases in appropriate requesting with a peer-delivered incidental teaching procedure for adults with developmental disabilities who served as either a peer tutor or peer learner during a lunch-making routine. The experimenters used a combination of instructing, prompting, and modeling to train peer tutors to observe peers' initiations (e.g., reaches) toward an item, subsequently place the desired object out of reach, prompt the learner to verbally request the item, and deliver the object contingent upon requests. As a result of training, appropriate requests increased and generalized to peers and staff during untrained activities. Furthermore, these requests were maintained even after termination of the training. Farmer-Dougan suggests that this is likely attributed to initiations contacting naturally occurring reinforcement contingencies, that is, access to the item and social interactions from peers.

Incidental teaching procedures were originally designed to increase the complexity of language, specifically requests, by delivering learner-specified items contingent upon target language. By design, incidental teaching procedures are well suited to teach requests or responses that are maintained by primary or tangible sources of reinforcement. To improve responding maintained by generalized social reinforcers via incidental teaching, instructors would likely need to systematically fade control from primary reinforcers to social reinforcers or incorporate techniques to actively program for generalization to social reinforcers (Stokes & Baer, 1977).

One notable example is the work of McGee and Daly (2007) who taught three children with autism to use age-appropriate social responses (e.g., "all right") during play using incidental teaching procedures and stimulus-fading techniques. In early stages of instruction, the instructors withheld access to a preferred item, and when the child initiated for a preferred item, the adult provided a social comment (e.g., "You can play with the toy next time"), prompted the child to engage in a targeted social response, and provided contingent access to the preferred item. After facilitating participants' independent social responding using prompt-fading procedures, the teachers provided a social comment during a time when the child already had access to a preferred item in the last fading step. If the child responded with a social phrase, the experimenters provided praise and continued access to the item. Following this teaching sequence, the experimenters evaluated the generalized use of social phrases, across teachers and settings. All three participants demonstrated generalization to a different free-play activity, and two of the three participants demonstrated generalization with a novel teacher. These findings suggest that control of social responses was transferred from primary reinforcers to social reinforcers.

Selecting behaviors that may be maintained by natural maintaining contingencies may also allow for language to come under the control of natural social reinforcement contingencies and not necessarily access to preferred items alone (Stokes & Baer, 1977). McGee, Almeida, Sulzer-Azaroff, and Feldman (1992) taught typical preschoolers to function as a peer tutor and implement incidental teaching strategies to increase social interactions of a child with autism (i.e., "target child") during play periods. Peer tutors were provided with a target child's highly preferred items to encourage social initiations. When the target child initiated toward an item, the peer tutor prompted the child to request the item and delivered the item contingent upon the request. The target children increased requests to peers during play, and the results suggest there were positive, collateral changes in reciprocal social interactions. That is, children with autism increased their initiations and responses to peer tutors, although there were no programmed contingencies for responses, and peer tutors increased their initiations and responses to children with autism, although their initiations were not targeted. This spread of effects from incidental teaching to other social behaviors suggests that responding came under the control of peer social interactions. Furthermore, peer tutors rated the children with autism as "more likable" on a Likert-type rating scale with pictorial representations of response options following the intervention. These results highlight the benefit of incorporating peers within social interventions and suggest a framework to improve social-emotional reciprocity and the relationship between individuals with autism and their peers.

11.2.3 Training Change Agents

Given the effectiveness of incidental training procedures, caregivers and instructors should be provided with the skills to implement these instructional procedures in the child's natural setting, such as the home and school environment. Training packages that consist of a combination of instructions and performance feedback have been successfully used to train caregivers in the home setting (Hsieh, Wilder, & Abellon, 2011), preschool teachers and paraprofessionals in the school setting (Kohler, Anthony, Steighner, and Hoyson, 2001), therapists in the clinic setting via telepractice (Neely, Rispoli, Gerow, & Hong, 2016), and peer tutors within a play context (McGee et al., 1992).

Although there are effective instructional methods to train change agents to implement incidental teaching techniques, one difficulty that instructors may face is identifying the types of environmental arrangements that are likely to influence child response. Kohler et al. (2001) noted that all four of the teachers that participated in the training evaluation had difficulty identifying techniques to facilitate social interactions for preschoolers with ASD. However, once this critical step was acquired, social interactions increased. Thus, future research may consider training programs designed to specifically improve change agents' discrimination of effective versus ineffective environmental arrangements by categorizing learner affective behavior as favorable or unfavorable dependent upon the strategy employed.

11.2.4 Clinical Implications

Incidental teaching is facilitated by first arranging the environment to evoke learner initiations under the control of naturally occurring stimuli, often by restricting access to preferred items. However, any arrangement which entices the learner to indicate an interest is suitable and may also include (a) offering small or inadequate portions of preferred items, (b) providing choice-making opportunities, (c) creating situations in which the learner needs assistance, and (d) creating unexpected situations (McCormick, 2014).

Regardless of the strategy employed, the social teacher (e.g., instructors, parents, peers, clinicians) should take care to ensure that the environmental arrangement introduces a naturally occurring cue and arranges a positive reinforcement contingency (e.g., access to an activity or item) rather than a negative reinforcement contingency where the child responds to terminate a demand. For example, an instructor may briefly interrupt play by removing a toy with which the child is engaging, the child requests the toy, and the instructor returns the toy. If the toy is removed in a manner that is analogous to turn-taking or other naturally occurring situations, when brief interruptions in play are components of engagement with the item, then this is consistent with the process of incidental teaching since the instructor is teaching the learner to engage in a response that *provides access* to preferred stimuli and is congruent with the natural environment. However, if the play is obtrusively interrupted, the instructor is then teaching the learner to engage in a response that *returns access* to preferred stimuli. In both contingencies, requests may increase under respective antecedent conditions, but a potential disadvantage in the latter is that the learner may begin to avoid the instructor if this is the primary type of teaching interaction. Similarly, previous research suggests that when instructors prompt responding (e.g., naming toy color) upon initiation of toy play, rates of toy play decrease, suggesting that adding a response requirement at the beginning of a target response may function as a punisher (Heal & Hanley, 2011).

In summary, the research base suggests a multitude of strategies to entice requests and prompt elaborations; the correct strategy is dependent upon the individual learner and their current preferences and conditions. Thus, a critical feature of incidental teaching is that instructor must notice and respond to the learner's behavior at each stage of the teaching process. The instructor must discriminate between effective and ineffective environmental arrangements based upon learner responding. To notice and respond to each child initiation, careful attention to the learner is required. Additionally, the instructor must assess the learner's skill set and current response to set an appropriate criterion for target responses during any given incidental teaching interaction. For example, it would be incorrect to prompt a learner to vocally request using adjective-noun phrases if the learner's repertoire does not include single words; rather, the instructor might start with one-word requests if the learner has a vocal repertoire. Similarly, the specific social behaviors targeted for teaching are dependent on the child's current repertoire and general knowledge of the domains and progressions of social behavior in typical and atypical development (McGee, Feldman, & Morrier, 1997).

11.3 Key Recommendations and Conclusion

While the theory and the procedures are relatively simple, the implementation of incidental teaching can be somewhat difficult and effortful. Our recommendations are set within the context of evidence-based practice in applied behavior analysis as described by Slocum et al. (2014). That is, research evidence is integrated with client values and clinical experience and wisdom. We have divided our recommendations into four specific areas of our experience that tend to be points of difficulty for clinicians serving children with autism.

11.3.1 Big Picture and Little Picture

Merriam-Webster's Dictionary defines the "big picture" as something "that gives the entire perspective" (Big picture, n.d.). With respect to treatment, Leaf (2016) cautioned clinicians to be mindful of the big picture when addressing the details (little picture) of treatment. In the case of social skills, the big picture is the development and maintenance of meaningful and fulfilling social relationships; the little picture is comprised of the momentary goals within a teaching interaction. In actuality, incidental teaching can both sabotage and help achieve the big picture goals. On one hand, each individual behavior that is taught can contribute to the development of relationships; on the other hand, because teaching is a relationship itself, unskilled management of the incidental teaching interaction can create poor relationships. For example, imagine if Devon's cousins required him to ask for the controller and spent several minutes correcting his pronunciation before they gave him the controller and his father also repeatedly asked for clearer pronunciation when prompting his bids during playtime. Typically, this type of interaction is done with the best of intentions and can be appropriate under certain conditions. For example, his interest in playing could be used to increase the accuracy of his articulations. But the goal in the example given is not to improve articulation; it is to increase social interactions and nurture his relationship with his family. In this case, the response demand may be greater than the value of the reinforcer (i.e., too much talking to get the ball), or it could alter the value of the reinforcer (i.e., too much talking delays the onset of the event, and it ceases to be a reinforcer). At the same time, there is the potential for embarrassment and social stigma on the part of the cousins or Devon. In fact, such circumstances are more likely to function as an aversive event and cause Devon to *move away* from the social interaction with his cousins. The big picture is lost over the little picture. In Devon's case, it might be more helpful to work on articulation in other instructional contexts where social behaviors and outcomes are not the primary goals.

Along the same lines, imagine two siblings on the floor playing with a block activity together and steadily increasing interactions and prolonging engagement. The big picture goal of any incidental teaching interaction in this scenario would be to continue and expand the interactions. In this case, the clinician must be mindful of what opportunities would most likely maintain the flow of interaction and not produce interruption. For example, the clinician could offer the sibling a bucket of additional figurines that would interest both children and be easily incorporated into the activity. The sibling could make access to the figurines contingent on an elaborated social response. Such management of contingencies has shown to be facilitative, rather than impeding of social outcomes (McGee et al., 1992).

It is often helpful to have a team to maintain perspective as to the validity of the ongoing procedures and outcomes of the teaching process. Stakeholders in the child's life constitute the social partners, informants, and collaborators for the child's well-being (e.g., family, peers, teachers, supervisors, community members) and can provide a rich source of perspective in balancing the social validity of the momentary and long-term goals (Fawcett, 1991; Lucyshin, Dunlap, & Albin, 2002; Wolf, 1978).

11.3.2 Learners with ASD Have Restricted Activities and Interests

The genesis of incidental teaching was with children who had language difficulties. Those children also had relatively typical interests and activities that functioned as reinforcers. ASD is a pervasive disorder. Not only are communication and social domains affected, but learners with ASD also have atypical, limited and uncommon activity engagement and preferences. This can present several challenges within the incidental teaching context, the first being that there has to be a preference (i.e., a potential reinforcer) that the instructor can use to help the learner progress. In the case of learners with ASD, this may mean that specific procedures will be needed to expand activities and interests (Alai-Rosales, Zueg, & Baynham, 2008; Leaf et al., 2012).

Second, although incidental teaching is a specific set of instructional procedures, it is important to note that several extensions have been specifically developed for individuals with ASD and come under the umbrella category of "Naturalistic Developmental Behavioral Interventions" (Schreibman et al., 2015). Each of these naturalistic procedures was developed in specific contexts (e.g., ages, settings, populations) and incorporated with specialized procedures regarding the instructional conditions (e.g., availability, arrangement, and presentation of antecedent stimuli), the response forms (e.g., progressions, extensions, and configurations), and consequences (e.g., timing, progression, and topographies). Furthermore, they are specific to ASD and are empirically validated (Schreibman et al., 2015). In every case, the naturalistic models were developed in ways that specifically addressed the unique motivational arrangments required for children with atypical and resticted interests.

Finally, due to the pervasive nature of the disorder, it is likely that incidental teaching will constitute one of many instructional arrangements over the course of a learner's clinical or education experiences. That is, the learner's success will depend on concurrent instructional programming across domains, settings, formats, and models. The particular progressions and selections should be dependent on the child's interests, progress and well-being (Alai-Rosales & Zueg, 2010).

11.3.3 Happy Progress

Happy progress is perhaps our most important recommendation. Incidental teaching is in the class of instructional strategies that are considered "sensitive and responsive interactional practices" (Division for Early Childhood, 2014, p. 14). The Council for Exceptional Children, Division for Early Childhood (2014), offers practices to support socially responsive interactions. These fit both pragmatically and conceptually with what we have presented here in the context of incidental teaching. They recommend that instructors observe and respond contingently to the range of a child's affective responses and adjust instruction accordingly, that instruction is arranged to increase learner initiations in the context of naturally occurring activities, that the consequences are natural and related to the child's interests and preferences, and that the instruction progresses in tandem with the child's growing skills. Throughout the chapter, we have illustrated through our conceptualizations, examples, and evidence the support for these recommendations as they relate to incidental teaching. We end this chapter by recommending "happy progress" as the criteria for determining the ongoing success of incidental teaching procedures. "Happy progress" means the arrangement of positive reinforcement contingencies, clearly signaled by the learner's happy and un-coerced initiations, consequated by natural, response-specific reinforcers, and occurring in the context of progressively more complex competence across behaviors, social partners, and situations over time.

References

Ala'i-Rosales, S., Zeug, N. M., & Baynham, T. Y. (2008). The development of interests in children with autism: A method to establish baselines for analyses and evaluation. *Behavioral Development Bulletin, 14*(1), 3. http://doi.org/10.1037/h0100502

Ala'i-Rosales, S., & Zeug, N. (2010). Three important things to consider when starting intervention for a child diagnosed with autism. *Behavior Analysis in Practice, 3*(2), 54–55.

American Psychiatric Association. (2013). *Diagnostic and statistical manual of mental disorders* (5th ed.). Washington, DC: Author. doi:10.1176/appi.books.9780890425596

Behavior Analyst Certification Board. (2017). BACB fifth edition task list. Retrieved from https://bacb.com/wp-content/uploads/2017/01/170113-BCBA-BCaBA-task-list-5th-ed-english.pdf.

Big picture. (n.d.). In *Merriam Webster Online*, Retrieved April 14, 2017, from https://www.merriam-webster.com/dictionary/big%20picture

Brown, L., Branston-McClean, M. B., Baumgart, D., Vincent, L., Falvey, M., & Schroeder, J. (1979). Using the characteristics of current and subsequent least restrictive environments in the development of curricular content for severely handicapped students. *Research and Practice for Persons with Severe Disabilities, 4*, 407–424.

Catania, C.A. (2013). *Learning* (5th ed.). Cornwall-on-Hudson, NY: Sloan Pub children who have autism. Early Education & Development, 11, 423–446. Co.

Davison, M., & Nevin, J. (1999). Stimuli, reinforcers, and behavior: An integration. *Journal of the Experimental Analysis of Behavior, 71*(3), 439–482. http://doi.org/10.1901/jeab.1999.71-439

Division for Early Childhood. (2014). DEC recommended practices in early intervention/early childhood special education 2014. Retrieved from http://www.dec-sped.org/recommendedpractices

Dyer, K., & Peck, C. A. (1987). Current perspectives on social/communication curricula for students with autism and severe handicaps. *Education and Treatment of Children, 10*, 338–351.

Etzel, B. C., & LeBlanc, J. M. (1979). The simplest treatment alternative: The law of parsimony applied to choosing appropriate instructional control and errorless-learning procedures for the difficult-to-teach child. *Journal of Autism and Developmental Disorders, 9*, 361–382. https://doi.org/10.1007/BF01531445

Farmer-Dougan, V. (1994). Increasing requests by adults with developmental disabilities using incidental teaching by peers. *Journal of Applied Behavior Analysis, 27*, 533–544. http://doi.org/10.1901/jaba.1994.27-533

Fawcett, S. B. (1991). Social validity: A note on methodology. *Journal of Applied Behavior Analysis, 24*, 235–239. http://doi.org/10.1901/jaba.1991.24-235

Green, C. W., & Reid, D. H. (1996). Defining, validating, and increasing indices of happiness among people with profound multiple disabilities. *Journal of Applied Behavior Analysis, 29*, 67–78. http://doi.org/10.1901/jaba.1996.29-67

Haring, T. G. (1992). The context of social competence: Relations, relationships, and generalization (chapter 12). In S. L. Odom, S. R. McConnell, & M. A. McEvoy (Eds.), *Social competence of young children with disabilities: Issues and strategies for intervention*. Baltimore, MD: Brookes Publishing.

Hart, B. M., & Risley, T. R. (1968). Establishing use of descriptive adjectives in the spontaneous speech of disadvantaged preschool children. *Journal of Applied Behavior Analysis, 1*(2), 109–120. https://doi.org/10.1901/jaba.1968.1-109

Hart, B., & Risley, T. R. (1974). Using preschool materials to modify the language of disadvantaged children. *Journal of Applied Behavior Analysis, 7*(2), 243–256. http://doi.org/10.1901/jaba.1974.7-243

Hart, B., & Risley, T. R. (1975). Incidental teaching of language in the preschool. *Journal of Applied Behavior Analysis, 8*, 411–420. https://doi.org/10.1901/jaba.1975.8-411

Hart, B., & Risley, T. R. (1980). In vivo language intervention: Unanticipated general effects. *Journal of Applied Behavior Analysis, 13*, 407–432. http://doi.org/10.1901/jaba.1980.13-407

Hart, B., & Risley, T. R. (1982). *How to use incidental teaching for elaborating language*. Austin, TX: Pro-ed.

Heal, N. A., & Hanley, G. P. (2011). Embedded prompting may function as embedded punishment: detection of unexpected behavioral processes within a typical preschool teaching strategy. *Journal of Applied Behavior Analysis, 44*), 127–131. http://doi.org/10.1901/jaba.2011.44-127

Hsieh, H.-H., Wilder, D. A., & Abellon, O. E. (2011). The effects of training on caregiver implementation of incidental teaching. *Journal of Applied Behavior Analysis, 44*, 199–203. http://doi.org/10.1901/jaba.2011.44-199

Johnston, J. M. (2014). *Radical behaviorism for ABA practitioners*. New York, NY: Sloan Publishing, LLC.

Johnson, J., Rahn, N., & Bricker, D. (2015). *An activity-based approach to early intervention*. Baltimore, MD: Paul Brookes.

Kaiser, A. P., Hancock, T. B., & Nietfeld, J. P. (2000). The effects of parent-implemented enhanced milieu teaching on the social communication of children who have autism. *Early Education and Development, 11*, 423–446. https://doi.org/10.1207/s15566935eed1104_4

Kanner, L. (1943). Autistic disturbances of affective contact. *The Nervous Child, 2*, 217–250.

Koegel, R. L., Bimbela, A., & Schreibman, L. (1996). Collateral effects of parent training on family interactions. *Journal of Autism and Developmental Disorders, 26*, 347–359. https://doi.org/10.1007/BF02172479

Koegel, R. L., O'Dell, M. C., & Koegel, L. K. (1987). A natural language teaching paradigm for nonverbal autistic children. *Journal of Autism and Developmental Disorders, 17*, 187–200. https://doi.org/10.1007/BF01495055

Koegel, R. L., & Williams, J. A. (1980). Direct versus indirect response-reinforcer relationships in teaching autistic children. *Journal of Abnormal Child Psychology*, *8*, 537–547. https://doi.org/10.1007/BF00916505

Kohler, F. W., Anthony, L. J., Steighner, S. A., & Hoyson, M. (2001). Teaching social interaction skills in the integrated preschool: An examination of naturalistic tactics. *Topics in Early Childhood Special Education*, *21*, 93–103. doi:10.1177/027112140102100203

Laski, K. E., Charlop, M. H., & Schreibman, L. (1988). Training parents to use the natural language paradigm to increase their autistic children's speech. *Journal of Applied Behavior Analysis*, *21*, 391–400. http://doi.org/10.1901/jaba.1988.21-391

Leaf, J. B. (2016, April). The future of research. In J. B. Leaf, *Preserving quality ABA and the effective implementation of autism treatment*. Symposium conducted at the Meeting of Center for the Advancement of Behavior Analysis, Seal Beach, CA.

Leaf, J. B., Oppenheim-Leaf, M. L., Leaf, R., Courtemanche, A. B., Taubman, M., McEachin, J., et al. (2012). Observational effects on the preferences of children with autism. *Journal of Applied Behavior Analysis*, *45*, 473–483. http://doi.org/10.1901/jaba.2012.45-473

Lovaas, O. I., Koegel, R., Simmons, J. Q., & Long, J. S. (1973). Some generalization and follow-up measures on autistic children in behavior therapy. *Journal of Applied Behavior Analysis*, *6*, 131–165. http://doi.org/10.1901/jaba.1973.6-131

Lucyshyn, J. M., Dunlap, G., & Albin, R. W. (Eds.). (2002). *Families and positive behavior support: Addressing problem behavior in family contexts*. Baltimore, MD: Paul H. Brookes.

McCormick, L. (2014). Specialized instructional strategies. In M. J. Noonan & L. McCormick (Eds.), *Teaching young children with disabilities in natural environments* (pp. 149–175). Paul H. Brookes Publishing.

McGee, G. G., Almeida, M. C., Sulzer-Azaroff, B., & Feldman, R. S. (1992). Promoting reciprocal interactions via peer incidental teaching. *Journal of Applied Behavior Analysis*, *25*, 117–126. http://doi.org/10.1901/jaba.1992.25-117

McGee, G. G., & Daly, T. (2007). Incidental teaching of age-appropriate social phrases to children with autism. *Research and Practice for Persons with Severe Disabilities*, *32*, 112–123. https://doi.org/10.2511/rpsd.32.2.112

McGee, G. G., Feldman, R. S., & Morrier, M. J. (1997). Benchmarks of social treatment for children with autism. *Journal of Autism and Developmental Disorders*, *27*, 353–364. https://doi.org/10.1023/A:1025849220209

McGee, G. G., Jacobs, H. A., & Regnier, M. C. (1993). Preparation of families for incidental teaching and advocacy for their children with autism. *OSERS, News in Print*, *5*, 9–13.

McGee, G. G., Krantz, P. J., Mason, D., & McClannahan, L. E. (1983). A modified incidental-teaching procedure for autistic youth: Acquisition and generalization of receptive object labels. *Journal of Applied Behavior Analysis*, *16*, 329–338. http://doi.org/10.1901/jaba.1983.16-329

McGee, G. G., Krantz, P. J., & McClannahan, L. E. (1985). The facilitative effects of incidental teaching on preposition use by autistic children. *Journal of Applied Behavior Analysis*, *18*, 17–31. http://doi.org/10.1901/jaba.1985.18-17

McGee, G. G., Krantz, P. J., & McClannahan, L. E. (1986). An extension of incidental teaching procedures to reading instruction for autistic children. *Journal of Applied Behavior Analysis*, *19*, 147–157. http://doi.org/10.1901/jaba.1986.19-147

McGee, G. G., Morrier, M. J., & Daly, T. (1999). An incidental teaching approach to early intervention for toddlers with autism. *Journal of the Association for Persons with Severe Handicaps*, *24*, 133–146. doi:10.2511/rpsd.24.3.133

McGee, G. G., Morrier, M. J., & Daly, T. (2001). The Walden early childhood programs. In S. L. Harris & J. S. Handleman (Eds.), *Preschool education programs for children with autism* (2nd ed.). Austin, TX: Pro-Ed.

McLean, M. E., Bailey, D. B., & Wolery, M. (2004). *Assessing infants and preschoolers with special needs* (3rd ed.). New York, NY: Macmillan.

National Autism Center. (2015). *Findings and conclusions: National standards project phase 2*. Randolph, MA: Author.

Neely, L., Rispoli, M., Gerow, S., & Hong, E. R. (2016). Preparing interventionists via telepractice in incidental teaching for children with autism. *Journal of Behavioral Education*, *25*, 393–416. https://doi.org/10.1007/s10864-016-9250-7

Noonan, M. J., & McCormick, L. (2014). *Teaching children with disabilities in natural environments: Methods and procedures*. Pacific Grove, CA: Paul H. Brookes Publishing Co..

O'Brien, M., Porterfield, J., Herbert-Jackson, E., & Risley, T. R. (1979). *The toddler center* (pp. 29–47). Baltimore, MD: University Park Press.

Odom, S. L., McConnell, S. R., & McEvoy, M. A. (Eds.). (1992). *Social competence of young children with disabilities: Issues and strategies for intervention*. Baltimore, MD: Paul H. Brookes.

Rogers-Warren, A., & Warren, S. F. (1980). Mands for verbalization facilitating the display of newly trained language in children. *Behavior Modification*, *4*, 361–382. https://doi.org/10.1177/014544558043006

Sackett, D. L., Rosenberg, W. M. C., Gray, J. A. M., Haynes, R. B., & Richardson, W. S. (1996). Evidence based medicine: What it is and what it isn't. *British Medical Journal*, *312*(7023), 71–72. http://doi.org/10.1136/bmj.312.7023.71

Schreibman, L., Dawson, G., Stahmer, A. C., Landa, R., Rogers, S. J., McGee, G. G., … Halladay, A. (2015). Naturalistic developmental behavioral interventions: Empirically validated treatments for autism spectrum disorder. *Journal of Autism and Developmental Disorders*, *45*, 2411–2428. https://doi.org/10.1007/s10803-015-2407-8

Skinner, B. F. (1957). *Verbal behavior*. Englewood Cliffs, NJ: Prentice-Hall. https://doi.org/10.1037/11256-000

Slocum, T. A., Detrich, R., Wilczynski, S. M., Spencer, T. D., Lewis, T., & Wolfe, K. (2014). The evidence-based practice of applied behavior analysis. *The Behavior Analyst Today, 37*(1), 41–56. http://doi.org/10.1007/s40614-014-0005-2

Stokes, T., & Baer, D. (1977). An implicit technology of generalization. *Journal of Applied Behavior Analysis, 10*, 349–367. doi:10.1901/jaba.1977.10-349

Sundberg, M. L., & Partington, J. W. (1998). *Teaching language to children with autism or other developmental disabilities*. Danville, CA: Behavior Analysts.

Taubman, M., Leaf, R., & McEachin, J. (2011). *Crafting connections: Contemporary applied behavior analysis for enriching social lives of persons with autism spectrum disorder*. New York, NY: DRL Books.

Warren, S. F., McQuarter, R. J., & Rogers-Warren, A. K. (1984). The effects of mands and models on the speech of unresponsive language-delayed preschool children. *The Journal of Speech and Hearing Disorders, 49*, 43–52. https://doi.org/10.1044/jshd.4901.43

Wolf, M. M. (1978). Social validity: The case for subjective measurement or how applied behavior analysis is finding its heart. *Journal of Applied Behavior Analysis, 11*, 203–214. https://doi.org/10.1901/jaba.1978.11-203

Pivotal Response Treatment: Empirically Supported Strategies to Target Social Competencies and Motivation in Individuals with ASD

12

Ty Vernon

Pivotal response treatment (PRT) is a comprehensive intervention package for treating the core social communication vulnerabilities associated with autism spectrum disorder (ASD). PRT is recognized as an empirically validated treatment (National Research Council, 2001; National Standards Project, 2008; Simpson, 2005). These treatment strategies target a number of pivotal developmental areas—key domains that, when targeted, also yield improvements in a broad array of skills.

PRT was originally conceptualized as the Natural Language Paradigm (Koegel, O'Dell, & Koegel, 1987b), as the origin of many of its component parts was rooted in research aimed at facilitating communicative speech. Using motivational principles (Koegel, Koegel, Harrower, & Carter, 1999b), researchers determined that the use of specific therapeutic strategies had a profound effect on behavioral learning paradigms. Specifically, when used to target social communication skills, the resulting language acquisition data was found to be superior when compared to a more structured applied behavior analysis approach (Mohammadzaheri, Koegel, Rezaei, & Bakhshi, 2015).

The communication impairments present in ASD are often perceived to be the most challenging and are generally prioritized by intervention programs (Rogers & Vismara, 2008). Tremendous strides have been made in the areas of early detection and early language intervention, bringing the state of the science to a place in which the majority of children who are diagnosed with ASD are expected to develop some level of communicative phrase speech (Wodka, Mathy, & Kalb, 2013). This change represents a paradigm shift in the understanding of the disorder—children with ASD are no longer perceived as uneducable, and expectations for long-term outcomes have increased significantly. At the same time, a better understanding of the range of cognitive abilities among those with ASD has emerged, encapsulated by the growing use of terms to capture cognitively advanced individuals, such as "high-functioning autism." As shifts in expectations occurred, so have priorities for intervention efforts. Now that effective intervention strategies exist that enable most children to acquire spoken language (Koegel, 2000), efforts have begun to address other seemingly insurmountable targets—the acquisition of play skills, social skills, and interpersonal competence to function effectively within natural environments and contexts.

12.1 Social Competence

Social competence is a nebulous concept that is perhaps more easily recognized by one's social partners than defined operationally (Waters &

T. Vernon, PhD (✉)
Koegel Autism Center, University of California Santa Barbara, Santa Barbara, CA, USA
e-mail: tyvernon@ucsb.edu

J.B. Leaf (ed.), *Handbook of Social Skills and Autism Spectrum Disorder*, Autism and Child Psychopathology Series, DOI 10.1007/978-3-319-62995-7_12

Sroufe, 1983). It encompasses a range of skills and insights that allow a person to effectively engage with and be positively perceived by their social partners. The developmental expectations associated with sufficient social competence increase significantly from birth through adulthood as the sophistication of interpersonal bids and responses aligns with unfolding cognitive capacities. The development of social cognition skills (e.g., perspective-taking, theory of mind, empathy) allows individuals to move beyond self-serving instrumental interactions and prioritize the needs of social partners during an encounter (Hala, 2013). This *other* focus creates opportunities for the development of parent-child bonds, close friendships, and romantic relationships.

Social competence acquisition is not a passive developmental progression. Rather, it is an active transactional process, as ongoing exchanges between a person and one's social environment mutually influence one another over time (Sameroff, 2009). For example, in early childhood, a parent's initiation of playful exchanges with a child fosters their toddler's willingness to make eye contact, direct smiles and laughter, and make verbal initiations. In turn, the child's positive social responses alter the parent's future desire to engage in similar exchanges. Over time, both parties jointly build crucial social momentum—a transactional, mutually influential dance that strengthens connection and social benefit for both members of the family. As a child develops and enters new social contexts, analogous transactional exchanges occur among same-aged peers.

Unfortunately, the transactional acquisition of social competence can become derailed if social responsiveness is compromised in one or both parties (Vernon, 2014). This poses a particular challenge to children with ASD, as their responsiveness to social bids and the quality and frequency of their social bids are often severely impacted. These limitations restrict the parent-child and peer-to-peer interactions that can take place, causing significant downstream developmental consequences (Jones & Klin, 2009).

When a person's level of social competence falls below a minimum threshold, this person is no longer perceived as an interested or desirable social partner by peers. For example, if a person is either (a) failing to make social bids or (b) employing the use of developmentally immature or inappropriate social strategies, peers are likely to ignore or outright reject this individual, precluding him or her from accessing the very social opportunities needed to help them to improve his or her social functioning. The presence of a social disorder, such as ASD, significantly decreases this baseline level of social competence, greatly limiting the likelihood that social traction and momentum can be established on its own.

There is growing recognition that intentional efforts to improve the acquisition of social competence can be highly effective. Specific skills can be broken down into component parts and taught through behavioral learning strategies. Incentivizing the acquisition of skills can be highly effective for motivating children to learn and use new skills within an interpersonal context. When delivered early in development, it is likely that early social vulnerabilities can be corrected, providing them with essential prerequisites that will allow them to be accepted by peers and successfully enter into a transactional, self-sustaining social learning context. PRT is an example of a highly effective intervention paradigm for promoting early social competencies for children with ASD to foster desirable long-term outcomes.

12.2 PRT Overview

PRT strategies initially target language development by overlaying motivational strategies on a three-step behavioral learning contingency (Koegel, O'Dell, & Koegel, 1987b). A child is presented with a preferred stimulus (often a favorite toy or object) and a prompt to make a verbal request. If the child makes a verbal attempt for the object, it is contingently delivered. This exchange strengthens the child's association between language use and desired outcomes, which in turn drives language acquisition. The use of motivational procedures—namely, child selection of intervention materials, use of simple bids to attract child attention, the combination of previously mastered and novel learning tasks, use of natural/logically related reinforcers, and the immediate reinforcement of any reasonable effort to respond—drives skill development but also has another benefit. There appear to be collateral gains in other, untargeted areas of development. Increasing motivation appeared to build developmental momentum and facilitate growth in multiple areas simultaneously. Specifically, in addition to language gains, there were often improvements to problem behaviors, eye contact, directed facial expressions, and overall engagement to both social partners and their environment (e.g., Vernon, Koegel, Dauterman, & Stolen, 2012).

12.2.1 Child Choice

Emphasizing a play-based therapeutic environment and allowing a child to select the play materials and activities have been demonstrated to maximize engagement and learning (Kaiser, Hancock, & Nietfeld, 2000; Koegel, Dyer, & Bell, 1987a), which is an extension and augmentation of early task variation research (Dunlap, 1984; Dunlap & Koegel, 1980). When the qualities of intervention stimuli leverage child attention and interest, it creates a situation in which a child is willing to attempt anything to continue to have access to the play materials. This moment is when intervention can most effectively promote the use of language as a social communicative tool. When such activities are paused, a prompt is used to guide the child to verbally request the activity.

Extended into the realm of social skills interventions, an older child's interests serve as a natural area of expertise. Embedding these interests within a play activity allows a child to take advantage of their pre-existing thematic knowledge and be perceived by peers as an expert on a particular topic. Additionally, the focus on these topics effectively obscures the true purpose of the activity (i.e., targeting social skills) from the children with ASD, reducing performance anxiety. Research suggests that these arrangements significantly increase participating children's engagement and social bids (Baker, Koegel, & Koegel, 1998; Koegel et al., 2014a).

12.2.2 Shared Control

After an activity has been identified, it is important to establish shared control over the stimulus materials. A child with unlimited access to a particular toy or activity does not have an incentive to make verbal requests, as the use of such a bid would not result in a change in her or his current experience. In contrast, if the child's parent or clinician can playfully gain shared control over the activity, the child now has an incentive to make a verbal request to the adult. Recently, emphasis has been placed on using child-preferred activities that require the presence of a social partner (i.e., the activity is only possible with the help of another person), thus strengthening the role of adults as essential play partners (Vernon, Koegel, Dauterman, Stolen, 2012). In PRT-based social skills interventions, the use of cooperative arrangements leverages the use of shared control (Koegel, Werner, Vismara, & Koegel, 2005). By dividing the materials of a mutually engaging activity between two playmates, opportunities are created for a child with ASD and a peer to work collaboratively to complete the activity. They must ask each other for access to each other's materials and work together to complete an art piece, construction project, or board game.

12.2.3 Child Attention and Clear Learning Opportunities

It is essential that a child is attending to the relevant stimuli prior to creating a learning opportunity. Parents and clinicians are encouraged to take action to entice the child's attention. This can be accomplished by moving into the child's line of sight, holding out a desired object, or providing a noncontingent preview of an activity (initial free access to sample a potentially motivating activity). Once a child's attention is obtained, an opportunity can be presented.

Children with ASD appear to have challenges attending to the most relevant aspects of their environment. When attempting to prompt for a child's language attempt, efforts should be made to limit the verbiage used. If a child is exposed to constant language use during a session (i.e., a narration of their play), he/she will likely be less responsive to verbal prompts to speak because the salience of those bids is reduced. When a child is initially acquiring language, adults are encouraged to limit their language use to single-word prompts used only when signaling a child to make a request. These simple prompts ensure that a clear expectation for a verbal response is established.

12.2.4 Use of Maintenance and Acquisition Tasks

During intervention efforts, a careful balance of developmental skill acquisition and the maintenance of motivation must be achieved. Exclusive exposure to challenging new skills will quickly erode motivation to continue in an intervention session. On the other hand, overexposure to mastered or nearly mastered tasks will likely create a high level of engagement but will be unlikely to result in meaningful skill acquisition. Used in combination, child responsiveness and correct responding are improved (Dunlap, 1984). PRT balances both types of learning trials to create highly motivated learners.

12.2.5 Natural Reinforcement

Early attempts to address social communication deficits relied on repeated presentation of discrete learning trials with small edibles and praise used as reinforcers. While progress was accomplished, intervention sessions were often laborious, and intrinsic task motivation was minimal. The use of "natural," functionally related reinforcement represented a paradigm shift in autism intervention efforts. A natural extension of the child choice paradigm, reinforcement no longer relied on arbitrary stimulus materials and instead became intrinsically rooted in the learning activity itself (Koegel & Williams, 1980; Williams, Koegel, & Egel, 1981). In early language learners, children became motivated to repeat verbal prompts and initiate language on their own. When applied to social skill instructional efforts, reinforcement exists naturally in social contexts that have successfully incorporated a child's interests and choices. Games with embedded themes provide a natural opportunity for a child to discuss and hear content related to these elements of interest. Likewise, social interventions targeting key conversational strategies can be facilitated through discussions of favorite topics. In this arrangement, the opportunity to both share information about a preferred topic and have a social partner reciprocate this interest provides sufficient reinforcement to practice a challenging conversational tool or strategy (Koegel, Ashbaugh, Koegel, Detar, & Regester, 2013).

12.2.6 Immediate Reinforcement of Reasonable Attempts

In skill learning paradigms, motivation to persist in learning is directly related to perceived predictability of reinforcement. When strict response requirements are imposed, it is highly likely that skill attempts will fall short of these criteria. PRT emphasizes reinforcement of any effortful attempt at a target skill, ensuring consistent access to reinforcement (Koegel, O'Dell, & Dunlap, 1988). Motivation is emphasized over perfection, and these loose target criteria actually promote more timely mastery of challenging developmental tasks. When used in peer-facilitated PRT sessions, peers learned to reinforce reasonable efforts at responding—thus altering the responsiveness of the social environment to promote the social and play skills of children with ASD (Kuhn, Bodkin, Devlin, & Doggett, 2008; Pierce & Schreibman, 1997).

12.3 Embedded Social Reinforcement

In more recent PRT empirical investigations, efforts were made to directly target social engagement and social skills. Rather than desiring social engagement to increase as a collateral gain, PRT procedures were modified to place social interaction at the forefront of the learning exchange. Children with ASD were conceptualized not as devoid of engagement, but rather as preferring engagement with specific thematic interests and sensory stimulation over social interaction (Vernon, 2014; Vismara & Lyons, 2007). Through the analysis of their preferred interests, the underlying characteristics of preferred activities and objects could be better understood. These traits could then be extracted and used in the development of a comparable social activity. Emphasis was placed on activities in which the presence of another person was essential to the experience (Koegel, Vernon, & Koegel, 2009). The social partner served to either enhance the nature of a previously nonsocial interest or create a new experience containing elements with known motivational qualities. Opportunities were still presented using the same three-part contingency, but this time access to preferred objects and nonsocial activities was replaced with access to a motivating social exchange. Social interaction became the primary reinforcer, blurring the boundaries between existing forms of motivation and social motivation.

The results of these investigations were very encouraging; core early social skills, such as verbal initiations, eye contact, and directed facial expressions, increased significantly (Koegel et al., 2009). By enhancing the social motivational components of the learning opportunity, there was a direct elicitation of social behaviors that are essential prerequisites to later social learning—namely, close attention to one's social behaviors, response to verbal input, and sustained levels of engagement.

Even more profound effects were made when parents were trained in these intervention methods. Data collected on parent social behaviors indicated that they significantly benefited as well (Vernon et al., 2012). Parent positive affect and synchronous engagement (i.e., mutually directed facial expressions) increased during these exchanges. To better understand the direction of the parent and child gains, time-window sequential analyses were conducted in which the time-windows immediately following the onset of each parent and child social behavior were examined for a corresponding response from the other party (Vernon, 2014). These analyses revealed that the onset of child social behaviors (e.g., verbal initiations, eye contact, positive affect) was directly driving parent social behaviors. Parent social behaviors were also evoking, in kind, child social responses. The resulting reciprocal interactions provided evidence of a powerful transactional exchange that persisted even after the parent education program concluded. These recent developments in the PRT research literature created a pivot point in which social motivation is identified as a viable early intervention target. It is now conceptualized that the foundation of social competence lies in sustained immersion in one's social environment, which relies on a foundation of social motivation. These new PRT procedures are intended to maximize one's inclination to seek out and engage in social contact, which then facilitates the growth of language, social skills, emotional developmental, and social cognition.

12.4 Social Initiations

Historically, motivation to speak was achieved by teaching the value of language to effectively and efficiently achieve instrumental needs—fulfilling basic survival needs of hunger and thirst, obtaining desired toys, and rejecting undesired activities. However, some core behavioral and developmental challenges remain. The first is the risk of prompt dependence. Many children become a passive agent of their environment, able to respond predictably to verbal prompts but are significantly less likely to initiate contact on their own. Children must be able to successfully self-advocate for their needs without dependence on external prompts and reminders. Additionally, social competence requires the use of language for more than just the attainment of personal needs. There is also a need to socially connect to simply share experiences. Once the foundation of language is laid, there appears to be a tremendous value in promoting its use for purely social bids.

Initiations appear to be another pivotal area of development. Evidence suggests that they are greatly diminished or even absent in children with ASD (Fredeen & Koegel, 2006) and they may serve as a predictor of long-term outcome (Koegel, Koegel, Shoshan, & McNerney, 1999a). Being an active agent in one's life is crucial, as it ensures that the individual can effectively self-advocate, self-promote, and self-govern. PRT strategies that are designed to promote self-initiations combine motivational and prompt-fading procedures. Specifically, after children have demonstrated reliable repetition of a verbal prompt, this motivation to respond is then used to facilitate an initiation through the use of time delay (i.e., "wait and see") and visual prompt procedures. Instead of the anticipated verbal prompt, a language opportunity is created by nonverbally enticing the child with the activity of interest and waiting for a more spontaneous verbal bid. Momentum from several verbal prompts can often be used to increase the likelihood that the same verbal bid will be used even in the absence of a subsequent prompt. After spontaneous language use is predictably obtained, the priority of intervention can then shift toward targeting more social uses of language.

12.4.1 Question-Asking Initiations

One of the challenges in prompting social language with individuals with autism is a decreased perceived sense of intrinsic motivation stemming from social interaction. Engaging in verbal communication for purely social purpose (i.e., drawing one's attention to an object of interest, sharing personal perspectives and experiences, and inquiring about the perspectives and experiences of others) is generally conducted because there is a perceived reward value in social contact. Unfortunately, this inherent reward value is often diminished in individuals with autism spectrum disorders (Koegel & Egel, 1979; Koegel, O'Dell, & Dunlap, 1988b). The remedy appears to lie in leveraging existing motivation. Because there is value in obtaining desired nonsocial outcomes (e.g., asking for objects), this asset is utilized to promote social inquiry. Specifically, the lines between instrumental and social requests are merged into a procedure that reinforces inquiries with highly desired objects. Ultimately, question-asking procedures have been directly linked to increases in the variety of inquiries employed by children with ASD (Koegel, Bradshaw, Ashbaugh, & Koegel, 2014a).

In these procedures, child-preferred objects are placed in an opaque container or otherwise hidden (e.g., bag, box, or behind one's back), and a prompt is delivered for the child to ask, "What's that?" (Koegel, Camarata, Valdez-Menchaca, & Koegel, 1997). The child's response to this prompt is reinforced with the revealing and labeling of the desired object, along with the opportunity to interact with the stimuli. These procedures are repeated several times with additional items in the container, which promotes the inherent reward value of asking questions. As a child gains mastery of this skill, these procedures are expanded to include the use of neutral and unfamiliar objects, so that the child is learning to make inquiries to acquire the names of a variety of new materials.

After mastery of the "What's that?" question is acquired, additional progress can be made with the introduction of additional question types (Koegel et al., 2014a). Preferred objects can be hidden around the room, requiring the use of a "Where is it?" question to learn their location. "Whose is it?" questions can be used to divide up desired materials, with particular emphasis placed on "It's yours" responses to ensure that the child is compelled to keep asking (Koegel, Koegel, Green-Hopkins, & Barnes, 2010). "When do we get to…" questions can be used to create opportunities to engage in favorite activities immediately (e.g., "Right now!") or after a brief time delay (e.g., "In five seconds"). Eventually, "What's happening?" prompts can also be paired with ongoing desired actions (e.g., pull tabs on pop-up books) to promote commenting on their environment (Koegel, Carter, & Koegel, 2003). As cognitive development continues, "why" questions can also be prompted to provide key information of interest to individuals as the primary reinforcer.

12.5 Peer Interaction

Peer interactions are the key to social competence at older ages. The PRT components are used to structure peer gatherings and ensure that both parties positively receive the social opportunities present in these interactions. The component of child-preferred stimuli is expanded to encompass mutually reinforcing activities, as the interest of both parties must be considered. Finding the overlap in interests ensures that motivation is maximized to increase investment in the exchange, even in the face of less than optimal interactions between the children. As previously noted, thematic interests have been successfully incorporated into popular children's activities to create activities with mutual appeal (Baker et al., 1998; Koegel et al., 2005). Adult facilitation is utilized to heighten child attention to the social bids of others, and prompting is used to ensure that efforts to socialize are reinforced. When possible, the materials of a playdate activity are divided among the children, mimicking the shared control setup present in an adult-facilitated PRT session. Children are incentivized to initiate requests to one another to gain access to desired play materials, thus creating multiple opportunities to increase both initiations and responses to same-aged peers.

12.6 Self-Management

As social motivation, language sophistication, and cognitive development converge, the stage is set for self-monitoring social exchanges. This is the developmental precipice of a third pivotal area of development—the area of self-monitoring, management, and regulation. Typically developing individuals constantly engage in ongoing self-regulation as a means to ensure that one's presentation is positively received.

For individuals with more limited monitoring skills, self-management procedures can be explicitly taught (Koegel & Koegel, 1990; Koegel, Koegel, Hurley, & Frea, 1992; Koegel, Koegel, & Ingham, 1986; Koegel, Koegel, Ingham, & Van Voy, 1988a). Children with ASD are provided with a definition of a key skill and are taught methods for monitoring their use of these skills. These particular skills are generally not intrinsically rewarding since they have not spontaneously emerged on their own. Therefore, motivation is heightened by introducing opportunities to receive child-selected incentives for attempting the use of the self-management procedures. After a few initial attempts at the new skill, efforts are received for access to the child-preferred object. When used for social development, this tool is particularly useful for targeting social conversation skills.

12.6.1 Self-Management in Conversation

When applying self-management to social conversation, the complexities of conversation are initially simplified and broken down into component parts (Doggett, Krasno, Koegel, & Koegel, 2013). The constant word stream emanating from conversational partners is divided into two primary components—questions and statements. Questions are defined as any attempt to obtain information from the other person, while a statement is used to share experiences, thoughts, and perspectives. Because of the infinite possibilities of questions involved in every conversational exchange, efforts are made to restrict response options during these teaching trials. The conversational facilitator introduces the concept of question asking by making a leading statement—that is, a statement that intentionally omits a desired piece of information and creates the basis for an obvious question. Leading statements such as "I went somewhere really fun yesterday," "I spent time with someone really fun this morning," or "I ate something really tasty for lunch" increase conversational expectations by guiding the recipient toward a particular follow-up question. After the question is asked, the individual records their use of the skill, and the conversation continues with more information and another leading statement. After sufficient opportunities for practice, the individual acquires enough of the specified number of practice opportunities to warrant access of their selected incentive. As a more advanced skill, empathetic questions can be used to express interest and concern to a social partner, resulting in improvements in perceived social desirability (Koegel, Ashbaugh, Navab, & Koegel, 2016).

Once questions to leading statements are mastered, efforts are shifted to reduce the prompt signal qualities of the statements made. "Neutral" statements are offered that more closely resemble typical conversational bids while the individual is still encouraged to make an appropriate inquiry. The individual is taught that every statement lends itself to multiple possible questions.

After question asking is sufficiently mastered, efforts are shifted to target statements. Statements are introduced as methods for sharing similar experiences or interests, providing syndications of empathy, or sharing personal information to serve as new conversational content. Again, the individual is encouraged to self-manage the use of statements in response to conversational bids. After hearing a particular social bid "I got a flat tire the other day," "I found 20 dollars on my walk to work," or "I love seafood so much," the individual is encouraged to think of an appropriate statement to make. Again, the leading nature of the statements is faded over time to more closely replicate everyday conversations.

Once these two components are mastered in isolation, efforts are then made to teach self-management of a more complex conversational framework (Koegel, Park, & Koegel, 2014b). Individuals are taught to respond to a particular question, add a few details (statements), and then ask a thematically related question to return the conversational "volley" to their partner. This structure is intended to facilitate conversations for individuals who dominate conversations with excessive, extraneous details, as well as those who make minimal contributions to social exchanges—bringing both parties to a middle ground to provide balance to the conversation. Participants are instructed that everyday conversations are far less rigid, but this framework becomes a rough guide to help structure conversation and make it more predictable. In turn, the capacity to sustain a conversation opens the door to deeper, sustainable relationships with others as the individual ages.

12.7 Conclusion

The ultimate goal of comprehensive PRT strategies is to use motivational procedures to promote self-sustaining social developmental skill use. Historically, this intervention package was used as a language intervention, leveraging the use of motivational and behavioral strategies to rapidly promote the acquisition and complexity of this foundational social competency. These principles have since been applied to target other skills associated with social success, including the use of spontaneous social initiations, play skills with peers, conversational bids and responses, and self-monitoring of social performance.

Social competence relies on adequate interpersonal immersion, which is maintained by comfort and expertise in the use of age-appropriate engagement strategies. A foundation of motivation to use verbal communication strategies initially elicits the use of single word and multi-word phrase speech. Next, strategies are used to promote the use of self-initiated language to create active social agents that can advocate for their own social needs. Emphasis is then placed on promoting question-asking strategies to merge instrumental and interpersonal communicative goals. Once the ability to make social inquiries and comments is established, self-management strategies are used to transfer skill acquisition responsibilities away from adult facilitators and promote self-monitoring social learners. PRT is intended to establish and foster the necessary level of social competence needed for acceptance in one's interpersonal environment, thus allowing them to access immersive experiential learning, which can then serve to facilitate future social development.

References

Baker, M. J., Koegel, R. L., & Koegel, L. K. (1998). Increasing the social behavior of young children with autism using their obsessive behaviors. *Journal of the Association for Persons with Severe Handicaps*, *23*, 300–308.

Doggett, R. A., Krasno, A. M., Koegel, L. K., & Koegel, R. L. (2013). Acquisition of multiple questions in the context of social conversation in children with autism. *Journal of Autism and Developmental Disabilities*, *43*(9), 2015–2025. doi:10.1007/s10803-012-1749-8

Dunlap, G. (1984). The influence of task variation and maintenance tasks on the learning and affect of autistic children. *Journal of Experimental Child Psychology, 37*(1), 41–64. doi:10.1016/0022-0965(84)90057-2

Dunlap, G., & Koegel, R. L. (1980). Motivating autistic children through stimulus variation. *Journal of Applied Behavior Analysis, 13*(4), 619–627. doi:10.1901/jaba.1980.13-619

Fredeen, R. M., & Koegel, R. L. (2006). The pivotal role of initiations in habilitation. In R. L. Koegel & L. K. Koegel (Eds.), *Pivotal response treatment for autism: Communication, social, and academic development*. Baltimore, MD: Brookes Publishing Company.

Hala, S. (2013). *The development of social cognition*. New York City, NY: Psychology Press.

Jones, W., & Klin, A. (2009). Heterogeneity and homogeneity across the autism spectrum: The role of development. *Journal of the American Academy of Child & Adolescent Psychiatry, 48*(5), 471–473.

Kaiser, A. P., Hancock, T. B., & Nietfeld, J. P. (2000). The effects of parent-implemented enhanced milieu teaching on the social communication of children who have autism. *Early Education and Development, 11*, 423–446.

Koegel, L. K. (2000). Interventions to facilitate communication in autism. *Journal of Autism and Developmental Disorders, 30*(5), 383–391. doi:10.1023/A:1005539220932

Koegel, L. K., Camarata, S., Valdez-Menchaca, M. C., & Koegel, R. L. (1997). Setting generalization of question-asking by children with autism. *American Journal on Mental Retardation, 102*(4), 346–357.

Koegel, L. K., Carter, C. M., & Koegel, R. L. (2003). Teaching children with autism self initiations as a pivotal response. *Topics in Language Disorders, 23*(2), 134–145.

Koegel, L. K., Koegel, R. L., & Ingham, J. C. (1986). Programming rapid generalization of correct articulation through self-monitoring procedures. *Journal of Speech and Hearing Disorders, 51*(1), 24–32.

Koegel, L. K., Koegel, R. L., Green-Hopkins, I., & Barnes, C. (2010). Brief report: Question-asking and collateral language acquisition in children with autism. *Journal of Autism and Developmental Disorders, 40*(4), 509–515. doi:10.1007/s10803-009-0896-z

Koegel, L. K., Koegel, R. L., Hurley, C., & Frea, W. D. (1992). Improving social skills and disruptive behavior in children with autism through self-management. *Journal of Applied Behavior Analysis, 25*(2), 341–353. doi:10.1901/jaba.1992.25-341

Koegel, L. K., Koegel, R. L., Shoshan, Y., & McNerney, E. (1999). Pivotal response intervention II: Preliminary long-term outcome data. *Research and Practice for Persons with Severe Disabilities, 24*(3), 186–198. doi:10.2511/rpsd.24.3.186

Koegel, R. L., & Egel, A. L. (1979). Motivating autistic children. *Journal of Abnormal Psychology, 88*(4), 418–426. doi:10.1037/0021-843X.88.4.418

Koegel, R. L., & Koegel, L. K. (1990). Extended reductions in stereotypic behavior of students with autism through a self-management treatment package. *Journal of Applied Behavior Analysis, 23*(1), 119–127. doi:10.1901/jaba.1990.23-119

Koegel, R. L., & Williams, J. A. (1980). Direct versus indirect response-reinforcer relationships in teaching autistic children. *Journal of Abnormal Child Psychology, 8*, 537–547.

Koegel, R. L., Bradshaw, J. L., Ashbaugh, K., & Koegel, L. K. (2014a). Improving question-asking initiations in young children with autism using pivotal response treatment. *Journal of Autism and Developmental Disorders, 44*(4), 816–827. doi:10.1007/s10803-013-1932-6

Koegel, R. L., Dyer, K., & Bell, L. K. (1987). The influence of child-preferred activities on autistic children's social behavior. *Journal of Applied Behavior Analysis, 20*(3), 243–252. doi:10.1901/jaba.1987.20-243

Koegel, R. L., Koegel, L. K., Ingham, J. C., & Van Voy, K. (1988). Within-clinic versus outside-of-clinic self-monitoring of articulation to promote generalization. *Journal of Speech and Hearing Disorders, 53*(4), 392–399.

Koegel, R. L., O'Dell, M. C., & Koegel, L. K. (1987). A natural language teaching paradigm for nonverbal autistic children. *Journal of Autism and Developmental Disorders, 17*(2), 187–200. doi:10.1007/BF01495055

Koegel, R. L., Vernon, T. W., & Koegel, L. K. (2009). Improving social initiations in young children with autism using reinforcers with embedded social interactions. *Journal of Autism and Developmental Disorders, 39*(9), 1240–1251. doi:10.1007/s10803-009-0732-5

Koegel, R. L., Werner, G. A., Vismara, L. A., & Koegel, L. K. (2005). The effectiveness of contextually supported play date interactions between children with autism and typically developing peers. *Research and Practice for Persons with Severe Disabilities, 30*, 93–102.

Koegel, R. L., O'Dell, M., & Dunlap, G. (1988). Producing speech use in nonverbal autistic children by reinforcing attempts. *Journal of Autism and Developmental Disorders, 18*(4), 525–538. doi:10.1007/BF02211871

Koegel, L. K., Ashbaugh, K., Koegel, R. L., Detar, W. J., & Regester, A. (2013). Increasing socialization in adults with Asperger's syndrome. *Psychology in the Schools, 50*(9), 899–909.

Koegel, L. K., Ashbaugh, K., Navab, A., & Koegel, R. L. (2016). Improving empathic communication skills in adults with autism spectrum disorder. *Journal of Autism and Developmental Disorders, 46*(3), 921–933.

Koegel, L. K., Koegel, R. L., Harrower, J. K., & Carter, C. M. (1999). Pivotal response intervention I: Overview of approach. *Journal of the Association for Persons with Severe Handicaps, 24*, 174–185.

Koegel, L. K., Park, M. N., & Koegel, R. L. (2014b). Using self-management to improve the reciprocal social conversation of children with autism spectrum disorder. *Journal of Autism and Developmental Disorders, 44*(5), 1055–1063.

Kuhn, L. R., Bodkin, A. E., Devlin, S. D., & Doggett, R. A. (2008). Using pivotal response training with peers in special education to facilitate play in two children with autism. *Education and Training in Developmental Disabilities*, *43*(1), 37–45.

Mohammadzaheri, F., Koegel, L. K., Rezaei, M., & Bakhshi, E. (2015). A randomized clinical trial comparison between pivotal response treatment (PRT) and adult-driven applied behavior analysis (ABA) intervention on disruptive behaviors in public school children with autism. *Journal of Autism and Developmental Disorders*, *45*(9), 2899–2907.

National Autism Center. (2008). *National standards project*. Randolf, MA: Author.

National Research Council – Committee on Educational Interventions for Children with Autism. (2001). *Educating children with autism*. Washington, DC: National Academy Press.

Pierce, K., & Schreibman, L. (1997). Multiple peer use of pivotal response training to increase social behaviors of classmates with autism: Results from trained and untrained peers. *Journal of Applied Behavior Analysis*, *30*(1), 157–160.

Rogers, S. J., & Vismara, L. A. (2008). Evidence-based comprehensive treatments for early autism. *Journal of Clinical Child & Adolescent Psychology*, *37*(1), 8–38.

Sameroff, A. (2009). *The transactional model*. Washington, DC: American Psychological Association.

Simpson, R. L. (2005). Evidence-based practices and students with autism spectrum disorders. *Focus on Autism and Other Developmental Disabilities*, *20*(3), 140–149. doi:10.1177/10883576050200030201

Vernon, T. W., Koegel, R. L., Dauterman, H., & Stolen, K. (2012). An early social engagement intervention for young children with autism and their parents. *Journal of Autism and Developmental Disorders.*, *42*(12), 2702–2717. doi:10.1007/s10803-012-1535-7

Vernon, T. W. (2014). Fostering a social child with autism: A moment-by-moment sequential analysis of an early social engagement intervention. *Journal of Autism and Developmental Disorders.*, *44*(12), 3072–3082.

Vismara, L. A., & Lyons, G. L. (2007). Using perseverative interests to elicit joint attention behaviors in young children with autism: Theoretical and clinical implications to understanding motivation. *Journal of Positive Behavior Interventions*, *9*, 214–228.

Waters, E., & Sroufe, L. A. (1983). Social competence as a developmental construct. *Developmental Review*, *3*, 79–97.

Williams, J. A., Koegel, R. L., & Egel, A. L. (1981). Response-reinforcer relationships and improved learning in autistic children. *Journal of Applied Behavior Analysis*, *14*(1), 53–60. doi:10.1901/jaba.1981.14-53

Wodka, E. L., Mathy, P., & Kalb, L. (2013). Predictors of phrase and fluent speech in children with autism and severe language delay. *Pediatrics*, *131*(4), e1128–e1134.

13 Helping Young Children with Autism Spectrum Disorder Develop Social Ability: The Early Start Denver Model Approach

Sally J. Rogers, Giacomo Vivanti, and Marie Rocha

13.1 Introduction

The *Early Start Denver Model* (ESDM) incorporates both a set of teaching procedures and a defined teaching content representing empirical knowledge derived from decades of research in developmental psychology (i.e., cognitive, social, emotional, linguistic, and communicative development) and learning science. Integrating research involving both typical learning and developmental and atypical developmental and learning patterns seen in autism spectrum disorder (ASD), the ESDM brings together the principles used by applied behavior analysis, allied health professions, and early childhood intervention into a comprehensive intervention for young children with ASD and their families. A variety of controlled and single subject design studies has demonstrated that some of its strongest effects occur in the social-communicative domain. How ESDM conceptualizes social-communicative development in ASD from empirical research, and how it translates those concepts into a manualized intervention that improves children's social communication, is the topic of this chapter.

Dr. Rogers and Dr. Rocha were partially supported by ACE MH R01 100030-05 to Dr. Rogers and IES R324A150211. Rogers was also supported by IDDRC 5U54HD079125-02 awarded to Dr. Abbeduto.

S.J. Rogers (✉) • M. Rocha
University of California, Davis MIND Institute, 2825 50th street, Sacramento, CA 95817, USA
email: sjrogers@ucdavis.edu

G. Vivanti
Drexel Autism Institute, Drexel University, Philadelphia, PA, USA

13.2 Overview and Theoretical Basis

Beginning at birth, human infants display a marked inclination toward social interaction. Behaviors and motives foundational to all human societies (e.g., social cohesiveness, participating in shared activities, helping, and cooperating to achieve shared goals) have their roots in early emerging social skills and the social experiences that they afford.

This far-reaching propensity for social participation and communication reflects a complex interplay of biobehavioral mechanisms shaped by evolutionary pressures that favored sociability because of its adaptive value (Bjorklund & Beers, 2016; Pagel, 2012). Rather than being equipped with extensive "hardwired" knowledge, like most animal offspring, human babies acquire knowledge through interaction with other people, an evolutionary adaptation that affords the advantage of flexible and context-dependent learning. Early emerging sociability facilitates learning both directly via the observation and acquisition of new behaviors and by engaging others, as children's motivation to participate in social

J.B. Leaf (ed.), *Handbook of Social Skills and Autism Spectrum Disorder*, Autism and Child Psychopathology Series, DOI 10.1007/978-3-319-62995-7_13

exchanges elicits attention, engagement and a "pedagogical attitude" in other people.

As abnormalities in socialization are the most distinctive and enduring feature of ASD, efforts to ameliorate symptoms of ASD require an understanding of the processes governing early social development. In the following sections, we will review recent research in the area, with a focus on typical social development and its derailment in ASD.

13.3 Early Social Development in Typical Development

The motivation to engage with and the ability to make sense of social interactions reflect a set of "system preferences" and dedicated neurocognitive facilities that are active from birth. Newborns pay more attention to people's faces, voices, and movements compared to nonsocial stimuli, and prefer physical contact with people rather than with inanimate objects (Cooper & Aslin, 1990; Dawson, Meltzoff, Osterling, Rinaldi, & Brown, 1998; Gliga & Csibra, 2007). Furthermore, throughout early development, children tend to experience social exchanges as more rewarding than solitary activities, actively seeking social interaction and taking pleasure in it. This early emerging social motivation, subserved by a network of brain areas including the amygdala and orbital and ventromedial regions of the prefrontal cortex, allows children to rapidly accumulate a wealth of knowledge from and about the social world, which further shapes their ability to navigate their social environment (Chevallier, Kohls, Troiani, Brodkin, & Schultz, 2012).

The inclination to engage with social stimuli supports and is supported by early emerging neurocognitive processes that enable children to decode people's behavior. These include the social perception neural circuit, which is located in the temporal lobe of the brain and responds selectively to biological motion (e.g., a person walking or clapping hands) versus nonsocial motion (e.g., windscreen-wiper movement; Pelphrey, Shultz, Hudac, & Vander Wyk, 2011).

Additionally, infants are equipped with systems specialized in the detection and processing of people's communicative goals (Csibra & Gergely, 2009). These systems, which encompass the subcortical and cortical structures of the so-called social brain, support the rapid processing of ostensive signals such as direct gaze and other nonverbal cues, conveying the feeling of being the target of another person's attention and future action (Frith & Frith, 2010; Senju & Johnson, 2009). Reading the communicative intent of others' behavior is a critical component of both social cognition (e.g., making sense of others' actions) and social communication (e.g., understanding and sharing meanings with other people).

Similarly, beginning in the first year of life, infants read a person's gaze toward a specific object as indicating that that object is the target of the person's attention, and use gaze cues to guide and coordinate another's and one's own attention toward a shared attentional focus (e.g., looking at the caregiver and pointing to a bird in the sky; Carpenter, Nagell, Tomasello, Butterworth, & Moore, 1998). This early emerging ability to initiate and respond to joint attention, supported by neural pathways that work in parallel in posterior and anterior brain regions, enable the child to perceive the other and the self as sharing the same visual and emotional experience (Bruner, 1975; Mundy, 2016).

Finally, starting from the first hours of life and throughout the lifespan, children display a unique capacity for imitation, which supports skill acquisition and promotes feelings of social-affective relatedness and psychological intimacy between the imitator and the model (Hurley & Chater, 2005; Nadel, 2014). Neural underpinning of imitative behavior involves several interconnected neural systems, including the specialized brain network called the "mirror neuron system" (Ferrari & Rizzolatti, 2014; Rizzolatti, Fadiga, Fogassi, & Gallese, 2002). The brain regions in this network respond in a similar way to the execution of a given action as well as to the observation of a similar motor act performed by others, thus allowing the observer to understand others' actions as if he or she would be doing the same action (Rizzolatti & Craighero, 2004). Similar "mirror properties" have been documented in different brain areas that activate in response to both the observation and the experience of particular emotions and sensations (Thioux & Keysers, 2010). This process, foundational to empathy (Keysers, 2011), enables children to be affected by the emotions and moods of people around them long before they engage in explicit reasoning about others' feelings.

The social-cognitive and social-affiliative processes described above shape and are shaped by the child's participation in joint play and care routines, during which adult and child are engaged in a coordinated and mutually reinforcing "choreography" that involves reciprocal imitation, sharing of affect, and turn taking. Repeated engagement in such joint activities provides the child with a wealth of opportunities to register and appreciate the correspondence and contingencies between their own and others' actions, thus building knowledge and neural specialization in social interactions.

Such iterative processes, where early preparation for sociability leads infants to participate in learning experiences that contribute to strengthen and refine the pathways of the social brain, enable children to become increasingly skilled and sophisticated at processing social information and navigating their social environment throughout the lifespan (Banaji & Gelman, 2013).

13.4 Early Social Development in ASD

Children with ASD show atypical patterns of social development that affect all the processes described above. During the first 18 months of life, infants developing ASD appear to be less responsive to their name being called (Miller et al., 2017), less interested in social scenes and faces (Chawarska, Macari, & Shic, 2013; Jones & Klin, 2013), less socially engaged (Bolton, Golding, Emond, & Steer, 2012), less inclined to imitate others (Rowberry et al., 2015), and less likely to initiate and respond to joint attention (Yoder, Stone, Walden, & Malesa, 2009). Additionally, a number of studies involving older children with ASD have documented fewer prosocial behaviors (e.g., helping, showing concern for a person displaying distress), reduced empathy, and fewer expressions of pleasure in social situations (Chevallier et al., 2012; Colombi et al., 2009; Newbigin, Uljarević, Vivanti, & Dissanayake, 2016). These early disruptions in social development are likely to affect behavioral organization and brain specialization in an iterative way. The diminished tendency to observe and imitate other people, to seek out and play with adults and peers, and to participate in joint activity routines negatively affect the opportunities to learn from and about the social environment (Dawson & Bernier, 2007; Nuske, Vivanti, & Dissanayake, 2016; Rogers & Dawson, 2010a; Vivanti, Hocking, Fanning, & Dissanayake, 2016). This, in turn, is likely to result in diminished neural and behavioral expertise about the social world, affecting both social and nonsocial dimensions of development. For example, difficulties in following others' pointing or gaze direction (i.e., deficits in response to joint attention) are associated with later difficulties in the language domain (Mundy, 2016), and reduced social attention is associated with difficulties in learning novel actions (Vivanti et al., 2011, 2016).

Additionally, as children with ASD are less likely to engage in social initiations directed toward their caregivers (e.g., making eye contact, vocalizing, gesturing, and bringing objects to show them), and more focused on objects and their sensory properties, their behavior is less likely to generate opportunities to learn from the caregivers' responses. This might result in a virtual "deprivation" from social experiences, which further exacerbates social difficulties (Dawson, 2008; Jones, Carr, & Klin, 2008).

While the biology of social impairments in ASD is far from being fully understood, it is likely that early social disruptions reflect differences in the "built-in" neurocognitive processes that underpin the social-affiliative and social-cognitive abilities observed in typical infants. For example, functional and structural abnormalities have been documented across areas of the social brain (see Schultz, Volkmar, & Chawarska, 2006, for a review) and in the mirror system – although there is no specific or universal neural signature distinguishing autism from other conditions.

Because of these early abnormalities, children with ASD might be less biased to engage in activities that provide the input needed for the specialization of the neural networks that support the experience-expectant development of the social brain (Schultz, 2005; Vivanti & Rogers, 2014).

Lack of social specialization at the brain level might result in the recruitment of other, nonsocial brain areas to process social stimuli. For example, several studies found that individuals with ASD might understand emotions relying on surface perceptual features (e.g., examining changes in the mouth angle to infer happiness), and explicit rules (e.g., mouth open means surprise; Deruelle, Rondan, Salle-Collemiche, Bastard-Rosset, & Da Fonseca, 2008; Ozonoff, Pennington, & Rogers, 1991). Consistent with behavioral findings, neuroimaging studies have reported enhanced activity in visual processing areas and reduced activity in the social brain areas during emotion and social understanding tasks for individuals with ASD (Dapretto et al., 2006; Harms, Martin, & Wallace, 2010; Nuske, Vivanti, & Dissanayake, 2013; Samson, Mottron, Soulieres, & Zeffiro, 2012). Engagement of "compensatory" nonsocial strategies might prevent individuals with ASD from experiencing the implicit "embodied" understanding of others' behavior that makes the social world intuitively graspable, meaningful, and rewarding long before children have an explicit theory of others' minds (Klin, Jones, Schultz, & Volkmar, 2003; Senju, 2012). Although the iterative processes linking initial biological abnormalities to the differences in social behavior characterizing ASD are not fully clear, there is consensus in the field that early emerging social deficits act as a barrier to participation in cultural practices and social learning experiences, thus representing a critical target for treatment.

13.5 The Earliest Social Relationship: Infant Attachment

Development of remediation strategies requires an appreciation of both the areas of weakness and the strengths of children with ASD in the social domain. Importantly, not all facets of sociability are disrupted for individuals with ASD, as illustrated by the literature focusing on attachment patterns in this population. The concept of "attachment," introduced by John Bowlby (1969) to describe the visceral and enduring affective bond between child and caregivers, involves a set of behavioral manifestations, including selective proximity-seeking, distress, and decreased exploratory behavior upon separation from the caregiver and relief upon reunion. Attachment quality is classified as "secure" when a child shows concern during episodes of separation from the caregiver and is quickly comforted by reunion, or "insecure" when this pattern is not observed (Ainsworth, Blehar, Waters, & Wall, 1978). Attachment quality has been found to predict various aspects of later well-being, such as emotion regulation (Dalsant, Truzzi, Setoh, & Esposito, 2015) and response to stressful events (Maunder, Lancee, Nolan, Hunter, & Tannenbaum, 2006). Historically, some theorists stated that ASD was caused by disturbed attachment processes (Mahler, 1952; see also Bowlby, 1969) or assumed that ASD indicated an absence of any attachments (Caparulo & Cohen, 1977; Rutter, 1983; see also Hobson, 1995).

Nevertheless, empirical work in the area has challenged the notion that the social symptoms of ASD must interfere with attachment formation. Early work by Sigman and Ungerer (1984), and subsequent research documented that children with ASD respond differently to caregivers versus strangers (Kasari, Sigman, & Yirmiya, 1993), make efforts to seek and maintain proximity with caregivers after a separation (Sigman & Mundy, 1989), engage in more proximity-seeking and less explorative behavior in the presence of a stranger (Dissanayake & Crossley, 1996), and show behavioral patterns that are, in the majority of cases, consistent with a classification of "secure attachment" (Rogers, Ozonoff, & Maslin-Cole, 1991; Rutgers et al., 2004). Additionally, the number of children with ASD showing insecure/disorganized attachment is higher compared to the normal population, but similar to mental-age matched children without ASD who have other conditions (Naber et al., 2007). Therefore,

ASD symptoms do not preclude the establishment of secure attachments in ASD, and children with ASD can form a secure social-affiliative bond with their caregivers. However, the impairments in joint attention, communication imitation, and sharing of emotions likely prevent children with ASD of taking full advantage of the social learning opportunities inherently woven into attachment-driven episodes of child–caregiver proximity (Vivanti & Nuske, 2016). Intervention strategies must therefore take into account such complex patterns of intact and impaired dimensions of social-affiliative development. This involves both capitalizing on the opportunities offered by the capacity for social-emotional bonding with significant others, and addressing the social deficiencies that hinder the opportunities for social development and social learning afforded by attachment relationships.

13.6 Peer Relations

Although often overlooked, peer relations are as important as child-adult bonding experiences to an individual's social development and to our understanding of ASD treatment (Dunn & McGuire, 1992; Vivanti, Duncan, Dawson, & Rogers, 2017). Peers provide opportunities for developing and practicing social behaviors that adults cannot provide, because interacting with peers who have similar cognitive, language and motor skills, preferences for activities and materials, and emotional reactions gives children unique insight into their own and others' contributions to social exchanges. From infancy onward, typically developing children show a spontaneous interest toward their peers, and by toddlerhood are capable and motivated to participate in joint activities organized around shared goals (e.g., building a big tower with blocks) without adult instruction (Sanefuji, Ohgami, & Hashiya, 2006). During these play exchanges, they coordinate their actions and share their emotion with their play partners (e.g., taking turns in adding blocks to the tower, and smiling to one another to share the suspense when the last block is added to the stack), using gestures, facial expressions, body postures, and reciprocal imitation to communicate, negotiate, and achieve shared goals (Tomasello & Hamann, 2012).

The opportunity to practice complex social and cooperative behaviors during play routines with peers supports the development of social-cognitive and social emotional skills such as empathy and mentalizing. For example, research indicates that children who grow up with siblings of a similar age show more advanced understanding of others' thoughts and feelings compared to those who do not have siblings, likely because they have more opportunities to practice and refine their social and emotional knowledge through peer play (McAlister & Peterson, 2007). Additionally, going to high quality child care environments that facilitate engagement in joint activities with peers has positive effects on social and communication development (National Institute of Child Health and Human Development Early Child Care Research Network, 2000, 2003). Finally, play routines with peers are foundational to the ability to form and maintain friendships, a factor that is critically associated with well-being across the lifespan (Majors, 2012).

Many children with ASD are inclined to initiate primarily to adults and rarely to peers (Thiemann-Bourque, 2013). Their diminished propensity and ability to imitate, take turns, and share experiences with peers make it difficult for them to learn, practice social behaviors, and develop friendships, further exacerbating their social difficulties. Interaction with peers is particularly difficult for children with ASD for a number of reasons.

Compared to adults, peers might be less inclined to socially engage with a child who does not initiate, does not respond to their initiations, or whose initiations are atypical (e.g., positioning themselves too far or too close, not using gaze, not knowing how to get the other persons' attention first). Additionally, even when engaged in a play activity with a peer, children with ASD might be overly directive, or unable to follow the peer's lead, and might struggle with sharing materials, taking turns, adapting to changes demanded by the activity (e.g., switching roles during a chasing game), or dealing with frustration if a peer does not respond in the desired way. Unlike adults, peers might not attempt to adjust their behavior to address these difficulties by patiently waiting for the child's responses, scaffolding the child's language, clarifying or simplifying the game rules, and/or adapting their communications and actions to facilitate the interaction. As a consequence, peer interactions can place exceptional demands on attending to and understanding others' actions and communications, dealing with frustration, and being flexible and responsive to rapidly changing situations. Interventions must therefore include strategies to address the many barriers to successful peer interactions.

13.7 Social-Emotional Foundations of Learning and Cognition, and Implications for Treatment

The literature reviewed thus far suggests that targeting early disruptions in social behaviors might counteract the cascading effects of social impairments for individuals with ASD. According to this model, building a repertoire of social behaviors for children with ASD during early childhood might confer beneficial effects across different developmental domains. While early approaches to intervention focused on modifying the topography of social behaviors according to the same procedures used to modify any other behavior, there is an increasing appreciation of the relevance of social-emotional and social-pragmatic dimensions of sociability in intervention literature (Smith & Iadarola, 2015).

Empirical research on language (Akhtar & Tomasello, 2000) and imitation (Over & Carpenter, 2012) has supported the notion that learning new words and behaviors in ASD is "gated" by the social-emotional engagement between them and her/his social partners. For example, young children are more likely to imitate adults and peers with whom they feel emotionally connected (Nielsen, Simcock, & Jenkins, 2008; Vivanti et al., 2016), and more likely to learn a new language if they play with someone who speaks that language, rather than if they are merely being exposed to the language through TV (Kuhl, 2007). Additionally, when children learn new words and new actions they do so by first understanding their social partner's goal to share new information (Tomasello, 2010). This body of literature is not easily accommodated within operant conditioning accounts of language and socialization, and supports the relevance of the social-pragmatic dimension of communication and the role of preverbal social-emotional engagement in the acquisition of language and socialization skills (Bloom, 2002; Kuhl, 2000, 2014; Parish-Morris, Hirsh-Pasek, & Golinkoff, 2013; Tomasello, 2003).

According to this perspective, preverbal affective and cognitive connectedness between infants and their social partners during participation in sociocultural practices such as play and daily routines is a prerequisite for, rather than a consequence of, the acquisition of social and communication skills. The framework of affective engagement, desire to share meanings, and preverbal understanding of others' communicative goals, in which early development takes place, is not just the context in which children learn to socialize – rather it is an active ingredient in the process of social development. Intervention strategies informed by this literature highlight the importance of social-emotional connectedness and understanding of self, others', and mutual goals to facilitate the acquisition of social skills in young children with ASD. Consistent with this framework, the ESDM aims to build a social-pragmatic and social-emotional foundation for the development of social behaviors so that complex behaviors such as word use are not simply memorized and emitted "on demand," but rather, built on the social infrastructure of joint attention, shared emotions and goals, and use of communicative acts for multiple pragmatic functions during meaningful and rewarding daily routines (Rogers, Charman, & Stone, 2006; Rogers & Dawson, 2010a, 2010b; Vivanti, Dawson, & Rogers, 2017).

13.8 Procedures for Fostering Social Development and Learning Within ESDM

Inside the ESDM, one begins with a child by creating dyadic exchanges that provide a great deal of pleasure for the child. Imagine this scenario involving bubble play with 24-month-old, Jason, a quiet, self-contained, and isolated child recently diagnosed with ASD, without speech or conventional communicative gesture:

> Therapist Terri picks up a bottle of bubbles and holds them out towards Jason, who is fiddling with some DUPLOS®. "Jason, want bubbles?," she asks while extending the bottle toward him. He looks at the bottle, turns toward her, extends his hand, and begins to approach. "Yes, you want bubbles!" she says, and opens the bubbles and blows a large stream of them toward Jason, who approaches and bats at them with pleasure, to which Terri shares happy emotion and excited comments. As soon as the bubbles have disappeared she blows another large stream, with active, happy child response. Terri blows a third time as soon as the bubbles have disappeared, with a happy response from him again. Now, when the bubbles disappear, Terri continues to hold the bubbles and look expectantly at Jason, waiting. He tries to initiate the bubble routine – he approaches, and looks directly at her eyes, to which she immediately responds, "Oh, you want bubbles. Bubbles! Sure." and blows them again. This scenario is repeated 2-3 times with great pleasure and shared smiles between the two. Since Jason is still highly motivated for the bubbles, on his next initiation (i.e., approach, look, and reach to the bubbles bottle), she hands him the closed bottle, saying, "You want bubbles! Here are the bubbles!" He takes them, looks at them, tries to open, and looks perplexed. She extends her hand and says, "You want help?" takes the bubbles, since he does not offer them, saying, "I'll help you" while opening the bubbles and then blows a big stream. "Here are the bubbles." This scenario occurs two more times, and by the third time Jason immediately offers her the bubbles with eye contact to request her help. "More bubbles, or book?" she asks as she offers both objects. Jason reaches for the book. "You want the book!" she says as she hands it to him while leading him to a beanbag chair. "Sit down" she says as she helps him sit in the chair while she sits in front and holds the book between them.

In this exchange, we see the core aspects of social learning well represented. The child becomes very aware of the responsive adult and begins attending to the adult and initiating social communications, as well as responding to adult requests. The child quickly learns that the partner responds contingently, and the child and partner become engaged in back and forth communication involving both action and emotional communications. The interaction is balanced; the child is sometimes the leader and sometimes the responder, as is the adult. Control of the activity is shared; the child has some control over the adult and the adult has some control over the child. Shared smiles and eye contact are used for multiple purposes: sharing emotion (an early developing joint attention act), requesting, and reciprocal contingent motor acts permeate this episode. These are the foundations of social learning and growth that permeate the ESDM of treatment.

At the same time, excellent behavioral teaching is present. The child is highly motivated, the adult is focused on teaching, the adult creates very clear three part contingencies (i.e., antecedent – behavior – consequence chains) which quickly build up the desired behavior. Because the learning goal is based on the child's current performance and represents a very small step forward (Vygotsky's, 1962 Zone of Proximal Development), the child learns easily, within a few repetitions. The adult uses successful prompt strategies, rapid prompt fading, and quickly begins to chain two responses together (e.g., giving object followed by a verbal gaze for request). Multiple trials are delivered to a highly motivated child and new behaviors are quickly built up from the child's baseline skills. In the following section we will describe how the ESDM therapist derives the intervention content and teaching procedures to build social skills and knowledge for each individual child.

13.8.1 Assessment Procedures and Treatment Goals

In the ESDM, as in all other high quality interventions, the therapist is working from a very specific set of short-term treatment objectives that have been developed from a careful assessment of the child's behavioral repertoire. In ESDM treatment, a trained ESDM therapist evaluates each child by administering the ESDM Curriculum Checklist

(Rogers & Dawson, 2010a, 2010b) before treatment begins and then readministers the checklist every 12-weeks throughout treatment. Using this comprehensive measurement tool, the therapist can assess each child's skills across all developmental domains including receptive communication, expressive communication, social skills, play skills, cognitive skills, fine motor skills, and adaptive skills. Each domain includes a developmental sequence of skills listed from less mature to more mature. The curriculum assessment is an essential component of the ESDM treatment and was designed as a tool to allow early intervention professionals to capture the child's current level of abilities and to develop appropriate treatment objectives. The child's skills are assessed by the therapist from child performance in typical play and care activities during a combination of interactive, observational, and parent interview procedures. This information is then used to create a set of behavioral targets for the next 12 weeks of ESDM treatment.

Let's look at a short example of how a therapist may use child observations and parent discussion during the assessment to create individualized and developmentally appropriate social communicative goals for a child named Alex.

13.8.2 Observation

During a curriculum assessment, the therapist provides many opportunities for Alex to request a toy or favorite food when it is held outside of his reach. The therapist observes that Alex will consistently reach toward the item to gain access. The therapist also observes that Alex rarely uses eye contact and never uses a point or speech to make a request. The therapist records these observations on the checklist.

13.8.3 Parent Interview and Discussion

The therapist asks Alex's mom if the requesting behavior that they observed during the assessment is similar to what she sees at home. His mother says yes. The therapist also asks specifically if he uses eye contact or pointing to make requests at home. Alex's mother says that he only makes eye contact to request fruit snacks and never points. The therapist records this response on the checklist. The therapist can see from the developmental sequence of skills on the checklist that eye contact and pointing are slightly more mature requesting behaviors than reaching. The therapist shares with his mother that since Alex is already using a reach to make requests, she would like to see him use eye contact more consistently and for him to learn to point. The therapist asks Alex's mother if she would like to target these behaviors during the next 12 weeks. Alex's mother agrees.

> Resulting Social Communicative Treatment Goal: When Alex desires an object out of reach, he will make eye contact with his partner and then either point or gesture with or without vocalization to his desired object to request toys and favorite foods, 75% or more of requests, both at home and at preschool, with parent and with therapist.

In the curriculum, requesting behaviors are listed in the expressive communication domain. This domain and all other domains in the curriculum checklist were derived from extensive literature reviews on the development of young children. In addition to being divided into multiple domains, the curriculum is divided into four levels with each level corresponding to a developmental age period (i.e., 12–18 months, 18–24 months, 24–36 months, and 36–48 months) in which infants and toddlers typically acquire these skills. Skills that children learn earlier in development are listed earlier in the checklist for each domain. One of the unique features of this curriculum is that the level of each skill in the curriculum checklist reflects the typical learning profile of young children with autism. Thus, each level contains more advanced visual motor skills than social communication skills.

The curriculum is administered in a play- and routine-based, natural interactive style using a wide array of age appropriate objects. In a routine-based assessment, many skills may be assessed within a single activity. The assessment is usually administered in 1–1.5 h and an ideal setting is in the home or a treatment room with a small table and chairs, an open carpeted floor area, a comfortable chair for the parent, and materials that will be needed to evoke the skills on the Curriculum Checklist. In between activities, the therapist will note which curriculum items were observed and which ones were probed but not observed.

Here is an example of a scenario that you might see during a 5 min period of an ESDM assessment:

> Therapist, Walter, has set out a bucket shaped shape sorter on the floor in front of the child, Mario. Mario took the top off the sorter, picked up the bucket, and dumped out the pieces. Mario then started putting the pieces in the bucket. Walter narrates his play by saying, "in" or "drop" with an excited voice as Mario puts in the shapes. Walter asked Mario to hand him a shape with an outstretched hand. Mario did not respond so Walter repeated, "Give me one" while pointing at his outstretched hand. Mario gives him the shape. Walter joins in the activity and starts putting shapes in the bucket. There is one shape left and Walter holds the shape in front of Mario but out of reach. Mario gives Walter eye contact and Walter gives him the shape and Mario puts it in the bucket. Now that all the pieces are in the bucket, Walter holds the bucket in the air and says "Ready, set, dump." Walter and Mario share smiles as the shapes fall to the floor. Walter and Mario repeat the routine of dumping the shapes three times and on the third time, Walter pauses after "Ready, set..." until Mario says "dah." Walter excitedly says "dump!" and quickly dumps the shapes out allowing Mario free access the shapes. After Walter lets Mario put a few more shapes in, Walter puts the lid on the sorter. Mario must now try to put the shapes in using the shape sorter holes. At first, Mario tries to put a shape in the wrong hole. Walter then points to the right hole and says, "It goes here." Mario does not respond. Walter repeats the instruction with a point and when Mario does not respond again, he uses a gentle physical prompt to guide Mario to put the shape in the hole. When Walter realizes that putting the shape in is difficult for Mario, he lightly helps him turn the piece around so it falls in. Walter repeats the sequence of pointing to where the shape goes and helping Mario, if he needs it, to follow his point and put the shape in the sorter. Mario starts looking around the room and Walter senses that he is losing interest in the shape sorter. Walter takes the lid off the shape sorter and says, "Let's clean up." Mario starts to stand up and Walter holds the bucket in front of him with the lid off, hands Mario one shape and says "Mario, time to clean up." Mario puts the shape in and Walter quickly puts in the other shapes. While Mario approaches his mother for a hug, Walter takes a few minutes to record the behaviors he observed during the activity. He takes the opportunity to check in with Mario's mother about behaviors she sees at home. He asks her if he plays with shape sorters at home. She says that he does but he always takes the lid off and does not place shapes through the sorter without help.
>
> Here is a list of curriculum skills that Walter assessed during the shape sorter activity:

1. Follows a proximal point to object or location
2. Gives object as verbally requested when paired with an adult's outstretched hand
3. Performs a one-step routine involving body actions paired with verbal/gesture cue
4. Produces five or more consonants in spontaneous vocalizations
5. Responds to preferred objects, and activities via gaze, reach, smiles and movements
6. Places one to two shapes in a shape sorter
7. Sits in a chair or facing adult during pleasurable activities without difficulty for 1–2 min
8. Uses pincer grasp and a three finger grasp as appropriate to toy
9. Completes play task and puts away

When the curriculum assessment is readministered every 12 weeks, it provides an opportunity for the therapist to identify new behavioral targets and to assess the generalization of skills acquired during the 12 week period. In order to use the tool as a measure of generalization, it is helpful to administer the assessment in a setting and with materials that are not typically used for treatment.

From the very beginning of a child's ESDM treatment, parents and family members play an active role and a therapist initiates a partnership with the parents during the initial curriculum assessment. It is important that the therapist ask parents about skills that are not observed during the assessment to find out if they are happening in other settings, such as the home. There are separate columns in the assessment to delineate which information was collected from observation and which information was collected through parent report. The therapist may also ask the parent to assist by joining activities, to see if the child responds differently with a familiar adult. For example, if the child does not respond when the therapist calls his/her name, the therapist may ask the parent to try calling the child's name. The initial assessment is also an opportunity to identify which ESDM strategies parents may already be using and which strategies would be most beneficial for them to learn. To do this, the therapist may ask a parent to do a short play activity with the child so s/he can get an idea of how they interact together at home. In addition to interviewing parents on the child's behavior repertoire, day care providers and preschool teachers can be another useful source of information if they are available.

Another way that parents are actively involved in the assessment is by sharing information about the daily routines of the child and what behaviors they value highly and which behaviors are less important to them. For example, for one family it may be very important that their child greets them when they come home, but it may not be important to them that their child uses an open cup. ESDM program goals are individualized and it is extremely important that any behavioral targets that are chosen are relevant for each family.

When a therapist develops treatment objectives it is important that each behavior that s/he would like the child to learn is clearly stated using descriptive language. In addition, an objective should describe under what circumstances the behavior is expected to occur and what the criteria are for meeting this objective.

Here is an example of an objective for Mario. When an adult calls child by name within 5 ft of the child, child will respond to his name with eye contact and orientation to the adult at the first or second call 80% of opportunities in 1 h for four out of five consecutive treatment sessions across three or more adults and settings.

Once treatment objectives are developed, you have a list of target skills, or behaviors, that you want the child to learn during therapy – this is your destination. But how will you get there? In order to create a road map to the destination, each objective needs a set of teaching steps. These teaching steps are critical as they are the "road map" to your final destination. The teaching steps describe which teaching strategies you will use to teach each skill (e.g., how you and the child are going to get from where you are to where you are going). Here are teaching steps developed for Mario to reach the objective above:

1. Child turns and looks at the adult when unoccupied 50% of opportunities (Base line skill).
2. Child turns and looks at adult when unoccupied and adult is within 2 ft of child 80% of opportunities.
3. Child turns and looks at adult when unoccupied and adult is within 5 ft of child 80% of opportunities.
4. Child turns and looks at adult when occupied and adult is within 5 ft of child 50% of opportunities.
5. Child turns and looks at adult when occupied and adult is within 5 ft of child 80% of opportunities.
6. Child turns and looks at adult when adult is within 5 ft of the child 80% of opportunities across three or more adults and settings (target).

13.8.4 Treatment Procedures

The flexible format of the ESDM treatment allows for a variety of ways to individualize the intervention and fit it to individual children and families' needs and preferences, including children's individual learning styles. While the naturalistic approach described throughout this chapter is the default teaching approach used in ESDM, it can be adapted in a Response-to-Intervention (RTI) approach for children whose learning rates or behavioral challenges indicate a need other types of reinforcers, more structure and repetitions of trials, more visual strategies, or alternative communication systems. These adaptations are specified in a pair of Decision Trees, one for language usage, and the other for learning rates, illustrated in Rogers and Dawson, 2010a, 2010b.

A second aspect of this flexibility is the environmental flexibility in terms of locations. Teaching opportunities take place throughout a child's day, in multiple settings (e.g., home, preschool, park). A third is the focus on teaching within activities and routines that are a part of everyday life for young children (e.g., mealtime, circle time, bath, bedtime, books, outdoor play).

A fourth is who is "teaching." Teaching can take place in one-to-one treatment with a trained therapist, during daily routines at home with parents, or with peers during play dates or in group settings. Developing children's skills with peers and in group and community interactions opens the door to a wider range of settings. Sibling group activities, peer group activities, restaurants, parks, birthday parties, church, the grocery store, doctor or dentist offices, and hair salons are all teaching contexts for the ESDM. We coach parents and others who are with a child regularly in ESDM strategies so that everyone who interacts with a child is able to create learning opportunities through engaging social interaction. In the next section, we will first describe the ways in which children's social abilities are developed within 1:1 interactions between children and adults (e.g., parents, other caregivers, and therapists). We will next discuss how peer interaction skills are supported within playdates and within interactions with siblings at home. Finally, we will describe the delivery of the ESDM within group environments in day care and preschool settings

13.8.4.1 Developing Children's Social Abilities Within 1:1 Interactions with Adults

The vignette at the start of this section portraying therapist Terri, child Jason, and the bubbles provided an example of the interactive style used within the ESDM, whatever its delivery type. As one can see in that example, Terri neither directs Jason through the activity, nor does she follow each of his leads without providing any direction. In this vignette, we see several aspects of the ESDM in use that define key elements of the interactive style that prepare children for social participation. The interaction is dyadic – both the child and the adult have roles, they take turns, and their turns are quite evenly balanced. The adult is a person – with choices, feelings, opinions, and preferences, and so is the child. The two need to negotiate their interactions in a way that both of their goals is met. Both partners have decision-making power. The child "voices" her/his goals, choices of activities, requests for help, emotional pleasure, and readiness for change. The adult has some decision-making power as well – in what activities will be offered, what locations will be used, and what child behaviors will result in goal achievement. The child and the adult share roles of leader and follower, share affect, send and receive communicative signals back and forth, share taking turns in the activity, and share decisions about what they will do together.

The activity has a certain structure – a four-part joint activity routine (JAR) (developed from Bruner, 1975, 1977) – which involves a (1) "set-up" social-communicative negotiation as the activity is chosen, (2) "theme" the joint development of a theme, or topic, that both share, (3) "variations" several variations and elaborations on the theme, and a (4) "closing transition" shared decision about the closing and transition to the next activity. In this structure, we see a basic conversational structure that will serve the child well with peers, older children, and adults. In these ways, the ESDM differs from interventions that primarily focus on adult responsivity by following children's leads, as well as from adult directed interventions, which require child responsivity by following adult leads.

In ESDM joint activities, the shared "topic" is an activity from the everyday life of a young child. Its structure is a social-communicative agreement about the topic: "the set-up" lands on an action carried out back and forth between the partners ("the theme", with turntaking), addition of "variations" by either partner that adds interest (attention), adds new ideas and language, and keeps the activity fresh and interesting, and a negotiated "closing and transition" to the next activity. Each phase is marked by adult communication and that marks the actions, objects, intentions, and agents. This joint, interactional activity structure, which scaffolds language development in toddlers moving from preverbal to verbal communication, is used to scaffold the basic social and communication framework that characterizes human interaction from infancy to adulthood – the "conversational" framework that includes agreed upon topics, reciprocal exchanges on a topic that allow for sharing control of interactions, and negotiating different desires via agreed upon topic endings and changes so that both partners have their needs met. These are the basic social principles of the interactional style, so essential for language learning, that are used in the ESDM.

The following section elaborates on emotional quality of the interactions, and adult management of activities.

13.8.4.2 Child Emotions

An important focus of the ESDM is creating positive emotional experiences for children during interactions with others. Therapists create routines using highly preferred objects and activities that include social and communicative actions. Working to draw the child's attention to social stimuli, the therapist uses strategies to foster the child's motivation to continue such activities. In the ESDM, a teaching event involves a typical early childhood activity, with multiple teaching trials, involving multiple objectives, from different developmental domains, embedded in each activity. Because the activities are typical interactions for adults and young children, an untrained observer may not notice the complex infusion of teaching opportunities that the adult is creating through the integration of developmental and behavioral strategies. Some activities may focus more heavily on skills in one or two domains (e.g., an activity that involves playing catch with a ball may focus on multiple gross motor objectives) while others can easily address objectives in four or more domains (e.g., mealtime: fine motor, social, communication, self-feeding, handwashing). However, it is a requirement of the ESDM approach that one or more of a child's social interaction/communication objectives are taught during every single teaching activity, so playing catch would also be teaching related communication.

13.8.4.3 Managing Activity Structure

The ESDM uses Joint Activity Routines (JARs) as the default structure for teaching. These may occur with or without objects. In activities without objects, called Sensory Social Routines (SSRs), the primary focus of the activity is on the social partner. Some examples of SSRs are chase, peek-a-boo, songs, and finger plays.

The basic teaching scenario involves a child and adult engaged in an activity that the child chooses or accepts. The adult uses a naturalistic teaching approach, in which both the child and adult engage in the activity, using a turn taking structure. The child's goals for the activity – whatever the child wants to do with the material – is the theme of the activity and the source of child motivation. As the child chooses the activity and seeks to attain his or her goal, the adult inserts an antecedent stimulus to evoke a target behavior dictated by the child's treatment plan. The child's performance of the targeted behavior, in response to the antecedent, is consequated, reinforced by the continuation of the activity (e.g., child imitates motor movements during a song and the adult continues the song), by comments, and often, positive emotional exchanges. Adult support for child performance follows a least-to-most prompting hierarchy unless otherwise specified, to encourage child initiative. Rather than repetition of one target behavior across multiple trials, various targets are addressed inside the four parts of each activity. The set-up, variations, and closing/transition phases allow for the insertion of antecedents and consequences for other target behaviors. Young children tend to enjoy repeating actions within an activity and children in the ESDM are free to repeat the activity as they wish, as long as the therapist feels there is continued learning value. Here is an example of a social objective being taught within a joint activity routine without objects (i.e., a SSR):

Child objective: When playing five different social games with others (e.g., chase, red rover, duck-duck-goose, obstacle course, and slide), Xavier will both initiate a game using appropriate verbal and nonverbal communication once every 15 min, and will also respond to a partner's initiation within 5 s.

Set-up: The therapist looks at the child, smiles, makes the hand gesture, and says. "I'm going to get you." The child looks at the therapist and smiles, showing interest.

Theme: The therapist repeats the phrase and starts to move toward the child. The child runs away but allows the therapist to catch the child by the arms; the adult says, "Got you!" Then the therapist puts the child down and they repeat the sequence two more times. The theme is adult chasing the child.

Variation: The therapist looks at the child and says, "Now chase me!" and starts slowly running away.

The child looks and smiles and the therapist repeats, "Chase me" using a hand gesture to try to encourage the child to come towards him. The child eventually chases the therapist, catches him, and is prompted to say, "got you!" The adult immediately repeats the whole scenario, chasing and catching the child (this is the presumed reinforcer for the child) and they proceed to take turns chasing and catching each other.

Closing/Transition: While the therapist is chasing the child, the child stops and picks up a book. Sensing that the child is losing interest, the therapist asks the child, "Are you done with chase?" and the child says, "All done chase." The therapist then says, "Okay we are all done chase. Let's read your book" and starts walking towards a bean bag chair in another part of the room. The child follows the therapist while holding the book and then sits on the beanbag.

In this example, you can see the therapist developing the cores of social competence – dyadic relations and reciprocity, intentional communication, appropriate play skills, core pragmatic functions of communication, with the pleasure of the chase game as the reinforcer for child engagement throughout the whole activity. This kind of activity is the delivery mode for the ESDM across all types of delivery (e.g., in 1:1 treatment, with caregivers/family members at home in everyday routines, with peers in playdates and preschool).

These joint activity routines are embedded in the natural routines that occur throughout a child's day at home, at preschool, or at day care. If treatment is occurring in a treatment room, then natural activities involving toy play, books, social play, meals, hygiene routines, gross motor play, art, and chores are simulated inside the treatment room. Materials used are the everyday materials found in homes, preschools, and day care centers. Joint activity routines are typically 5–10 min in length and include the following types of activities:

1. Books
2. Object play (e.g., art, construction toys, musical activities and instruments, toys that teach cognitive skills, symbolic play, water play, balls, and other physical activities involving objects)
3. Sensory-social play routines in which there are no objects, like songs, dancing, and social games, swings, slides, or play routines like the bubbles above in which the adult has an object that stimulates high levels of pleasure and motivation, social communication exchanges and attention to the partner
4. Meals
5. Chores
6. Outdoor play-ball play, hide and go seek
7. Dressing and hygiene routines (e.g., handwashing, dressing, bath time, toileting)

13.9 Developing Peer Interactions in Playdates

The flexible format of the ESDM also allows a parent or therapist to create opportunities for learning peer interaction skills during playdates. As with all ESDM intervention, playdates may take place in a variety of settings including the family home or community settings.

13.9.1 When to Start

Level 1 of the ESDM curriculum checklist includes social behaviors that children engage in during activities with adults, as these behaviors tend to develop earlier than social behaviors with peers in young children. In addition, given the atypical patterns of social development observed in children with autism, it is particularly important that children have a solid platform of social behaviors with adults on which to build social interactions with peers. In Level 2, social skill behaviors with peers are included and continue through Level 4. At any time during an ESDM program, a child may have opportunities to interact with peers, but a child's objectives would not focus on peer interaction behaviors until after Level 1 social skills have been mastered. Thus, playdates that incorporate ESDM teaching typically begin once a child has objectives from Level 2 in the social skills domain.

Here is an example of a social skills objective for Level 2. This objective is written specifically for playdates with peers. Keep in mind that oftentimes the behaviors targeted during playdates are skills that were already mastered with adults, but additional practice and support is necessary for the skill to generalize to peers across different settings:

> *Child objective*: During play routines with peers, when a peer offers Virginia a toy or snack by holding it out towards her (within 2 ft of her face) and makes a verbal offer (e.g., "Here Ginny"), Virginia will take the object from the peer within 3 s on 80% of opportunities for 2 consecutive playdates across 10 different objects, and two different peers, both in home and at school.

13.9.2 Getting Started

Once behavioral objectives including social skills with peers have been agreed upon by the parents and therapist during the curriculum assessment process, parents will be asked to take a key role in organizing playdates. During parent coaching sessions, with the support of an ESDM therapist, parents will be asked to think of appropriate peer playmates. These playmates may be family members, neighbors, family friends, or classmates. Ideally, peer playmates are children that will have an ongoing relationship with the child and continue to interact with the child in other settings. It is also beneficial to choose children who are developmentally mature, socially skilled, and who listen and follow adult directions well. Before playdates commence, a therapist will also discuss other topics during parent coaching including how to approach parents to set up playdates, choosing a time and setting, who will facilitate the playdates, planning activities, and how to prepare the child. The level of detail in the discussion for each of these topics will depend on who will facilitate or lead the playdates (e.g., the parent or the therapist). If the parent will facilitate the playdate, the discussion of each of these topics will be more in-depth.

13.9.3 Facilitating Playdates

Whether a peer playdate is facilitated by the parent or therapist, careful planning is critical to its success. One factor to consider is the duration of the playdate. It is important that the playdate is long enough to provide many learning opportunities but not so long that either child loses motivation or becomes frustrated. We usually recommend that playdates are 30–60 min and may start out shorter and get longer over time. It is important that playdates always end on a positive note and sometimes this means keeping them shorter until there are multiple successful playdates in a row. The second important factor to consider is which activities to choose. Each activity should be semistructured (e.g., activities that require turn taking or close-ended activities), motivating for both children (this is important to assess ahead of time if possible), relatively short (e.g., 5–10 min), and organized with cooperative arrangements (e.g., set up activities in ways that promote sharing materials and face-to-face interactions). Also, multiple activities should be planned for every playdate. The preparation of the child with ASD for both the activities and the social behaviors expected during the playdate is also important and can be achieved through priming or practicing the activity and social behaviors before the playdate. Priming may occur a few days before the playdate or earlier that same day. When a child knows what is expected and how to respond to environmental stimuli, this promotes success. Additionally, when a child knows how to do an activity well, this creates an opportunity for the child with ASD to be the expert who can assist the peer.

Once the playdate begins, the facilitator may be very involved in the transitions between activities (e.g., "Come to the table, it's time for a snack") but during activities, a facilitator should try to stay in the background of the activity, reducing the likelihood that children will become dependent on her/him and increasing the likelihood of spontaneous interactions between peers. When support is needed (e.g., a peer offers a toy to the child and the child does not respond), the facilitator will use prompting strategies, usually least-to-most, to support the social behaviors that are being taught. The adult provides invisible support, sitting behind the child and assuring that the children are face-to-face.

13.9.4 Playdates with Siblings

If a sibling is chosen for playdates, the potential benefit is great because of the daily social interactions that occur between children in the same household. However, sometimes siblings are not an ideal choice for a playmate because they are too young or because they already have a history of problem behavior with the child or with the parent if the parent is the facilitator. Depending on the child, a therapist may suggest starting playdates with a different peer or with the therapist as the facilitator rather than the parent. No matter what systematic plan the parents and therapist agree on, the plan should be clearly described in the teaching steps and progress monitored through data collection. If the sibling has a history of problem behaviors during interactions with the child (e.g., ignoring, grabbing, pushing), a behavior intervention plan should be developed right away to maximize the likelihood of positive and rewarding play interactions for both children.

13.10 ESDM Delivery in Groups

When children with ASD are enrolled in group settings such as childcare or preschool programs, the presence of peers can decrease solitary time and increase the number and the duration of social learning episodes, as children will have more opportunities to observe others' actions and communicate, initiate, imitate, share, cooperate, problem solve, and receive feedback about the effects of their behavior. However, for these beneficial effects to occur, it is necessary to design intervention procedures that involve (1) a careful selection of individualized learning objectives that can be addressed within the constraints and opportunities of group activities, and (2) a set of strategies to target such objectives through peer interaction.

ESDM strategies can be effectively used to target social skills within group settings, with one adult delivering instruction to small groups of children (Vivanti et al., 2014, 2016). This delivery format, called Group ESDM (G-ESDM; Vivanti et al., 2017), capitalizes on the widespread availability of preschool programs in the community, the culturally universal tradition of educating young children in group settings, and the social and learning opportunities provided by peers (either typically developing peers, or peers who also have an ASD diagnosis).

G-ESDM objectives focus on behaviors that enable the child's active participation in cooperative activities, such as giving and sharing materials with peers, turn taking, helping, as well as communicating, verbally and nonverbally about the actions needed to achieve the shared goals and the emotions associated with that experience. To facilitate this process, the adults set up activities that bring children together within the same space and lend themselves to social exchanges, such as art table activities, "sensory" games such as games with rice and shaving cream, group music and movement routines such as "Ring-around-the Rosie" and parachute games. Additionally, activities are designed so that children are face-to-face and can easily share and pass materials, help each other, and imitate one another. In this context, the adult actively monitors the quantity and quality of social reciprocity and communication, redirecting the children to the activity, encouraging communication as needed, prompting social behaviors according to a least-to-most prompting hierarchy, repairing communication breakdowns, and facilitating conflict resolution. For example, if a child with ASD and three peers spontaneously gather in the same area to play with Play-doh, the adult will join in as a play partner, modeling, prompting, and facilitating the flow of the game and targeting behaviors such as giving/receiving items, showing, imitating, sharing affect, requesting, and commenting on what each other is doing throughout the activity. Additionally, using simple language and actions, the adult narrates the shared play activity (e.g., saying "roll, roll, roll!"), draws children's attention to each other, (e.g., saying "ready, set, go!" to highlight each child's turn), and helps peers to initiate and maintain interactions and ensure that attempts to interact are noticed and responded to quickly and appropriately.

Using the same techniques, social behaviors taught during joint activities with peers can be targeted outside of the intervention or educational setting, in daily routines and common environments where peers are present (e.g., playgrounds, swimming pools, shopping malls, friends' birthday parties). For example, during a family party involving a child with ASD and her/his peers, several goals can be targeted, such as (1) cooperating with peers in filling an inflatable swimming pool with water and toys; (2) practicing taking and waiting for their turn during a ball game or other games in the pool; (3) using verbal and nonverbal communication to comment about the ongoing activities, emotions, and sensations associated with being in the pool; (4) during snacks, passing bowls and cups to peers, serving food to each other, handing out drink bottles, helping each other to clean up spills; (5) assist each other during the hand washing process (e.g., turning on the tap).

13.11 Challenges Presented by Additional Disabilities or Impairments

Given the primary nature of social difficulties in ASD, it is often the case that parents, teachers, and interventionists assume that all of a child's social problems stem from ASD. Unfortunately, this is an example of "diagnostic overshadowing," the tendency for the presence of one disorder to overshadow the presence of other conditions that may be contributing or accountable for the specific difficulty being considered. Since ASD often occurs with other disorders, the professionals on the ESDM diagnostic or treatment teams must consider the possibility that additional difficulties are contributing to a child with ASD's social difficulties and learning, and address these within the child's individual treatment plan. Additional social challenges may occur related to (1) significant difficulties in parent-child relationships; (2) lack of understanding or use of speech; (3) presence of severe attention problems; (4) extreme lack of interest in other children; (5) difficulties with regulation of anger and aggression; and (6) children with significantly impaired cognitive abilities. While there is no room in this chapter to expand on all of these topics, we will expand on two: parent-child relationship difficulties and significant cognitive impairments, given the challenges that these often raise for therapists in terms of choosing activities, identifying appropriate learning targets, managing the conflicts that can arise with children and parents, and assuring enough repetitions for learning.

13.12 Significant Difficulties in Parent-Child Relationships

While young children with ASD and young children who have parent-infant relationship problems may share a variety of symptoms, the symptoms are present for different reasons and differential diagnosis is an important first step. However, there are certainly children and parents for which both sets of problems are present. Fortunately, the Parent Early Start Denver Model (P-ESDM) approach has a variety of commonalities with common practice in infant mental health work, providing the clinician with a toolkit for addressing both sets of difficulties.

Young children with disorganized attachment patterns and those with an avoidant attachment style may both demonstrate behaviors that may raise questions for parents about ASD. In disorganized attachment patterns, stereotypies, avoidance of eye contact, lack of approach to parents for help or comfort, and discomfort with cuddling are some of the symptoms that overlap with ASD symptoms. Parents of avoidant children may also report poor eye contact, lack of use of the parent for help and comfort, and a seeming indifference to the presence of parents and their coming and goings.

There was a time when ASD was considered a primary disorder of attachment, with the assumption that children with ASD did not show preference for the parents, seeking of comfort or help, security in the presence of the parent, responsiveness to their comings and goings, proximity seeking, or pleasure in affectionate exchanges.

However, a line of studies that extends almost 20 years and spans the globe has demonstrated that young children with ASD may show secure or insecure attachment patterns. Although the percentage of securely attached children with ASD is lower than in typically developing children of the same age or the same mental age, this situation is also true of children with other types of developmental disorders (Rogers et al., 1991). Furthermore, secure attachment in ASD demonstrates characteristics with other aspects of development in ASD that mirror those seen in typical development, involving communication, learning, and social patterns. Finally, attachment security in ASD is related to parental responsivity and sensitivity to child cues, just as it is in typical development (Capps, Sigman, & Mundy, 1994; Oppenheim, Koren-Karie, Dolev, & Yirmiya, 2012). Thus, attachment security appears to be a valid construct in ASD. However, children with ASD may express their attachment security somewhat differently than typically developing toddlers (Rogers et al., 1991). Of particular importance here is stereotypy, which a child with ASD may use to signal positive excitement or pleasure at reunion with a parent rather than signaling distress and agitation.

Parent-child relationship difficulties may often be communicated through parents' descriptions of what is happening in their own lives. Parental separations, severe anxiety disorder, depression, and/or open, angry conflicts may be accompanyed by marked changes in child behavior including sleep and poor eating, sadness or avoidance, increased crying and clinging, increased irritability or anxiety and fearfulness, and low energy or fatigue for children with ASD just as in young children without ASD.

When a family and child are struggling with both ASD and relationship difficulties, ESDM practice would assign a team leader who is trained in both parent-child difficulties and ESDM, as well as providing opportunities for regular reflective supervision with another clinician, typically as part of the peer supervision provided by all ESDM team leads. A thorough understanding of the parent-child and family dynamics can be gathered through the regular ESDM activities of home visits, routine-based assessment practices, parent discussions, and coaching. The provision of weekly or biweekly parent-child coaching should be part of all ESDM treatment deliveries and provides a vehicle for focusing on the development of sensitive, responsive parenting and whatever barriers may be at play. Parent descriptions of their own mental health difficulties may lead to referral for individual treatment as well. Here is a case description in which both sets of problems were present and both were addressed successfully within the ESDM treatment.

13.12.1 Case Presentation

LM, aged 27 months, whose parents were from middle East, was referred for intensive treatment and ESDM parent coaching by his diagnostic team. As a newborn, he suffered from early feeding difficulties and was hospitalized twice during his first year for illenesses. He was the only child of his parents, who lived far away from their own families and did not have much contact with them. His mother described him during his first year as a pleasant, easy infant who gave her much pleasure, though feeding and sleeping were always challenges for her. She described him as changing in the second year of his life, losing his few words, withdrawing, becoming difficult, irritable, and generally either isolated or angry. The parent's goals for treatment included developing some communication, reducing tantrums and anger, improving feeding and sleeping problems, and helping to find ways to play with him and with toys. They had bought the ESDM parent manual but did not see how to go about the activities with their son.

In the first parent-child contact, while both parents were present, the father carried out all the parent-child interactions. He carried LM, a small, slender, quiet 2-year-old, in and out of the room, played with him in physical games on the floor, worked with the therapist to carry out the ESDM play interactions involved in the curriculum assessment, took care of the child's runny nose, clothing, dirty diapers, and all food and snacks.

The mother did not approach or touch the child, and the child did not look at or approach his mother. The mother described the child as frequently angry and stated that she was afraid of him, that his habit of kicking, biting, hitting, and throwing things when angry had injured her. In the second assessment visit, in which these same interactional patterns continued, the therapist at one point engaged the child in a block stacking task right beside the mother, and, after setting up a routine of handing blocks to the child to stack, handed a block to the mother instead, who visibly drew back. With encouragement, the mother handed him the block, which he took easily and stacked, and this new routine continued. When reflecting on the activity (a set part of ESDM coaching is reflection after each activity), the mother voiced her anxiety about being hurt.

The following week, the mother came alone with LM, reporting that the father had to return overseas to his parents' home to deal with the death of his father and the need to manage family affairs. The mother carried him into the room kicking and screaming, but as soon as she put him down he calmed and sought out a toy. After some talking time, to learn about the situation at home, I asked the mother to play a little to help him get ready for the session, so she went to him and immediately began to move him, setting off another tantrum. She backed away and sat on the floor, near me. I observed how it seemed like he did not like to be physically directed, to which she agreed. This was the first treatment session, and the topic was "Get Into the Spotlight," so we discussed the idea of getting her child's attention by being near him in his activities, helping him, showing interest and approval, imitating him with toys, but not giving him any directions, instructions, or demands (see Rogers et al., 2012 for the topics and activities in the parent manual). Since he was now engaged in a sorting box quite contently, she tentatively moved closer to him from the side. I encouraged her to hand him a block that had fallen out of his reach, and she picked up the block and placed it in front of him. He picked it up and put it in its slot. I commented, "You helped him, and he took it." (ESDM coaching practice prioritizes using descriptive language, which draws attention to the relationships between parent behavior and child behavior, rather than praise, e.g., "nice!", which marks the therapist's authority and approval).

I encouraged her to comment about what he was doing, so she began to narrate his activities. As she did, he looked at her once or twice. Since she was beside him, I encouraged her to move more in front of him so he could see her better. She did, also offering him another block from out of his reach. He took it from her hand and put it in. They sat there together for a few minutes, the mother commenting, describing, handing blocks over, helping if one fell off, pointing to the correct hole if he was having trouble finding it. LM looked comfortable, relaxed, receptive, and looked more and more to his mother as she provided well synchronized responses. In her reflection afterward, she commented on how surprised she was that he allowed her to participate. I commented that he looked very comfortable, that he seemed to enjoy her presence and engagement. She smiled and seemed very pleased. I started to offer snacks to LM in the course of our sessions, and he responded by taking them and eating finger foods and spoon foods. I very quickly shifted this over to his mother to carry out and she was delighted to see him eating, which soon included using a spoon and a cup (he had mostly been bottle-fed up to this point). She then shared a significant problem that she was having – getting him out of the car seat when she arrived home with him. He was furious when she turned off the car and tried to lift him from the seat, and he fought furiously against being removed. She was worried that she could not get a flailing, aggressive child out of the seat safely. We discussed how much he disliked being physically managed in general, and I asked her what activities might motivate him to leave the car. She said he loved their iPad, but they had been told that he should have no screen time, so they did not let him have it. I wondered what would happen if she removed the iPad from the glove compartment of her car when she returned home and told him he could play with it when they got inside the house. She imagined that and thought it might be helpful.

At the start of the following week's session, he walked into the treatment room on his own for the first time, carrying a little train, with a smile. I asked the mother how the car seat routine went, and she said it had gone very well, from the start. When she offered a favorite object which he seldom got, like a train or the iPad, he reached out to take it, and she lifted him out, put him down, and held his hand while he walked to their destination holding a favorite object. She then went on to tell me that she had also successfully used a transition object to get him into the car in the morning, and onto the changing table. He responded very positively to these, and the tantrums and upsets were greatly reduced that week. He was also eating solids during mealtimes at the table (i.e., actually sitting on the table, because in the past he had rejected being put in his highchair and she was afraid to trigger that reaction). I commented on how skillfully she had worked with him, thought through various challenges, found a way to communicate with him about what was coming next in a way he could understand. She beamed and commented on how quickly he learned, and we both agreed that he was a capable little boy. She also reported that he had started to count and say letters, which she had him demonstrate to me. Her confidence was growing in her child's ability to learn and her ability to teach him and understand what he was communicating.

In the weeks that followed, we continued to work on topics in the parent manual, with its emphasis on following children's leads, imitating and helping, narrating and approving, taking turns without taking over, parallel play, giving choices and opportunities to communicate, and understanding nonverbal communicative behavior. All these practices involve parental sensitivity and responsivity, and these went well for mother and child. LM developed several gestures quickly, including pointing to request, head shakes for protest, waves for greetings, and began to babble and approximate some words. He also showed increased approaches to his mother for help and comfort, increasing proximity to her, giving and showing things to her, and showed pleasure in touch and cuddles with her. His tantrums were few and far between. Eating at the table became well established. The father came back from his absence to a very different situation than he had left. When I asked him what it was like to have his son now routinely going to his mother for help and comfort instead of to him, he spoke about how happy he was to see the bond that had developed between the two of them.

13.13 Children with Significant Cognitive Impairments

A very common question asked of ESDM trainers is whether it is appropriate to use the ESDM with children who are chronologically older, but not developmentally older, than the recommended ages. The common response to this is that we do not consider the ESDM as an appropriate treatment for children with ASD who may be 9 years of age but with language and play skills that are at a 2-year-old's level, and the reasons for these are several. First, the style of interaction that the ESDM uses is very much based on research concerning characteristics of adult-toddler interactions that facilitate language learning, cooperative social behavior, age-appropriate toy play, and play with other young children. This is the developmental orientation of the ESDM – using those pathways that we know contribute to learning in typical development to address needs of children with atypical development, as long as evidence demonstrates that these pathways also exist in ASD. This is not only a developmental approach, it is also a functional approach – teaching young children with ASD to function in everyday environments and activities as their same aged peers do, in order to prepare them for age based environmental expectations.

For school-aged children with ASD, their peers are school aged children, their primary environments are those of older children, and their age defines different expectations of peers, adults, and various environments. Their competences and their needs are assessed in terms of how they function in these environments. For school-aged children with both severe intellectual impairments and ASD, there is little evidence that a developmental approach will improve their outcomes. On the contrary, the literature is full of examples of the successful use of learning science – applied behavior analysis – to teach these children useful functional skills that support their ability to participate and interact with same age mates in various types of activities. Assessments need to examine children's communication, motor, self-care, cognitive, social, and behavioral skills and needs to determine what strengths they have to build on and what skills can be taught successfully now that will result in more personal independence and effective and pleasurable social communication interactions in everyday environments with peers and adults.

For young children who have severe cognitive impairments, as well as ASD, how does the clinician determine when to take a developmental route and when to take a more functional route? A straightforward answer has to do with the developmental needs of the child vis-á-vis his or her age. The key determinant is whether the developmental approach would lead one to be using materials, ways of interacting, or activity routines that are inappropriate for the child's chronological age. If that is the case, then the developmental approach needs to be adapted to use age appropriate materials and adapted activities, given the focus in the ESDM and the approach to children and adults with disabilities in general, which is to support their inclusion and participation in everyday environments within their community, social network, and family.

13.14 Evidence Supporting Efficacy of ESDM

More than 15 papers on the effects of using the ESDM to improve outcomes for young children with ASD have been published to date, including papers from Australian, Italian, Canadian, and American authors. Papers have examined the effects of the ESDM delivered at high intensity (i.e., 1:1 for 1–2 years), parent-implemented ESDM taught via parent coaching for a limited number of hourly sessions, telehealth delivered parent coaching, and the ESDM delivered in group day care settings. Fourteen of the 15 papers have reported positive effects on overall development, language, adaptive behavior, and/or behavior problems. The studies with the most rigorous designs involve three randomized controlled trials (RCT; i.e., Dawson et al., 2010, Rogers et al., 2012, Vismara et al., 2016), a comparative study (i.e., Vivanti et al., 2014) using a high quality community intervention as the contrast, and three studies using single subject designs (i.e., Vismara et al., 2009, 2012, 2013).

Of the three published RCTs, two found positive effects of the ESDM compared to community treatment. In the first published ESDM outcome papers, Dawson et al. (2010, 2012) reported on the outcomes of 48 children randomized into 20 h of 1:1 home based, interventionist-delivered ESDM plus twice monthly parent coaching and daily parent practice, compared to children receiving typical community care. The ESDM group averaged 15 h of ESDM intervention, and the community group averaged 18 h of community intervention, over the 24 months of treatment. The study demonstrated multiple significant gains made by the ESDM group compared to the community group, including significantly higher IQ gains, adaptive behavior scores, language gains, and symptom reduction. In addition, an important finding involved electrophysiological differences of the groups post-treatment compared to an age matched group with typical development (Dawson et al., 2012). This study demonstrated atypical brain responses to looking at objects versus faces in the community treatment group when compared to the typical group, but typical brain responses to faces compared to objects when the ESDM group was compared to the typical group. A follow-up of these two groups over several years post-treatment showed that the ESDM group continued to demonstrate several areas of enhanced function compared to the community controls in social communication ability as measured by the ADOS, communication and social ability as measured by the Vineland, and differences approaching significance in IQ scores (Estes et al., 2015).

The second RCT, carried out by Rogers et al. (2012), examined the effects of a very low intensity parent coaching intervention using the ESDM techniques compared to community interventions. In this study, the ESDM group received 1.5 h of treatment and the community group averaged 3.7 h of treatment. Both groups of parents increased their child coaching skills similarly and both groups of children demonstrated similar acceleration of developmental rates and language gains. The ESDM did not result in enhanced parent or child performance when compared to community treatment. However, it produced the same amount of growth in both parents and children with only 40% of the amount of intervention hours used by the community group for the same outcomes, and the ESDM parents demonstrated significantly stronger working alliances with therapists than the comparison group.

The third RCT was conducted by Vismara et al. (2016) and involved low intensity telehealth parent coaching and parent implementation of the ESDM delivered to 14 families. Parents received a 1.5 h coaching session weekly for 12 weeks, and had access to a website with: (a) a goal-tracking program to record daily practice of the P-ESDM topics, child behaviors taught, and activities used; (b) modules with text instruction, video examples, practice exercises, and frequently asked questions; and (c) a resource center of website links and tool kits, among other things. Child and parent outcomes were compared to 10 families randomized to the community treatment comparison group. These families also received a 1.5 h telehealth session weekly that did not involve coaching, and access to the information on the website that was not specific to the ESDM. Results demonstrated a significant effect of the experimental treatment on parent fidelity of implementation of the ESDM. There were no significant differences in child social communication in the two groups. The importance of these findings relates to the often replicated studies that consistently demonstrate a positive relationship between more responsive parenting and more advanced language learning in young children over time (Pickles, Harris, & Green, 2015).

Two other RCT studies are currently in analysis. A study of 30 children and parents in a parent coaching study comparing two versions of the ESDM parent coaching model, and a multisite study of the 97 children involved in an intensive ESDM treatment compared to community intervention are currently being prepared for publication.

In addition to these three RCTs, Vivanti et al. (2014) conducted a well-controlled study of 57 Australian children with ASD ages 18–60 months of whom 27 received 12 months of 15 or more hours per week of ESDM delivered in a group situation with staff ratios of one adult to three children. The ESDM group was compared to a carefully matched group of 30 children receiving 15 h or more of early intervention for 12 months delivered by high quality public preschools that used a combination of empirically based intervention approaches. In this study, as in the earlier Dawson et al. 2010 study, there was a significant advantage in several areas including overall developmental rate and receptive language scores for the ESDM group.

The parent coaching version of the ESDM was also tested in a series of studies using single subject designs (i.e., Vismara et al., 2009, 2012, 2013). Vismara et al. (2009) reported on eight parents and children, aged 12–26 months, who received 1 h of parent coaching per week for 12 weeks. The study demonstrated that the majority of parents mastered the ESDM strategies in six 1 h sessions and maintained these through a 12 week follow-up and children demonstrated increases in social communication. Vismara et al. (2012) reported on nine parents and children ages 16–38 months who received 1 h per week of parent coaching via telehealth for 12 weeks. Fidelity as measured by a rating tool was achieved in an average of 6 h (weeks) and child social communication increased as parent fidelity increased. Vismara et al. (2013) involved eight parents and children 18–45 months of age. Parents received telehealth coaching for 1.5 h per week plus access to a self-guided website. Parents achieved fidelity in an average of 7 weeks and child social communication increased in concert with increases in parent fidelity.

Additional ESDM studies involving pre-post designs have been published by colleagues in Italy (parent coaching; Colombi et al., 2016) and Australia (day care center; Vivanti, Paynter, Duncan, Fotergill, et al., 2014). Since pre-post designs do not provide strong tests of efficacy, the results will not be reviewed in detail, but suffice it to say that both papers supported the findings from the more ESDM rigorous studies in their reports of developmental acceleration (Italy) and improvement in child language, cognition, and behavior problems (Australia).

13.15 Areas of Future Research

From the above data, it appears that the ESDM approach is an efficacious intervention that particularly enhances social-communicative functioning for young children with ASD. Whether it is also an effective intervention when used in typical public community settings has not been as strongly demonstrated. Most of the studies to date have involved university-based intervention studies, and the few that are more community based (e.g., Colombi et al., 2016) have not used designs that allow one to assess effectiveness. Those studies need to be done, and we are currently engaged in one such study of the parent coaching model. RCTs of community delivered ESDM are needed to assess the effectiveness of this intervention approach for community wide adoption.

Other studies need to examine the effects of the ESDM on more molecular constructs than IQ, autism severity, and language maturity. We have focused on these broad outcomes in our initial studies because our goal has always been to make significant differences in the developmental trajectories and outcomes of children with ASD, and language and IQ are the best predictors of poor versus better outcomes in ASD in later life (for a review see Magiati, Tay, & Howlin, 2014). However, these are umbrella constructs that reflect changes in many areas of child skill and knowledge, and we need to understand the developmental changes, or mechanisms, that underlie these improvements in key behavior constructs in order to understand how to best target intervention in terms of efficiency and economy. In addition to seeking a more molecular understanding of the ESDM intervention effects, we want to understand other aspects of learning and change that are affected by the ESDM: attention, social preference and social reward, emotional arousal and regulation, abstract concept formation, relationship aspects like emotional contagion, intersubjectivity and knowledge of other minds, and self-formation.

We need to look closely at characteristics of children who respond with more acceleration and those who respond with less acceleration, as well as which children need adaptation of the approach as described in the ESDM decision tree. And just as importantly, we need to understand whether those adaptations improve child learning rates. Finally, we need to test aspects of the intervention, like the decision tree, in a sequenced intervention design to determine whether our heuristic process based on clinical knowledge holds up to empirical assessment. Recent psychometric analysis has supported the curriculum tool, or at least a briefer version of it, as a useful tool that correlates significantly with both standard developmental measures and standard ASD symptom and severity measures.

13.16 Clinical Implications and Recommendations

From the above description of how an integrated intervention that encompasses both developmental science and learning science approaches the opportunity to support the social development of young children with ASD, several points have likely emerged for the reader. One involves the many domains of skills, development, and learning that underlie children's progress in learning to be responsive social partners with others. Of great importance is the skilled use of both intentional verbal communication and its nonintentional coordination with nonverbal communicative cues in the gestural, postural, and affective domains. Another involves a skilled and flexible repertoire of age-appropriate social and object oriented games, vocabulary, and use of learning and play materials, and activities of all types that allow children to participate in the same activities as other children at similar skill levels. A third is the ability to engage reciprocally with others during all these activities, watching what others do, imitating them flexibly, seeing other's goals and adding to them, being able to follow a partner as well as to lead, requesting to join in, inviting others to join, catching others' affective displays and mirroring them back, and sharing emotion messages and materials with others. A fourth involves knowledge of what others think, feel, and experience at an age-appropriate level so that one can appreciate the other's perspective. Doubtless there are more. There is no one discipline of training that adequately prepares a single professional with the expertise to assess social participation in all these ways and develop appropriate treatment plans. The complexity of social development is best supported by a treatment team that spans many different areas of expertise (e.g., communication, motor development and praxis, early cognitive development, early childhood education, behavior analysis, and countless others).

(1) One implication and recommendation is for interdisciplinary input in developing treatment plans and assessing treatment progress in the social domain.

The second clinical implication and recommendation follows closely with the first. In order to develop an adequate treatment plan for social development for an individual child, a wide range of developmental and behavioral skills need to be assessed, built upon, and brought together in moment-by-moment interactions with other children.

(2) The interdisciplinary knowledge needed to develop an individualized plan for supporting social development requires comprehensive assessment data of a child's current abilities across the many domains of development.

The last clinical implication and recommendation addressed here involves the contexts in which children develop their social abilities. In American life today, the give and take of family life represent the first social environment of all children, beginning with parents, and adding older and younger siblings and other relatives to the mix as infants become toddlers. Peer groups of same age mates in preschool, play groups and playdates, and recreational and church groups represents the second social environment of preschoolers. If we are to prepare young children with ASD for life in the community at age 5, at 15, and at 25, we need to begin at home and in other contexts with same age mates, where the expectations, practices, and cultural rules are most clearly expressed. We cannot recreate these contexts in artificial settings, and what we teach children in artificial settings, including in therapy and specialized settings, may not be helpful to them in natural contexts. This is why the ESDM emphasizes working together with parents and family members in homes and other community settings. This is why we encourage families to seek inclusive settings for their children, and within those settings, we work very hard to support children indirectly (i.e., invisible supports), so that their primary partners in interactions are the children and adults who belong to those settings. We believe that the needed learning for an individual child can be embedded in the ongoing daily activities and interactions of everyday life in everyday settings, as long as it is facilitated by a partner in those settings, with enough learning opportunities to support rapid learning.

(3) The implication and recommendation is to embed the individual treatment plan for social development for a young child with ASD into social contexts, routines, and activities of family life as well as contexts that contain community age mates and the adults supervising and teaching them, supported as needed by additional adults who support adequate learning opportunities through indirect rather than direct interactions.

References

Ainsworth, M. D. S., Blehar, M. C., & Waters, E. (1978). Wall S Patterns of attachment: A psychological study of the strange situation.Hillsdale, NJ. : Lawrence Erlbaum Associates.

Akhtar, N., & Tomasello, M. (2000). The social nature of words and word learning. In *Becoming a word learner: A debate on lexical acquisition* (p. 115). Oxford, UK: Oxford University Press.

Banaji, M. R., & Gelman, S. A. (2013). *Navigating the social world: What infants, children, and other species can teach us*. New York: Oxford University Press.

Bjorklund, D. F., & Beers, C. (2016). The adaptive value of cognitive immaturity: Applications of evolutionary developmental psychology to early education. In *Evolutionary perspectives on child development and education* (pp. 3–32). Cham, Switzerland: Springer International Publishing.

Bloom, P. (2002). Mindreading, communication and the learning of names for things. *Mind & Language*, *17*(1-2), 37–54.

Bolton, P. F., Golding, J., Emond, A., & Steer, C. D. (2012). Autism spectrum disorder and autistic traits in the Avon longitudinal study of parents and children: Precursors and early signs. *Journal of the American Academy of Child and Adolescent Psychiatry*, *51*(3), 249–260.

Bowlby, J. (1969). *Attachment and loss: Attachment*. NY: Basic Books.

Bruner, J. S. (1975). The ontogenesis of speech acts. *Journal of Child Language*, *2*(1), 1–19.

Bruner, J. S. (1977). Early social interaction and language acquisition. In H. R. Schaffer (Ed.), *Studies in mother-infant interaction* (pp. 271–289). New York: Academic Press.

Caparulo, B. K., & Cohen, D. J. (1977). Cognitive structures, language, and emerging social competence in autistic and aphasic children. *Journal of the American Academy of Child Psychiatry*, *16*(4), 620–645.

Capps, L., Sigman, M., & Mundy, P. (1994). Attachment security in children with autism. *Development and Psychopathology*, *6*(02), 249–261.

Carpenter, M., Nagell, K., Tomasello, M., Butterworth, G., & Moore, C. (1998). Social cognition, joint attention, and communicative competence from 9 to 15 months of age. *Monographs of the Society for Research in Child Development*, *63*, i–174.

Chawarska, K., Macari, S., & Shic, F. (2013). Decreased spontaneous attention to social scenes in 6-month-old infants later diagnosed with autism spectrum disorders. *Biological Psychiatry*, *74*(3), 195–203.

Chevallier, C., Kohls, G., Troiani, V., Brodkin, E. S., & Schultz, R. T. (2012). The social motivation theory of autism. *Trends in Cognitive Sciences*, *16*(4), 231–239.

Colombi, C., Liebal, K., Tomasello, M., Young, G., Warneken, F., & Rogers, S. J. (2009). Examining correlates of cooperation in autism: Imitation, joint attention, and understanding intentions. *Autism*, *13*(2), 143–163.

Colombi, C., Narsizi, A., Ruta, L., Cigala, V., Gagliano, A., Pioggia, G., & Muratori, F. (2016). Implementation of the Early Start Denver Model in an Italian community. *Autism*, 1–8. http://doi.org/10.1177/1362361316665792

Cooper, R. P., & Aslin, R. N. (1990). Preference for infant-directed speech in the first month after birth. *Child Development*, *61*(5), 1584–1595.

Csibra, G., & Gergely, G. (2009). Natural pedagogy. *Trends in Cognitive Sciences*, *13*(4), 148–153.

Dalsant, A., Truzzi, A., Setoh, P., & Esposito, G. (2015). Maternal bonding in childhood moderates autonomic responses to distress stimuli in adult males. *Behavioural Brain Research*, *292*, 428–431.

Dapretto, M., Davies, M. S., Pfeifer, J. H., Scott, A. A., Sigman, M., Bookheimer, S. Y., & Iacoboni, M. (2006). Understanding emotions in others: Mirror neuron dysfunction in children with autism spectrum disorders. *Nature Neuroscience*, *9*(1), 28–30.

Dawson, G. (2008). Early behavioral intervention, brain plasticity, and the prevention of autism spectrum disorder. *Development and Psychopathology*, *20*(03), 775–803.

Dawson, G., & Bernier, R. (2007). Social brain circuitry in autism. In D. Coch, G. Dawson, & K. Fischer (Eds.), *Human behavior and the developing brain*. New York: Guilford Press.

Dawson, G., Meltzoff, A. N., Osterling, J., Rinaldi, J., & Brown, E. (1998). Children with autism fail to orient to naturally occurring social stimuli. *Journal of Autism and Developmental Disorders*, *28*(6), 479–485.

Deruelle, C., Rondan, C., Salle-Collemiche, X., Bastard-Rosset, D., & Da Fonseca, D. (2008). Attention to low-and high spatial frequencies in categorizing facial identities, emotions and gender in children with autism. *Brain and Cognition*, *66*, 115–123.

Dissanayake, C., & Crossley, S. A. (1996). Proximity and sociable behaviours in autism: Evidence for attachment. *Journal of Child Psychology and Psychiatry*, *37*(2), 149–156.

Dunn, J., & McGuire, S. (1992). Sibling and peer relationships in childhood. *Journal of Child Psychology and Psychiatry*, *33*(1), 67–105.

Ferrari, P. F., & Rizzolatti, G. (2014). Mirror neuron research: The past and the future. *Philosophical Transactions of the Royal Society of London. Series B, Biological Sciences*, *369*(1644), 20130169–20130169.

Frith, U., & Frith, C. (2010). The social brain: Allowing humans to boldly go where no other species has been. *Philosophical Transactions of the Royal Society, B: Biological Sciences*, *365*(1537), 165–176.

Gliga, T., & Csibra, G. (2007). Seeing the face through the eyes: A developmental perspective on face expertise. *Progress in Brain Research*, *164*, 323–339.

Harms, M. B., Martin, A., & Wallace, G. L. (2010). Facial emotion recognition in autism spectrum disorders: A review of behavioral and neuroimaging studies. *Neuropsychology Review*, *20*(3), 290–322.

Hobson, R. P. (1995). *Autism and the development of mind*. East Sussex, UK: Lawrence Erlabum.

Hurley, S., & Chater, N. (2005). *Perspectives on imitation: From neuroscience to social science*. Cambridge, MA: MIT Press.

Jones, W., Carr, K., & Klin, A. (2008). Absence of preferential looking to the eyes of approaching adults predicts level of social disability in 2-year-old toddlers with autism spectrum disorder. *Archives of General Psychiatry*, *65*(8), 946–954.

Jones, W., & Klin, A. (2013). Attention to eyes is present but in decline in 2-6-month-old infants later diagnosed with autism. *Nature*, *504*(7480), 427–431.

Kasari, C., Sigman, M., & Yirmiya, N. (1993). Focused and social attention of autistic children in interactions with familiar and unfamiliar adults: A comparison of autistic, mentally retarded, and normal children. *Development and Psychopathology, 5*(03), 403–414.

Keysers, C. (2011). *The empathic brain*. Amsterdam: Social Brain Press.

Klin, A., Jones, W., Schultz, R., & Volkmar, F. (2003). The enactive mind, or from actions to cognition: Lessons from autism. *Philosophical Transactions of the Royal Society of London B: Biological Sciences, 358*(1430), 345–360.

Kuhl, P. K. (2000). A new view of language acquisition. *Proceedings of the National Academy of Sciences, 97*(22), 11850–11857.

Kuhl, P. K. (2007). Is speech learning "gated" by the social brain? *Developmental Science, 10*, 110–120.

Kuhl, P. K. (2014). Early language learning and the social brain. *Cold Spring Harbor symposia on quantitative biology*, vol. 79, pp. 211–220.

Magiati, I., Tay, X. W., & Howlin, P. (2014). Cognitive, language, social, and behavioral outcomes in adults with autism spectrum disorders: A systematic review of longitudinal follow-up studies in adulthood. *Clinical Psychology Review, 34*, 73–86.

Mahler, M. S. (1952). On child psychosis and schizophrenia: Autistic and symbiotic infantile psychoses. *The Psychoanalytic Study of the Child, 7*, 286. Retrieved from http://psycnet.apa.org/psycinfo/1953-07936-001

Majors, K. (2012). Friendships: The power of positive alliance. In *Positive relationships* (pp. 127–143). Dordrecht, The Netherlands: Springer.

Maunder, R. G., Lancee, W. J., Nolan, R. P., Hunter, J. J., & Tannenbaum, D. W. (2006). The relationship of attachment insecurity to subjective stress and autonomic function during standardized acute stress in healthy adults. *Journal of Psychosomatic Research, 60*(3), 283–290.

McAlister, A., & Peterson, C. (2007). A longitudinal study of child siblings and theory of mind development. *Cognitive Development, 22*(2), 258–270.

Miller, M., Iosif, A. M., Hill, M., Young, G. S., Schwichtenberg, A. J., & Ozonoff, S. (2017). Response to name in infants developing autism spectrum disorder: A prospective study. *The Journal of Pediatrics, 183*, 141.

Mundy, P. C. (2016). *Autism and joint attention: Development, neuroscience, and clinical fundamentals*. New York: Guilford Publications.

Naber, F. B., Swinkels, S. H., Buitelaar, J. K., Bakermans-Kranenburg, M. J., van IJzendoorn, M. H., Dietz, C., … van Engeland, H. (2007). Attachment in toddlers with autism and other developmental disorders. *Journal of Autism and Developmental Disorders, 37*(6), 1123–1138.

Nadel, J. (2014). *How imitation boosts development: In infancy and autism spectrum disorder*. Oxford, UK: Oxford University Press.

Newbigin, A., Uljarević, M., Vivanti, G., & Dissanayake, C. (2016). Brief report: Empathic responsiveness of high functioning children with autism to expressed and anticipated distress. *Journal of Autism and Developmental Disorders, 46*(10), 3338–3343.

NICHD Early Child Care Research Network. (2000). The relation of child care to cognitive and language development. *Child Development, 71*(4), 960–980.

NICHD Early Child Care Research Network. (2003). Does amount of time spent in child care predict socio-emotional adjustment during the transition to kindergarten? *Child Development, 74*(4), 976–1005.

Nielsen, M., Simcock, G., & Jenkins, L. (2008). The effect of social engagement on 24-month-olds' imitation from live and televised models. *Developmental Science, 11*(5), 722–731.

Nuske, H. J., Vivanti, G., & Dissanayake, C. (2013). Are emotion impairments unique to, universal, or specific in autism spectrum disorder? A comprehensive review. *Cognition & Emotion, 27*(6), 1042–1061.

Nuske, H. J., Vivanti, G., & Dissanayake, C. (2016). Others' emotions teach, but not in autism: An eye-tracking pupillometry study. *Molecular Autism, 7*(1), 36.

Oppenheim, D., Koren-Karie, N., Dolev, S., & Yirmiya, N. (2012). Maternal sensitivity mediates the link between maternal insightfulness/resolution and child-mother attachment: The case of children with Autism Spectrum Disorder. *Attachment and Human Development, 14*, 567–584.

Over, H., & Carpenter, M. (2012). Putting the social into social learning: Explaining both selectivity and fidelity in children's copying behavior. *Journal of Comparative Psychology, 126*(2), 182–192.

Ozonoff, S., Pennington, B. F., & Rogers, S. J. (1991). Executive function deficits in high-functioning autistic individuals: Relationship to theory of mind. *Journal of Child Psychology and Psychiatry, 32*(7), 1081–1105.

Pagel, M. (2012). *Wired for culture: Origins of the human social mind*. New York: WW Norton & Company.

Parish-Morris, J., Hirsh-Pasek, K., & Golinkoff, R. M. (2013). From coo to code: A brief story of language development. In P. D. Zelazo (Ed.), *The Oxford handbook of developmental psychology* (vol. 1, pp. 867–908). New York: Oxford University Press.

Pelphrey, K. A., Shultz, S., Hudac, C. M., & Vander Wyk, B. C. (2011). Research review: Constraining heterogeneity: The social brain and its development in autism spectrum disorder. *Journal of Child Psychology and Psychiatry, 52*(6), 631–644.

Pickles, A., Harris, V., & Green, J. (2015). Treatment mechanism in the MRC preschool autism communication trials; implications for study design and parent-focussed therapy for children. *Journal of Child Psychology and Psychiatry, 56*, 162–170.

Rizzolatti, G., & Craighero, L. (2004). The mirror-neuron system. *Annual Review of Neuroscience, 27*, 169.

Rizzolatti, G., Fadiga, L., Fogassi, L., & Gallese, V. (2002). From mirror neurons to imitation: Facts and speculations. *The Imitative Mind: Development, Evolution, and Brain Bases, 6*, 247–266.

Rogers, S. J., Charman, T., & Stone, W. (2006). Evidence-based intervention for language development in young children with autism. In *Social and communication development in autism spectrum disorders: Early identification, diagnosis, and intervention* (p. 14379). New York, NY: Guilford.

Rogers, S. J., & Dawson, G. (2010a). *Early Start Denver Model curriculum checklist for young children with autism*. New York: Guilford Press.

Rogers, S. J., & Dawson, G. (2010b). *Early start Denver model for young children with autism: Promoting language, learning, and engagement*. New York/London: Guilford Press.

Rogers, S. J., Ozonoff, S., & Maslin-Cole, C. (1991). A comparative study of attachment behavior in young children with autism or other psychiatric disorders. *Journal of the American Academy of Child and Adolescent Psychiatry, 30*(3), 483–488.

Rowberry, J., Macari, S., Chen, G., Campbell, D., Leventhal, J. M., Weitzman, C., & Chawarska, K. (2015). Screening for autism spectrum disorders in 12-month-old high-risk siblings by parental report. *Journal of Autism and Developmental Disorders, 45*(1), 221–229.

Rutter, M. (1983). Cognitive deficits in the pathogenesis of autism. *Journal of Child Psychology and Psychiatry, 24*(4), 513–531.

Samson, F., Mottron, L., Soulieres, I., & Zeffiro, T. A. (2012). Enhanced visual functioning in autism: An ALE meta-analysis. *Human Brain Mapping, 33*(7), 1553–1581.

Sanefuji, W., Ohgami, H., & Hashiya, K. (2006). Preference for peers in infancy. *Infant Behavior & Development, 29*, 584–593.

Schultz, R. T. (2005). Developmental deficits in social perception in autism: The role of the amygdala and fusiform face area. *International Journal of Developmental Neuroscience, 23*(2), 125–141.

Schultz, R. T., Volkmar, F. R., & Chawarska, K. (2006). The social brain in autism. In *Understanding autism: From basic neuroscience to treatment* (pp. 323–348). In S. Moldin, J.C.R. Rubenstein (Eds.), New York: Taylor Francis.

Senju, A. (2012). Spontaneous theory of mind and its absence in autism spectrum disorders. *The Neuroscientist, 18*(2), 108–113.

Senju, A., & Johnson, M. H. (2009). The eye contact effect: Mechanisms and development. *Trends in Cognitive Sciences, 13*(3), 127–134.

Sigman, M., & Mundy, P. (1989). Social attachments in autistic children. *Journal of the American Academy of Child and Adolescent Psychiatry, 28*(1), 74–81.

Sigman, M., & Ungerer, J. A. (1984). Attachment behaviors in autistic children. *Journal of Autism and Developmental Disorders, 14*(3), 231–244.

Smith, T., & Iadarola, S. (2015). Evidence base update for autism spectrum disorder. *Journal of Clinical Child & Adolescent Psychology, 44*(6), 897–922.

Thiemann-Bourque, K. (2013). Peer-mediated intervention. In *Encyclopedia of autism spectrum disorders* (pp. 2152–2161). New York, NY: Springer.

Thioux, M., & Keysers, C. (2010). Empathy: Shared circuits and their dysfunctions. *Dialogues in Clinical Neuroscience, 12*(4), 546–552.

Tomasello, M. (2003). *Constructing a language: A usage-based theory of language acquisition*. Cambridge, MA: Harvard University Press.

Tomasello, M. (2010). *Origins of human communication*. Cambridge, MA: MIT press.

Tomasello, M., & Hamann, K. (2012). Collaboration in young children. *The Quarterly Journal of Experimental Psychology, 65*, 1–12.

Vivanti, G., Dawson, G., & Rogers, S. J. (2017). Early learning in autism. In *Implementing the group-based early start denver model for preschoolers with autism* (pp. 1–12). Cham, Switzerland: Springer International Publishing.

Vivanti, G., Duncan, E., Dawson, G., & Rogers, S. J. (2017). Facilitating learning through peer interactions and social participation. In *Implementing the group-based early start denver model for preschoolers with autism* (pp. 87–99). Cham, Switzerland: Springer International Publishing.

Vivanti, G., Hocking, D. R., Fanning, P., & Dissanayake, C. (2016). Social affiliation motives modulate spontaneous learning in Williams syndrome but not in autism. *Molecular Autism, 7*(1), 40.

Vivanti, G., McCormick, C., Young, G. S., Abucayan, F., Hatt, N., Nadig, A., … Rogers, S. J. (2011). Intact and impaired mechanisms of action understanding in autism. *Developmental Psychology, 47*(3), 841.

Vivanti, G., & Nuske, H. J. (2016). Autism, attachment, and social learning: Three challenges and a way forward. *Behavioural Brain Research, 325*, 251.

Vivanti, G., Paynter, J., Duncan, E., Fothergill, H., Dissanayake, C., & Rogers, S. J. (2014). Effectiveness and feasibility of the Early Start Denver Model implemented in a group-based community childcare center. *Journal of Autism and Developmental Disorders, 44*, 3140–3153.

Vivanti, G., & Rogers, S. J. (2014). Autism and the mirror neuron system: Insights from learning and teaching. *Philosophical Transactions of the Royal Society, B: Biological Sciences, 369*(1644), 20130184.

Vygotsky, L. S. (1962). *Thought and language*. Cambridge, MA: MIT Press.

Yoder, P., Stone, W. L., Walden, T., & Malesa, E. (2009). Predicting social impairment and ASD diagnosis in younger siblings of children with autism spectrum disorder. *Journal of Autism and Developmental Disorders, 39*(10), 1381–1391.

14 Video-Based Instruction for Learners with Autism

Kevin M. Ayres, Jason Travers, Sally B. Shepley, and Rachel Cagliani

14.1 Video-Based Instruction

Video-based instruction (VBI) emerged in the literature in 1987 when Harring, Kennedy, Adams, and Pitts-Conway evaluated video as a component of intervention for teaching shopping skills to adults with developmental disabilities. In this study, the authors reported the positive effects of VBI to promote generalization. By using video to present models, these researchers offered practitioners an alternative to live action models and provided a new means to model behaviors that are not otherwise easily modeled in vivo (or at least not modeled repeatedly). In the three decades since that publication, there have been more than 40 studies evaluating aspects of VBI as well as a half dozen narrative literature reviews or meta-analyses. Moving from videotapes (Alcantara, 1994) and videodisks (Wissick, Lloyd, & Kinzie, 1992) to DVDs and portable DVD players (Mechling, Gast, & Fields, 2008), smartboards (Yakubova & Taber-Doughty, 2013) and mobile devices (Cihak, Fahrenkrog, Ayres, & Smith, 2010), as well as "wearables" and augmented reality (Cihak et al., 2016) access to video has evolved.

The growth of research on VBI likely reflects the increasing ubiquity of mobile technology and corresponding high degree of social validity. Learning by imitating video is not peculiar to autism or special education. The practice has existed for a long time but has not often been referred to as VBI; entire television networks have succeeded on the premise that VBI can be enjoyable and help people learn new skills (e.g., Food Network). The high degree of social validity, ease of use, and, most importantly, efficacy provide the foundation and rationale for using video as an instructional tool. Examining online resources (e.g., YouTube.com©) to locate video models to solve household problems (e.g., repairing a doorbell) is commonplace. The focus of this chapter, however, is on the application of VBI to support learning by individuals diagnosed with autism.

This chapter provides background on research with practical implications for teachers and therapists who wish to use VBI. The discussion is organized first around the rationale and practical considerations for using VBI broadly. This

K.M. Ayres (✉) • R. Cagliani
School of Education, The University of Georgia, Athens, GA, USA
e-mail: kayres@uga.edu; Cagliani rrepstein@gmail.com

J. Travers
Department of Special Education, The University of Kansas, Lawrence, KS, USA
e-mail: Travers jason.travers@ku.edu

S.B. Shepley
College of Education, University of Kentucky, Lexington, KY, USA
e-mail: Shepley sally.shepley@uky.edu

J.B. Leaf (ed.), *Handbook of Social Skills and Autism Spectrum Disorder*, Autism and Child Psychopathology Series, DOI 10.1007/978-3-319-62995-7_14

includes the logic for using video as a component of instruction along with discussion about variables known to impact or theorized to impact VBI. Following this, the chapter's focus shifts to provide a concrete background on the research, application, and considerations for using video to teach social skills and functional life skills. Within this context, the goal is for the reader to increase their understanding of why and when to use video along with an improved knowledge of how to implement VBI with learners diagnosed with autism.

14.1.1 Rationale

When a low-tech solution is possible, why choose high tech? The best reason to use high-tech solutions is to help achieve better outcomes or provide a more efficient or expedient result. Much of the rationale for using VBI revolves around logistical factors more than evidence of increased efficiency. Some of the seminal work in this area continues to help provide sound reasoning for incorporating video into instruction.

Haring, Kennedy, Adams, and Pitts-Conway (1987) argued that one of the barriers to programming for generalization by training multiple exemplars (Stokes & Baer, 1977) involves the inefficiency of this procedure for some skills. In particular, the authors considered the range of community-based settings one might need to sample to achieve generalized responding. Recognizing that response generalization is a critical goal for instructional programming for individuals diagnosed with autism, the authors proffered that using some form of simulation in the form of actors portraying the skills in several natural environments might provide the level of multiple exemplar training needed for generalized responding.

If one were to conduct an ecological inventory focused on identifying the different ways to dry one's hands in the bathrooms of stores, restaurants, and other community gathering places, they would find an array of systems from air dryers to different towel dispensers. Sampling each of these on training trips would be ideal but may not be logistically feasible. Incorporating video modeling into training may allow learners to sample a wider range of exemplars than they could on a single training trip and still result in generalization (e.g., Haring et al., 1987).

Beyond providing quality examples of a variety of stimuli, VBI can also narrow or focus the instructional universe in a way that cannot be done in the natural environment. Sherer et al. (2001) suggested that instructional arrangements that include video may enhance attention on critical stimuli because video may make them more salient. Moreover, instructors have greater control over the presentation of stimuli in a video because they do not have to worry about the natural variations that may occur spontaneously in the natural environment. This isolation and control also allow the instructor certainty over the quality of the model. With a high-quality model, an instructor can recycle the material and ensure that assistants or parents teaching the same skill use the same model. This may provide a level of continuity for instruction and improve acquisition in contrast to seeing two or three different models of a chained task and inconsistent adherence to a task analysis.

14.1.2 Considerations for Producing in Videos for Instruction

Learning from VBI requires, at a minimum, two prerequisite skills. First, the learner must have the visual acuity to see what is depicted on the screen. Some researchers have documented that for some learners, larger screens (and therefore larger images) are more efficient (Mechling & Ayres, 2012). Second, the learner must also demonstrate generalized imitation. If the learner has not already demonstrated generalized imitation, then VBI will not likely produce desired effects for the individual. McCoy and Hermansen (2007) synthesized 34 studies that evaluated the use of video modeling for individuals diagnosed with autism. Their review specifically looked at the different types of models that are often used in video modeling including adult models, peer models, point-of-view models, self-models, and a mix of models. Included studies had at least one participant diagnosed with autism aged 2–36 years. The review highlighted that individuals without imitation and attending skills may experience difficulty with video modeling and that further research should be conducted with individuals without these potential prerequisite skills. To date, the authors of this chapter are unaware of any empirical studies demonstrating the efficacy of teaching imitation via video.

If the learner can imitate, then several other factors should be considered prior to producing video(s). These are summarized in Fig. 14.1. A primary consideration is whether to produce a video or search for an existing video to use as the model. Some publishers have released high-quality video models intended for teaching functional life skills to individuals diagnosed with developmental disabilities. These provide teachers and therapists with simple, ready-made curricular materials that can be included in instruction. Such videos may also be more appealing due to convenience but may also be less effective. For example, Mechling, Ayres, Foster, and Bryant (2013) compared the efficacy of custom-made videos to commercially produced videos to teach chained tasks to high school students diagnosed with autism. The researchers reported that while all students responded to both video formats, the use of customized videos reliably led to better improvements in performance. Therefore, interventionists may consider commercially made (or generic videos from sources like Youtube.com©) but recognize that they may achieve greater gains with videos customized to their context.

An additional consideration relates to the viewer's perspective, irrespective of whether creating custom videos or using commercially produced or borrowed content. For example, some researchers have evaluated the efficacy of VBI shot from the perspective of the person doing the action. This is frequently referred to as point-of-view (POV) video instruction (see Mason, Davis, Boles, & Goodwyn, 2013 for a meta-analysis of POV video modeling). In contrast, some researchers have used video shot from the perspective of a bystander. Ayres and Langone (2007) reported results of a study comparing instruction of gross motor tasks with POV and what the researchers referred to as third-person video modeling. Very few differences were observed in terms of rate of acquisition, errors, or time in instruction, which led the researchers to conclude that either format may be a viable choice for gross motor tasks. They cautioned, however, that POV may not provide sufficient information for social skills (e.g., facial expressions that should be imitated).

Another variation in third-person video modeling includes using the learner as their own model. Referred to as video self-modeling (VSM), the interventionist creates a video of the person performing the task and edits out all prompts and disfluencies to produce an example for use in instruction. The rationale for using VSM rests partially on Bandura's social learning theory (Bandura, 1977) that suggested individuals were more likely to imitate models that were similar to themselves. Mason, Davis, Ayres, Davis, and Mason (2016) reported the results of a meta-analysis evaluating the efficacy of VSM for teaching students diagnosed with autism. They noted particularly strong effects when teaching social and communication skills. One benefit of producing VSM examples is that it can be done in the context of initial instruction itself as the teacher or therapist probes responding and prompts through the sequence of a skill. A meta-analysis by Bellini and Akullian (2007) highlighted that robust effects occurred across intervention, maintenance, and generalization when video modeling was used to teach functional skills. Taken together, these meta-analyses provide sufficient evidence for using VSM in a range of contexts.

Among the final set of choices discussed here regarding video production is whether to include narration to the video. Smith, Ayres, Mechling, and Smith (2013) noted that much of the research regarding VBI and video modeling had overlooked that participants may have been responding to narration included in the video examples rather than imitating the video. They evaluated the additive effect of narration to video on the acquisition of multistep chained tasks by middle school-aged students diagnosed with autism. They reported that video modeling with narration

Fig. 14.1 Preliminary, preproduction, and postproduction considerations for video-based instruction

Preliminary Consideration	
Visual Acuity	· Does the learner have necessary visual acuity to see what is depicted on screen?
Generalized Imitation	· Does the learner have a generalized repertoire of imitation behavior?
Pre-production Considerations	
Produce or Select Video	· Will you create a video for the student, or search and select an existing video that models the target behavior?
Identify the Perspective the Video Will Use	· Is a bystander perspective appropriate for the target behavior? · Is point-of-view (POV) perspective appropriate for the target behavior? · Is video self-modeling appropriate for the modeled target behavior?
Decide Whether Narration Will Be Used	· Will narration likely contribute to improved performance of the modeled target behavior?
Post-production Considerations	
Identify Whether Video Modeling or Video Prompting is Appropriate	· Will playing a video that models the entire (chained) response more likely evoke imitation of the target behavior? · Will short clips that model each step of an entire (chained) response more likely evoke imitation of the target behavior?
Identify Who Will Be The Instructional Agent	· Will a teacher, therapist, paraprofessional, parent, sibling, caregiver, or similar individual be responsible for implementing the intervention procedures? · Can the learner be taught to deliver his or her own instructor using a self-instructional process?
Prepare a List of Steps for Applying the Intervention	· Will you obtain a practice guide that outlines procedures for video modeling or for video prompting? · Will you rely on procedures from a specific study to generate the list of steps for applying the intervention? · How and who will data be collected to evaluate the effectiveness of the intervention? · How will data be collected to ensure the proper intervention procedures are followed? · Who will interpret the data and make decisions about adjustments to the video(s), instructional agent(s), and/or steps for applying the intervention?

was more efficient for two of the participants than the video that did not include narration. Smith et al. found that narration was not required for the other two participants to acquire the skills, but the participants expressed a preference for videos that included narration. From a practical standpoint, this would indicate that including narration of the steps in a multistep video is likely beneficial and at least provides consistent models of the vocabulary associated with certain tasks.

14.2 Procedural Considerations for Delivering Video-Based Interventions

Although the factors discussed next do not capture all possible variables one might consider when producing video for instruction, a summary of key features will be helpful to various professionals when preparing and producing video(s) for instruction. After the video for instructional use has been created, professionals should decide how to incorporate the video into instruction. Integration of video into instruction generally follows one of two broad categories, video modeling and video prompting, but sometimes may include procedures from both categories. Professionals also will need to decide who will deliver the intervention (i.e., follow the prescribed set of procedures). The majority of research on video modeling and VBI has used teachers or therapists as intervention agents, but parents and/or caregivers also may be appropriate depending on the targeted skill. An additional option is to teach the learner to control delivery of instruction from the instructional video. Following a brief description of the differences between video modeling and video prompting, we will address the issue of who leads instruction.

14.2.1 Video Modeling

Video modeling describes the process of displaying a video in its entirety prior to asking a learner to imitate what they saw. This application of VBI represents the simplest form from a teaching standpoint: prepare video, press play, and ask the learner to imitate. Researchers have documented the efficacy of video modeling across a wide range of skills, ages, and ability levels. They have further explored multiple means of presenting models including continuous video modeling (Mechling, Ayres, Purrazzella, & Purrazzella, 2014) and chunking (Sigafoos et al., 2007). In comparisons of video modeling to video prompting, video prompting is generally reported to be more effective and efficient (Cannella-Malone et al., 2006); however, some researchers have reported results showing that video modeling is superior (Taber-Doughty et al., 2011). In general, video modeling may have some advantages when introducing a skill for the first time because the learner has an opportunity to see the entire sequence of steps uninterrupted.

14.2.2 Video Prompting

Video prompting may have specific benefits for learners who have difficulty attending to longer videos because, during video prompting, each discrete step of the video is shown as needed. Typically, the therapist incorporates the video into a systematic prompt-fading intervention like least-to-most prompting (e.g., Smith, Ayres, Mechling, Alexander et al., 2013) or constant time delay (e.g., Graves, Collins, Schuster, & Kleinert, 2005). The learner only sees the portion of the video that is relevant to the behavior that is needed at that point in time. For example, if a learner has independently worked through 5 steps of a 12-step task analysis and pauses on the sixth step, the therapist would then show only the few seconds of video relevant to that step. This can pose some logistical challenges if the teacher has, for example, filmed a 90-s video and the student requires a prompt at the sixth step which falls at the 45th second of the video. The teacher has to fast forward the video to the appropriate place. Alternatively, if the teacher films each step separately or cuts the video into steps, then he or she may be able to navigate directly to the segment the students needs.

14.2.3 The Instructor

While a teacher or therapist can deliver instruction with video modeling or video prompting, over the past decade more work has emerged focused on teaching learners to deliver their own instruction (see Smith, Shepley, Alexander, & Ayres, 2015 for a review of this literature). As individuals diagnosed with autism access new environments (e.g., vocational settings), the demands and expectant behaviors will change from the way they were initially taught. Therefore, instead of anticipating each and every variation of a behavior and trying to teach as many discrete tasks as possible at school, instructors should focus their curriculum on self-instructional behaviors so learners can begin to teach themselves across environments. Once a student learns to self-instruct, they have acquired a pivotal skill allowing them greater independence (Ayres, Shepley, Douglas, Shepley, & Lane, 2015). Explicit instruction of self-instruction can lead to generalized use of the self-instructional process and independent initiation of self-instruction when encountering novel tasks (Smith et al., 2016). Learners also have the autonomy to pursue learning things that are of high interest to them.

Although multiple websites (e.g., YouTube.com©) provide ample collections of video that many people use to self-instruct, some students diagnosed with autism require explicit instruction in locating and using video from online resources or published curricula. In cases where the internet or other resources do not meet the learner's needs, researchers have identified ways to help students create their own instructional supports for the purposes of self-instruction by filming others performing the task (Shepley, Smith, Ayres, & Alexander, 2017). One advantage for learners in creating their own self-instructional materials is that they no longer have to rely on others to provide the raw material. For example, an adult learning a new job from a fellow employee or job coach can use a mobile device to video any tasks he or she may need to reference later.

Regardless of who delivers instruction, understanding the methods and means to using video in a variety of contexts will assist practitioners with designing better instruction for their students. The remainder of this chapter focuses on VBI in specific contexts: first, social skills and second, more life skills. The reasons for using video in the different contexts vary and some of the challenges within those settings also vary. Exploring the research in these domains and seeing how to translate the research to practice will permit therapists to provide efficient and evidence-based instruction that meets the needs of their students.

14.3 Video-Based Instruction for Social Skills

Social skills are difficult to teach because seemingly minute changes in the environment can significantly change what responses are socially appropriate or inappropriate. Something as benign as riding an elevator can be exceptionally complicated, as the social conventions vary considerably according to the situation. When standing alone in an elevator, it may be perfectly okay to blow one's nose. However, the presence of another person means blowing your nose is socially inappropriate. Similarly, where one stands in the elevator depends heavily on the number of people in the elevator at that time. In most cultures, it is socially inappropriate to stand immediately next to the only other person in the elevator. When only two unfamiliar people are in the elevator, they stand as far apart as possible because this is considered socially appropriate. However, as more people enter and exit the elevator, the socially appropriate proximity of fellow riders changes. Other unwritten rules of elevator etiquette also vary and include the direction riders should face, where they should look, whether conversations are appropriate and what topics can be discussed, asking people what floor they need versus moving to allow them access to the buttons, etc. Importantly, most people have acquired elevator etiquette and a vast array of social skills via a rich history of social experiences. Indeed, few people have received explicit instruction for elevator etiquette, asking to play a game with peers, approaching a person to ask for a date, or countless other social skills for various and nuanced social situations.

Whether initiating conversations (Nikopoulos & Keenan, 2004), recognizing and responding to socially inappropriate behavior of others (Spivey & Mechling, 2016), complimenting others (Macpherson, Charlop, & Miltenberger, 2015), or engaging in play activities (MacDonald, Clark, Garrigan, & Vangala, 2005), VBI has been found to be an effective method for supporting social skills acquisition and performance for learners diagnosed with autism and other developmental disabilities. VBI is ideal for teaching social skills because it allows for the incorporation of various elements that highlight key social cues.

14.4 Video-Based Instruction for Social Skills Acquisition and Performance

Communication is inherently a social behavior, and given that children diagnosed with autism often have poorly developed social and communication skills, communication is often a priority of intervention teams. VBI has been an effective social communication support for learners diagnosed with autism, and much of the research in this area has focused on preschool and elementary school children diagnosed with autism. Manding (e.g., requesting) is perhaps the most fundamental communication skill (Sundberg & Partington, 1998). Any request is a mand regardless of whether the individuals makes it via speech, voice output devices, or other symbolic means (e.g., writing, gesture, picture exchange) that is reinforced by consequences specific to the request (Skinner, 1957). For example, a child might see a preferred item and vocalize while looking and reaching toward the item. A caregiver or teacher might recognize this requesting behavior and respond by retrieving and delivering the item to the child. Access to the item contingent on vocalizing and gesturing (or crying, tantruming, engaging in self injury, etc.) will likely reinforce requesting, making similar responses more likely to occur in the future.

VBI can support the acquisition and generalized use of manding. Plavnick and Ferreri (2011) used a functional analysis to confirm participants were engaging in problem behavior to gain access to preferred items or activities (i.e., requesting), then enlisted video models for appropriate requests. These researchers found acquisition, mastery, and generalization of requesting were better when VBI was clearly linked to functional communication when compared to VBI for communication skills that were unrelated to behavior function. Cihak, Smith, Cornett, and Coleman (2012) found VBI promoted more rapid acquisition and consistent requesting among four preschool children diagnosed with developmental delays, including autism, when combined with picture exchange communication system (PECS; Bondy & Frost, 2002) compared to PECS alone. Essentially, Cihak et al. used video modeling as a means of priming requests prior to introducing contrived opportunities to request (consistent with the first phase of the PECS protocol). These and similarly focused studies (e.g., Jones, Lerman, & Lechago, 2014; Plavnick & Vitale, 2016; Wilson, 2013) indicate VBI can be an effective means for teaching young children diagnosed with autism to make requests.

In a somewhat novel study, MacManus, MacDonald, and Ahearn (2015) combined VBI with a series of scripted pretend play activities for three preschool children diagnosed with autism. The researchers used 3-min videos of play sets replete with related action figures based on child interests (e.g., superheroes and villains) and scripted series of actions and phrases to be followed by the learner. The researchers measured adherence to the scripts as well as impromptu generalizations when specific elements were missing (e.g., using a different hero or villain when the scripted one was unavailable; using novel statements during play). The participants increased engagement in play, used more vocalizations, and demonstrated stimulus and response generalization, thereby illustrating the efficacy of video-based instruction for teaching complex play skills often observed in peers without social and play deficits.

Children diagnosed with autism are often described as having significant difficulty transitioning between activities (Lequia, Wilkerson, Kim, & Lyons, 2015). This difficulty often manifests as noncompliance that varies in topography and severity (e.g., aggression to others or self, elopement, tantrums). However convenient it may be to limit transitions and restrict access to unfamiliar activities, such accommodations may have the inadvertent effect of increasing frequency and intensity of severe behavior occasioned by transitions. A common strategy is to utilize personnel to assist with and reinforce transitions, but this resource-intensive tactic is not always feasible. VBI may provide a practical and effective remedy for this common problem. Indeed, researchers have used priming techniques in videos to explain and demonstrate students' successful transition behavior and have found them to be an inexpensive, unobtrusive, and reliable way to improve transitions.

Schreibman, Whalen, and Stahmer (2000) used video models depicting appropriate transitions in the homes and community that often accompanied problem behavior with three young children diagnosed with autism. Parents implemented the intervention and, over time (i.e., 12–40 sessions), decreased disruptive transitions to zero occurrences. Participants learned to predict the upcoming transition(s) and the associated reinforcing consequences that typically accompanied (e.g., ending the mall trip at the toy store). In a different study aimed at enhancing transitions, Cihak et al. (2010) used video models of students diagnosed with autism engaging in ten transitions associated with the daily activity schedule. Rather than relying on a visual schedule, the researchers provided students with an iPod® with the transition videos and prompted them to view the transition video associated with the next destination/activity. They incorporated additional prompts contingent on transition errors until the participant diagnosed with autism arrived at the correct destination. Within 8 to 14 sessions, all four participants learned to transition to locations throughout the school, but withdrawal of the intervention resulted in increased difficulty with transitions, suggesting that video models for transitions may function as an important accommodation worthy of prolonged or permanent use.

14.4.1 Play and Other Complex Social Skills

Engagement in play offers children opportunities to develop various social skills vital for realizing long-term social outcomes. For example, play in young children affords opportunities to communicate and other foundational skills such as commenting, taking turns, cooperation, problem-solving, and developing friendships. As children mature, these and other skills become increasingly important to all aspects of education, including extracurricular activities. However, children diagnosed with autism often do not acquire or use these sorts of social skills without explicit instruction. The features associated with VBI (outlined in previous sections) suggest it can be used in various ways to support social skill development among learners diagnosed with autism in the elementary school years, and several studies support this conclusion. For example, an important play-based social skill relates to attempts to persistently solicit peers to join a preferred activity (e.g., to play a game of tag). Grosberg and Charlop (2014) explained that learners diagnosed with autism may quickly give up recruiting peers to play an outdoor game after being rebuffed, but typical peers usually persist until they identify and are joined by companions. Accordingly, these authors used VBI to teach four elementary school-aged children diagnosed with autism to engage in persistent social initiations of play with peers. Videos showed a model soliciting a peer to play a game, with some videos showing the first and second peers approached declining to join, followed by the model asking a third peer who agreed to play. Results indicated the participants learned to persist in soliciting peers to join them in play activities and that the skill is generalized to different peers and settings.

Social conventions evolve over time and are highly contextual. Thus, appropriate social skills in preschool and elementary school may eventually be deemed inappropriate for adolescents and adults. Relationship dynamics change during adolescence and throughout adulthood, and obtaining desired outcomes (e.g., employment, friendships, marriage) often is dependent on acquiring knowledge and skills about nuanced social situations with acquaintances, close friends, extended and immediate family members, and intimate partners. The nuances of social situations are complicated by the need for complex social skills, such as chained behaviors, that may not always contact reinforcing contingencies (Plavnick, Sam, Hume, & Odom, 2013). Though few studies are available that explicitly examined VBI as an intervention to teach social skills to adolescents and young adults diagnosed with autism, it is worth distinguishing older from younger learners because appropriate social skills evolve over time.

Plavnick et al. (2013) used VBI to promote complex social skills among four adolescent participants diagnosed with autism. Specifically, these researchers developed a small library of 15 videos (i.e., three different clips for each of the five targeted social skills) and implemented VBI to teach participants to (1) invite a peer to join in an activity, (2) ask peers if they could join their activity, (3) ask about the interests of peers, (4) offer assistance to peer or adult, and (5) maintain conversations. Results indicated rapid acquisition and maintenance of targeted social skills for all four participants. These skills were also taught in a replication study (i.e., Plavnick, Kaid, & MacFarland, 2015) that produced similar results, indicating that several complex social skills can be taught to adolescents diagnosed with autism using VBI.

Chan and John (2012) suggested video modeling could be used to teach sexuality-related skills, including appropriate dating behavior, as well as aspects of privacy and modesty. Though no studies are available to guide the development of procedures, some sources are available that describe intervention procedures for supporting health sexuality education (Travers & Whitby, 2014; Whitby & Travers, 2014). Travers and Tincani (2010) describe decision-making guidelines along with a rationale for providing sexuality education to learners diagnosed with autism. Also, individuals diagnosed with autism may be at increased risk for sexual exploitation (Travers, Tincani, Whitby, & Boutot, 2014), and video modeling may be an effective means of teaching individuals diagnosed with autism to reject unwanted advances, recognize dangerous behavior of others, and seek help if victimized. The demonstrable benefits of VBI and establishment of video modeling as an evidence-based practice (Wong et al., 2015), along with the need for systematic and explicit instruction for complex social behavior, suggest sexuality-related curricula, and VBI may well complement to generate positive sociosexual outcomes for adolescents and adults diagnosed with autism, though researchers should investigate what types of VBI, procedures, and skills are most amenable to this type of intervention.

VBI has been used in isolation or complementary to other interventions (e.g., PECS) to promote various social skills in preschool-aged children diagnosed with autism, including basic communication skills (e.g., requesting), imaginary play skills, and increasing appropriate transitions from/to activities. VBI also has supported acquisition and generalization of more complex social skills for elementary school children, including persistent solicitation of peers to join a preferred activity. Video instruction also can be useful for teaching elementary school students diagnosed with autism leisure skills such as motion-activated video games (e.g., Nintendo Wii™; Spriggs, Gast, & Knight, 2016) and promoting conversation skills (Charlop, Gilmore, & Chang, 2008; Charlop & Milstein, 1989).

14.5 Video-Based Instruction in Life Skills

A primary goal of life skills instruction is to assist individuals to become more independent, thus having more opportunities to participate in their community. Life skills instruction may include teaching personal hygiene (e.g., applying deodorant), job skills (e.g., individualized according to employer), and daily living skills (e.g., housekeeping). Many of these tasks require large or expensive materials (e.g., stove), making it impossible for an instructor to model in vivo without "undoing" a step. For example, if the instructor models how to turn on a gas burning stove, they then must turn off the flame to allow the learner to imitate this step. This exact performance may be imitated by the learner diagnosed with autism, leading the instructor to implement additional error correction procedures. VBI eliminates this barrier while also allowing the instructor to program for multiple variations of materials used across environments when teaching life skills.

Life skills instructors should consider the specific set of materials and the individual's environment when developing interventions. There will likely be a substantial number of variations when teaching a specific life skill from one individual to the next. Laundry is one skill that varies based on the specific materials and environment. Some washers and dryers require digital setting adjustments, while others have a dial for each setting. Additionally, the skills required to wash clothes in a home are much different than washing clothes in a laundromat or group laundry facility. The variability among materials and settings requires an accompaniment of specific models. The ability to individualize models based on specific settings and materials allows the learner to view the life skills tasks in the natural environment, thus allowing instructors to program for generalization across settings, materials, and people (Charlop-Christy, Le, & Freeman, 2000).

VBI is different from other forms of modeling in that it allows prompting and directions to take place in a non-stigmatizing way when delivered via common forms of modern technology. This technology could benefit the majority of adults diagnosed with autism who are unemployed or cannot receive proper accommodations at their workplace. According to the Institute of Education Sciences National Longitudinal Transition Study-2 (NLTS-2; Newman et al., 2011), less than half of surveyed of young adults diagnosed with autism had worked for pay within 2 years of when data were collected. Additionally, 9.9% of individuals diagnosed with autism were fired from a job within 2 years of when the data were collected. These numbers clearly indicate a need for additional technologies to support individuals with autism in the workforce.

Cimera and Cowan (2009) reported that individuals diagnosed with autism require the most costly vocational rehabilitation services when compared to services for other individuals diagnosed with disabilities, indicating a need for vocational rehabilitation counselors who specialize in autism. Similarly, job coaches effectively reduce barriers and enhance employer accommodations, but such services are expensive and difficult to obtain (Schartz, Hendricks, & Blanck, 2006). VBI may provide some solution to the high costs associated with limited access to job training for adults diagnosed with autism (Wilczynski, Trammell, & Clarke, 2013). For example, Sauer, Parks, and Heyn (2010) examined the use of cueing systems (an umbrella term encompassing VBI, used to describe assistive technology that delivers prompts to independently complete tasks) as a job training tool for individuals diagnosed with cognitive disabilities. Results indicated that video prompts as a cueing system were valuable teaching tools for individuals diagnosed with cognitive disabilities in the workforce. Similarly, Burke et al. (2013) successfully increased adults diagnosed with autism ability to perform shipping tasks at their workplace using video modeling delivered through a tablet. The participants in the study and their caregivers considered the intervention to be socially valid and worthy of recommendation to other individuals diagnosed with autism in the workforce.

In addition to VBI saving resources when instructing life skills, a video can serve as a more appropriate model when targeted tasks are often viewed as private. Regardless of age and relationship to the individual diagnosed with autism, a live model of toilet training could be perceived as unethical, yet toilet training is a critical life skill that will increase access to future social and vocational environments.

Drysdale, Lee, Anderson, and Moore (2015) used video modeling to teach the steps for using the restroom including traveling to the restroom, undressing, sitting on the toilet, eliminating in the toilet, redressing, and flushing. The young boys diagnosed with autism included in the study acquired all of the steps for independent toileting within 8 days. Additionally, the use of video modeling required less prompting from a caregiver or therapist compared to when video modeling was not used.

There is evidence to support that VBI is an effective intervention to support daily living and vocational skills instruction for individuals diagnosed with autism. Along with its effectiveness, VBI can serve as a much needed support for adults diagnosed with autism as they begin to enter the workforce. Practitioners interested in using VBI to teach life skills should consider ways to implement the procedures for their learners diagnosed with autism. Often, VBI is one element of a larger instructional package to teach these skills; therefore it is important to consider additional components to accompany VBI, such as various prompt-fading strategies including least to most and time delay.

14.5.1 Component of Systematic Instruction

The majority of studies using VBI evaluated videos as a stand-alone, independent variable, in which the participant learns to complete a life skills task from viewing a video model or a series of video prompts. Although video modeling is an evidence-based practice for individuals diagnosed with autism (Wong et al., 2015), the procedures used do not always incorporate errorless teaching techniques. Instructors therefore may need to provide additional prompts and implement prompt-fading strategies for a learner to achieve the mastery criterion for a task. Specifically, a video may be used as a component of systematic instruction (such as least-to-most prompts or time delay) to ensure the learner correctly completes the life skills task. For example, Smith, Ayres, Mechling, Alexander et al. (2013) used a video model in the prompt hierarchy to teach high school students with disabilities to perform vocational office tasks. This procedure saved resources related to training instructors to implement the model and the need for two full sets of office supplies while also fading the use of prompts entirely until learners acquired the skills independently. In another variation, Mechling et al. (2008) used VBI and least-to-most prompting as a treatment package. Participants were first shown a video prompt depicting a single step of a cooking task, and, if unsuccessful, researchers prompted the participants to view the video again using least-to-most prompting. Likewise, Mechling, Gast, and Seid (2010) evaluated a third way to incorporate VBI into a least-to-most prompt hierarchy that was controlled by the participants. Three different prompts (i.e., picture, picture + audio, and video + audio) for each step of the cooking tasks were loaded onto a mobile device. Participants could select the prompt necessary to each complete step, and all participants self-faded their use of prompts from most intrusive (video prompt) to least intrusive (picture only) until they performed the tasks independently.

For some individuals, time delay procedures, where the instructor delivers the controlling prompt required to evoke a correct response as opposed to progressing through a prompt hierarchy, may be a more efficient use of instructional time for many individuals diagnosed with autism (Ault, Wolery, Gast, Doyle, & Eizenstat, 1988). Therefore, if a learner diagnosed with autism has a history of correctly responding to model prompts, an instructor should consider supplementing live modeling with video modeling. For example, Graves et al. (2005) used constant time delay paired with video prompts to instruct high school-aged students to perform three cooking tasks, each at different stations within a typical kitchen (e.g., stove, microwave, countertop). Initially the participants were given the task direction, "Cook the _____," and viewed a video of the entire cooking task. Following the video model, video prompts of each step played following a 0-s delay. The delay was faded to 5 s until all participants performed the cooking tasks independently. At the completion of the study, all videos, including the priming video model, were removed from instruction and participants performed the tasks independently.

When teaching life skills to individuals diagnosed with autism, the goal of response prompting strategies is to fade the prompt until the learner is independently responding to the discriminative stimulus, whether that be a task direction (e.g., "clean the window") or naturally occurring environmental stimuli (e.g., a smudgy window). However, in some circumstances, such as when an individual has infrequent opportunities to engage in tasks or if they have difficulty with short-/long-term memory, they may indefinitely be dependent on a video prompt. If taught to deliver their own controlling prompt (i.e., video), learners diagnosed with autism can self-instruct through novel tasks and transitions, thus still increasing their independence with activities of daily living. In such cases, videos may be better characterized as an accommodation rather than a problem of prompt dependence.

14.5.2 Self-Instruction

Evidence supports the efficacy of teaching individuals to self-instruct using videos. Smith et al. (2015) conducted a review of independent self-instruction on chained tasks. They found 19 studies that met criteria over a 34-year span. While not part of the researchers' inclusion criteria, all included chained tasks which were considered life skills. Eight studies used video as the controlling self-instructional prompt, six of which were presented on handheld devices. The authors summarized ways in which researchers instructed self-instructional strategies, drawing attention to the fact that the learner has not generalized these strategies until they are completely free of instructor support, including any prompts to refer back to technology and error correction procedures.

When presented with an unknown task, ideally a learner would seek out his or her needed technology (e.g., an iPhone®) and navigate to the specific video model or prompts required to complete the skill. Yet, every study included in Smith et al. (2015) either included verbal directions to use technology (e.g., "Use the video to help you make popcorn"), handed the participant the self-instructional materials following the task direction, or had the self-instructional materials prearranged to the specific prompt (e.g., video displayed on device screen so participant only had to press play). Future researchers and practitioners should teach this pivotal skill to a criterion, plan for generalization from the outset, and assess for maintenance of self-instruction behaviors. This involves instructors carefully choosing what information to include in the task direction they present.

Smith et al. (2016) appear to be the first to examine independent and generalized initiation of a self-instructional prompt for high school students diagnosed with autism spectrum disorder (ASD). Following the task directive to complete a novel cooking, office, or party preparation task, the researchers used progressive time delay to deliver a verbal directive to "use the iPhone." All participants independently generalized initiation of retrieving the phone from their pocket in at least one environment. These findings suggest professionals should consider including initiation of a prompt as the first step in the task analysis to teach students diagnosed with autism to self-instruct. For example, if a student has demonstrated success with video models delivered via an iPhone®, the steps to self-instruct would include taking the iPhone® out of his or her pocket (or retrieving from set location), pressing the home button, swiping left to unlock, etc., until the student has accessed a video model corresponding to the target task.

Spriggs, Knight, and Sherrow (2015) taught high school students diagnosed with autism to self-instruct through three novel tasks (a combination of vocational, academic, and daily living) using video models embedded within a visual activity schedule on an iPad®. This combination of two visual strategies, schedules and video modeling, allowed learners to acquire multiple novel skills while self-instructing. Using an inexpensive application for Apple® devices (i.e., My Pictures Talk), researchers used least-to-most prompting to teach students to navigate the iPad® to the set app, select and view the first video, then perform the modeled tasks. Upon completion of a single task, participants advanced to the next video by swiping left or pressing a green arrow. Although the participants in this study only completed three tasks, practitioners could embed as many tasks as needed into a visual activity schedule to complete in a given environment.

Although most self-instructional studies using video technologies were conducted in school settings (Smith et al., 2015), it is critical to instruct these skills in the natural environment as well, such as an employment setting for vocational tasks (Kellems & Morningstar, 2012), a public university for pedestrian skills (Mechling & Seid, 2011), or an actual apartment for daily living tasks (Mechling & Stephens, 2009; Mechling et al., 2008). To plan for generalization across environments during the initial acquisition of self-instructional skills, practitioners could use Spriggs et al.'s (2015) methodology and combine it with procedures used by Smith et al. (2016). This would consist of teaching learners diagnosed with autism to initiate their device, navigate the media library, select the visual activity schedule corresponding to the current or directed environment (e.g., kitchen, Home Depot, walk to post office), and view a series of novel tasks/transitions presented as video models within the schedule. The technology could then serve as an instructional resource for the learner replete with videos organized by environment that learners independently access when all or some of the steps are unknown.

The use of video models to teach self-instruction of life skills is a relatively new innovation reported in the research literature. If this form of technology is effective for a learner diagnosed with autism, we may not necessarily need to fully fade the prompt but instead view the mobile device as a prosthetic that they need to access their environment (Ayres et al., 2015). On the other hand, unnecessary dependence on the device (i.e., always viewing a video model, regardless of past history of independence) can conflict with goals of increasing task completion, efficiency, and accuracy. Accordingly, researchers should identify and evaluate strategies to teach learners to discriminate between situations when video support is and is not needed (i.e., distinguishing between, "I do not know how to complete this task, therefore I must self-instruct" and "I have done this many times and do not need video support").

14.6 Conclusion

Technology affords teachers and therapists' unprecedented resources to deliver instructional prompting and supports in any setting and in accordance with individual needs. Moreover, the intuitive design of mobile device hardware and applications, as well as increasingly ubiquitous nature of mobile technology, generates high social validity for VBI across various contexts. Teaching with video is not, however, without key considerations and procedures – simply making and showing a video to a learner diagnosed with autism will not likely bring desired changes in behavior. As with any teaching approach that uses any medium (e.g., books, journal articles), adherence to effective procedures for implementation is just as important as the content being conveyed. Education and related professionals should therefore consider the current evidence when designing instructional interventions, including those that incorporate VBI.

As we have outlined in this chapter, educators must make several decisions regarding the form and content of their video prior to and following video production. Having made these decisions, educators can proceed to integrate video with systematic prompt-fading procedures to support independence and, perhaps, advance toward self-instruction. Whether teaching social skills or chained life skills, ample evidence exists to support using VBI for learners diagnosed with autism (Wong et al., 2015). Furthermore, given the size of the literature base, educators can easily locate a range of options regardless of the instructional domain.

As technology changes and possibilities expand, teachers and therapists will likely be initiating new applications for VBI before researchers are able to evaluate them. Being mindful of collecting data and attending to the overall quality of instruction will ensure that these novel applications support the learning needs of students. With the growth of augmented reality and wearable computers, the near future possibilities for VBI and video-based supports could bring about significant changes in how individuals diagnosed with autism and other disabilities interact with their environments. However, teacher reliance on any single instructional technique, including VBI, will not likely result in meeting the unique instructional needs of all students. Thus, VBI should be accompanied by a range of evidence-based practices to support the social, behavioral, communicative, and functional skills that often comprise educational programming for learners diagnosed with autism. And although VBI has many logistical advantages (e.g., recycling instructional material), teachers and therapists still must individualize instruction when using this intervention method. One way to achieve this via VBI is to incorporate different types of VBI for different students and/or for different skills. By packaging evidence-based practices with variations of VBI for different skills and learners, education professionals will better position themselves to positively impact their students by increasing social and life skills in current and future environments.

References

Alcantara, P. R. (1994). Effects of videotape instructional package on purchasing skills of children with autism. *Exceptional Children, 61*, 40–55.

Ault, M. J., Wolery, M., Gast, D. L., Doyle, P. M., & Eizenstat, V. (1988). Comparison of response prompting procedures in teaching numeral identification to autistic subjects. *Journal of Autism and Developmental Disorder, 4*, 627–636.

Ayres, K. M., & Langone, J. (2007). A comparison of video modeling perspectives for students with autism. *Journal of Special Education Technology, 22*, 15–30.

Ayres, K. M., Shepley, S. B., Douglas, K., Shepley, C., & Lane, J. (2015). Mobile technology as a prosthesis: Using mobile technology to support community engagement and independence. In T. Cardon (Ed.), *Technology and the treatment of autism spectrum disorder*. New York: Springer International Publishing. doi:10.1007/978-3-319-20872-5

Bandura, A. (1977). *Social learning theory*. Upper Saddle River, NJ: Prentice Hall.

Bellini, S., & Akullian, J. (2007). A meta-analysis of video modeling and video self-modeling interventions for children and adolescents with autism spectrum disorders. *Exceptional Children, 73*, 264–267.

Bondy, A., & Frost, L. (2002). *A picture's worth: PECS and other visual communication strategies in autism*. Bethesda, MD: Woodbine House.

Burke, R. V., Allen, K. D., Howard, M. R., Downey, D., Matz, M. G., & Bowen, S. L. (2013). Tablet-based video modeling and prompting in the workplace for individuals with autism. *Journal of Vocational Rehabilitation, 38*, 1–14.

Cannella-Malone, H., Sigafoos, J., O'Reilly, M., de la Cruz, B., Edrisinha, C., & Lancioni, G. E. (2006). Comparing video prompting to video modeling for teaching daily living skills to six adults with developmental disabilities. *Education and Training in Developmental Disabilities, 41*, 344–356.

Chan, J., & John, R. M. (2012). Sexuality and sexual health in children and adolescents with autism. *The Journal of Nurse Practitioners, 8*, 306–315.

Charlop, M. H., Gilmore, L., & Chang, G. T. (2008). Using video modeling to increase variation in the conversation of children with autism. *Journal of Special Education Technology, 23*, 47–66.

Charlop, M. H., & Milstein, J. P. (1989). Teaching autistic children conversational speech using video modeling. *Journal of Applied Behavior Analysis, 22*, 275–285.

Charlop-Christy, M. H., Le, L., & Freeman, K. A. (2000). A comparison of video modeling with in vivo modeling for teaching children with autism. *Journal of Autism and Developmental Disorders, 30*, 537–552.

Cihak, D. F., Fahrenkrog, C. D., Ayres, K. M., & Smith, C. (2010). The use of video modeling via a video iPod® and a system of least prompts to improve transitional behaviors for students with autism spectrum disorders in the general education classroom. *Journal of Positive Behavior Interventions, 12*, 103–115.

Cihak, D. F., Moore, E. J., Wright, R. E., McMahon, D. D., Gibbons, M. M., & Smith, C. (2016). Evaluating augmented reality to complete a chain task for elementary students with autism. *Journal of Special Education Technology, 31*, 99–108.

Cihak, D. F., Smith, C. C., Cornett, A., & Coleman, M. B. (2012). The use of video modeling with the picture exchange communication system to increase independent communicative initiations in preschoolers with autism and developmental delays. *Focus on Autism and Other Developmental Disabilities, 27*, 3–11.

Cimera, R., & Cowan, R. (2009). The costs of services and employment outcomes achieved by adults with autism in the US. *Autism, 13*, 285–302.

Drysdale, B., Lee, C., Anderson, A., & Moore, D. (2015). Using video modeling incorporating animation to teach toileting to two children with autism spectrum disorder. *Journal of Developmental and Physical Disabilities, 27*, 149–165.

Graves, T. B., Collins, B. C., Schuster, J. W., & Kleinert, H. (2005). Using video prompting to teach cooking skills to secondary students with moderate disabilities. *Education and Training in Developmental Disabilities, 40*, 34–46.

Grosberg, D., & Charlop, M. (2014). Teaching persistence in social initiation bids to children with autism through a portable video modeling intervention. *Journal of Developmental and Physical Disabilities, 26*, 527–541.

Haring, T. G., Kennedy, C. H., Adams, M. J., & Pitts-Conway, V. (1987). Teaching generalization of purchasing skills across community settings to autistic youth using videotape modeling. *Journal of Applied Behavior Analysis, 20*, 89–96.

Jones, J., Lerman, D. C., & Lechago, S. (2014). Assessing stimulus control and promoting generalization via video modeling when teaching social responses to children with autism. *Journal of Applied Behavior Analysis, 47*, 37–50.

Kellems, R. O., & Morningstar, M. E. (2012). Using video modeling delivered through iPods to teach vocational tasks to young adults with autism spectrum disorders. *Career Development and Transitions for Exceptional Individuals, 35*, 155–167.

Lequia, J., Wilkerson, K. L., Kim, S., & Lyons, G. L. (2015). Improving transition behaviors in students with autism spectrum disorders: A comprehensive evaluation of interventions in educational settings. *Journal of Positive Behavior Interventions, 17*, 146–158.

MacDonald, R., Clark, M., Garrigan, E., & Vangala, M. (2005). Using video modeling to teach pretend play to children with autism. *Behavioral Interventions, 20*, 225–238.

MacManus, C., MacDonald, R., & Ahearn, W. H. (2015). Teaching and generalizing pretend play in children with autism using video modeling and matrix training. *Behavioral Interventions, 30*, 191–218.

Macpherson, K., Charlop, M. H., & Miltenberger, C. A. (2015). Using portable video modeling technology to increase the compliment behaviors of children with autism during athletic group play. *Journal of Autism and Developmental Disorders, 45*, 3836–3845.

Mason, R. A., Davis, H. S., Ayres, K. M., Davis, J. L., & Mason, B. A. (2016). Video self-modeling for individuals with disabilities: A best-evidence, single case meta-analysis. *Journal of Developmental and Physical Disabilities, 28*, 623–642.

Mason, R. A., Davis, H. S., Boles, M. B., & Goodwyn, F. (2013). Efficacy of point-of-view video modeling: A meta-analysis. *Remedial and Special Education, 34*, 333–345.

McCoy, K., & Hermansen, E. (2007). Video modeling for individuals with autism: A review of model types and effects. *Education and Treatment of Children, 30*, 183–213.

Mechling, L. C., & Ayres, K. M. (2012). A comparative study: Completion of fine motor office related tasks by high school students with autism using video models on large and small screens. *Journal of Autism and Developmental Disabilities, 42*, 2364–2373. doi:10.1007/s10803-012-1484-1

Mechling, L. C., Ayres, K. M., Foster, A. L., & Bryant, K. J. (2013). Comparing the effects of commercially available and custom-made video prompting for teaching cooking skills to high school age students with autism. *Remedial and Special Education, 34*, 371–383.

Mechling, L. C., Ayres, K. M., Purrazzella, K., & Purrazzella, K. (2014). Continuous video modeling to prompt completion of multi-component tasks by adults with moderate intellectual disability. *Education and Training in Autism and Developmental Disabilities, 49*, 3–16.

Mechling, L. C., Gast, D. L., & Fields, E. A. (2008). Evaluation of a portable DVD player and a system of least prompts to self-prompt cooking task completion by young adults with moderate intellectual disabilities. *The Journal of Special Education, 42*, 179–190.

Mechling, L. C., Gast, D. L., & Seid, N. H. (2010). Evaluation of a personal digital assistant as a self-prompting device for increasing multi-step task completion by students with moderate intellectual disabilities. *Division on Autism and Developmental Disabilities, 45*, 422–439.

Mechling, L. C., & Seid, N. H. (2011). Use of hand-held personal digital assistant (PDA) to self-prompt pedestrian travel by young adults with moderate intellectual disabilities. *Educational Training in Autism and Developmental Disabilities, 46*, 220–237.

Mechling, L. C., & Stephens, E. (2009). Comparison of self-prompting of cooking skills via picture-based cookbooks and video recipes. *Education and Training in Developmental Disabilities, 44*, 218–236.

Newman, L., Wagner, M., Knokey, A. M., Marder, C., Nagle, K., Shaver, D., Wei, X., with Cameto, R., Contreras, E., Ferguson, K., Greene, S., and Schwarting, M. (2011). *The post-high school outcomes of young adults with disabilities up to 8 years after high school. A report from the national longitudinal transition study-2 (NLTS2). (NCSER 2011–3005).* Menlo Park, CA: SRI International.

Nikopoulos, C. K., & Keenan, M. (2004). Effects of video modeling on social initiations by children with autism. *Journal of Applied Behavior Analysis, 37*, 93–96.

Plavnick, J. B., & Ferreri, S. J. (2011). Establishing verbal repertoires in children with autism using function based video modeling. *Journal of Applied Behavior Analysis, 44*, 747–766.

Plavnick, J. B., Kaid, T., & MacFarland, M. C. (2015). Effects of a school-based social skills training program for adolescents with autism spectrum disorder and intellectual disability. *Journal of Autism and Developmental Disorders, 45*, 2674–2690.

Plavnick, J. B., Sam, A. M., Hume, K., & Odom, S. L. (2013). Effects of video-based group instruction for adolescents with autism spectrum disorder. *Exceptional Children, 80*, 67–83.

Plavnick, J. B., & Vitale, F. A. (2016). A comparison of vocal mand training strategies for children with autism spectrum disorder. *Journal of Positive Behavior Interventions, 18*, 52–62.

Sauer, A., Parks, A., & Heyn, P. (2010). Assistive technology effects on the employment outcomes for people with cognitive disabilities: A systematic review. *Disability and Rehabilitation: Assistive Technology, 6*, 377–391.

Schartz, H., Hendricks, D. J., & Blanck, P. (2006). Workplace accommodations: Evidence based outcomes. *Work, 27*, 345–354.

Schreibman, L., Whalen, C., & Stahmer, A. C. (2000). The use of video priming to reduce disruptive transition behavior in children with autism. *Journal of Positive Behavior Interventions, 2*, 3–11.

Shepley, S. B., Smith, K. A., Ayres, K. M., & Alexander, J. L. (2017). The use of video modeling to teach individuals with disabilities to film a video on an iPhone. *Education and Training in Autism and Developmental Disabilities, 52*, 158–169.

Sherer, M., Pierce, K. L., Paredes, S., Kisacky, K. L., Ingersoll, B., & Schreibman, L. (2001). Enhancing conversation skills in children with autism via video technology: Which is better, "self" or "other" as a model? *Behavior Modification, 25*, 140–158.

Sigafoos, J., O'Reilly, M., Cannella, H., Edrisinha, C., de la Cruz, B., Upadhyaya, M., … Young, D. (2007). Evaluation of a video prompting and fading procedure for teaching dish washing skills to adults with developmental disabilities. *Journal of Behavioral Education, 16*, 93–109.

Skinner, B. F. (1957). *Verbal behavior*. New York, NY: Appleton-Century Crofts.

Smith, K. A., Ayres, K. M., Alexander, J. A., Ledford, J., Shepley, C., & Shepley, S. B. (2016). Initiation and generalization of self-instructional skills in adolescents with autism and intellectual disability. *Journal of Autism and other Developmental Disabilities, 46*, 1196–1209.

Smith, K. A., Ayres, K. M., Mechling, L., Alexander, J. L., Mataras, G., & Shepley, S. B. (2013). The effects of a system of least prompts with video prompting to teach office tasks to individuals with moderate intellectual disability. *Career Development and Training for Exceptional Individuals, 38*, 39–49.

Smith, K. A., Shepley, S. B., Alexander, J. L., & Ayres, K. M. (2015). The independent use of self-instruction for the acquisition of untrained multi-step tasks: A review of the literature. *Research in Developmental Disabilities, 40*, 19–30.

Smith, M., Ayres, K. M., Mechling, L., & Smith, K. (2013). A comparison of the effects of video modeling with narration versus video modeling without narration on the functional skill acquisition of adolescents with autism. *Education and Training in Autism and Developmental Disabilities, 14*, 165–179.

Spivey, C. E., & Mechling, L. C. (2016). Video modeling to teach social safety skills to young adults with intellectual disability. *Education and Training in Autism and Developmental Disabilities, 51*, 79–92.

Spriggs, A. D., Gast, D. L., & Knight, V. F. (2016). Video modeling and observational learning to teach gaming access to students with ASD. *Journal of Autism and Developmental Disorders*. Advance online publication doi: 10.1007/s10803-016-2824-3.

Spriggs, A. D., Knight, V., & Sherrow, L. (2015). Talking picture schedules: Embedding video models into visual activity schedules to increase independence for students with ASD. *Journal of Autism and Developmental Disabilities, 45*, 3846–3861.

Stokes, T. F., & Baer, D. M. (1977). An implicit technology of generalization. *Journal of Applied Behavior Analysis, 10*(2), 349–367. http://doi.org/10.1901/jaba.1977.10-349

Sundberg, M. L., & Partington, J. W. (1998). *Teaching language to children with autism and other developmental disabilities: Augmentative communication*. Concord, CA: AVB Press.

Taber-Doughty, T., Bouck, E. C., Tom, K., Jasper, A. D., Flanagan, S. M., & Bassette, L. (2011). Video modeling and prompting: A comparison of two strategies for teaching cooking skills to students with mild intellectual disabilities. *Education and Training in Autism and Developmental Disabilities, 46*, 499–513.

Travers, J., & Tincani, M. (2010). Sexuality education for individuals with autism spectrum disorders: Critical issues and decision making guidelines. *Education and Training in Autism and Developmental Disabilities, 45*, 284–293.

Travers, J. C., Tincani, M., Whitby, P. J. S., & Boutot, E. A. (2014). Sexuality education for persons with severe disabilities: A self-determination philosophical approach. *Education and Training in Autism and Developmental Disabilities, 49*, 232–247.

Travers, J. C., & Whitby, P. J. S. (2014). Sexuality and relationships for individuals with autism spectrum disorders. In M. Tincani & A. Bondy (Eds.), *Adults with autism spectrum disorder: Evidence-based and promising practices*. New York: Guilford Press.

Whitby, P. J. S., & Travers, J. C. (2014). Let's talk about sex: Sexuality education for learners with developmental disabilities. In J. Hart (Ed.), *Friendship 101: Developing social skills among children and youth with autism and developmental disabilities*. Arlington, VA: Council for Exceptional Children.

Wilczynski, S. M., Trammell, B., & Clarke, L. S. (2013). Improving employment outcomes among adolescents and adults on the autism spectrum. *Psychology in the Schools, 50*, 876–887.

Wilson, K. P. (2013). Teaching social-communication skills to preschoolers with autism: Efficacy of video versus in vivo modeling in the classroom. *Journal of Autism and Developmental Disorders*, *43*, 1819–1831.

Wissick, C. A., Lloyd, J. W., & Kinzie, M. B. (1992). The effects of community training using a videodisc-based simulation. *Journal of Special Education Technology*, *11*, 208–221.

Wong, C., Odom, S. L., Hume, K. A., Cox, A. W., Fettig, A., Kucharczyk, S., … Schultz, T. R. (2015). Evidence-based practices for children, youth, and young adults with autism spectrum disorder: A comprehensive review. *Journal of Autism and Developmental Disorders*, *45*, 1951–1966.

Yakubova, G., & Taber-Doughty, T. (2013). Brief report: Learning via the electronic interactive whiteboard for two students with autism and a student with moderate intellectual disability. *Journal of Autism and Developmental Disorders*, *43*, 1465–1472.

15 Visual Learning Strategies to Promote Independence and Appropriate Social Behavior

Thomas S. Higbee and Tyra P. Sellers

15.1 Introduction

As noted in other chapters in this text, individuals with autism spectrum disorder (ASD) often present with behavioral challenges that make it difficult for them to interact effectively with the social world. They may also have difficulty completing multistep tasks and sustaining attention for extended periods of time. The interventions described in this chapter, photographic activity schedules (hereafter called, activity schedules) and social scripting/script fading, were specifically designed to help individuals with ASD overcome these challenges. In this chapter, we will introduce these two techniques, briefly review the research supporting their effectiveness, and then offer suggestions for how they can be used, both together and separately, to improve the lives of individuals with ASD and their families.

T.S. Higbee (✉) • T.P. Sellers
Department of Special Education & Rehabilitation, Utah State University, Logan, UT, USA
e-mail: tom.higbee@usu.edu

15.2 Photographic Activity Schedules

Photographic activity schedules are a visual cueing technique that, when paired with a physical prompting procedure called *graduated guidance* (described later), can help individuals with ASD learn to complete progressively longer sequences of behavior without adult assistance. Activity schedules were pioneered by Pat Krantz, Lynn McClannahan, Greg MacDuff, and their colleagues, at the Princeton Child Development Institute (PCDI; McClannahan & Krantz, 2010). Since their original formulation, other researchers have refined and added complexity to the types of activities that can be taught using activity schedules.

As an intervention, activity schedules are composed of two primary components: (1) a visual schedule and (2) a physical prompting/prompt fading procedure called *graduated guidance*. While activity schedules can take many forms, the simplest and most common version is a small, three-ring binder with multiple pages that contain pictures, either photos or icons, representing specific activities, one to a page. More complex forms of schedules for advanced learners may include written labels for activities instead of pictures/icons where all activities are listed on a single page in list form on either a sheet of paper or an electronic device. Learners are taught to follow activity schedules using

J.B. Leaf (ed.), *Handbook of Social Skills and Autism Spectrum Disorder*, Autism and Child Psychopathology Series, DOI 10.1007/978-3-319-62995-7_15

specific prompting techniques that do not require the use of verbal instructions or verbal prompting. Specifically, learners are taught to follow the visual schedule using a most-to-least prompting hierarchy, in order to prevent errors, where the instructor guides the learner to complete the activity schedule sequence by physically prompting the learner from behind. As the purpose of teaching a learner to follow an activity schedule is to reduce dependence on adult prompts, the instructor avoids the use of any verbal instructions and verbal or gestural prompts while teaching the learner to follow the schedule. If physical prompting alone is not sufficient to produce independent schedule-following behavior, reinforcement can be added to the teaching procedures for specific behaviors where the learner may be having difficulty. Please see McClannahan and Krantz (2010) for suggestions about how and when to use external reinforcers and how and when to remove them.

As the learner begins to follow the schedule, the instructor gradually reduces the amount of physical support provided (and external reinforcement if used) until the learner can complete the schedule without support. The sequence of activities in the schedule changes from session to session to ensure that the learner is learning to follow the schedule rather than simply memorizing a sequence of activities. The final page of the schedule usually contains a picture/icon/text representing a terminal reinforcer such as a preferred snack or activity. As learners acquire the ability to follow schedules, more complex features such as choices between multiple activities and visual cues to use electronic timers to complete timed activities can be included as well as cues to initiate social interactions using social scripts (detailed in the sections that follow). Detailed procedures for setting up basic activity schedules and common teaching procedures can be found in McClannahan and Krantz (2010).

15.2.1 Summary of Research

Researchers have repeatedly demonstrated that activity schedules can be an effective means of promoting independent behavior for individuals with ASD. In an early study on activity schedules, MacDuff, Krantz, and McClannahan (1993) used a basic activity schedule to teach a series of tasks to four children with ASD. In the study, the activity schedule cued the participants to complete three work tasks (e.g., worksheets) and three leisure activities (e.g., watching television). Instructors taught participants to follow the schedules through the use of graduated guidance. As a result of the schedule and prompting procedures, all four participants increased levels of on-task behavior across all six tasks.

Bryan and Gast (2000) also used activity schedules and graduated guidance to increase the on-task behavior of four students with ASD between the ages of 7 and 9 years in an elementary school resource classroom. Results indicated that the schedules and graduated guidance procedure increased on-task behavior during academic activities with all participants during both teaching and generalization activities. When the authors removed the graduated guidance, participant responding continued at criterion levels. However, when the activity schedule book was removed, participant responding deteriorated, indicating that the activity schedule was controlling participant responding.

Watanabe and Sturmey (2003) explored the use of incorporating choice into activity schedules with adults with ASD. In their study, three adults with ASD had learned to use activity schedules to complete work tasks in a vocational setting. When researchers allowed these individuals to choose the order of the work tasks and create their own activity schedules, engagement increased significantly when compared to baseline conditions. These data suggested that adding choice elements to activity schedules can increase engagement.

Machalicek et al. (2009) used activity schedules with correspondence training to teach three school-aged children with ASD to play appropriately on the playground. In addition to a one-page visual schedule of activities, pictures of the activities were attached to playground structures, and children were taught to match pictures from the activity schedule to the pictures on the playground equipment. In a deviation from standard activity schedule teaching procedures, participants were also taught, using verbal and physical prompting, to review the schedule of activities prior to starting play. Results of the study indicated that all three children learned to follow the schedules and that appropriate play increased and problem behavior decreased as a result of the intervention.

More recently, Akers, Higbee, Pollard, Pellegrino, and Gerencser (2016) used an activity schedule to promote appropriate play on a school playground for three preschoolers with ASD. In this study, children who had previously engaged in repetitive play on the playground learned to use an activity schedule to complete a series of appropriate playground activities. Results showed that all participants showed significant increases in the number of appropriate playground activities completed when the activity schedule was present.

15.2.2 Implications for Researchers

Many important research questions remain surrounding the use of activity schedules. The primary one has to do with the extent to which activity schedules can be removed or faded once they are in place. To date, few published cases of activity schedules being successfully removed or faded exist (Akers, Higbee, Gerecser, & Pellegrino, in press, being a notable exception). Generally, when the activity schedule is removed, learner responding returns to pre-intervention levels. It is possible that, in some cases, the presence of the activity schedule could be stigmatizing to the individual learner or that it may overly constrain behavior to the activity sequence specified on the schedule. Thus, there may be utility in investigating methods of systematically fading visual schedules. For those learners for whom the schedule cannot be completely faded, perhaps the schedule could be modified to a format that is more typical of age peers such as a planner or smartphone-based schedule. Future researchers may wish to investigate these and other topics including the use of activity schedules to cue more complex forms of social behavior (described later).

15.2.3 Implications for Clinical Application

Based on the available research, it appears that activity schedules are a useful tool for practitioners who wish to promote increasingly complex series of behaviors for individuals with ASD. Before teaching an individual with ASD to follow an activity schedule, it is important that the practitioner ensures that the learner has the necessary prerequisites for learning to follow a schedule. Key prerequisite skills are (1) demonstrating picture-object correspondence skills so that when shown a picture of an activity, the learner can find the appropriate materials for that activity, (2) tolerating physical prompting, and (3) demonstrating the ability to independently complete the activities included in the schedule (this is more critical for a beginning learner as novel activities can be introduced into the schedule once the learner acquires basic schedule-following behavior). If any of these prerequisite skills are missing, the practitioner should work with the learner until these skills are acquired before beginning an activity schedule.

When creating a beginning activity schedule, the practitioner should select moderately-preferred closed-ended activities (i.e., with a clear beginning and ending) that can be completed in a relatively brief period of time and that the learner already knows how to complete. In initial training stages, the focus is on learning how to follow the schedule rather than on the activities themselves. The learner should be taught the subsequent schedule-following sequence: (1) obtain the schedule book, (2) open to the first activity page, (3) touch the picture/icon representing the activity, (4) obtain the materials necessary for completing the activity, (5) complete the activity, (6) return the materials to their original location, (7) return to the schedule book and turn the page to the next activity, (8) repeat steps 3–7 until the last page is reached and the terminal reinforcer obtained, and (9) close the schedule book and return it to its original location if necessary. The individual should be taught to complete these steps using physical prompts delivered from behind (and external reinforcers if necessary). Over the course of teaching sessions, the instructor should reduce the amount of physical support provided (and external reinforcers delivered) until the learner completes the schedule independently.

Data collection for activity schedules usually involves measuring learner performance during each individual step of following the schedule mentioned in the previous paragraph. This can be accomplished in several ways. A simple method of data collection is to score each schedule component as being completed independently or with prompting and then calculating a percentage of independence by dividing the number of independently completed steps by the total number of steps. With some learners, it may be advantageous to record the level of prompting required to perform each step. How often data are collected will vary depending on the circumstances of the learning environment. While it may be helpful in beginning phases to take data during every teaching session, this may not be practical in all settings. A more practical alternative strategy might be to alternate between teaching sessions and data collection/probe sessions at a ratio of two to three teaching sessions for every data collection/probe session. In this kind of a system, the instructor could use a 3-s time delay procedure to determine which steps of the activity schedule require physical prompting and at what level. This information from the data collection/probe session could then be used to determine the level of prompting used during the next two to three teaching sessions (see Gerencser, Higbee, Akers, & Contreras, 2017, for more information about this data collection system).

Once a learner is reliably following a basic activity schedule with closed-ended activities, more advanced schedule features can be included. For example, choice opportunities can be included in the schedule in addition to preselected activities. The most basic choice preparation involves replacing the single picture on an activity schedule page with a piece of Velcro® and labeling the page as a "choice" page. On the facing (left) page, two pictures of available activities are attached with Velcro. The learner is allowed to select from these two activities by moving one of the pictures from the facing page to the activity schedule page and then touching the picture and proceeding as normal to retrieve the materials and complete the activity. If the individual does not select one of the two activities independently, the instructor can use physical prompts to facilitate a selection response. These prompts should then be faded over time as the learner begins making an active choice. A more complex form of choice making can be incorporated by creating a "choice board" that is located near where the learner completes the activity schedule. An example of a "choice board" is a poster board with strips of Velcro where multiple pictures of available activities can be attached. When the learner is ready to make choices from a wider variety of activities, pictures of these activities can be placed on the choice board and a choice page with a piece of Velcro where a picture can be attached and can be included in the activity schedule book. The learner is taught, via physical prompting, to go to the choice board, select the picture of an activity, place the picture on the choice page of the activity schedule book, touch the picture, and then proceed as normal to obtain the materials and complete the activity.

A second advanced feature of activity schedules is the inclusion of open-ended activities. The inclusion of activities that do not have a predetermined end point is accomplished by training the learner to use a specially prepared kitchen timer to set the end point for the activity. A simple push-button digital kitchen timer works best for this purpose. The "minute" button of the timer is color-coded with either a small red sticker or with red paint. The "start/stop" button of the timer is color-coded green in the same fashion. Stickers representing the number of minutes for a given activity (e.g., three red dots = 3 min) are placed on the picture followed by a green sticker to symbolize the "start" button. The learner is taught, via physical prompting, to touch the first red sticker on the picture and then push the red button on the timer. Next, the learner is prompted to touch the second red sticker on the picture and then push the red button again on the timer. When the process has been completed for all red stickers, the student is prompted to touch the green sticker and then push the green "start" button. The learner is then prompted to begin engaging in the activity. When the timer alarm sounds, the individual is guided from behind back to the timer and prompted to press the "stop" button to deactivate the alarm. The learner is then prompted to replace the materials from the activity and return to the schedule book and turn the page as normal. Across all teaching procedures in activity schedules, if physical prompting alone is not sufficient to produce participant responding, reinforcement can be added for independent completion of activity schedule steps. If the instructor is not able to fade physical prompts for setting and using the timer after a few sessions, booster sessions to practice only setting, activating, and deactivating the timer can be conducted outside of activity schedule sessions. Once the leaner can reliably use the timer, a wide variety of age-appropriate open-ended activities can be included in the schedule.

Finally, visual or auditory prompts can also be included in the schedule to promote social initiations with either adults or peers. This is accomplished through the use of social scripting/script fading, the topic of the next section.

15.3 Social Scripts and Script Fading to Promote Social Interactions

Social scripts and script fading are an effective intervention to teach a variety of social language to children with autism. Social scripts are visual or auditory cues that prompt an individual to engage in a contextually appropriate vocal response (McClannahan & Krantz, 2005). The scripts typically consist of statements or questions that are taught using textual or auditory scripts, physical or vocal prompts with time delay, and prompt fading (McClannahan & Krantz, 2005). The scripts are then systematically faded from back to front through a series of predetermined steps by removing the text or the recorded message. For example, a full script might include "Do you want to play with me?" The first step in fading might entail cutting off the word "me" for a text script or recording an audio script to say "Do you want to play with." Script fading continues until the physical script materials are completely removed, stimulus control is systematically transferred to some other stimuli (e.g., a place mat or play materials), or the scripts are faded to a small version of the script material (e.g., a small piece of the script card with no text or with the first letter of the script). Individuals can be taught several different scripts for a given social situation to promote varied responding and use of combined and novel responses.

Researchers have evaluated the effects of social scripts and script fading on teaching individuals to initiate social interactions with comments or questions during general social activities (Brown, Krantz, McClannahan, & Poulson, 2008; Krantz & McClannahan, 1993; Sarokoff, Taylor, & Poulson, 2001; Stevenson, Krantz, & McClannahan, 2000) and play activities (Gantz, Kaylor, Bourgeois, & Hadden, 2008; Ganz et al., 2012; Garcia-Albea, Reeve, Brothers, & Reeve, 2014; Groskreutz, Peters, Groskreutz, & Higbee, 2015; Ledbetter-Cho et al., 2015; Reagon & Higbee, 2009; Wichnick, Vener, Keating, & Poulson, 2010a). Argott, Townsend, Sturmey, and Poulson (2008) used scripts and script fading to teach children to make empathetic statements, and Wichnick, Vener, Pyrtek, and Poulson (2010b) focused on teaching responses to peer initiations. Another common use of scripts is to teach manding behavior. A mand is defined as a verbal response that is under the control of the relevant establishing operation and reinforced by a specific, relevant consequence (Skinner, 1957). Specifically, researchers have also investigated the use of scripts and fading to teach manding for food (Betz, Higbee, Kelley, Sellers, & Pollard, 2011; Brodhead, Higbee, Gerencser, & Akers, 2016; Sellers, Kelley, Higbee, & Wolfe, 2016), manding for social attention (Krantz & McClannahan, 1998; MacDuff, Ledo, McClannahan, & Krantz, 2007; Pollard, Betz, & Higbee, 2012), and manding for help (Dotto-Fojut, Reeve, Townsend, & Progar, 2011).

In a recent literature review, Akers, Pyle, Higbee, Pyle, and Gerencser (2015) synthesized the results of 16 studies that evaluated the effects of social scripts and fading procedures with individuals with autism ranging in age from 2 through 15 years old. Based on the criteria set forth by the What Works Clearinghouse (2008), the authors concluded that social scripts and fading is an empirically supported treatment (Akers et al., 2015). In addition, the authors applied standards for determining if social scripts and fading is an evidence-based practice (Wong et al., 2015) and determined that social scripts and fading meets the criteria to be considered as such (Akers et al., 2015). Higbee and Brodhead (2016) generally described social script and fading research and provided guidelines for using the intervention in clinical programming for individuals with autism. Following the synthesis by Akers and colleagues (2015), there have been several articles published evaluating the effects of social scripts and script fading with children with autism. The following sections include a review of the research, areas for continued investigation, and, finally, implications for using social scripts and script fading in clinical practice.

15.3.1 Summary of Research

In one of the earliest studies evaluating the use of social scripts and script fading, Krantz and McClahannan (1993) focused on increasing peer interactions during scheduled art activities using text-based scripts with four preteen aged children with autism. Researchers provided an initial vocal prompt to complete the art activity and to "talk a lot." Printed scripts were used to prompt participants to initiate comments or questions to their peers about past or upcoming activities or items in the school environment. Scripts were faded from end to beginning by removing words, until only the quotation marks remained. All participants acquired the scripted responses and increased unscripted responses. In addition, increased peer interactions generalized to a novel teacher, setting, and materials and maintained at 2-month post-intervention checks.

Following the study by Krantz and McClahannan (1993), researchers have continued to evaluate the effects of scripts and script fading on increasing children with autisms' ability to initiate social language in the form of comments and questions. Stevenson, Krantz, and McClannahan (2000) embedded auditory scripts (specifically, language master cards) into photographic activity schedules in the classroom with four children with autism, ages 10–15 years, to teach initiating comments and questions to an adult communication partner. The scripts focused on topics such as favorite snacks and games. Participants were physically prompted to place the scripts into the language master machine, following which they repeated the social script that they heard. Scripts were faded by systematically removing the recorded language from the end to the beginning and then fading the physical stimuli (language master machine and then the cards). All four participants mastered the scripts and increased scripted and unscripted interactions.

Ganz, Kaylor, Bourgeois, and Hadden (2008) used text-based scripts with three children with autism, ages 7–12 years, in a private school for children with autism to increase initiating comments to peers during preferred leisure activities. The participants mastered the scripts, but responding decreased for two during fading and ceased for all when the scripts were removed. Argott, Townsend, Sturmey, and Poulson (2008) implemented text-based scripts (with the addition of an auditory script for one participant) and fading to teach empathetic statements and questions to instructors with three adolescents in a private school for students with autism. Instructors presented a combination of gestures (e.g., yawning, rubbing eyes, clapping) and facial expressions (e.g., smiling, squinting eyes, grimacing) in the presence of related scripts, and participants were taught to ask an empathetic question (e.g., "Are you ok?") or make an empathetic statement (e.g., "You look tired."). Scripts were faded out completely for all participants. Participants increased scripted and unscripted statements, generalized to untrained social cues and an untrained instructor, and maintained responding at a 6-week follow-up. Wichnick et al. (2010a) evaluated the effects of auditory scripts and fading on peer initiations with three young children within a private day program and school for children with autism within a structured play context. All participants acquired the scripted responses, reached the terminal fading step, and increased not only the use of unscripted language but also novel responses. These results generalized to untrained toy sets but only following complete fading of the script material from the training toy sets.

Groskreutz et al. (2015) implemented text-based scripts and fading with three participants with autism in a public preschool classroom to increase play-based commenting with an adult. All participants engaged in the targeted commenting following complete fading of the script material, increased use of novel commenting, and generalized responding to untrained play activities and materials. In another study, researchers taught four boys, attending a private school for children with autism, to initiate conversations during play activities (Garcia-Albea et al., 2014). Specifically, the researchers successfully used auditory scripts and fading, paired with multiple exemplar training (i.e., a wide range of training stimuli), to increase initiating conversations and to produce responding with untrained stimuli for all participants.

In addition to using social scripts and fading to teach social initiations, researchers have used social scripts to teach children with autism to respond to bids for social interactions. Wichnick et al. (2010b) explored using audio scripts and fading to teach three young children with autism to respond to their peers' comments or questions during a structured play activity. The study was conducted at a private school for individuals with autism and targeted response statements such as "That's cool!" Following acquisition, the scripts were systematically faded, and all participants increased the use of unscripted responses, as well as novel responses. Generalization and maintenance were not assessed.

Ledbetter-Cho et al. (2015) focused on increasing peer-to-peer initiations and responses using text-based scripts in a play context with three young children at a university-based autism clinic. All participants mastered the scripts and increased scripted, unscripted, and novel initiations and responses with peers. The data were aggregated across initiations and responses, so it is not possible to know the effects on the individual social communication types. Results generalized to untrained toys, setting, and peers and maintained at follow-up.

Another type of social interaction is manding for things such as food, attention, help, and information. Betz et al. (2011) used auditory scripts to train three young children with autism to mand for snack items from an instructor using several different mand frames (i.e., scripted language requiring the child to insert the desired item, such as "May I please have________?"). An interesting component of that study was that the researchers included a small colored sticker on the auditory script device that was then shifted to the placemat, in an attempt to facilitate transfer of stimulus control. All participants acquired the mand frames and increased scripted, unscripted, and novel mand frames. In addition, the results generalized to a more typical snack setting and maintained at follow-up. Two other studies (Brodhead et al., 2016; Sellers et al., 2016) successfully used text-based scripts to teach several mand frames during a structured snack activity to young children in a university-based autism preschool.

Social scripts and fading have also been successfully applied to teaching children with autism to mand for attention from adults. Krantz and McClannahan (1998) embedded textual scripts into an activity schedule to teach three children to make bids for attention (e.g., "Look!" and "Watch me.") from instructors. All three participants increased the use of the scripted mands for attention, as well as unscripted mands. These results generalized to untrained communication partners and untrained activity schedule tasks. In a later study, MacDuff et al. (2007) used auditory scripts, fading, and items placed in unexpected locations (e.g., a toy on the wall of a hallway) to teach bids for joint attention to adults in an autism clinic setting. All participants increased mands for joint attention (i.e., pointing, making eye contact, and stating "See?"), and responding generalized to untrained environments and maintained at follow-up. In an extension of that study, Pollard et al. (2012) used similar procedures with text-based scripts to successfully increase mands for joint attention (e.g., "Look, it's a ________.")

with three young children with autism at a university-based preschool. Results generalized to an untrained conversation partner, stimuli, and a new environment and maintained at follow-up.

Researchers have also applied scripts and fading to teach adolescents with autism to mand for assistance from an adult during a vocational task (Dotto-Fojut et al., 2011). Specifically, the researchers trained the participants to approach an adult when they encountered a problem during a vocational task in the classroom. The researchers implemented text-based scripts to teach the participants to indicate the problem (e.g., some item was broken or missing) and to mand for assistance in the form of a question (e.g., asking if there was more of an item). All participants acquired the targeted language, and results generalized to untrained work materials and maintained at follow-up.

While most of the research on scripts and fading have used researchers or instructors as the implementers, at least two studies have specifically evaluated the effects of the procedures when implemented by other individuals, such as parents and peers. Reagon and Higbee (2009) implemented auditory scripts to increase play-based comments with three young children with autism in the home setting. An important component of this study was that parents were taught to implement the prompting and fading procedures. All participants increased the use of play statements following script fading, maintained similar levels at a 2-week follow-up, and increased play statements with untrained play materials. The blank audio device remained in place for two participants. Ganz et al. (2012) evaluated the use of typical peers as implementers. The researchers used text-based scripts to increase peer-to-peer questions, praise statements, and requests for help with a middle-school student with autism during a craft activity in her public school classroom. The training peer was provided with presession coaching on how to implement the procedures. Participant responding increased over baseline with the training peer. Responding remained slightly above baseline with the training peer, but did not generalize to a peer who was not associated with the script training and fading.

The majority of studies using scripts present the scripts in the context of an activity in conjunction with, but separate from, the relevant items in the activity. However, researchers in two studies (i.e., Brown et al., 2008; Sarokoff et al., 2001) investigated the effects of strategically incorporating the scripts into the packaging of the relevant stimuli in an attempt to facilitate stimulus control and script fading. Sarokoff et al. (2001) implemented text-based social scripts and fading with two children with autism, ages 8 and 9 years, in the context of having a snack and playing video games in the classroom. The physical scripts were embedded onto the relevant physical stimuli (i.e., placed on the video game case). Scripts were fully faded for both participants, and both increased the use of scripted and unscripted responses. Results generalized to untrained stimuli and peers and maintained at 1- and 3-month probes. Similarly, Brown et al. (2008) embedded text scripts into the relevant stimuli (i.e., snack items, video cases, and sports equipment) in a mock store to increase peer conversations in the context of a shopping activity with three students with autism, ages 7–14 years. The scripts were fully faded for all participants. Scripted and unscripted responses increased for all participants and the results generalized into community stores.

15.3.2 Implication for Researchers

There are several specific areas that researchers might consider to continue to investigate the effects of using scripts and script fading to increase social communication skills of individuals with autism. The vast majority of the studies focusing on scripts and script fading have been conducted with young children and adolescents. Implementing scripts and script fading with adults with autism may require specific considerations (e.g., a lengthy learning history, possible stigmatizing effects of script materials); therefore, replicating and expanding research to an older participant population is warranted. Because the purpose of social scripts and the fading thereof is to increase the independent use of social communication, researchers should continue to investigate methods to ensure that the language will be functional for the individuals in natural settings, such as family members in homes, sales clerks and servers in community contexts (e.g., stores, parks, doctors' offices), teachers and peers in schools, and coworkers and bosses in vocational settings. More research is needed demonstrating that effects generalize to natural change agents and that this technology is effective when implemented by para-educators, peers, parents, siblings, and job coaches. Finally, given that the increases in social communication fail to sustain once the script materials are completely removed for some individuals, it is important that researchers continue to investigate effective methods to ensure transfer of stimulus control to stimuli present in the natural relevant context.

15.3.3 Implications for Clinical Application

There are several resources that clinicians can turn to when designing clinical programming using social scripts and fading. Optimally, practitioners can access empirical articles, many of which describe the procedures in technological detail that can then be used to design a clinical protocol. Clinicians can refer to the book *Teaching Conversation to Children with Autism: Scripts and Script Fading* (McClahannan & Krantz, 2005), written by two researchers and experts on this topic. The book describes types of scripts, prerequisites to consider, getting ready to teach using scripts and script fading, strategies for effective teaching, and how to collect data. The authors also include sections for strategies specific to learner characteristics, such as non-readers, beginning readers, and accomplished readers. The book includes an appendix section with resources for practitioners, including progress report templates and data sheets. Readers are also referred to the Akers et al. (2016) synthesis article and the Higbee and Brodhead (2016) article, as both provide practitioner recommendations, based on the reviewed research. Specific considerations for clinicians when planning to implement scripts and script fading with individuals with autism are outlined below.

Before getting started, there are several things to consider aimed at increasing the likelihood that the script intervention will be successful. Clinicians need to critically evaluate the learner, the available technology (e.g., auditory versus text scripts), the type of social language targeted for increase, and the natural context in which the social language should ultimately occur. Preplanning the intervention with careful consideration of these variables will allow educators to implement procedures systematically and evaluate the decision steps if optimal results are not obtained.

One of the first decisions to make is what type of script to implement: auditory or text based. It is best to make the choice based on the critical features of each technology and the current skills of the individual. This may be an obvious consideration, but auditory scripts require that the learner's hearing is sufficient to hear the prerecorded message. Auditory scripts require the learner to have a fairly developed echoic repertoire, as the learner is required to listen to and repeat the prerecorded message. The learner must also possess the fine motor skills to activate the device, which typically involves pressing a small button. It is possible that clinicians could use devices that mitigate the need for fine motor skills such as large, flat switches that are easy to activate. Features of the device could be enhanced to increase discrimination, such as using a marker or sticker to make the activation button a bright color. Learners may initially need some level of physical prompting to activate the device, so individuals who find physical prompting aversive may require a different script type or pre-training to tolerate the prompts. Because auditory scripts do not require visual discrimination skills, provided that the individual can find the device and activate it, auditory scripts might be appropriate for learners who have not yet mastered visual discrimination skills or who have a visual impairment. Some learners may engage in problem behavior when presented with printed materials, such as icons or text, in which case, auditory scripts might be a viable solution.

Text-based scripts do not require that the individual be able to read. Instead, the printed words serve as discriminative stimuli to evoke a particular vocal response. Individuals who cannot read, or who do not read fluently, will likely need pre-teaching to produce the correct vocal response in the presence of the individual words and phrases that make up the scripts. Pre-teaching can be conducted in a discrete trial format with prompt delay and fading. For text scripts to effectively control the vocal responses, the individual must be able to attend to and scan the text. Text-based scripts can be implemented without physical prompting for many individuals; therefore, text-based scripts might be an optimal technology for individuals who do not respond well to physical prompts or who have a history of becoming dependent on physical prompts.

The next consideration is the type of social communication targeted for acquisition and increase. Knowing the form of communication response will help practitioners in subsequent decisions, such as determining the specific language to be targeted, the relevant teaching context and implementers, and mastery criteria. Scripts and fading have been successfully used to teach and increase a wide variety of social language, including initiating comments and questions, responding to comments and questions, and manding for things such as attention, food, and help. Practitioners should identify social language deficits to target increasing social communication that will be meaningful to the individual and will increase independence. For example, if the individual has a strong vocal verbal repertoire and social communication skills but only asks communication partners questions about narrow topics that are interesting to the individual, scripts might be used to teach and strengthen asking a variety of social questions. Despite the clinical goal, it may be beneficial to start very young individuals with autism, or novel script users, with scripts related to manding for highly preferred items. Doing so allows the learner to contact frequent and valuable reinforcement for engaging in the scripted responses. Once the individual acquires scripts for manding for preferred items, then scripts can be used to target other social communication types, such as commenting, questioning, or more complex manding.

When deciding on the exact content of the scripts, the learner's current vocal repertoire and age should be taken into consideration. The language targeted should be developmentally appropriate for the individual, and context within it will be used. One strategy for determining appropriate language content is to observe the responses produced by the individual's peers engaging in the targeted social activity. It may be beneficial to create initial scripts that are at a level just below the individual's current level to increase the likelihood that the learner will acquire the scripts quickly and contact frequent reinforcement. Once the simpler script versions have been acquired, more complex scripts can be introduced. For example, if a learner already has the response "Wow!" and typically communicates in single-word utterances, perhaps targeting simple two-word scripts such as "Wow! Cool." would be an appropriate place to start. Once the two-word scripts are mastered, more complex scripts such as "Wow! That's cool." and then "Wow! That's super cool, dude!" could be introduced. On the other hand, if a learner typically speaks in complete sentences, clinicians might start with complex scripts.

With the script type, social language category, and specific script language selected, the next consideration is the teaching context. This includes not only the physical setting, but other important elements, such as the materials, the social activity/context, and the implementers. It may be best for practitioners to take a backward approach here, first considering the terminal context in which that language is intended for functional use and working back from there if necessary. It may be the case that doing so results in the decision to teach the scripts in the natural context versus in a more controlled context. For example, consider a middle-school student who communicates in complete sentences, has difficulty navigating social situations that require problem-solving and question asking, and does not engage in problem behavior. Specifically, when his favorite lunch option is not readily available in the lunchroom, instead of asking if there is more of the particular item in the kitchen or for alternative choices, he simply goes without lunch. In this case, it may be possible to implement the scripts in the relevant context (i.e., the lunchroom when his favorite items are not available), as opposed to teaching them in an instructional setting and working toward generalization. On the other hand, some individuals may require initial teaching in a more structured setting with limited distractions. If not teaching in the natural context, it is important to approximate the natural setting in order to promote generalization. It is worth noting that it may take several steps to get from a very structured, distraction-free setting to a more natural context by systematically adding in more relevant features of the terminal environment.

Clinicians should carefully consider and plan the activities, materials, and implementers used to teach the relevant social scripts. Because the goal of social scripts and fading is to increase independent social communication in a specific context, it is important to ensure that the relevant features of that context are established as discriminative stimuli and any necessary relevant motivating operations are in place. Again, planning from the ultimate goal backward can facilitate a more streamlined approach to outlining the steps. If the goal is to increase social commenting to same-age peers during free play, it may be best to teach within the context of that activity, with the peers, and the materials common to that activity. If that is not possible, knowing the goal allows practitioners to plan successive approximations to get to the terminal goal (e.g., structured play with adults → structured play with peers → unstructured play with adults and peers → unstructured play with peers). It may be the case that some educators do not have access to the relevant environment or natural change agents. However, if the terminal goal is known, the practitioner can work to approximate the conditions under which the scripted language is intended to be used and create a plan for those with access to the relevant environment to follow. For example, if the goal is to have an individual engage in social communication with a server at a favorite restaurant, an educator in a school setting might create a mock restaurant in the classroom to teach and practice the skill. Following mastery, the educator might have novel adults from the school (e.g., unfamiliar teachers, paraprofessionals, or administrative staff) act as the server. The educator can then train the parents to implement the procedure at the target restaurant.

When the practitioner has made all of the preparatory considerations, it is time to think about the specifics of how to teach and fade the scripts. The most common strategy for teaching scripts employs a time delay, to allow for independent responses to emerge and contact reinforcement, most-to-least vocal or physical prompting, and reinforcement for correct responses. At least two studies embedded scripts onto the relevant materials to promote transfer of stimulus control from the script materials to the items present in the context (i.e., Brown et al., 2008; Sarokoff et al., 2001), and another used colored stickers to aid in transferring control from the auditory script buttons to a placement in the context of snack (i.e., Betz et al. 2011). Therefore, practitioners might consider incorporating the labels of relevant items, or pairing the scripts directly with the relevant materials, as a bridge to transferring stimulus control.

Auditory and text-based scripts can essentially be faded in the same manner, by removing text or language from the end of the script. For text-based scripts, fading typically involves physically cutting off the end of the scripts, either word by word or based on a percentage of the script. Auditory script fading requires that the script be rerecorded, omitting language from the end of the script. For example, in either case, the script "Will you play with me please?" would be faded to "Will you play with me," "Will you play with," "Will you play," and so forth. Practitioners should set mastery criteria, based on relevant learner information, for initiating the fading steps (e.g., independent responding on 80% of opportunities across two sessions). This will ensure that progress toward independent response production can be monitored. Fading too quickly may result in increased errors, less contact with reinforcement, increased prompting, and moving back steps which prolongs the training time. Practitioners could also "probe ahead" by periodically testing out more advanced fading steps and, if the student responds correctly, skipping the unnecessary steps.

Data collection is critical to determine progress toward the terminal goal and to move forward with prompt and script fading. To demonstrate that social scripts are effective at increasing the targeted social language, it is important to collect baseline data before introducing script training. That is, educators may elect to collect data on frequency (or percent of opportunity if the response requires a specific discriminative stimulus for it to occur, as with responding to a greeting or answering a question) of the targeted response over several days to demonstrate the individual's current performance level. During script training, data can be recorded on prompts used, independent responses using the scripted language, and the fading steps. Clinicians should also consider tracking responses that are contextually appropriate, but were not expressly taught. For example, a student may begin to modify some of the language of a script, combine two or more scripts, or emit novel responses (i.e., language not expressly taught). Following script training and fading, data should continue to be collected to demonstrate that effects sustain outside of the training context and over an appropriate period of time. If training did not occur in the natural context, data should be taken in the presence of the relevant variables. For example, if the scripts were trained in the classroom but are relevant to the playground, data should be collected during playground activities to demonstrate that the desired effects were obtained in the relevant natural context.

15.4 Combining Social Scripts and Photographic Activity Schedules to Promote Complex Social Play

In previous sections of this chapter, we have described how photographic activity schedules and social scripting/script fading can be used to promote independence and spontaneous language use by individuals with autism. In this final section, we will describe how these two techniques can be combined to promote complex social play. The most basic manner in which activity schedules and social scripting/script fading can be combined is to simply add scripts to an individual activity schedule to cue a social initiation or exchange. Recently, however, researchers have begun to investigate more complex strategies for promoting interaction among children with autism and their peers using these techniques.

15.4.1 Brief Summary of Research

Betz, Higbee, and Reagon (2008) investigated the use of a "joint" activity schedule to promote interactive game play between three pairs of preschoolers with autism. All participants had previously learned to follow independent activity schedules. The authors created a schedule that cued participants to play a series of closed-ended preschool games that involved turn taking (e.g., Crocodile Dentist™, Kerplunk™, etc.). At the top of each activity schedule page was a picture of one of the two children, indicating who was responsible for obtaining and returning the materials, as well as who would choose the game if it was a choice page. Type-written scripts were also included on the activity schedule page so that participants could initiate play with simple statements such as "Play with me." The schedule was composed of two pages of pre-chosen activities and two pages where the responsible child could select a game from a choice board. Standard graduated guidance procedures (McClannahan & Krantz, 2010) were followed to teach participants to follow the schedule. Results indicated that the joint activity schedules significantly increased levels of joint engagement between participants, defined as both participants playing the game together or completing a component of the schedule appropriately, as well as the total number of games played during a session. Participants' engagement maintained at high levels when activities were re-sequenced and when new games were introduced. When researchers removed the activity schedule for one participant pair, responding returned to baseline levels, indicating that the activity schedule was controlling the participants' behavior.

Brodhead, Higbee, Pollard, Akers, and Gerencser (2014) extended the work of Betz et al., (2008) by investigating the use of activity schedules and social scripts to teach three pairs of young children with autism to play hide-and-seek. Because the game of hide-and-seek requires participants to play different roles, namely, the "hider" and the "seeker," the authors used two separate schedule books instead of the single book used by Betz and colleagues. The books were sequenced so that when one child was on a "hider" page, the other was on a "seeker" page. There were two types of "hider" pages. On a fixed location page, there was a picture of a location within the participants' classroom that represented where the child should hide as well as a typewriting script that said "Oh, no!" that the child was taught to tear off and stick to a Velcro watch band that each child wore while playing. In this way, the child could take the script with them to the hiding location and follow it when they were found by the seeker. Choice pages were identical to fixed location pages except that there were pictures of two potential locations to hide on the left-facing page and the hider could select a hiding location by moving one of the pictures to the right page and then proceeding as normal. Seeker pages contained the type-written script, "Go hide." followed by the numbers 1–20 with a circle around each number that the participant could use to cue him/herself to count to 20. The seeker page also contained a movable script that said, "I found you." that could be attached to the Velcro watch band and taken while looking for the other participant. Finally, there was a detachable piece of cardstock with two pictures of potential hiding locations attached that the participant could take out of the book and use to prompt him/herself where to look for the other participant. During a given session, participants each had two turns to play the role of hider and two turns to play the role of seeker. The final page of the book contained the script "Thanks for playing" for both participants. Participants were pre-taught the various hiding locations used in the study, and researchers verified that each participant could go to each hiding location when shown the picture before the study began. Participants were also pre-taught the type-written words used in the scripts.

During baseline, none of the participants engaged in any of the hiding or seeking behaviors. When the linked activity schedules were introduced and the students were taught to follow them using typical activity schedule training procedures, physical prompting with graduated guidance, all three pairs of participants rapidly learned to play the game with high levels of accuracy and independence. They continued to play accurately when the order of who was playing what role changed as well as when novel locations were introduced. While the authors were able to fade many of the scripts used in the study, when they removed the schedule completely, all participants stopped playing, and their response patterns returned to what they had been during baseline sessions. No systematic attempts were made to fade the schedule.

In a third study in this research line, by Akers et al. (in press), the authors sought to build upon the work of Brodhead et al. (2014) by using activity schedules to teach young children with ASD to play hide-and-seek with three typically developing peers. Aside from expanding the number of children involved, Akers et al. also investigated whether or not the activity schedule could be systematically faded once the children learned to follow it.

In Akers et al.' (in press) study, three preschool-aged children with ASD along with a group of typically developing preschoolers were taught to play hide-and-seek using activity schedules that included type-written social scripts. As with Brodhead et al. (2014), there were two schedules used in the study. The "hider schedule" was composed of a single page that had seven pictures of potential hiding locations along with a type-written script underneath each picture. Participants who were hiding were taught to choose any of the pictures, tear it off the page, then go to the location specified on the picture, and stay there until they were found by the seeker. Once found by the seeker, they would follow the predetermined script for that session. Three different scripts were taught, and these scripts were rotated across sessions in an attempt to promote varied responding on the part of the children. The "seeker schedule" included a picture of one of the children, to indicate whose turn it was to play the seeker role, followed by type-written scripts that stated "My turn" and "Go hide" to signal to the other participants that they should select a picture from the hider binder and go to their respective hiding locations. Below the scripts were a set of numbers with circles around them that the students could touch to prompt themselves to count to 20. The last feature of the page was the script "Ready or not, here I come!" that the seeker stated to cue the other children that seeking would begin. On the left-facing page of the binder was a strip of cardboard that had pictures of all of the potential hiding places on the right side and pictures of each of the children who would be hiding on the left side along with four frowny-face icons. The seeker was taught to go to the first location and check to see if a child was hiding there. If there was a child, the seeker moved his/her picture to the right side of the strip covering that location and stated the script that was written below the picture. Three scripts were rotated across sessions to promote variable responding on the part of the seeker. If no child was found in the hiding location, the seeker was taught to move one of the frowny-face icons to the right side of the strip on top of the location to indicate that the location had been searched but no child found. The seeker proceeded to the next location and repeated the process until all three children were found. Everyone then returned to the schedule books, the hiders replaced the location pictures in the hider binder, and the seeker turned the page to see whose turn would be next. This process continued until all four children had a turn to be the seeker.

Standard physical prompting and graduated guidance procedures were used with all children, including the typically developing peers, to teach them how to follow the schedule to play hide-and-seek together. All children learned to follow the schedules to play hide-and-seek in 14 sessions or less. During a no-schedule probe session, participants' responding returned to near baseline levels for two participants and decreased slightly for the third participant. Based on this result, the systematic fading of the schedule began. The authors systematically removed portions of the hider and seeker binders across multiple sessions based on student responding (see Akers et al., in press, for a detailed description of the fading steps and procedures). For two of the three participants, the experimenters were able to remove all visual supports, including scripts, except a single page that indicated the order that the children would play the role of the seeker. The third participant continued to require the use of the circles with numbers in them to count all the way to 20 plus a modified seeker strip that only contained pictures of the three children who were hiding as he would not consistently seek out all three children when the seeker strip was removed. With these reduced supports in place, all three children were able to play hide-and-seek in a novel environment and in a 2-week follow-up session.

15.4.2 Implications for Researchers

Researchers have shown that activity schedules with embedded social scripts can be used to teach complex sequences of behavior including social games such as hide-and-seek and that, at least in some cases, these visual supports can be completely faded or reduced. The full potential of visual support systems such as activity schedules remains to be determined, however, and researchers should continue to explore how these visual supports can be used to promote complex social behavior. Given that relatively little is known about the fading of activity schedules, as researchers develop more complex activity schedules, they should also explore ways that these schedules can be faded when appropriate. Additionally, according to the research literature, all of the participants in the complex activity schedule studies reviewed here were already fluent followers of individual activity schedules before they were taught to follow the more complex schedules. Researchers may wish to explore whether or not the ability to follow an individual schedule is a necessary prerequisite skill set in order to follow more complex schedules. Researchers may also wish to compare the use of activity schedules and social scripting to other evidence-based training procedures, such as video modeling, to see which procedures are more effective and efficient for teaching a given set of skills.

15.4.3 Implications for Practitioners

This recent line of research on the use of activity schedules and social scripting/script fading to promote complex social behavior with young children suggests that these techniques might be useful tools for the behavior analytic practitioner who is teaching clients to engage in complex social play. Given that all of the participants in the studies described in this section were fluent independent activity schedule followers before being taught to follow more complex schedules, practitioners, until research informs otherwise, should ensure that their learners master basic activity schedules and scripts before attempting to use complex schedules like those described here. It is interesting to note that the teaching procedures used in these complex activity schedule studies were the same procedures that are typically used to teach basic activity schedule following: physical prompting and graduated guidance. Thus, while visual support systems designed to promote more complex behavior may need to be more complex, the general teaching procedures used to promote more simple sequences of behavior appear to be sufficient to teach complex behavior as well.

15.5 Summary

As described both within this chapter and the other chapters in this book, behavioral researchers have developed many effective techniques for helping individuals with ASD learn to more effectively participate in the social world. The two techniques described in this chapter, photographic activity schedules and social scripting/script fading, are flexible and effective tools that practitioners can use to help individuals with autism learn to independently complete complex, multistep tasks and communicate effectively in social situations. Both strategies take advantage of strengths displayed by many individuals with ASD to facilitate additional learning and community participation. While much research has already been conducted on these specific techniques, used individually or together, more work needs to be done to determine new skills and environments in which these intervention tools can be effectively used.

References

Akers, J. S., Higbee, T. S., Gerencser, K. R., & Pellegrino, A. J. (in press). An evaluation of group activity schedules to promote social play in children with autism. *Journal of Applied Behavior Analysis*. (2017) 50(3): 567–581

Akers, J. S., Higbee, T. S., Pollard, J. S., Pellegrino, A. J., & Gerencser, K. R. (2016). An evaluation of photographic activity schedules to increase independent playground skills in young children with autism. *Journal of Applied Behavior Analysis, 49*, 1–6.

Akers, J. S., Pyle, N., Higbee, T. S., Pyle, D., & Gerencser, K. R. (2015). A synthesis of script fading effects with individuals with autism spectrum disorder: A 20-year review. *Review Journal of Autism and Developmental Disorders, 3*(1), 1–17.

Argott, P., Townsend, D. B., Sturmey, P., & Poulson, C. L. (2008). Increasing the use of empathic statements in the presence of a non-verbal affective stimulus in adolescents with autism. *Research in Autism Spectrum Disorders, 2*(2), 341–352.

Betz, A. M., Higbee, T. S., Kelley, K. N., Sellers, T. P., & Pollard, J. S. (2011). Increasing response variability of mand frames with script training and extinction. *Journal of Applied Behavior Analysis, 44*(2), 357–362.

Betz, A., Higbee, T. S., & Reagon, K. A. (2008). Using joint activity schedules to promote peer play in preschoolers with autism. *Journal of Applied Behavior Analysis, 41*, 237–241.

Brodhead, M. T., Higbee, T. S., Gerencser, K. R., & Akers, J. S. (2016). The use of a discrimination-training procedure to teach mand variability to children with autism. *Journal of Applied Behavior Analysis, 49*(1), 34–48.

Brodhead, M. T., Higbee, T. S., Pollard, J. S., Akers, J. S., & Gerencser, K. R. (2014). The use of linked activity schedules to teach children with autism to play hide-and-seek. *Journal of Applied Behavior Analysis, 47*(3), 645–650.

Brown, J. L., Krantz, P. J., McClannahan, L. E., & Poulson, C. L. (2008). Using script fading to promote natural environment stimulus control of verbal interactions among youths with autism. *Research in Autism Spectrum Disorders, 2*(3), 480–497.

Bryan, L. C., & Gast, D. L. (2000). Teaching on-task and on-schedule behaviors to high-functioning children with autism via picture activity schedules. *Journal of Autism and Developmental Disorders, 30*, 553–567.

Dotto-Fojut, K. M., Reeve, K. F., Townsend, D. B., & Progar, P. R. (2011). Teaching adolescents with autism to describe a problem and request assistance during simulated vocational tasks. *Research in Autism Spectrum Disorders, 5*(2), 826–833.

Ganz, J. B., Kaylor, M., Bourgeois, B., & Hadden, K. (2008). The impact of social script and visual cues on verbal communication in three children with autism spectrum disorders. *Focus on Autism and Other Developmental Disabilities, 23*(2), 79–94.

Ganz, J. B., Heath, A. K., Lund, E. M., Camargo, S. P., Rispoli, M. J., Boles, M., & Plaisance, L. (2012).

Effects of peer-mediated implementation of visual scripts in middle school. *Behavior Modification, 36*(3), 378–398.

Garcia-Albea, E., Reeve, S. A., Brothers, K. J., & Reeve, K. F. (2014). Using audio script fading and multiple-exemplar training to increase vocal interactions in children with autism. *Journal of Applied Behavior Analysis, 47*(2), 325–343.

Gerencser, K. R., Higbee, T. S., Akers, J. S., & Contreras, B. P. (2017). An evaluation of interactive computerized training to teach parents to implement a photographic activity schedule. *Journal of Applied Behavior Analysis, 50*(3), 567–581.

Groskreutz, M. P., Peters, A., Groskreutz, N. C., & Higbee, T. S. (2015). Increasing play-based commenting in children with autism spectrum disorder using a novel script-frame procedure. *Journal of Applied Behavior Analysis, 48*(2), 442–447.

Higbee, T., & Brodhead, M. (2016). Promoting independence, verbal behavior and social skills in individuals with autism through activity schedules and script fading. *International Journal of Behavior Analysis & Autism Spectrum Disorders, 1*(2), 1–8.

Krantz, P. J., & McClannahan, L. E. (1993). Teaching children with autism to initiate to peers: Effects of a script-fading procedure. *Journal of Applied Behavior Analysis, 26*(1), 121–132.

Krantz, P. J., & McClannahan, L. E. (1998). Social interaction skills for children with autism: A script-fading procedure for beginning readers. *Journal of Applied Behavior Analysis, 31*(2), 191–202.

Ledbetter-Cho, K., Lang, R., Davenport, K., Moore, M., Lee, A., Howell, A., … O'Reilly, M. (2015). Effects of script training on the peer-to-peer communication of children with autism spectrum disorder. *Journal of Applied Behavior Analysis, 48*(4), 785–799.

MacDuff, J. L., Krantz, P. J., & McClannahan, L. E. (1993). Teaching children with autism to use photographic activity schedules: Maintenance and generalization of complex response chains. *Journal of Applied Behavior Analysis, 26*, 89–97.

MacDuff, J. L., Ledo, R., McClannahan, L. E., & Krantz, P. J. (2007). Using scripts and script fading procedures to promote bids for joint attention by young children with autism. *Research in Autism Spectrum Disorders, 1*(4), 281–290.

McClannahan, L., & Krantz, P. (2010). *Activity schedules for children with autism, second edition: Teaching independent behavior*. Bethesada, MD: Woodbine House.

McClannahan, L. E., & Krantz, P. J. (2005). *Teaching conversation to children with autism: Scripts and script fading (topics in autism)*. Bethesda, MD: Woodbine House.

Machalicek, W., Shogren, K., Lang, R., Rispoli, M., O'Reilly, M. F., Franco, J., & Sigafoos, J. (2009). Increasing play and decreasing the challenging behavior of children with autism during recess with activity schedules and task correspondence training. *Research in Autism Spectrum Disorders, 3*(2), 547–555.

Pollard, J. S., Betz, A. M., & Higbee, T. S. (2012). Script fading to promote unscripted bids for joint attention in children with autism. *Journal of Applied Behavior Analysis, 45*(2), 387–393.

Reagon, K. A., & Higbee, T. S. (2009). Parent-implemented script fading to promote play-based verbal initiations in children with autism. *Journal of Applied Behavior Analysis, 42*(3), 659–664.

Sarokoff, R. A., Taylor, B. A., & Poulson, C. L. (2001). Teaching children with autism to engage in conversational exchanges: Script fading with embedded textual stimuli. *Journal of Applied Behavior Analysis, 34*(1), 81–84.

Sellers, T. P., Kelley, K., Higbee, T. S., & Wolfe, K. (2016). Effects of simultaneous script training on use of varied Mand frames by Preschoolers with autism. *The Analysis of Verbal Behavior, 32*(1), 15–26.

Skinner, B. F. (1957). *Verbal behavior*. New York: Appleton-Century-Crofts.

Stevenson, C. L., Krantz, P. J., & McClannahan, L. E. (2000). Social interaction skills for children with autism: A script-fading procedure for nonreaders. *Behavioral Interventions, 15*(1), 1–20.

What Works Clearing House, 2014 Clearinghouse, W. W. (2008). *WWC procedures and standards handbook*. Washington, DC: Institute of Education Sciences. Retrieved 1 Jan 2009.

Watanabe, M., & Sturmey, P. (2003). The effect of choice-making opportunities during activity schedules on task engagement of adults with autism. *Journal of Autism and Developmental Disorders, 33*, 535–538.

Wichnick, A. M., Vener, S. M., Keating, C., & Poulson, C. L. (2010a). The effect of a script fading procedure on unscripted social initiations and novel utterances among young children with autism. *Research in Autism Spectrum Disorders, 4*(1), 51–64.

Wichnick, A. M., Vener, S. M., Pyrtek, M., & Poulson, C. L. (2010b). The effect of a script fading procedure on responses to peer initiations among young children with autism. *Research in Autism Spectrum Disorders, 4*(2), 290–299.

Wong, C., Odom, S. L., Hume, K. A., Cox, A. W., Fettig, A., Kucharczyk, S., … Schultz, T. R. (2015). Evidence-based practices for children, youth, and young adults with autism spectrum disorder: A comprehensive review. *Journal of Autism and Developmental Disorders, 45*(7), 1951–1966.

16 Peer Mediation Interventions to Improve Social and Communication Skills for Children and Youth with Autism Spectrum Disorders

Debra M. Kamps, Rose Mason, and Linda Heitzman-Powell

16.1 Social and Communication Characteristics in Autism Spectrum Disorders (ASD)

Social skills deficits are a core characteristic of ASD and impact social communication development and outcomes across the life span (American Psychiatric Association, 2013; Scheeren, Koot, & Begeer, 2012). The Diagnostic and Statistical Manual (DSM-V) indicates social communication deficits as a major criteria for ASD including (1) persistent deficits in social communication and social interaction across multiple contexts; (2) deficits in nonverbal communicative behaviors used for social interaction (e.g., abnormalities in eye contact and body language or deficits in understanding and use of gestures, lack of facial expressions); and (3) deficits in developing, maintaining, and understanding relationships and making friends. Paul, Miles Orlovski, Chuba Marcinko, and Volkmar (2009) described pragmatic differences in conversational language for persons with high-functioning ASD (HFA) to include problems related to "…the amount of information provided in conversation to satisfy listener needs, the degree to which topics are managed and reciprocated, the ability to respond to partner cues and engage in reciprocal exchanges" (Paul et al., 2009, p. 120).

The following narrative is designed to present literature reviews and exemplary studies with a focus on peer training and peer mediation interventions (PMIs) to address these issues and social deficits presenting in ASD. Studies including literature reviews were identified through a search of peer-reviewed journals through EBSCO publishing: Academic Search Complete, Google Scholar, JSTOR, PsycINFO, Education Resources Information Center (ERIC), Medline, Web of Science, and WorldCat. Key search words were *autism*, *social skills*, *peers*, or *peer mediation* with selected dates from 2003 to 2016. The literature described is not inclusive of all 203 studies yielded from the search, but rather a representative sample of the findings.

D.M. Kamps (✉)
Juniper Gardens Children's Project, University of Kansas, Kansas City, KS, USA
e-mail: dkamps@ku.edu

R. Mason
Assistant Professor, Department of Educational Studies, College of Education, Purdue University, Kansas City, KS, USA

L. Heitzman-Powell
University of Kansas Medical Center, Kansas City, KS, USA

J.B. Leaf (ed.), *Handbook of Social Skills and Autism Spectrum Disorder*, Autism and Child Psychopathology Series, DOI 10.1007/978-3-319-62995-7_16

The chapter sections include (a) defining PMIs, (b) models of PMIs, (c) evidence-based practices (EBP) and exemplary studies of PMIs, (d) summary of social skills intervention reviews, (e) summary of PMI literature reviews, (f) key findings, and (g) conclusions and future research.

16.2 Defining Peer-Mediated Interventions

PMIs are considered EBP by the National Professional Development Center on ASD (http://autismpdc.fpg.unc.edu/content/ebp-update) and the National Standards Project (http://www.nationalautismcenter.org) and found to be effective in remediating social and communication deficits for children with ASD. Wong et al. (2013) defined peer-mediated instruction and intervention as:

> …used to teach typically developing peers ways to interact with and help learners with ASD acquire new behaviors, communication, and social skills by increasing social opportunities within natural environments…peers are systematically taught ways of engaging learners with ASD in social interactions in both teacher-directed and learner-initiated activities. (p. 70)

The goals of PMIs are to increase social competence as a foundation for forming relationships. Guralnick (1990) defined social competence as the ability to successfully and appropriately select and carry out interpersonal goals. Stichter and Conroy (2006) defined peer-related social competence as the ability to engage in reciprocal interactions and form relationships with peers (as reported in Whalon, Conroy, Martinez, & Werch, 2015). Tager-Flusberg, Paul, and Lord (2005) suggest that communication programs typically have a social component given the social nature of communication (as cited in Reichow & Volkmar, 2010). PMI, thus, seems a logical and appropriate choice to build social competence and communication for children and youth with ASD. Recent reviews have summarized empirical evidence of PMIs (e.g., Wang, Parrila, & Cui, 2012) and social skill interventions (e.g., Reichow & Volkmar, 2010); thus, our understanding of the effectiveness of different models has greatly increased.

16.3 General Models of Peer-Mediated Interventions

DiSalvo and Oswald (2002) described three basic intervention approaches for PMI to increase social behaviors of children with ASD: (1) manipulation of the situation or contingencies to promote interaction, (2) peer instruction in initiation and social interaction strategies to promote interactions, and (3) target child instruction in initiation strategies, with a fourth option of a combination of approaches. The authors reported on various structures to support interaction including arrangements that structure the environment/contingencies and instruction for children and peers to include (a) integrated play groups (Wolfberg & Schuler, 1999); (b) peer buddy, peer tutoring, and peer network approaches (Haring & Breen, 1992; Garrison-Harrell, Kamps, & Kravitz, 1997; Kamps, Barbetta, Leonard, & Delquadri, 1994, Kamps, Dugan, Potucek, & Collins, 1999; Laushey & Heflin, 2000); (c) pivotal response training (PRT; Pierce & Schreibman, 1995, 1997) and peer initiation training (Goldstein, Kaczmarek, Pennington, & Shafer, 1992; Sainato, Goldstein, & Strain, 1992); (d) target child initiation training (Zanolli, Daggett, & Adams, 1996); and (e) group-oriented contingencies (Kohler et al., 1995; Odom & Strain, 1986). These models of PMI established early on have continued to be reported across numerous studies as effective for increasing social communication skills for participants with ASD.

Sperry, Neitzel, and Engelhardt-Wells (2010) recently prescribed a model for using PMIs based on behaviorism and social learning theory. Steps of this model include (1) selecting four to five peers that exhibit good social and communication skills, are well liked by peers, and have a positive social interaction history with the child with ASD, (2) training and supporting peers in understanding similarities and differences of children with ASD including specific children with whom they will be engaged, (3) training peers in specific strategies (e.g., playing behaviors, providing assistance, keeping interactions going, engaging in conversations) with direct instruction and practice to learn strategies, (4) implementing structured teaching sessions with the peers and the participants with ASD with prompting and feedback from the teacher/provider, (5) implementing PMI in naturalistic classroom and school settings (i.e., arranging schedules to include peer-mediated learning activities, having materials and visual cues available, identifying responsible staff, planning for prompting and reinforcement), and (6) extending initiations and opportunities across the day. These steps outlined in the model from Sperry and colleagues incorporate EBP from three decades of PMI research.

16.4 Evidence-Based Practices and Strategies Used in Peer-Mediated Intervention

Wong et al. (2013) recently published a synthesis of EBP for children and youth with ASD. From their review of literature published between 1990 and 2011, 27 practices were reported as providing sufficient evidence to be considered best practice. PMIs and social skills interventions were included. Interestingly, of those 27 practices, 9 other practices are routinely used as part of PMI strategies: modeling, naturalistic intervention, prompting, reinforcement, scripting, self-management, social narratives, structured play groups, and task analysis (see list of practices and definitions in the Wong report).

16.4.1 EBP and Strategies Used in PMI

The majority of studies on PMIs have included training peers, sometimes participants with ASD independently or concurrently, and teachers and interventionists to prompt specific skills or competencies in order to increase social and communication skills. The most effective approaches have used *behavioral techniques* such as positive reinforcement, modeling, shaping, fading, redirection, prompting, and extinction to teach peers and participants with ASD (Corbett et al., 2014, as cited in Chang & Locke, 2016; Camargo et al., 2014). Specific skill categories taught using PMIs have included (1) *social skills instruction* to increase knowledge of the rules of social engagement and interactions (Garfinkle & Schwartz, 2002; Laushey & Heflin, 2000; Licciardello, Harchik, & Luiselli, 2008; White, Koenig, & Scahill, 2010; Wood, Fujii, Renno, & Van Dyke, 2014); (2) teaching specific *social communication strategies* such as instructing peers and participants with ASD to use requests and share toys and games, comments about play/activities of self and others, niceties (e.g., saying please and thank you), and play organizers (e.g., joining in game rules) (Kamps et al., 2014; Odom, Chandler, Ostrosky, McConnell, & Reaney, 1992; Thiemann & Goldstein, 2004); (3) teaching communication partners and participants *joint attention* within naturally occurring activities and routines (Kasari, Freeman, & Paparella, 2006; Schertz, Odom, Baggett, & Sideris, 2013); and (4) pivotal responses targeted in *PRT* including giving clear instructions, using of child-selected stimulus materials, teaching self-initiations, interspersing maintenance items, using of natural reinforcers, and reinforcing attempts (Koegel, Koegel, Harrower, & Carter, 1999; Pierce & Schreibman, 1995). Several researchers have emphasized the importance of how and what peers are trained to do and the potential effects on outcomes. "Peer models may need more structured training to help them intentionally think about, plan, and create opportunities for social interactions to promote social initiations when they interact with children with ASD" (Chang & Locke, 2016, p. 8).

16.4.2 Settings for PMI

PMI studies generally include structured arrangements within social activities and naturally occurring social times that provide multiple opportunities for social interaction between participants with ASD and typically developing peers. These settings or social structures often include *social skills and play groups/center time* with classmates using age-appropriate toys and games (Hundert, Rowe, & Harrison, 2014; Kamps et al., 2014), *lunch groups* (Koegel, Fredeen et al., 2012), and *recess groups* (Lang et al., 2011; Mason et al., 2014), all including peer training and demonstrating positive outcomes in increasing social interaction and communicative behaviors for participants. In some studies, the activities were specifically designed and controlled to provide teaching opportunities and feedback such as pullout social groups or therapy sessions. In other studies, specific structures or routines were superimposed within the naturally occurring activity to prompt interactions with peers or arrange opportunities for peers to prompt and reinforce communication. Several studies have illustrated the generalized effects of having multiple structured activities such as organized games with rules and turn-taking procedures and peer networks for children with ASD in preschool settings (Goldstein et al., 1992; Strain & Bovey, 2011), elementary school settings (Garrison-Harrell et al., 1997; Kamps, Potucek, Gonzalez-Lopez, Kravits, & Kemmerer, 1997), and with only a few in secondary settings (Hughes et al., 2013).

16.4.3 Exemplary PMI Studies

Table 16.1 provides a description of 35 studies representing the PMI literature. The table describes participants and settings, specific strategies and contexts regarding PMI procedures, and outcomes. These studies were selected to exemplify a range of practices and strategies across the PMI literature, with an emphasis on well-defined procedures for practitioners, and based on publications over the last 10 years.

16.5 Summary of Social Skills Reviews

A number of reviews have focused on social skills interventions that included studies using peer training and PMI procedures. Seven of those reviews were selected as most relevant and are described in the following narrative. Summaries include the time period of included studies, number of studies and participants, intervention strategies, and findings.

Rao, Beidel, and Murray (2008) reviewed the literature investigating *social skills training* for children with HFA published in 2007 or earlier. Ten studies with 124 participants met the inclusion criteria of (a) 18 years or younger with ASD, (b) involving a social skills intervention that directly taught the children, and (c) use of a single-case experimental design with direct measure of the change in skills. Only three of the studies included peers for interaction or to facilitate skills (i.e., Barry et al., 2003; Bauminger, 2002; Kamps et al., 1992). Matson, Matson, and Rivet (2007) conducted a review of the *social skills treatment* literature during this same time period. The review included 79 studies and 360 participants, 20 of the studies reviewed included PMIs. The findings from both reviews described effective strategies similar to other literature reviews such as modeling and reinforcement and visual cuing and scripts (see reviews). In addition, unique procedures included *self-management* to build social behaviors and teach self-evaluation of skill use (Koegel, Koegel, Hurley, & Frea, 1992); *Social Stories*™ read by parents (Sansosti & Powell-Smith, 2006); *parent education* accompanying social skills groups (Solomon, Goodlin-Jones, & Anders, 2004); use of *community activities* to foster generalization of skills (Barnhill, Cook, Tebbenkamp, & Myles, 2002; Tse, Strulovitch, Tagalakis, Meng, & Fombonne, 2007); and use of a *curriculum teaching social cognition, emotional understanding*, and social interaction during group practice sessions with peers twice a week (Bauminger, 2002). Overall the reviewers (i.e., Matson et al., 2007; Rao et al., 2008) stated the need for more empirical evidence and clearer descriptions of intervention components. From a practical standpoint, a primary recommendation was designing social skills interventions to facilitate skill generalization outside of the treatment setting and with novel people through programmed practice in naturalistic settings with unfamiliar peers and long-term implementation

Table 16.1 Sample peer-mediated interventions: participant characteristic, procedures, and outcomes

Study authors	Participants/settings	Peer-mediated intervention description	Outcomes
Social skills groups/play groups/centers			
Boudreau and Harvey (2013)	$N = 3$ with ASD, 4–7 years old, peers in triad	*Video self-modeling of initiations to peer*, 6–9 video clips per participant, viewed just prior to playtime with peers	Increased spontaneous initiations to peers
Chung and Douglas (2015)	$N = 3$ with ASD, 10–12 years old, 2 peers each; one para, one SPED teacher, and one general education teacher each	Combined *(1) para training and peer prompting*: proximity to peers, speech-generating device (SGD) enhancement with peer/social interaction messages including greeting, requesting, and commenting and *(2) para self-monitoring* of prompts to peers, all implemented in general education classes (art and library)	Increased reciprocal peer interactions; increased use of SGD with peers in general education classes; increased initiations by students with ASD and peers; increased time in general education classes; increased proximity to peers
Hundert et al. (2014); procedures based on Laushey and Heflin (2000)	$N = 3$ preschool children with ASD with moderate ID; class-wide peers playing in dyads	Combined *(1) social scripts around themes based on child preferences*: "pirate treasure game," "calendar and weather," and grocery shopping – taught by researcher and in dyads using tokens to reinforce completion of eight steps for each play script – and *(2) peer buddies with all class members* taught to initiate (go over, look at person, ask); accept invitation (stop, look at person, say if you want to play); and maintain play with rules to "stay," "play," and "talk" to buddy	Increased in percentage of intervals of interactive play in training settings with the use of social scripts alone. Increases were not seen in the generalization setting – free play – until the peer buddies strategies were trained
Ganz and Flores (2008)	$N = 3$ with ASD, 4 years old; 1–2 peers in play group	Combined *(1) visual cues for thematic play* (ocean theme, birthday parties, farm animals); *(2) peer training* to (a) engage participant in play (get your friend's attention, talk to him, hand him a toy) and (b) play with the toys your friend is playing with (when your friend talks, you say something too); *(3) peer prompting* of participant to use scripts (hold script in front of a friend, hand over your hand to point to card, verbally model words, tell participant to say ____)	Increased in scripted phrases during play; increased in content-related comments; increased unscripted phrases for one participant; increased responses to peers for all participants but variability

(continued)

Table 16.1 (continued)

Study authors	Participants/settings	Peer-mediated intervention description	Outcomes
Gena (2006)	$N = 3$ preschool children with ASD and normal intelligence, 3–4 years old; 12 peers; free play	*Combined (1) initiation training for children with ASD* in five skills: asking questions, displaying affective behavior, giving commands, announcing information, and inviting classmates; *(2) shadow teacher prompting and social reinforcement* contingent on initiations and instruction following during play	Increased spontaneous initiations to peers during semi-structured play and free play; increased responses to peer initiations
Jung, Sainato, and Davis (2008)	$N = 3$ children with ASD 5–6 years old; 6 peers with DD but appropriate interaction skills; center time	*Peer training using high-probability social request sequences with embedded peer modeling.* Experimenter delivered requests first to the peer to model and then to the target child. Praise and gestural praise (tickles, hugs) were provided for compliance	Increased compliance for low-probability social requests following the use of high-probability requests with peer modeling; increased social interaction with trained peer and generalization peer
Kamps et al. (2014)	$N = 56$ kinder and first grade with moderate to high-functioning ASD (39 control group); 4–6 peer classmates each; 30 min small groups 3 × per week	Combined *(1) peer and child with ASD training* in social communication skills (share, request, comment about self, comment about others, niceties, turn-taking, and play organizers), *(2) prompting and reinforcement* for peer mediation and communication during play groups with two peers, and *(3) visual picture and text cues* used during training and play. School staff – delivered intervention	Increased communications (initiations and responses) during structured play groups; growth in initiations to peers during nontreatment social probes and natural settings; improved core language scores; improved teacher ratings. Both experimental and control groups improved in communication skills K to first grade
Katz and Girolametto (2013)	$N = 3$ with ASD, 4–5 years old; 2 peers each	*Participants with ASD and peers taught to use storyboards* – illustrated social skills – Let's play, my turn/your turn, do it again, asking for help; training sessions for all children; play sessions with teacher providing scaffolding of skill use; teachers taught and coached to facilitate interactions during play	Increased extended interactions (three or more turns of interactive engagement); increased ratings of social interaction skills (interacts well, takes turns, engages in extended interactions)
Koegel, Werner, Vismara, and Koegel (2005)	$N = 2$ with ASD, 8–9 years old; peers from classroom	*Play dates (home, park, beach, zoo, bowling alley) with contextual support* – adult-facilitated cooperative arrangements between the children with ASD and peers, i.e., mutually reinforcing, shared materials to complete activity	Increased reciprocal interactions; improved positive affect for participants with ASD and peers; increased invitations from peers for play dates

(continued)

Table 16.1 (continued)

Study authors	Participants/settings	Peer-mediated intervention description	Outcomes
Liber, Frea, and Symon (2008)	$N = 3$ with ASD; 6–9 years old; play areas with peers with disabilities	*(1) Training for participants with ASD to request peer play*: ten-step analysis for trains included ask peer to play, tell peer "let's play trains," give peer two pieces, tell peer "let's make a train," ask peer for train pieces, put pieces together with peer, ask peer for more pieces, move train around track, tell peer "your turn," tell peer "that was fun"; *(2) graduated time delay* to teach play sequence	Increased use of steps in play activity (correct and unprompted responses); increased play and requesting skills; anecdotal reports of increased quality of social interaction; generalization of skills to non-training setting
McGee and Daly (2007)	$N = 3$ with ASD, 4–5 years old; 4 typical peers from preschool class	*Incidental teaching using preferred toys*: phased teaching use of pivotal phrases: all right, you know what? and prompt fading	Increased use of phrases with teacher, some generalization to free play with peers, increased number of words spoken to peers
Parker and Kamps (2011)	$N = 29$ with ASD, 9 years old; 15 peers; 2–3 per session; after-school activities	*Task analysis* training for participants for games, cooking, and ordering in a restaurant; peer training to prompt TA; *peer and participant training to use social scripts* to communicate and interact during activities	Increased completion of steps in TA; increased in verbalizations directed to peers; increased activity engagement across tasks
Strain and Bovey (2011)	$N = 177$ preschoolers with ASD in intervention (117 control); peer classmates; inclusive classrooms	*LEAP (Learning Experiences and Alternative Program for Preschoolers and Parents)*: (1) full inclusion preschool class, (2) *peer training* and *peer mediation* in natural settings, (3) environmental arrangement to facilitate social opportunities, (4) *social skills and communication training for children with ASD and teaching until generalization occurs*, and (5) parent skills training and coaching	LEAP classroom children made twice the gains on measures of cognitive development and language development, reductions in autism severity, improved teacher ratings of social behavior, and reductions in problem behavior. All gains larger than for control group
Trottier, Kamp, and Mirenda (2011)	$N = 2$ students with ASD, 11 years old, ID; 3 peers each	*Peer (confederate) training to provide prompts to the students with ASD to use SGD during games*; peers taught to gain attention, gesture to devices to prompt communication phrase relevant to activities (Bingo page with 15 spoken messages; turn-taking game phrases, Star Wars matching game, etc.)	Increased spontaneous and prompted communications between students with ASD and peers

(continued)

Table 16.1 (continued)

Study authors	Participants/settings	Peer-mediated intervention description	Outcomes
Wolfberg, DeWitt, Young, and Nguyen (2015)	*N* = 48 children with ASD 5–10 years old; 54 typical peers in intervention and 90 unfamiliar peers; conducted in after-school programs	*Integrated play groups manualized training for children with ASD*: implemented by researchers using guided practice to (a) nurture play initiations (responding to ways to express interests and intentions to play); (b) scaffold play; (c) guide social communication to elicit attention, initiate, respond, and sustain reciprocal engagement; and (d) guide play with strategies to support experiences slightly beyond the child's present level	Increased symbolic and social play and parallel proximity and common focus play; decreased in isolated and onlooker-orientation play behaviors
Wood et al. (2014)	*N* = 13 children with ASD 7–11 years old; IQ > 70; observations at recess with peers	*(1)* "Building confidence" *cognitive behavior therapy*: coping with anxiety and friendship skills taught to children and parents and 32 sessions/90 min weekly; *(2) skill practice on play dates*; *(3) social coaching/priming* by parents, therapists, and service providers before peer activities at school; *(4) peer buddies* at school; *(5) rewards* for skill use across settings	Increased interactions and positive responses to peers' bids; reduced autism severity ratings by blind observers
Recess and lunch setting peer-mediated interventions			
Harper, Symon, and Frea (2008) Procedures based on Pierce and Schreibman (1995); Koegel PRT	*N* = 2 with ASD 8–9 years old, 1 at grade level, one 3 years old < grade level; 6 peers, triads: 2 peers and 1 participant	*Peer training in pivotal response training (PRT)*: gaining attention, varying activities, narrating play, reinforcing attempts, and turn-taking; trainer explained strategies and then modeled and role-played with other peers on the playground; trainer reviewed strategies each day before recess with peers	Increased initiations and turn-taking by children with ASD; increased number of recess activities; maintained after intervention was withdrawn; peers implemented with high fidelity
Kasari, Rotheram-Fuller, Locke, and Gulsrud (2012)	*N* = 60 with ASD mean age = 8 years old, IQ = 90; 45 in intervention; peers on playground	Combined *(1) peer training using direct instruction, modeling, and role-playing* to engage children on playground who were isolated – strategies included encouraging social interactions and game playing and conflict resolution – *(2) child training to initiate* and join in games with peers on the playground; skills individualized and taught to mastery using role-play and rehearsal	Peer training group showed more change in social network salience; both peer and child training reduced solitary play; improved teacher ratings of social skills for the peer group; no change in friendship nominations

(continued)

Table 16.1 (continued)

Study authors	Participants/settings	Peer-mediated intervention description	Outcomes
Koegel, Kuriakose, Singh, and Koegel (2012)	$N = 3$ kindergarteners with ASD, 1 year below grade level academically; playground	*Initiation training for children with ASD* using PRT and prompting and reinforcement: (1) facilitated social play with choice and task variation and interventionist inviting peers to play, encouraging the child to play, and prompting responses to peers; (2) facilitated social play with initiation training to begin games with peers, join in existing game, transition to a new game, and continue with turn-taking	Increased social engagement during facilitated play; increased generalization of initiations to recess with initiation training; increased positive affect ratings during facilitated play with generalization to recess following initiation training
Loftin, Odom, and Lantz (2008)	$N = 3$ with ASD, 9–10 years old; lunchroom and recess peers	Combined *(1) training for children with ASD to initiate and self-monitor using task analysis* of having conversations at lunch, skills taught 1:1 and then practiced in small groups and in cafeteria *and (2) peer training* to respond to participants	Increased social initiations, maintained after self-monitoring and reinforcement removed; increased social interactions; decreased repetitive behaviors
Macpherson, Charlop, and Miltenberger (2015)	$N = 5$ with ASD, 9–11 years old; low adaptive, social behaviors; athletic group play	*Portable video modeling (adults)* using compliments and compliment gestures, participants watched treatment video when they reached second base during kickball game and instructed to "do what he saw in video"	Increased use of compliments during kickball games using video modeling – both scripted and unscripted compliments increased; two maintained without VM after six intervention sessions
Mason et al. (2014)	$N = 3$ with ASD, 6–8 years old; 2 peers each; training in small groups, intervention at recess	Combined *(1) peer and student with ASD training*: modeling and role-playing examples to talk, share, and play nice with friends; *(2) visual picture and text cues* to prompt skill use; *(3) prompting of peers* to initiate and maintain interactions at recess; *(4) rewards* for all students for skill use	Increased communication acts (initiations/responses) by students with ASD at recess; continued interactions with peers reported by implementers for two of three participants

(continued)

Table 16.1 (continued)

Study authors	Participants/settings	Peer-mediated intervention description	Outcomes
McFadden, Kamps, and Heitzman-Powell (2014); some procedures based on Koegel PRT	$N = 4$ children with ASD, 6–8 years old; 2 with mild ID; kindergarten and second grade peers at recess	Combined *(1) peer and child with ASD training*: (a) class-wide lessons in playing together and having fun, complimenting and encouraging friends, talking about play and giving ideas, using names, and getting attention and (b) pre-recess huddle with 2–4 peers to role-play skills; and *(2) prompting, feedback, and reinforcement* by para during recess play (a) feedback every 5 min and (b) post-recess huddle to give points toward earning a class party	Increased spontaneous initiations to peers and total communication with peers during recess; increased commenting and requesting behaviors; increased responses by peers to children with ASD
Murdock and Hobbs (2011)	$N = 12$ children with ASD, 5–6 years old; 8 peers; preschool classes	*Social narratives and visual cues* (photographs with conversation bubbles) of play vignette – "picture me playing"/five story lessons and three practice pretend play sessions with peers	Increased instances of play dialogue with novel vignette; increased novel dialogue statements
Owen-DeSchryver, Carr, Cale, and Blakely-Smith (2008)	$N = 3$ students with ASD 7–10 years old, 2 with ID; 3–4 peers each; probes at lunch and recess	*Peer training* in phases (1) rational for friendships with students with special needs, (2) discussion of strengths about specific participants, and (3) guided discussion on play strategies, conversation topics, helping, and simple management for non-response or unusual behaviors	Increased peer initiations to children with ASD for trained and untrained peers; increased initiations and responses by the children with ASD to peers; increased peer responses to initiations
Reynolds, Gast, and Luscre (2016)	$N = 4$ students with ASD 5–6 years old, mild ID; 2 peers each small group; probes at recess	Self-management (SM) training with video modeling; use of *self-monitoring of initiations to peers* during lunch; graphing following lunch; *reinforcement* – pennies for initiations to peers	Increased initiations to peers during lunch; increased intervals of social interactions; increased initiations and interactions at recess/generalization
Sansosti and Powell-Smith (2008)	$N = 3$ students with ASD, 6–9 years old, low-average IQ	Training for participants with ASD *(1) video models of computer-based social stories with pictures* – to teach social communication – joining in and maintaining conversations; watched prior to recess with teacher prompt to use skills; *(2) prompting for peer confederate* to engage in activity upon request	Increased social communication skills (joining in) with the addition of peer prompting; maintenance of skills during follow-up; generalization for one participant

(continued)

Table 16.1 (continued)

Study authors	Participants/settings	Peer-mediated intervention description	Outcomes
Trembath, Balandin, Togher, and Stancliffe (2009)	*N* = 3 preschoolers with ASD; 6 peers (2 each); training in indoor and outdoor play, group activities, tea and lunch	*Peer training as* "special helpers" *using (1) naturalistic teaching* – skills presented in a story fashion included (a) show him what you are doing or something he can play, (b) wait to see if he wants to play, and (c) tell him what you are doing or tell him its name; and *(2) SGD device* showing partner how to use the talker	Increased frequency of communicative behaviors with peers with more during naturalistic + SGD for two of three participants; slight increases during generalization
Peer-mediated intervention in middle and high school settings/adolescents with ASD			
Hughes et al. (2013)	*N* = 3 high school students with ASD – high functioning to severe ID; one typical peer each; guitar class, art class, PE 90-minute blocks	*Peer training in social interaction and goal-setting*: (a) discussion of their nomination as strong peer model and benefits to participation, (b) description of participants' communication behaviors and interests, (c) ways to interact based on common interest and the class, (d) setting goals for a number of interactions to have with partner, and (e) the use of a self-monitoring sheet for recording goals and goal attainment	Increased peer initiations to students with ASD and generally beyond the set goal, increased time and minutes interacting between students and peers with variability in settings, strong social validity reports from peers, positive social validity from teachers
Koegel, Fredeen et al. (2012)	*N* = 3 students with ASD 11–13 years old, grade level academically; peers available during lunch in middle school	*Social clubs formed based on perseverative interests* (movie trivia club, comic book and gaming club, card games) of students with ASD with flyers distributed to recruit peers with snacks and refreshments during club meetings and club activities available during the lunch block in all phases	Increased percentage of intervals at lunch interacting and initiating with peers (no participants engaged in club activities prior to the special interest club)
Reilly et al. (2014)	*N* = 3 with ASD, 16–18 years old, mild ID; 11 peer trainers; 30 peers in general education class	Combined *(1) peer training to prompt students with ASD to ask novel questions using communication books* organized in a variety of topics (sports, school events, recreational interests) and to show interest in peers "what class do you have next?" what did you do last night?; *(2) participant training in the use of books prior to baseline*	Increased novel questions during generalization sessions, increased peer partner initiations, improved quality ratings of interactions by peers, increased reciprocity from peers with peer-directed questions

(continued)

Table 16.1 (continued)

Study authors	Participants/settings	Peer-mediated intervention description	Outcomes
Schmidt and Stichter (2012); based on curriculum by Stichter and Conroy (2006)	$N = 3$, 13 years old with ASD, seventh grade; 3 peers; small group instruction; skill use at lunch, generalization in middle school math class	Combined *(1) peer training curriculum*: direct instruction and modeling of skills; phase 1, initiate and continue topics, and phase 2, proximity wait for participant to initiate and reinforce; *(2) social competence intervention for participants with ASD*: 20 lessons in recognition and expression of facial expression, sharing ideas, turn-taking in conversation, recognition feelings and emotions (self and others), and problem-solving	Increased generalization of interaction with peers during lunch with "peer initiation phases"; some but less interaction during math class
Simpson and Bui (2016)	$N = 4$ children with ASD, low functioning; 24 second grade peers	Combined *(1) class-wide PMI shared reading buddies, visual cues*: stay with your buddy, read with your buddy, and talk with your buddy; *(2) peers provided rewards* (happy faces exchanged for edibles)	Increased responses to peers (but not initiations by students with ASD); increased initiations by peers; social validity high reported in peer statements and helping behaviors
White et al. (2010)	$N = 15$ with ASD, 11–14 years old, average IQ; 2 peer tutors in therapy group of 4 with ASD	*Social skills group for ASD with peer tutors as models*: manualized treatment based on cognitive behavior therapy using variety of skills, i.e., compliments, relaxation, initiating and maintaining conversations with peers, appropriate responding, social problem-solving, self-monitoring emotions and social skills, social rules and social cues, dealing with teasing and bullying	Improved parent ratings of social communication/social motivation, 13 of 15 no longer in the severe range of ASD, teachers and parents reported improvement in social initiation and participation in social activities

of social skills interventions to maintain skills and growth.

Reichow and Volkmar (2010) completed an extensive review of *social skills interventions* for individuals with ASD. The review included 66 studies published between 2001 and 2008, with a total of 513 participants, 186 of whom were preschoolers, 291 school-aged, and 36 older participants. Their review was completed using published guidelines for criteria to provide an EBP synthesis of the research (i.e., Reichow, Volkmar, & Cicchetti, 2008). Using these criteria, 13 reports indicated a strong rigor rating and 53 adequate ratings. Of interest is that 10 of the 35 studies with preschool-aged participants and 10 of the 31 studies with school-aged participants, for a total of only 30%, included a peer training or peer-mediated component, although several others measured social interactions with peers as an outcome. Interventions fell into eight primary categories with most indicated as having sufficient evidence for Reichow and colleagues to recommend continued use. Interventions included (1) *applied behavior analysis* (ABA) with different prompting and reinforcement schedules as well as imitation and modeling (recommended); (2) *naturalistic interventions* using behavioral methods and including antecedents and consequences (recommended for young children, insufficient for older); (3) *parent training* (recommended for young children); (4) *peer training* and mediation with liked aged peers (recommended); (5) *social skills groups* with participants with or without disabilities (tentative support); (6) *visual cues* as a primary component of interventions such as scripts, picture cues, and Social Stories™ (recommended); (7) *video modeling* with evidence showing it is usually effective but may need additional interventions to produce desired changes (tentative support); and (8) others (see review for specific citations). The authors concluded that a large number of studies reported evidence for the use of ABA procedures in combination with peer training as effective for preschoolers as well as school-aged children; however, it was difficult to apply the evidence-based criteria to studies because of variability in intervention procedures and the use of combined procedures.

Several social skills reviews published between 2014 and 2015 supported Reichow and Volkmar's (2010) findings (i.e., Camargo et al., 2014; Ferraioli & Harris, 2011; Kasari & Patterson, 2012; Wang et al., 2012). Wang et al. (2012) conducted a meta-analysis of single-case design studies targeting *social skills interventions* for individuals with ASD. Their review included 115 studies with 343 participants published from 1994 to 2012. Kasari and Patterson (2012) completed a review of 34 studies published from 2010 to 2012 investigating interventions targeting social impairment for children with ASD. Fifty-one participants in studies using single-case designs were included, and 695 participants in studies using group designs were included in the review. The interventions centered on improving three general areas: social skills knowledge, peer relationships for the older participants, and joint attention/joint engagement for the younger participants. Only 13 of the studies were clearly reported to include peers, peer training, or PMI as part of the intervention. Camargo et al. (2014) reviewed behaviorally based interventions to improve social interaction skills of children with ASD in inclusive settings. They defined behaviorally based interventions to include ABA procedures such as prompting, imitation, modeling, and reinforcement schedules and social interaction skills as those that enabled social exchanges such as turn-taking, sharing, initiating conversations, making comments, and otherwise reciprocal initiation and response sequences. Nineteen studies met their criteria for inclusion, with 55 participants with ASD. A variety of intervention types were described in the studies in the three reviews including many in Reichow and Volkmar's report: *prompting and reinforcement* (Gena, 2006); *peer imitation* (Garfinkle & Schwartz, 2002); *social skills groups with peers* (Banda, Hart, & Liu-Gitz, 2010; Gonzalez-Lopez & Kamps, 1997; Hughes et al., 2011); *Social Stories™* (Reichow & Sabornie, 2009; Schneider & Goldstein, 2010); *combined peer and child training* for social interaction (Kasari et al., 2012); *peer mediation at recess* (Harper et al., 2008); *play dates* (Jull & Mirenda, 2011; Koegel et al., 2005; Koegel, Kuriakose et al., 2012); *music therapy* (Kern & Aldridge, 2006); *teaching joint activity routines* (Betz, Higbee, & Reagon, 2008; Ferraioli & Harris, 2011); *augmentative communication systems* including the Picture Exchange Communication System (Charlop-Christy, Carpenter, Le, LeBlanc, & Kellet, 2002; Kravits, Kamps, Carnazzo, & Potucek, 2002; Sigafoos et al., 2009); *scripts and visual cues* (Krantz & McClannahan, 1998; Thiemann & Goldstein, 2004); and *video modeling* (Simpson, Langone, & Ayres, 2004; Tetreault & Lerman, 2010).

Wang and colleagues' (Wang et al., 2012) analysis showed a mean effect size of 1.36, across 839 dependent variables in the studies, indicating that, on average, socials skills interventions for individuals with ASD are effective. Camargo et al. (2014) indicated that behaviorally based interventions meet criteria for EBP for improving the social skills of children with ASD in inclusive settings. Kasari et al. (2012) stressed a need for future research to focus on the active ingredients of interventions such as dose (e.g., time in intervention) required to obtain an effect and the agent of change such as parents, peers, teachers, or siblings. Kasari et al. indicated moderate and large effects for studies with joint attention/engagement interventions and mixed results for studies addressing social skills. They reported added benefits from studies focusing on core deficits such as joint attention and engagement, social initiations and responses, and the development of friendships.

In a recent review, Whalon et al. (2015) conducted a meta-analysis of single-case design studies of school-based peer-related social competence interventions. A total of 37 studies published from 2000 to 2013 with 105 participants were reviewed. Primary criteria for inclusion were that at least one outcome variable measuring interactions (e.g., initiations or responses) or engagement with typically developing peers. Interventions were categorized as (1) *child-specific* or combined specific strategies such as video modeling paired with positive reinforcement and self-management on compliment-giving behaviors (Apple, Billingsley, & Schwartz, 2005); (2) *adult-mediated*, which most often consisted of direct instruction, practice with prompting, and contingent praise (Boudreau & Harvey, 2013; Licciardello et al., 2008); (3) *social narratives* (Chan & O'Reilly, 2008) or a behavioral learning strategy to teach cooperative participation in activities with peers (Bock, 2007); (4) *video modeling* or video self-modeling (Bellini, Peters, Benner, & Hopf, 2007; Buggey, 2012); and (5) *peer training* in which peers were taught skills such as sharing, suggesting ideas for play, joining in or maintaining play, initiating talk, and assisting or offering help (Harper et al., 2008; Katz & Girolametto, 2013; Koegel, Vernon, Koegel, Koegel, & Paullin, 2012; Kravits et al., 2002; Parker & Kamps, 2011). General findings were that children with ASD can benefit from social skills interventions with their peers in school settings, with moderate and strong effect sizes for adult-mediated, child-specific, PMIs, and multicomponent interventions and mixed effect sizes for social narratives and video modeling.

16.5.1 Summary

In summary, several comprehensive literature reviews have focused on social skills training and interventions for individuals with ASD. Many included components of peer training and PMIs, but not all. Arrangements included teacher- or peer-directed skills, as well as a combination of both elements. Overall, findings concluded that the evidence supports social skills training, including the use of peer training as an effective or, at least, promising intervention (Reichow & Volkmar, 2010; Whalon et al., 2015).

16.6 Summaries of Peer-Mediated Intervention Reviews

In the past 10 years, seven literature reviews have specifically focused on the use of peer training and PMI with children and adolescents with ASD. Many of these report the use of PMI as an effective intervention to improve social and communication outcomes for participants. The reviews are described in the following narrative and indicate the time period of included studies, number of studies and participants, intervention strategies, and general findings.

Two early reviews on PMI included Choi (2007) reporting on *peer training methods* for children and adolescents with ASD based on reviews of 45 studies and Chan et al. (2009) reporting on 42 studies, including 172 participants and 396 peers. Publication dates ranged from 1985 to 2008, with only five published between 2004 and 2008 (Chan et al., 2009). Choi concluded from the review and reported findings (McGrath, Bosch, Sullivan, & Fuqua, 2003) that it is more effective and efficient to teach children with ASD to be responsive to peers than to be the initiators of interaction. Similarly Chan et al. reported *peer initiation* to participants with ASD as the most common intervention (i.e., reported in 50% of the studies). Techniques for *instructing peers to maintain interactions* included prompting play and communication (Chung et al., 2007); repeating and expanding verbalizations and making requests (Sasso, Mundschenk, Melloy, & Casey, 1998); responding to children's attempts to communicate (Garrison-Harrell et al., 1997); and PRT (Koegel et al., 1999; Pierce & Schreibman, 1997). Peers provided academic prompting and tutoring, cooperative learning in several studies (Carter, Cushing, Clark, & Kennedy, 2005; Kamps, Leonard, Potucek, & Garrison-Harrell, 1995; Kamps et al., 1994; Kamps et al., 2002; Laushey & Heflin, 2000), and special friends or buddies and peer networks with members recruited based on common interests and hobbies (Haring & Breen, 1992; Hughes et al., 2002; Laushey & Heflin, 2000; Schleien, Mustonen, & Rynders, 1995). Peers were taught to provide contingent reinforcement in one third of the studies. Lee, Odom, and Loftin (2007) reported in the Chan review effects for using PMIs to decrease stereotypic behavior as well as improving play and social engagement. Several studies recommended the peer selection process which includes high status or popular peers and those with typically positive interaction skills as a way to promote generalization and reduce stigmatization (Sasso & Rude, 1987). Sasso and Rude (reported in Chan et al., 2009) concluded that while few studies collected treatment fidelity, when fidelity was used to shape the peers' intervention skills, better outcomes were noted. Thus, higher fidelity resulted in better outcomes. Their findings (Sasso & Rude, 1987) also reported social validity of PMIs from the peers' perspective (e.g., students reported they enjoyed participating, learned valuable skills, felt pride in involvement, etc.).

Zhang and Wheeler (2011) published a meta-analysis of PMIs for young children with ASD published between 1978 and 2006. Findings from 45 articles, with 118 children, were presented. Effect sizes (ES) were calculated and indicated that PMIs were highly effective for increasing the frequency and duration of social interactions for children with ASD ages 3–8 years old. Intervention strategies included peer modeling with video modeling, with the highest reported ES (i.e., 3.16); peer initiation training and group-oriented contingency as the most commonly used strategies; peer monitoring, peer networking, and peer tutoring used less frequently; and combined interventions (e.g., teaching initiations and responses) as the most frequently used approach and with the second largest ES (i.e., 1.89). Interventions implemented in the home settings for children under eight were somewhat more effective than those in school settings, although outcomes were effective in integrated and segregated school settings as well. Interventions that planned for generalization across behaviors and included active involvement of parents and siblings promoted stronger effects (Baker, Koegel, & Koegel, 1998; Tsao & Odom, 2006). Zhang and Wheeler also reported larger effect sizes for interventions measuring social responses than those targeting social initiations. They recommended investigations to understand how to promote positive social initiations for children with ASD and how to use peer modeling as a component of more interventions targeting social interactions.

Watkins et al. (2015) conducted a review of peer-mediated social interaction interventions in inclusive settings for children with ASD. Fourteen studies, restricted to those published between 2008 and 2014, with 44 participants were included. Only studies in which (a) peers shared context and activities, (b) the setting was an inclusive environment, and (c) an experimental design allowed analysis of the intervention effects for directly observed social behaviors were included in the review. Settings included general education classrooms, playgrounds, lunchrooms, or combinations of settings. The majority of studies included peers who met the criteria defined by Odom and Strain (1984) to include those with typical language and social skills, compliance with directions, good attendance and availability, and teacher recommendation. Effective procedures included peer initiation, prompting and reinforcing procedures, and proximity. PMI strategies included those referenced in prior reviews including (a) PRT techniques, (b) use of scripted phrases related to play themes (Ganz & Flores, 2008), (c) high-probability request sequences with peer modeling (Jung et al., 2008), (d) environmental modifications to incorporate preferences (Koegel, Fredeen et al., 2012), (e) visual supports (Hughes et al., 2011; Katz & Girolametto, 2013), (f) teacher prompting (Banda et al., 2010), (g) self-monitoring strategies (Hughes et al., 2013; Loftin et al., 2008), and (h) tangible reinforcement for skill use (Mason et al., 2014). Watkins and colleagues' findings indicated positive outcomes for the majority of studies. Further, of the nine studies that measured generalization, eight demonstrated generalization of skills. Strategies that promoted generalization included initiation, prompting, and reinforcing skills. An additional important finding was that outcomes for the participants with ASD were better when the participating peers expressed interest, demonstrated good language and social skills, and complied with instructions during intervention.

Chang and Locke (2016) conducted a review of studies utilizing group designs that evaluated the efficacy of PMIs for children with ASD. The review included five studies, which together included a total of 260 participants (i.e., Corbett et al., 2014; Kamps et al., 2014; Kalyva & Avramidids, 2005; Kasari et al., 2012; Roeyers, 1996). Methods across studies included structured peer training to teach peers to respond to and model target behaviors for the children with ASD and to help them play and reinforce social behaviors. Four studies included modeling by trainers and role-play or rehearsals with peers. Only one study (i.e., Kasari et al., 2012) provided separate training for the peers. The role of trainers during the social activities following training was to support and facilitate the interactions between children with ASD and their peers during indoor play activities at school or camp and at recess. Three studies showed implementation fidelity, and only one study showed reliable implementation by school staff (Kamps et al., 2014). General conclusions were that PMIs are effective and meet the standard criteria of EBP (Reichow et al., 2008). They further stressed the importance of measuring implementation fidelity in real-world settings including peers' fidelity of mediation.

Zagona and Mastergeorge (2016) conducted a review of PMIs for young children with ASD analyzing 17 studies published between 2004 and 2014 with 110 participants. The authors described a comprehensive model of PMIs to include the following steps: (1) selection of peers with the purpose of teaching them skills and strategies to sustain interactions with children with ASD, (2) play/structured activities to provide coaching, prompting, and reinforcement for peers during naturalistic activities, and (3) PMIs implemented in natural classroom settings noting classroom arrangements and availability of cooperative activities and materials. The authors provided rich descriptions of the use of successful PMIs for improving outcomes through social skills groups implemented across a variety of settings including lunch and recess (Loftin et al., 2008; Mason et al., 2014; Owen-DeSchryver et al., 2008); in middle schools, in cooking class (Ganz et al., 2012); at lunch (Collet-Klingenberg, Neitzel, & LaBerge, 2012); across multiple settings such as lunch and math (Schmidt & Stichter, 2012); and in separate rooms in inclusive schools (Trottier et al., 2011). Findings indicated that the majority of studies found an increase in social communication skills for participants with ASD following peer training. Also, PMIs were found to be more effective than when adults were the only trainers (Kasari et al., 2012 as reported in Zagona & Mastergeorge, 2016). Zagona and Mastergeorge (2016) stressed the importance of embedding peer training into everyday routines to promote generalization. An important conclusion from this review was that peer training creates opportunities for children with ASD to engage with receptive partners across a variety of contexts and activities particularly in inclusive settings. Inclusive settings may provide repeated and contextually appropriate opportunities for PMI to occur.

16.7 Key Findings and Recommendations

Peer training and PMIs are clearly supported by the evidence across multiple reviews (Camargo et al., 2014; Chan et al., 2009; Chang & Locke,

2016; Watkins et al., 2015; Whalon et al., 2015; Zagona & Mastergeorge, 2016; Zhang & Wheeler, 2011). A number of key findings supported from the research are outlined below.

First, typically developing peers are a recommended component to interventions addressing social competence for children and individuals with ASD (Camargo et al., 2014; Watkins et al., 2015). Chang and Locke (2016) suggest that the benefits of PMIs include typically developing peers that can model appropriate social behaviors, peers that are readily accessible in school settings to act as intervention agents, and peers that provide multiple opportunities for children with ASD to practice their new skills (Chan et al., 2009, as cited in Chang & Locke). Further, training multiple peers and practice with unfamiliar peers and settings is beneficial for promoting generalization of skills, but also peers trained for PMI may provide prompts to one another to interact with children with ASD and other disabilities (Kohler et al., 1995; McFadden et al., 2014; Rao et al., 2008). Researchers recommend basic guidelines with respect to the choice of peers. For example, peers who are skilled or highly socially competent, are popular, and who have an existing interest in the participants with ASD are more effective and willing to provide peer modeling (Locke, Rotheram-Fuller, & Kasari, 2012; Watkins et al., 2015). Only one study found social skills instruction without peers (i.e., teacher-directed) to be more effective than with PMIs (Kasari et al., 2016). The authors reported that teacher-directed skills training was especially effective for children with high rates of problem behaviors and low teacher perception of a close relationship at baseline. In some cases, using behavioral strategies to reinforce peers' interactions with children with ASD, as a means to motivate and increase their efforts, may be necessary (DiSalvo & Oswald, 2002). Likewise, teaching peers to initiate and maintain play with their classmates with ASD can improve the peers' ability to relate to all peers and thus may reinforce their efforts (Belchic & Harris, 1994 reported in DiSalvo & Oswald, 2002). Importantly, social validity for PMIs has been reported in several studies. Peers have reported improved self-concept, reduced fear of differences, increased tolerance, more accepting of friendships, and the rewarding nature of the peer mediation activities (Breen, Haring, Pitts-Conway, & Gaylord-Ross, 1985; Kamps et al., 1998; Locke et al., 2012; Peck, Donaldson, & Pezzoli, 1990; Pierce & Schreibman, 1995). Reichow and Volkmar (2010) suggested clearer descriptions of the peer selection process in research and greater inclusion of siblings as peer agents.

A second finding is that training children with ASD to respond and initiate to their peers can provide powerful changes in their ability to socialize and communicate. Many researchers recommend training for the participants with ASD which may occur concurrently with their peers (Kamps et al., 2014). Targeted skills selected for intervention will impact acquisition and generalization. For example, teaching initiation strategies have been widely used and may increase generalization of skills to novel settings for participants with ASD (Kasari et al., 2012; Koegel, Kuriakose et al., 2012; Taylor et al., 2005). Using choice and perseverative interests for individuals with ASD may provide a common ground for social interactions with peers, which may also improve motivation and outcomes (Boyd, Controy, Mancil, Nakao, & Alter, 2007: Koegel, Matos-Freden, Lang, & Koegel, 2012). A key is to understand if training for the participants with ASD needs to be conducted independently (Laugeson, Ellingsen, Sanderson, Tucci, & Bates, 2014), as a prerequisite for PMI, or to occur concurrently with peer training. The literature suggests benefits to training both peers and participants with ASD jointly (Kamps et al., 2014). In addition, an important consideration for the participants with ASD is the length of intervention and likely the need for social skills interventions spanning many years and stages in transitioning to different environments. Social behavior is more than just play skills or functioning in social groups with peers. Developing social competence continues to be a need for adolescents and young adults with ASD, and effective intervention can impact a lifelong trajectory of independence and community participation.

A third finding is that setting matters. Social skills interventions and PMIs conducted in the setting in which the students will use the skills promote higher maintenance and generalization (Bellini et al., 2007; Camargo et al., 2014). Inclusive settings may have added value for PMIs (Koegel, Kuriakose et al., 2012). In addition, implementation of PMIs may have more powerful effects and generalized outcomes when implemented in multiple general education settings (e.g., classroom, lunchroom, playground; Camargo et al., 2014; Harper et al., 2008; Kamps et al., 1997, 2002). Kasari and Patterson (2012) concur that the intervention setting matters, suggesting that toddlers may respond differently to different interventionists (i.e., therapists and parents) and settings and developmental differences may further impact responsiveness to treatment. They concluded there may be benefits to pairing different treatment deliveries and settings (e.g., parents and therapists or individual and group interventions). Zhang and Wheeler (2011) similarly suggested increasing the number of types of interventions implemented in home and community settings. In general, studies found that implementation in natural or real-world settings by community/school staff can significantly improve outcomes and generalization (Kaale, Smith, & Sponheim, 2012; Kasari & Patterson, 2012).

Fourth, a variety of EBPs are effective within PMIs to improve social outcomes for children with ASD. Examples include peer training, parent facilitated play dates, facilitated social play, initiation training, clubs in school settings based on perseverative interests, visual cues and social scripts, self-monitoring of skill use with peers, and video-based interventions such as video modeling with peers as a model, video self-modeling, and video feedback (Bellini & Akullian, 2007; Koegel, Park, & Koegel, 2014; Kourassanis, Jones, & Fienup, 2015; Reynolds et al., 2016; State & Kern, 2012). Recent advances in Augmentative and Alternative Communication systems and video modeling technology have improved communication skills for students with ASD (Macpherson et al., 2015; Strasberger & Ferreri, 2014); however, more studies are needed to incorporate peer mediation in the use of technology with students with ASD (Trottier et al., 2011). DiSalvo and Oswald (2002) recommend comparisons of peer effort to determine which strategies most effectively increase the attention of their partners with ASD and further that "Pinpointing when and how learning best occurs will lead to greater refinement of intervention approaches" (p. 205). Hughes et al. (2013) suggested that peer training includes a mechanism for peers to set goals and monitor interactions with the high schoolers with ASD independently of the researchers, which also allowed peers to determine or choose how much interaction to have during activities in the class. Their procedures produced high levels of social validity for peers and teachers alike.

Fifth, characteristics, functioning levels, and child-specific deficits need to be considered in selecting PMI. A number of researchers addressing children and youth with ASD recommend attention to learner characteristics and careful descriptions of interventions and implementation to determine which are best for which type of child (Kasari & Lawton, 2010; Watkins et al., 2015). Koegel, Matos-Freden et al. (2012) similarly suggested assessment of underlying causes of poor performance for the individual to inform intervention planning. For example, is the deficit likely a social avoidance function or does social attention function as a reinforcer for behaviors that may or may not be socially appropriate?

Rao et al. (2008) stated that researchers and practitioners need to attend to specific deficits and characteristics of participants in choosing social skills intervention (i.e., whether existing cognitive and language skills of participants meet the complexity of more complex training programs). Ferraioli and Harris (2011) and others (e.g., Chang & Locke, 2016) reported in their reviews that children with higher verbal skills are more likely to benefit from social skills instruction. Rao et al. further stated individual characteristics such as social anxiety and attention issues may further impact outcomes. Their findings suggest that mixed (i.e., heterogeneous) samples of children within the same social skills group may hinder outcomes for some.

Watkins et al. (2015) suggest that interventions best for students with a skill deficit include those with direct instruction of social interaction, peer prompting, and planned reinforcement. In contrast, intervention that targets the use of skills such as peer proximity, preferred interests, and increased peer initiations may be a better fit for participants with a performance deficit. Whalon et al. (2015) stated that social development of children with ASD is influenced by cognitive and communication skills (Constantino, 2011), and, yet, many times these characteristics are not provided in studies; thus, it is difficult to detect patterns between intervention effects and these variables.

Sixth, measuring outcomes for PMIs and improvements in social competence for persons with ASD is complex. ASD and core social, communication, and behavioral characteristics are complex, as is planning intervention including PMI. A variety of outcomes are possible with PMI such as (a) increased initiations, responses, and duration of social interactions; (b) improvements in language; (c) increased use of communication devices; (d) more positive peer nominations and social network membership; (e) less isolation on the playground; and (g) social and friendship benefits for both children with ASD and peers (Chang & Locke, 2016; Kasari, Locke, Gulsrud, & Rotheram-Fuller, 2011; Mason et al., 2014; Matson et al., 2007; Thiemann & Goldstein, 2004). In spite of being an EBP and strong outcomes with PMIs, better measurement is needed to individualize and monitor skills. Measures of the quality, as well as quantity, of interactions with peers are needed.

Kasari and Patterson (2012) recommend researchers (a) increase our understanding and measurement of outcomes that are meaningful and sustainable (e.g., improved social relationships, sustained social interactions) and (b) support deployment into community settings. Reichow and Volkmar (2010) similarly recommend the need to "...utilize measures that examine the ability of individuals with ASD to function within their social milieu" (p. 163). Several reviews concluded the need for measures of treatment fidelity, including fidelity of peers' behaviors, as well as generalization programming and assessment (Camargo et al., 2014).

16.8 Conclusions and Future Directions

Several conclusions can be made based on the evidence in the literature summarized in this chapter. PMIs are effective for improving social and communication outcomes for children and youth with ASD. A variety of EBPs can be incorporated within PMIs to increase their effectiveness. Interventions can be implemented in multiple settings with teachers, parents, and peers with and without disabilities. Research into the treatment fidelity, including peer fidelity, and conditions under which PMI maximizes learning for participants with ASD in the future studies can greatly enhance our understanding of the mechanisms underlying the positive outcomes.

PMI has been successfully implemented across a variety of settings and age groups. A large number of peer modeling and other peer inclusive strategies have been implemented in preschool settings (Reichow & Volkmar, 2010; Whalon et al., 2015). The Learning Experiences and Alternative Program for Preschoolers and Parents model (LEAP; Strain & Bovey, 2011), in particular, provides an evidence-based model for systemic enhancements in inclusive preschools using multiple peer and child-specific training strategies to dramatically improve the long-term outcomes for children with ASD. Behaviorally based PMIs have strongest outcomes (Camargo et al., 2014; Reichow & Volkmar, 2010). Research clearly suggests that early intervention for social behaviors may be as critical to future outcomes as early language intervention. "Early behavioral support for social skills of children with ASD in inclusive settings can promote quicker adaptation and social adjustment with typically developing peers, enhancing the quality of their relationships that can mitigate future challenges in adulthood and future independent living" (p. 2111, Camargo et al., 2014).

A large body of literature exists supporting PMIs in elementary school settings (see Reichow

& Volkmar, 2010; Watkins et al., 2015; Whalon et al., 2015). Social skills groups with peers, lunch and recess interventions, and peer buddy programs are reported effective with this age group. In addition, early studies demonstrated benefits for peer tutoring and cooperative learning arrangements to improve academic and social skills. Only a few recent studies have investigated effects of PMI for children with ASD in academic groups, and while academic gains have been noted, social outcomes have not been measured or have shown limited change (Kamps et al., 2016; Ledford & Wehby, 2015; Peturdottir, McComas, McMaster, & Horner, 2007).

16.8.1 Future Research

In spite of the positive nature and outcomes for PMI, much work needs to be done, particularly in the areas of generalization and sustainability of PMI in school and community settings. Measures of generalization to natural contexts within social skills interventions and PMIs, in particular, are limited and often not measured (Bellini et al., 2007). This suggests that programming for generalization of social and communication skills to novel peers and settings is still quite challenging and in need of further research. Whalon et al. (2015) suggest that many PMI investigations teach isolated skills or use isolated intervention strategies that only address a single aspect of social competence. Improvements are often in controlled rather than authentic settings with limited maintenance and generality. They further suggest that given the heterogeneity associated with ASD, assessment to determine and define target behaviors is needed, yet seldom reported. In addition, while peers report social validity for PMIs with their classmates with ASD, much is still unknown. Moving beyond tolerance of ASD and all disabilities to acceptance and the value to peers and subsequent societal and policy implications has yet to be explored.

All reviews pointed to the need for additional research on interventions addressing social- communication skills for adolescents and young adults with ASD (Camargo et al., 2014; Chang & Locke, 2016; Reichow & Volkmar, 2010; Walton & Ingersoll, 2013). Only a few studies have been implemented in secondary school and community settings (Hughes et al., 2013; Schmidt & Stichter, 2012), and many interventions addressing social behaviors for adolescents are done in clinical settings and in groups with other persons with ASD rather than using peer models (Schohl et al., 2014; White et al., 2013).

A final area for future research is adoption of PMI as common practice to support students with ASD in public schools. Peer network and PMI in schools were first reported in the literature three decades ago (Gaylord-Ross, Haring, Breen, & Pitts-Conway, 1984; Haring & Breen, 1992). However, this type of approach to increase social communication skills and relationships has yet to be widely accepted and is not a common school-based intervention. Dingfelder and Mandell (2011) recommended features of research to address the *research-to-practice* gap in autism intervention. They propose applying diffusion of innovation theory to plan for more successful dissemination, noting that, generally, interventions are not adopted or maintained because of a misfit between the intervention and the needs and capacities of the setting. In schools this is generally described as limited resources. They recommend a few strategies to address this issue. Intervention research should target ecologically valid outcomes that are relevant to the system and match the needs of stakeholders, that is, most salient to public practice. This would necessitate involving parents and teachers early in the research planning stages. Using outcome measures relevant to the system (e.g., schools, families) would maximize interest. Manualizing treatments and soliciting feedback from consumers while making modifications to better fit the environment (e.g., accessing resources within highly social times in schools and rotating peers as mediators) and individual students' needs might also increase the likelihood of adoption and sustainability (Kasari & Smith, 2013). Other suggestions would be to train teachers and peers to implement interventions as is typically the case with PMI and further assess (a) the fidelity of practitioners' and peers' use of the practices in natural settings and (b) their ability to use and generalize intervention components in routine practice across multiple contexts (Goldstein, 2002; Kamps et al., 1997; Kamps et al., 2014). Zagona and Mastergeorge (2016) stressed the importance of dynamic professional development with coaching and mentoring to facilitate peer support for engaging children with ASD, as well as promoting practitioner's awareness and the inherent value of including typical peers with children with ASD within a variety of contexts in and out the classroom (Kasari et al., 2012; Schmidt & Stichter, 2012).

Certainly, interventions that address social communication skills that are relevant to all children – not just children with ASD – may be more acceptable. In addition, PMIs that have an academic component or are complementary to academic goals would increase its use in school settings as well. Dingfelder and Mandell (2011) further suggest planning for self-regulation and stabilization of interventions by providing training, materials, and "incrementally facilitating independent use" (p. 605). Perhaps equally important in the adoption of PMIs and the inherent strategies is ensuring the practices fit within school-wide systems promoting universal prosocial skills and adaptive behaviors for all students, along with teacher support teams and targeted small group or intensive interventions for any students needing additional supports to succeed.

In summary, research over several decades has shown positive effects of PMIs for improving social communication skills for children and youth with ASD. Setting the bar high with a goal for all students, including those with ASD and other disabilities, to learn to socialize and communicate effectively and appropriately with their peers in school environments might promote more widespread adoption and sustainability of PMI practices. Further, a continued focus on social competence beyond school environments with attention to interventions for adolescents and adults with ASD can greatly impact their school life, future employment, and overall quality of life with long-term positive outcomes.

References

American Psychiatric Association. (2013). *Diagnostic and statistical manual of mental disorders (DSM-V-TR)*. Washington DC: Author.

Apple, A. L., Billingsley, F., & Schwartz, I. S. (2005). Effects of video modeling alone and with self-management on compliment-giving behaviors of children with high-functioning ASD. *Journal of Positive Behavior Interventions*, *7*(1), 33–46.

Baker, M., Koegel, R., & Koegel, L. (1998). Increasing the social behavior of young children with autism using their obsessive behaviors. *The Journal of the Association for Persons with Severe Handicaps*, *23*, 300–308.

Banda, D. R., Hart, S. L., & Liu-Gitz, L. (2010). Impact of training peers and children with autism on social skills during center time activities in inclusive classrooms. *Research in Autism Spectrum Disorders*, *4*(4), 619–625.

Barnhill, G. P., Cook, K. T., Tebbenkamp, K., & Myles, B. S. (2002). The effectiveness of social skills intervention targeting nonverbal communication for adolescents with Asperger syndrome and related pervasive developmental delays. *Focus on Autism and Other Developmental Disabilities*, *17*(2), 112–118.

Barry, T. D., Klinger, L. G., Lee, J. M., Palardy, N., Gilmore, T., & Bodin, S. D. (2003). Examining the effectiveness of an outpatient clinic-based social skills group for high-functioning children with autism. *Journal of Autism and Developmental Disorders*, *33*(6), 685–701.

Bauminger, N. (2002). The facilitation of social-emotional understanding and social interaction in high-functioning children with autism: Intervention outcomes. *Journal of Autism and Developmental Disorders*, *32*(4), 283–298.

Belchic, J., & Harris, S. (1994). The use of multiple peer exemplars to enhance the generalization of play skills to the siblings of children with autism. *Child and Family Behavior Therapy*, *16*, 1–25.

Bellini, S., & Akullian, J. (2007). A meta-analysis of video modeling and video self-modeling interventions for children and adolescents with autism spectrum disorders. *Exceptional Children*, *73*, 264–287.

Bellini, S., Peters, J., Benner, L., & Hopf, A. (2007). Meta-analysis of school-based social skills interventions for children with autism spectrum disorders. *Journal of Remedial and Special Education*, *28*, 153–162.

Betz, A., Higbee, T., & Reagon, K. (2008). Using joint activity schedules to promote peer engagement in preschoolers with autism. *Journal of Applied Behavior Analysis*, *41*(2), 237–241.

Bock, M. A. (2007). A social-behavioral learning strategy intervention for a child with Asperger syndrome: Brief report. *Remedial and Special Education*, *28*, 258–265.

Boudreau, J., & Harvey, M. T. (2013). Increasing recreational initiations for children who have ASD using video self-modeling. *Education and Treatment of Children, 36*, 49–60.

Boyd, B. A., Controy, M. A., Mancil, G. R., Nakao, T., & Alter, P. J. (2007). Effects of circumscribed interests on the social behaviors of children with autism spectrum disorders. *Journal of Autism and Developmental Disorders, 37*, 1550–1561.

Breen, C., Haring, T., Pitts-Conway, V., & Gaylord-Ross, R. (1985). The training and generalization of social interaction during break time at two job sites in the natural environment. *Journal of the Association for Persons with Severe Handicaps, 10*, 41–50.

Buggey, T. (2012). Effectiveness of video self-modeling to promote social initiations by 3-year-olds with autism spectrum disorders. *Focus on Autism and Other Developmental Disabilities, 27*, 102–110.

Camargo, S., Rispoli, M., Ganz, J., Hong, E., Davis, H., & Mason, R. (2014). A review of the quality of behaviorally-based intervention research to improve social interaction skills of children with ASD in inclusive settings. *Journal of Autism and Developmental Disorders, 44*, 2096–2116.

Carter, E. W., Cushing, L. S., Clark, N. M., & Kennedy, C. H. (2005). Effects of peer support interventions on students' access to the general curriculum and social interactions. *Research and Practice for Persons with Severe Disabilities, 30*, 15–25.

Chan, J. M., Lang, R., Rispoli, M., O'Reilly, M., Sigafoos, J., & Cole, H. (2009). Use of peer-mediated interventions in the treatment of autism spectrum disorders: A systematic review. *Research in Autism Spectrum Disorder, 3*, 876–889.

Chan, J. M., & O'Reilly, M. F. (2008). A Social Stories™ intervention package for students with autism in inclusive classroom settings. *Journal of Applied Behavior Analysis, 41*(3), 405–409.

Chang, Y., & Locke, J. (2016). A systematic review of peer-mediated interventions for children with autism spectrum disorder. *Research in Autism Spectrum Disorders, 27*, 1–10.

Charlop-Christy, M., Carpenter, M., Le, L., LeBlanc, L., & Kellet, K. (2002). Using the picture exchange communication system (PECS) with children with autism: Assessment of PECS acquisition, speech, social-communicative behavior, and problem behavior. *Journal of Applied Behavior Analysis, 35*, 213–231.

Choi, S. (2007). Peer training methods for children and adolescents with autism: A review. *International Journal of Pedagogies & Learning, 3*, 92–97.

Chung, K. M., Reavis, S., Mosconi, M., Drewry, J., Matthews, T., & Tasse, M. J. (2007). Peer-mediated social skills training program for young children with high-functioning autism. *Research in Developmental Disabilities, 28*, 423–436.

Chung, Y., & Douglas, K. (2015). A peer interaction package for students with autism spectrum disorders who use speech-generating devices. *Journal of Developmental and Physical Disabilities, 27*, 831–849.

Collet-Klingenberg, L., Neitzel, J., & LaBerge, J. (2012). Power-PALS (Peers Assisting, Leading, Supporting): Implementing a peer-mediated intervention in a rural middle school program. *Rural Special Education Quarterly, 3*, 3–11.

Constantino, J. N. (2011). Social impairment. In E. Hollander, A. Kolevzon, & J. T. Coyle (Eds.), *Textbook of autism spectrum disorders* (pp. 139–146). Washington, DC: American Psychiatric Publishing Inc.

Corbett, B. Swain, D., Coke, C., Simon, D., Newsom, C., Houchins-Juarez, N., Jenson, A., Wang, L., & Song, Y. (2014). Improvement in social deficits in autism spectrum disorders using a theatre-based, Peer-mediated intervention. *Autism Research, 7*, 4–16.

Dingfelder, H., & Mandell, D. (2011). Bridging the research-to-practice gap in autism intervention: An application of diffusion of innovation theory. *Journal of Autism and Developmental Disorders, 41*, 597–609.

DiSalvo, D. A., & Oswald, D. P. (2002). Peer-mediated interventions to increase the social interaction of children with autism consideration of peer expectancies. *Focus on Autism and Other Developmental Disabilities, 17*(4), 198–208.

Ferraioli, S. J., & Harris, S. L. (2011). Treatments to increase social awareness and social skills. *Evidence-based practices and treatments for children with autism.* In B. Reinchow, P. Doehring, D. V. Cicchetti, & F. R. Volmar (Eds.), *Evidence-based practices and treatments for children with autism* (pp. 171–196). New York: Springer.

Ganz, J., Heath, A., Lund, E., Camargo, S., Rispoli, M., Boles, M., & Plaisance, L. (2012). Effects of peer-mediated implementation of visual scripts in middle school. *Behavior Modification, 36*, 378–398.

Ganz, J. B., & Flores, M. M. (2008). Effects of the use of visual strategies in play groups for children with autism spectrum disorders and their peers. *Journal of Autism and Developmental Disorders, 38*(5), 926–940.

Garfinkle, A., & Schwartz, I. (2002). Peer imitation: Increasing social interactions in children with autism and other developmental disabilities in inclusive preschool classrooms. *Topics in Early Childhood Special Education, 22*(1), 26–38.

Garrison-Harrell, L., Kamps, D., & Kravitz, T. (1997). The effects of peer networks on social-communicative behaviors for students with autism. *Focus on Autism & Other Developmental Disabilities, 12*(4), 241–254.

Gaylord-Ross, R., Haring, T., Breen, C., & Pitts-Conway, V. (1984). The training and generalization of social interaction skills with autistic youth. *Journal of Applied Behavior Analysis, 17*, 229–247.

Gena, A. (2006). The effects of prompting and social reinforcement on establishing social interactions with peers during the inclusion of four children with autism in preschool. *International Journal of Psychology, 41*, 541–554.

Goldstein, H. (2002). Communication intervention for children with autism: A review of treatment efficacy.

Journal of Autism and Developmental Disorders, *32*(5), 373–396.

Goldstein, H., Kaczmarek, L., Pennington, R., & Shafer, K. (1992). Peer-mediated intervention: Attending to, commenting on, and acknowledging the behavior of preschoolers with autism. *Journal of Applied Behavior Analysis*, *25*, 289–305.

Gonzalez-Lopez, A., & Kamps, D. (1997). Social skills training to increase social interaction between children with autism and their peers. *Focus on Autism and Other Developmental Disabilities*, *12*, 2–14.

Guralnick, M. J. (1990). Social competence and early intervention. *Journal of Early Intervention*, *14*(1), 3–14. doi:10.1177/105381519001400101

Haring, T. G., & Breen, C. G. (1992). A peer-mediated social network intervention to enhance the social integration of persons with moderate and severe disabilities. *Journal of Applied Behavior Analysis*, *25*(2), 319–333.

Harper, C. B., Symon, J. B. G., & Frea, W. D. (2008). Recess is time-in: Using peers to improve social skills of children with autism. *Journal of Autism and Developmental Disorders*, *38*(5), 815–826.

Hughes, C., Copeland, S., Wehmeyer, M., Agran, M., Cai, X., & Hwang, B. (2002). Increasing social interaction between general education high school students and their peers with mental retardation. *Journal of Developmental and Physical Disabilities*, *14*, 387–402.

Hughes, C., Golas, M., Cosgriff, J., Brigham, N., Edwards, C., & Cashen, K. (2011). Effects of a social skills intervention among high school students with intellectual disabilities and autism and their general education peers. *Research & Practice for Persons with Severe Disabilities*, *36*(1), 46–61.

Hughes, C., Golas, M., Cosgriff, J., Reilly, C., Heilingoetter, J., Brigham, N., … Bernstein, R. (2013). A peer-delivered social interaction intervention for high school students with autism. *Practice for Persons with Severe Disabilities*, *38*, 1–16.

Hundert, J., Rowe, S., & Harrison, E. (2014). The combined effects of social script training and peer buddies on generalized peer interaction of children with ASD in inclusive classrooms. *Focus on Autism and Other Developmental Disabilities*, *29*, 206–215.

Jull, S., & Mirenda, P. (2011). Parents as play date facilitators for preschoolers with autism. *Journal of Positive Behavior Inerventions*, *13*, 17–30.

Jung, S., Sainato, D. M., & Davis, C. A. (2008). Using high-probability request sequences to increase social skills to students with autism to increase peer interactions in young children with autism. *Journal of Early Behavioral Education*, *7*, 335–357.

Kaale, A., Smith, L., & Sponheim, E. (2012). A randomized controlled trial of preschool-based joint attention intervention for children with autism. *Journal of Child Psychology and Psychiatry*, *53*, 97–105.

Kalyva, E., & Avramidids, E. (2005). Improving communication between children with autism and their peers through the "circle of friends"; a small-scale intervention study. *Journal of Applied Research in Intellectual Disabilities*, *18*, 253–261.

Kamps, D., Barbetta, P., Leonard, B., & Delquadri, J. (1994). Classwide peer tutoring: An integration strategy to improve reading skills and promote interactions among students with autism and regular education peers. *Journal of Applied Behavior Analysis*, *27*, 54–60.

Kamps, D., Gonzalez-Lopez, A., Potucek, J., Kravits, T., Kemmerer, K., & Garrison-Harrell, L. (1998). What do the peers think? Social validity of integrated programs. *Education and Treatment of Children*, *21*, 107–134.

Kamps, D., Heitzman-Powell, L., Rosenberg, N., Mason, R., Schwartz, I., & Romine, R. (2016). Effects of reading mastery as a small group intervention for young children with ASD. *Journal of Developmental and Physical Disabilities*, *28*, 703–722.

Kamps, D., Leonard, B., Vernon, S., Dugan, E., Delquadri, J., Gershon, B., … Folk, L. (1992). Teaching social skills to students with autism to increase peer interactions in an integrated first grade classroom. *Journal of Applied Behavior Analysis*, *25*, 281–288.

Kamps, D., Mason, R., Thiemann-Bourque, K., Feldmiller, S., Turcotte, A., & Miller, T. (2014). The use of peer networks to increase communicative acts of first grade students with autism spectrum disorders. *Focus on Autism and Other Developmental Disabilities*, *29*, 230–245.

Kamps, D., Potucek, J., Dugan, E., Kravits, T., Gonzalez-Lopez, A., Garcia, J., … Garrison-Kane, L. (2002). Peer training to facilitate social interaction for students with autism. *Exceptional Children*, *68*, 173–187.

Kamps, D., Potucek, J., Gonzalez-Lopez, A., Kravits, T., & Kemmerer, K. (1997). The use of peer networks across multiple settings to improve interaction for students with autism. *Journal of Behavioral Education*, *7*, 335–357.

Kamps, D. M., Leonard, B., Potucek, J., & Garrison-Harrell, L. (1995). Cooperative learning groups in reading: An integration strategy for students with autism and general classroom peers. *Behavioral Disorders*, *21*, 89–109.

Kamps, D., Dugan, E., Potucek, J., & Collins, A. (1999). Effects of cross aged peer tutoring networks among students with autism and general education students. *Journal of Behavioral Education, 9*, 97–115.

Kasari, C., Dean, M., Kretzmann, M., Shih, W., Orlich, F., Whitney, R., … King, B. (2016). Children with autism spectrum disorder and social skills groups at school: A randomized trial comparing intervention approach and peer composition. *Journal of Child Psychology and Psychiatry*, *57*, 171–179.

Kasari, C., Freeman, S., & Paparella, T. (2006). Multiple effects of joint attention intervention for children with autism: A randomized controlled intervention study. *Journal of Child Psychology and Psychiatry*, *47*, 611–620.

Kasari, C., & Lawton, K. (2010). New directions in behavioral treatment of autism spectrum disorders. *Current Opinion in Neurology, 23*(2), 137–143.

Kasari, C., Locke, J., Gulsrud, A., & Rotheram-Fuller, E. (2011). Social networks and friendships at school: Comparing children with and without ASD. *Journal of Autism and Developmental Disorders, 41*(5), 533–544.

Kasari, C., & Patterson, S. (2012). Interventions addressing social impairment in autism. *Current Psychiatry Reports, 14*, 713–725.

Kasari, C., Rotheram-Fuller, E., Locke, J., & Gulsrud, A. (2012). Making the connection: Randomized controlled trial of social skills at school for children with autism spectrum disorders. *Journal of Child Psychology and Psychiatry, 53*, 431–439.

Kasari, C., & Smith, T. (2013). Interventions in schools for children with autism spectrum disorder: Methods and recommendations. *Autism, 17*, 254–267.

Katz, E., & Girolametto, L. (2013). Peer-mediated intervention for preschoolers with ASD implemented in early childhood education settings. *Topics in Early Childhood Special Education, 33*(3), 133–143. doi:10.1177/0271121413484872

Kern, P., & Aldridge, D. (2006). Using embedded music therapy interventions to support outdoor play of young of children with autism in an inclusive community-based child care program. *The Journal of Music Therapy, 43*(4), 270–294.

Koegel, L., Koegel, R., Hurley, C., & Frea, W. (1992). Improving social skills and disruptive behavior in children with autism through self-management. *Journal of Applied Behavior Analysis, 25*, 341–353.

Koegel, L., Matos-Freden, R., Lang, R., & Koegel, R. (2012). Interventions for children with autism spectrum disorders in inclusive school settings. *Cognitive and Behavioral Practice, 19*(4), 401–412.

Koegel, L. K., Koegel, R. L., Harrower, J. K., & Carter, C. M. (1999). Pivotal response intervention I: Overview of approach. *Journal of the Association for Persons with Severe Handicaps, 24*, 174–185.

Koegel, L. K., Kuriakose, S., Singh, A. K., & Koegel, R. L. (2012). Improving generalization of peer socialization gains in inclusive school settings using initiations. *Behavior Modification, 36*(3), 361–377.

Koegel, L. K., Park, M. N., & Koegel, R. L. (2014). Using self-management to improve the reciprocal social conversation of children with autism spectrum disorder. *Journal of Autism and Developmental Disorders, 44*(5), 1055–1063.

Koegel, L. K., Vernon, T. W., Koegel, R. L., Koegel, B. L., & Paullin, A. W. (2012). Improving social engagement and initiations between children with autism spectrum disorder and their peers in inclusive settings. *Journal of Positive Behavior Interventions, 14*, 220–227. doi:10.1177/1098300712437042

Koegel, R., Fredeen, R., Kim, S., Danial, J., Rubinstein, D., & Koegel, L. (2012). Using perseverative interests to improve interactions between adolescents with autism and their typical peers in school settings. *Journal of Positive Behavior Interventions, 14*(3), 133–141.

Koegel, R., Werner, L., Vismara, L. A., & Koegel, L. K. (2005). The effectiveness of contextually supported play date interactions between children with autism and typically developing peers. *Research & Practice for Persons with Severe Disabilities, 30*(2), 93–102.

Kohler, F., Strain, P., Hoyson, M., Davis, L., Donina, W., & Rapp, N. (1995). Using a group-oriented contingency to increase social interactions between children with autism and their peers: A preliminary analysis of corollary supportive behaviors. *Behavior Modification, 19*, 10–32.

Kourassanis, J., Jones, E., & Fienup, D. (2015). Peer-video modeling: Teaching chained social game behaviors to children with ASD. *Journal of Developmental and Physical Disabilities, 27*, 25–36.

Krantz, P., & McClannahan, L. (1998). Social interaction skills for children with autism: A script-fading procedure for beginning reads. *Journal of Applied Behavior Analysis, 31*, 191–202.

Kravits, T., Kamps, D., Carnazzo, K., & Potucek, J. (2002). Increasing communication skills for an elementary-aged student with autism using the picture exchange communication system. *Journal of Autism and Developmental Disabilities, 32*, 225–230.

Lang, R., Kuriakose, S., Lyons, G., Mulloy, A., Boutot, A., Britt, C., … Lancioni, G. (2011). Use of school recess time in the education and treatment of children with autism spectrum disorders: A systematic review. *Research in Autism Spectrum Disorders, 5*, 1296–1305.

Laugeson, E., Ellingsen, R., Sanderson, J., Tucci, L., & Bates, S. (2014). The ABCs of teaching social skills to adolescents with autism spectrum disorder in the classroom: The UCLA PEERS program. *Journal of Autism and Developmental Disorders, 44*, 2244–2256.

Laushey, K. M., & Heflin, L. J. (2000). Enhancing social skills of kindergarten children with autism through the training of multiple peers as tutors. *Journal of Autism and Developmental Disorders, 30*, 183–193.

Ledford, J. R., & Wehby, J. H. (2015). Teaching children with autism in small groups with students who are at-risk for academic problems: Effects on academic and social behaviors. *Journal of Autism and Developmental Disorders, 45*, 1624–1635.

Lee, S., Odom, S. L., & Loftin, R. (2007). Social engagement with peers and stereotypic behavior of children with autism. *Journal of Positive Behavioral Intervention, 9*, 67–79.

Liber, D. B., Frea, W. D., & Symon, J. B. G. (2008). Using time-delay to improve social play skills with peers for children with autism. *Journal of Autism and Developmental Disorders, 38*, 312–323.

Licciardello, C. C., Harchik, A. E., & Luiselli, J. K. (2008). Social skills intervention for children with autism during interactive play at a public elementary school. *Education and Treatment of Children, 31*(1), 27–37.

Locke, J., Rotheram-Fuller, E., & Kasari, C. (2012). Exploring the social impact of being a typical peer model for included children with autism spectrum disorders. *Journal of Autism and Developmental Disorders, 42*, 1895–1905.

Loftin, R. L., Odom, S. L., & Lantz, J. F. (2008). Social interaction and repetitive motor behaviors. *Journal of Autism and Developmental Disorders, 38*, 1124–1135.

Macpherson, K., Charlop, M., & Miltenberger, C. (2015). Using portable video modeling technology to increase the compliment behaviors of children with autism during athletic group play. *Journal of Autism and Developmental Disorders, 45*, 3836–3845.

Mason, R., Kamps, D., Turcotte, A., Cox, S., Feldmiller, S., & Miller, T. (2014). Peer mediated interventions: Increasing communicative acts of students with autism spectrum disorders at recess. *Research in Autism Spectrum Disorders, 8*, 334–344.

Matson, J., Matson, M., & Rivet, T. (2007). Social-skills treatments for children with autism spectrum disorders: An overview. *Behavior Modification, 31*, 682–707.

McFadden, B., Kamps, D., & Heitzman-Powell, L. (2014). Social communication effects of peer-mediated recess intervention for children with autism. *Research in Autism Spectrum Disorders, 8*, 1699–1712.

McGee, G. G., & Daly, T. (2007). Incidental teaching of age appropriate social phrases to children with autism. *Research & Practice for Persons with Severe Disabilities, 32*(2), 112–123.

McGrath, A., Bosch, S., Sullivan, C., & Fuqua, R. (2003). Training reciprocal social interactions between preschoolers and a child with autism. *Journal of Positive Behavior Interventions, 5*, 47–54.

Murdock, L., & Hobbs, J. (2011). Picture me playing: Increasing pretend play dialogue of children with autism spectrum disorders. *Journal of Autism and Developmental Disorders, 41*, 870–878.

Odom, S., Chandler, L., Ostrosky, M., McConnell, S., & Reaney, S. (1992). Fading teacher prompts from peer-initiation interventions for young children with disabilities. *Journal of Applied Behavior Analysis, 25*, 307–317.

Odom, S., & Strain, P. (1984). Peer mediated approaches to promoting children's social interaction: A review. *American Journal of Orthopsychiatry, 54*, 544–557.

Odom, S., & Strain, P. (1986). A comparison of peer-initiation and teacher-antecedent interventions for promoting reciprocal social interaction of autistic preschoolers. *Journal of Applied Behavior Analysis, 19*, 59–71.

Owen-DeSchryver, J. S., Carr, E. G., Cale, S. I., & Blakely-Smith, A. (2008). Promoting social interactions between students with autism spectrum disorders and their peers in inclusive school settings. *Focus on Autism and Other Developmental Disorders, 23*, 15–28.

Parker, D., & Kamps, D. (2011). Effects of task analysis and self-monitoring for children with autism in multiple social settings. *Focus on Autism and Developmental Disorders, 26*, 131–142. doi:10.1177/1088357610376945

Paul, R., Miles Orlovski, S., Chuba Marcinko, H., & Volkmar, F. (2009). Conversational behaviors in youth with high-functioning ASD and Asperger syndrome. *Journal of Autism and Developmental Disorders, 39*, 115–125.

Peck, C. A., Donaldson, J., & Pezzoli, M. (1990). Some benefits nonhandicapped adolescents perceive for themselves from their social relationships with peers who have severe handicaps. *Journal of the Association for Persons with Severe Handicaps, 15*, 241–249.

Peturdottir, A., McComas, J., McMaster, K., & Horner, K. (2007). The effects of scripted peer tutoring and programming common stimuli on social interactions of a student with autism spectrum disorder. *Journal of Applied Behavior Analysis, 40*, 353–357.

Pierce, K., & Schreibman, L. (1995). Increasing complex social behaviors in children with autism: Effects of peer-implemented pivotal response training. *Journal of Applied Behavior Analysis, 28*, 285–295.

Pierce, K., & Schreibman, L. (1997). Multiple peer use of pivotal response training to increase social behaviors of classmates with autism: Results from trained and untrained peers. *Journal of Applied Behavior Analysis, 28*, 285–295.

Rao, P., Beidel, D., & Murray, M. (2008). Social skills interventions for children with Asperger's syndrome or high-functioning autism: A review and recommendations. *Journal of Autism and Developmental Disorders, 38*, 353–361.

Reichow, B., & Sabornie, E. (2009). Brief report: Increasing verbal greeting initiations for a student with autism via a Social Story™ intervention. *Journal of Autism and Developmental Diosorders, 39*, 1740–1743.

Reichow, B., & Volkmar, F. (2010). Social skills interventions for individuals with autism: Evaluation for evidence-based practices within a best evidence synthesis framework. *Journal of Autism and Developmental Disorders, 40*(2), 149–166.

Reichow, B., Volkmar, F., & Cicchetti, D. V. (2008). Development of an evaluative method of determining the strength of research evidence in autism. *Journal of Autism and Developmental Disorders, 38*, 1311–1318.

Reilly, C., Hughes, C., Harvey, M., Brigham, N., Cosgriff, J., Kaplan, L., & Bernstein, R. (2014). "Let's Talk!": Increasing novel peer-directed questions by high school students with autism to their general education peers. *Education and Training in Autism and Developmental Disabilities, 49*(2), 214–231.

Reynolds, B. M., Gast, D. L., & Luscre, D. (2016). Self-management of social initiations by kindergarten students with disabilities in the general education classroom. *Journal of Positive Behavior Interventions, 16*(3), 137–148.

Roeyers, H. (1996). The influence of nonhandicapped peers on the social interactions of children with a pervasive developmental disorder. *Journal of Autism and Developmetal Disorders*, *26*, 303–320.

Sainato, D. M., Goldstein, H., & Strain, P. S. (1992). Effects of self-evaluation on preschool children's use of social interactions strategies with their classmates with autism. *Journal of Applied Behavior Analysis*, *25*, 127–141.

Sansosti, F. J., & Powell-Smith, K. A. (2006). Using Social Stories™ to improve the social behavior of children with Asperger syndrome. *Journal of Positive Behavior Interventions*, *8*(1), 43–57.

Sansosti, F. J., & Powell-Smith, K. A. (2008). Using computer-presented Social Stories™ and video models to increase the social communications skills of children with high-functioning autism spectrum disorders. *Journal of Positive Behavior Interventions*, *10*(3), 162–178.

Sasso, G. M., Mundschenk, N. A., Melloy, K., & Casey, S. (1998). A comparison of the effects of organismic and setting variables on the social interaction behavior of children with developmental disabilities. *Focus on Autism and Other Developmental Disorders*, *13*, 2–16.

Sasso, G. M., & Rude, H. A. (1987). Unprogrammed effects of training high-status peers to interact with severely handicapped children. *Journal of Applied Behavior Analysis*, *20*, 35–44.

Scheeren, A., Koot, H., & Begeer, S. (2012). Social interaction style of children and adolescents with high-functioning autism spectrum. *Journal of Autism and Developmental Disorders*, *42*, 2046–2055.

Schertz, H., Odom, S., Baggett, K., & Sideris, J. (2013). Effects of joint attention mediated learning for toddlers with autism spectrum disorders: An initial randomized controlled study. *Early Childhood Research Quarterly*, *28*, 249–258.

Schleien, S., Mustonen, T., & Rynders, J. (1995). Participation of children with autism and nondisabled peers in a cooperatively structured community art program. *Journal of Autism and Developmental Disorders*, *25*, 397–413.

Schmidt, C., & Stichter, J. (2012). The use of peer-mediated interventions to promote the generalization of social competence for adolescents with high-functioning autism and Asperger's syndrome. *Exceptionality*, *20*, 94–113.

Schneider, N., & Goldstein, H. (2010). Using social stories and visual schedules to improve social appropriate behaviors with children with autism. *Journal of Positive Behavioral Intervention*, *12*, 149–160.

Schohl, K., Van Hecke, A., Carson, A., Dolan, B., Karst, J., & Stevens, S. (2014). A replication and extension of the PEERS intervention: Examining effects on social skills and social anxiety in adolescents with autism spectrum disorders. *Journal of Autism and Developmetal Disorders*, *44*, 532–545.

Sigafoos, J., Green, V., Payne, D., Son, S., O'Reilly, M., & Lancioni, G. (2009). A comparison of picture exchange and speech-generating devices: Acquisition, preference, and effects on social interaction. *AAC: Autmentative and Alternative Communication*, *25*, 99–109.

Simpson, A., Langone, J., & Ayres, K. M. (2004). *Embedded video and computer based instruction to improve social skills and plan for peer social interactions*. Austin, TX: Pro-Ed.

Simpson, L. A., & Bui, Y. (2016). Effects of a peer-mediated intervention on social interactions of students with low-functioning autism and perceptions of typical peers. *Education and Training in Ausitm and Developmental Disabilities*, *51*(2), 162–178.

Solomon, M., Goodlin-Jones, B. L., & Anders, T. F. (2004). A social adjustment enhancement intervention for high functioning autism, Asperger's syndrome, and pervasive developmental disorder NOS. *Journal of Autism and Developmental Disorders*, *34*(6), 649–668.

Sperry, L., Neitzel, J., & Engelhardt-Wells, K. (2010). Peer-mediated instruction and intervention strategies for students with autism spectrum disorders. *Preventing School Failure*, *54*, 256–264.

State, T. M., & Kern, L. (2012). A comparison of video feedback and in vivo self-monitoring on the social interactions of an adolescent with asperger syndrome. *Journal of Behavioral Education*, *21*(1), 18–33.

Stichter, J. P., & Conroy, M. A. (2006). *How to teach social skills and plan for peer social interactions*. Austin, TX: Pro-Ed.

Strain, P., & Bovey, E. (2011). Randomized, controlled trial of the LEAP model of early intervention for young children with autism spectrum disorders. *Topics in Early Childhood Special Education*, *31*, 133–154.

Strasberger, S., & Ferreri, S. (2014). The effects of peer assisted communication application training on the communicative and social behaviors of children with autism. *Journal of Developmental and Physical Disabilities*, *26*, 513–526.

Tager-Flusberg, H., Paul, P., & Lord, C. (2005). Language and communication in autism. In F. R. Volkmar, A. Klin, R. Paul, & D. J. Cohen (Eds.), *Handbook of autism and pervasive developmental disorders* (3rd ed.pp. 335–364). Hoboken, NJ: Wiley.

Taylor, B., Hoch, H., Potter, B., Rodriguez, A., Spinnato, D., & Kalaigian, M. (2005). Manipulating establishing operations to promote initiations toward peers in children with autism. *Research in Developmental Disabilities*, *26*, 385–392.

Tetreault, A., & Lerman, D. (2010). Teaching social skills to child with autism using point-of-view video modeling. *Education and Treatment of Children*, *33*, 395–419.

Thiemann, K., & Goldstein, H. (2004). Effects of peer training and written text cueing on social communication of school-age children with pervasive developmental disorder. *Journal of Speech, Language and Hearing Research*, *47*, 126–144.

Trembath, D., Balandin, S., Togher, L., & Stancliffe, R. J. (2009). Peer-mediated teaching and augmentative and alternative communication for preschool-aged children with autism. *Journal of Intellectual and Developmental Disability*, *34*(2), 173–186.

Trottier, N., Kamp, L., & Mirenda, P. (2011). Effects of peer-mediated instruction to teach use of speech-generating devices to students with autism in social game routines. *Augmentative and Alternative Communication*, *27*, 26–39.

Tsao, L., & Odom, S. (2006). Sibling-mediated social interactions intervention for young children with autism. *Topics in Early Childhood Special Education*, *26*, 106–123.

Tse, J., Strulovitch, J., Tagalakis, V., Meng, L., & Fombonne, E. (2007). Social skills training for adolescents with Asperger syndrome and high-functioning autism. *Journal of Autism and Developmental Disorders*, *37*, 1960–1968.

Walton, K., & Ingersoll, B. (2013). Improving social skills in adolescents and adults with autism and severe to profound intellectual disability: A review of the literature. *Journal of Autism and Developmental Disorders*, *42*, 594–615.

Wang, S., Parrila, R., & Cui, Y. (2012). Meta-analysis of social skills interventions of single-case research for individuals with autism spectrum disorders: Results from three-level HLM. *Journal of Autism and Developmental Disorders*, *43*, 1701–1716.

Watkins, L., O'Reilly, M., Kuhn, M., Gevarter, C., Lancioni, G., Sigafoos, J., & Lang, R. (2015). A review of peer-mediated social interaction interventions for students with autism in inclusive settings. *Journal of Autism and Developmental Disorders*, *45*, 1070–1083.

Whalon, K. J., Conroy, M. A., Martinez, J. R., & Werch, B. L. (2015). School-based peer-related social competence interventions for children with autism spectrum disorder: A meta-analysis and descriptive review of single case research design studies. *Journal of Autism Developmental Disorders*, *45*(6), 1513–1531.

White, S., Ollendick, T., Albano, A., Oswald, D., Johnson, C., Southham-Gerow, M., ... Scahill, L. (2013). Randomized control trial: Multimodal anxiety and social skill intervention for adolescents with autism spectrum disorder. *Journal of Autism and Developmental Disorders*, *43*, 382–394.

White, S. W., Koenig, K., & Scahill, L. (2010). Group social skills instruction for adolescents with high-functioning autism spectrum disorders. *Focus on Autism and Other Developmental Disabilities*, *25*, 209–219.

Wolfberg, P., DeWitt, M., Young, G., & Nguyen, T. (2015). Integrated play groups: Promoting symbolic play and social engagement with typical peers in children with ASD across settings. *Journal of Autism and Developmental Disorders*, *45*, 830–845.

Wolfberg, P., & Schuler, A. L. (1999). Fostering peer interaction, imaginative play and spontaneous language in children with autism. *Child Language Teaching and Therapy*, *15*, 41–52.

Wong, C., Odom, S., Hume, K., Cox, A., Fettig, A., Kucharczyk, S., ... Schultz, T. (2013). *Evidence-based practices for children, youth, and young adults with autism spectrum disorder*. Chapel Hill: The University of North Carolina, Frank Porter Graham Child Development Institute, Autism Evidence-Based Practice Review Group.

Wood, J., Fujii, C., Renno, P., & Van Dyke, M. (2014). Impact of cognitive behavioral therapy on observed autism symptom severity during school recess: A preliminary randomized, controlled trial. *Journal of Autism and Developmental Disorders*, *44*, 2264–2276.

Zagona, A., & Mastergeorge, A. (2016). An empirical review of peer-mediated interventions: Implications for young children with autism spectrum disorders. *Focus on Autism and Other Developmental Disabilities*, *17*, 198–207.

Zanolli, K., Daggett, J., & Adams, T. (1996). Teaching preschool age autistic children to make spontaneous initiations to peers using priming. *Journal of Autism and Developmental Disorders*, *269*(4), 407–422.

Zhang, J., & Wheeler, J. J. (2011). A meta-analysis of peer-mediated interventions for young children with autism spectrum disorders. *Education and Training in Autism and Developmental Disabilities*, *46*, 61–77.

Parent-Mediated Interventions for Social Communication in Young Children with ASD

17

Karis A. Casagrande and Brooke R. Ingersoll

17.1 Introduction

Autism spectrum disorder (ASD) is a lifelong, neurodevelopmental disability that is characterized by deficits in social communication and interaction, as well as by restricted and repetitive patterns of behaviors and interests (American Psychiatric Association, 2013). Social communication refers to both the verbal and nonverbal behaviors used to initiate and respond to social interactions. Deficits in early nonverbal social communication skills, such as gestures, social imitation, joint attention, and symbolic play, are some of the earliest emerging symptoms of ASD (Landa, Holman, & Garrett-Mayer, 2007; Mundy & Crowson, 1997; Woods & Wetherby, 2003; Zwaigenbaum, Bryson, & Garon, 2013). In addition, they are related to the development of more complex social, language, and cognitive skills (e.g., Mundy & Crowson, 1997; Werner, Dawson, Munson, & Osterling, 2005), making them an important target of early intervention.

In addition to their impact on child outcomes, social communication deficits are related to parent well-being in a number of ways. Increasing social communication and language skills has been found to reduce challenging behaviors for children with ASD (e.g., Carr & Durand, 1985; Koegel, Koegel, & Surratt, 1992), which are one of the strongest predictors of parent stress (Lecavalier, Leone, & Wiltz, 2006). Social deficits also contribute to the increased stress profile seen among parents of children with ASD compared to other developmental disabilities (Baker-Ericzén, Brookman-Frazee, & Stahmer, 2005; Davis & Carter, 2008). Parents have also expressed that the combination of challenging behaviors and lack of social responsiveness in ASD can lead to difficulty in developing strong bonds with their children (e.g., Hoppes & Harris, 1990). Furthermore, the severity of the social deficits in ASD is closely related to family functioning more broadly (Herring et al., 2006), indicating a unique and complex profile of family and child needs to be addressed. As a result, best practice guidelines in early intervention for children with ASD emphasize the need for parent involvement in comprehensive interventions that address social communication skills (e.g., Maglione, Gans, Das, Timbie, & Kasari, 2012; Schreibman et al., 2015; Zwaigenbaum et al., 2015).

There are many different ways to involve parents in the education of their child. Parent-mediated intervention, or PMI, is a specific form of parent involvement that provides systematic training in intervention strategies to help a parent accomplish specific goals or outcomes for their

K.A. Casagrande (✉) • B.R. Ingersoll
Department of Psychology, Michigan State University, East Lansing, MI, USA
e-mail: casagra3@msu.edu

J.B. Leaf (ed.), *Handbook of Social Skills and Autism Spectrum Disorder*, Autism and Child Psychopathology Series, DOI 10.1007/978-3-319-62995-7_17

child (Bearss, Burrell, Stewart, & Scahill, 2015). PMI is used in the treatment of a variety of childhood disorders and is typically focused on helping parents manage their child's behavior, improve the parent-child relationship, and increase specific developmental skills in the child. PMI can be used in combination with direct intervention, but it can also be considered a primary intervention strategy in its own right, particularly in the treatment of very young children. In this chapter, we will focus on parent-mediated interventions that target the development of social communication skills for young children with ASD. We begin by exploring the rationale for the use of parent-mediated intervention in the treatment of social communication deficits for young children with ASD. Next, we summarize the research on current parent-mediated social communication interventions and provide guidelines for researchers and practitioners in evaluating these interventions. Finally, we describe future directions for the field.

17.2 Rationale for Parent-Mediated Interventions

The importance of teaching parents to serve as intervention agents for their children with ASD was first highlighted by Lovaas, Koegel, Simmons, and Long (1973). They noted that children with ASD who received intensive early behavioral intervention, and returned to a home in which the parents were trained to carry out the intervention themselves, maintained their treatment gains, whereas children who returned to institutionalized settings that did not carry over the treatment methods lost the skills that they had acquired. Teaching parents to utilize intervention techniques is also associated with increased skill generalization. For example, one early study (i.e., Koegel, Schreibman, Britten, Burke, & O'Neill, 1982) compared the effects of training parents to implement behavior therapy with their child to therapist-implemented intervention. Although children in both groups made similar gains during treatment, children in the parent training group were more likely to respond appropriately to parent questions and directions during unstructured observations in the home.

Since these observations, a number of controlled studies have demonstrated that parents can learn to implement a range of evidence-based intervention strategies with a high degree of fidelity (e.g., Aldred, Green, & Adams, 2004; Kaiser & Roberts, 2013; Koegel, Bimbela, & Schreibman, 1996; Mahoney & Perales, 2003) and that the use of these strategies results in increased use of language targets (Kaiser & Roberts, 2013), vocabulary (Ingersoll, Wainer, Berger, Pickard, & Bonter, 2016; McConachie, Randle, Hammal, & Le Couteur, 2005), and developmental language level (Schertz, Odom, Baggett, & Sideris, 2013; Wetherby et al., 2014), as well as improved joint attention (Casenhiser, Shanker, & Stieben, 2013; Kasari, Gulsrud, Wong, Kwon, & Locke, 2010), imitation (Ozonoff & Cathcart, 1998; Vismara et al., 2016), play skills (Kaiser & Roberts, 2013; Kasari, Gulsrud, Paparella, Hellemann, & Berry, 2015), symptom severity (Aldred, Green, Emsley, & McConachie, 2012; Solomon, Van Egeren, Mahoney, Huber, & Zimmerman, 2014), and social-emotional functioning (Mahoney & Perales, 2003, 2005) for their child with ASD.

PMI also has the potential to greatly increase treatment intensity compared to direct service delivery models. While early intensive intervention results in the most optimal outcomes (Dawson, 2008), the majority of children with ASD receive services through the school system and not through outside early intervention sources (Bilaver, Cushing, & Cutler, 2016). Additionally, over 90% of children in Bilaver et al. (2016) survey received no intensive intervention services prior to or during preschool. Given the high number of recommended hours of intervention for young children with ASD (25 h/week, Myers & Johnson, 2007), training parents allows for increased therapeutic contact throughout a child's day and greatly increases the number of early intervention hours a child receives. This model can also greatly increase the reach of professionals in providing support for families and children with ASD, as it requires fewer hours of direct contact with families. For example, parents of children with pervasive and developmental disabilities who were given 1 h of instruction in responsive teaching (RT) reported using the intervention techniques for an average of 15 h/week (Mahoney & Perales, 2005) allowing professionals to serve a greater number of families.

PMI can also reduce a number of other barriers that parents of children with ASD face in obtaining services. For example, parents of children with ASD may have difficulty transporting their child to appointments (Zeman, Swanke, & Doktor, 2011), experience high out-of-pocket costs for care (Järbrink, Fombonne, & Knapp, 2003), and often miss work or experience a loss of income (Montes & Halterman, 2008) with clinic-based services. PMI can be implemented within the home or remotely at the parent's convenience and requires fewer hours of professional contact, reducing these barriers. PMI also has the capacity to increase access to services and to reach underserved communities where intensive intervention service providers may not be available to meet the needs of the community (Meadan, Meyer, Snodgrass, & Halle, 2013; Suppo & Floyd, 2012). In addition to increasing access to care, PMIs have the potential to reduce overall cost of care when used as early interventions (e.g., Chasson, Harris, & Neely, 2007).

Finally, although the emphasis of PMI has been on improving child outcomes and improving access to care, there has been an increasing focus on its impact on broader family functioning (Karst & Van Hecke, 2012; Strauss et al., 2012; Wainer, Hepburn, & Griffith, 2016). Parents of children with ASD generally experience increased stress, decreased self-efficacy, poor family relationships, and a higher rate of mental health issues compared to parents of children with other developmental disabilities (see Karst & Van Hecke, 2012 for a review), suggesting the increased need for intervention packages that address family-level functioning. Training parents in intervention techniques has been shown to improve both parent mental health and the quality of parent-child interactions, resulting in more positive family interactions (Koegel et al., 1996; Strauss et al., 2012; Webster, Feiler, Webster, & Lovell, 2004). Parents participating in PMI have experienced increased positive perceptions of their child, increased confidence and self-efficacy, and decreased stress (Coolican, Smith, & Bryson, 2010; Estes et al., 2014; Ingersoll et al., 2016; Turner-Brown, Hume, Boyd, & Kainz, 2016). Further, parents who participate in parent training programs report more optimism about their own ability to influence their child's development (Koegel et al., 1982), which may help parents maintain their efforts with their child over time (NRC, 2001).

17.3 Current Research on Parent-Mediated Social Communication Interventions for Children with ASD

Although the rationale for parent-mediated social communication interventions is strong, its evidence base is somewhat less clear. A number of single-case design studies and randomized controlled trials have demonstrated positive effects of PMI on child social communication and parent outcomes, leading a number of technical review panels to conclude that PMI is an evidence-based intervention practice for children with ASD, including the National Research Council (NRC, 2001), National Standards Project (NSP; Wilczynski et al., 2009), Autism Intervention Research Network on Behavioral Health (AIR-B; Maglione et al., 2012), and National Professional Development Center for ASD (NPDC-ASD; Wong et al., 2015). At the same time, there have been several recent RCTs that have found either modest or null effects of PMI on child outcomes (e.g., Carter et al., 2011; Rogers, Estes et al., 2012; Turner-Brown et al., 2016), and two recent systematic reviews were unable to draw strong conclusions about the overall effectiveness of PMI for improving children's social communication skills given limits in methodology and high variability across studies (Beaudoin, Sébire, & Couture, 2014; Oono, Honey, & McConachie, 2013). Differences in conclusions between systematic reviews are primarily related to review methodology. For example, several reviews which report consistent positive findings focus primarily on single-subject designs evaluating PMIs for social communication skills (Lang, Machalicek, Rispoli, & Regester, 2009; Meadan, Ostrosky, Zaghlawan, & Yu, 2009; Patterson, Smith, & Mirenda, 2012), whereas reviews reporting mixed findings focused exclusively on randomized controlled trials of more broad PMIs (Beaudoin et al., 2014; Oono et al., 2013). Given the variability in findings, it is important to consider important factions that may impact the effectiveness of PMI for improving child social communication skills and family functioning. Below we consider four such factors: the intervention approach taught to parents, the social communication skills targeted, the format and intensity of the parent training model, and parent variables that may influence outcomes.

Table 17.1 presents an overview of 14 PMIs for young children with ASD that address social communication as a primary target of intervention; the table includes a brief description of the intervention approach, training format, and suggested intensity. We included only studies in which there was a detailed intervention description or manual, two or more peer-reviewed publications per intervention package, and at least one experimental study for each intervention. Table 17.2 breaks down the evidence base for each intervention package, summarizing the study design and outcomes.

17.3.1 Intervention Approach

PMIs follow a wide range of theoretical approaches, drawing from behavioral, naturalistic, and developmental traditions. Developmental approaches to intervention are based on research indicating that children develop social communication within the context of socially meaningful, affect-laden, and child-directed interactions (e.g., Bruner, 1983; Gerber, 2003; Prizant & Wetherby, 1998). Half of PMIs for social communication included in Table 17.1 fit into this category, including but not limited to Hanen's More than Words (HMW; Sussman, 2012), Play and Language for Autistic Youngsters (PLAY Project; Solomon et al., 2014), Preschool Autism Communication Trial (PACT; Green et al., 2010), and responsive teaching (RT; Mahoney & MacDonald, 2007). Generally, these developmental interventions focus on improving the parent-child relationship and increasing parental responsivity to communicative attempts from the child, which provides more subtle opportunities for skill development. Common techniques in developmental interventions include using extended wait time, contingent imitation, and environmental arrangement to evoke more complex skills, rather than the structured prompts seen in behavioral approaches. Additionally, all developmental interventions in Table 17.2 include the use of video review to help parents identify communication cues from their child that they may have missed during live interactions.

A newer class of intervention, Naturalistic Developmental Behavioral Intervention (NDBI), has blended behavioral, naturalistic, and developmental strategies given the number of elements shared across approaches (see Schreibman et al., 2015 for a review). NDBIs comprise the second half of the PMIs seen in Table 17.1. Pivotal Response Training (PRT; Koegel et al., 1989), Parent-Implemented Enhanced Milieu training (P-EMT, Kaiser et al., 2007), and Parent-implemented Early Start Denver Model (P-ESDM; Rogers, Dawson et al., 2012) were some of the earlier models. More recent NDBIs include the Early Social Interaction Parent-Implemented Intervention (ESI-PII; Wetherby & Woods, 2006), Project ImPACT (Ingersoll & Dvortcsak, 2010), and JASPER (Kasari et al., 2010).

In contrast to traditional behavioral approaches where teaching occurs in a structured learning environment, teaching episodes in NDBIs are chosen based on the child's interests and occur in naturalistic settings, such as routines and play. While the learning environment is loosely structured and child driven, teaching opportunities follow the behavioral tradition of explicit prompting and contingent reinforcement. Additionally, reinforcements in NDBIs are a natural

Table 17.1 Overview of parent-mediated social communication interventions for young children with ASD

Intervention	Detailed description	Brief description	Approach	Format	Suggested dosage	Suggested practice
Early Social Interaction Parent-Implemented Intervention (ESI-PII)	Wetherby and Woods (2006)	Modified version of the SCERTS curriculum designed to teach toddlers social communication, play, and emotion regulation	NDBI	Individual and group parent-child sessions (or group-only format)	Biweekly individual sessions and nine group sessions over 9–12 months (group format is one weekly session over 9 months)	25 h/week
Family Implemented TEACCH for Toddlers (FITT)	Turner-Brown et al. (2016)	Modified version of the TEACCH model to support development of language, social communication, and play in toddler at risk for ASD	Eclectic	20 individual parent-child sessions and 4 small group parent-only sessions	24 weekly 1.5-h sessions	*Not specified*
Focused Playtime Intervention (FPI)	Siller, Hutman, and Sigman (2013): supplemental materials	Intervention aimed at increasing child language through increased responsive parental communication	Developmental	Individual parent-child sessions	12 weekly 1.5-h sessions over 3 months	Daily (no specific amount)
Hanen's More than Words (HMW)	Sussman (2012); Girolametto, Sussman, and Weitzman (2007): Appendix A	Teaches increased parental responsiveness and sensitivity during everyday routines in order to foster the development of social communication, imitation, and play.	Developmental	Eight group parent-only sessions with three individual parent-child sessions	11 weekly 2.5-h group and 1.5-h individual sessions	*Not specified*
Improving Parents As Communication Teachers (Project ImPACT)	Ingersoll and Dvortcsak (2010)	Intervention designed to target social engagement, language, imitation, and play through a blend of developmental and naturalistic behavioral techniques	NDBI	Individual parent-child sessions (or group format)	24 biweekly 1-h sessions (group format is three weekly 3-h sessions and six weekly 45-min sessions)	30 min/day

(continued)

Table 17.1 (continued)

Intervention	Detailed description	Brief description	Approach	Format	Suggested dosage	Suggested practice
Milton and Ethel Harris Research Initiative Treatment (MEHRIT)	Casenhiser et al. (2013)	Intervention designed to increase social interaction and communication following the guidelines of the DIR model	Developmental	Individual parent-child sessions	Weekly 2-h sessions over 12 months	3 h/day
Parent-implemented Early Start Denver Model (P-ESDM)	Rogers, Dawson, and Vismara (2012)	Integrates developmental, naturalistic, and behavioral methods to increase parental responsivity and improve child social communication and other developmental skills	NDBI	Individual parent-child sessions	12 weekly 1-h sessions	Not a requirement
Parent-Implemented Enhanced Milieu Training (EMT)	Kaiser, Hancock, and Trent (2007)	Naturalistic intervention designed to teach language using the child's interests and initiations in everyday contexts	NDBI	Individual parent-child sessions	24 biweekly 30-min sessions	*Not specified*
Parent-Implemented Joint Attention, Symbolic Play, Engagement, and Regulation (P-JASPER)	Kasari et al. (2010): Appendix A	Naturalistic, developmental intervention targeting foundational social communication skills including joint attention, imitation, gesture, and play	NDBI	Individual parent-child sessions	24 biweekly 45-min sessions	*Not specified*
Pivotal Response Training (PRT; previously Natural Language Paradigm, NLP)	Koegel et al. (1989), Koegel, Koegel, Bruinsma, Brookman, and Fredeen (2003)	Naturalistic intervention to create child change by targeting pivotal areas of development such as motivation, responsivity, self-management, and social initiation	NDBI	Individual parent-child sessions (or group format)	Highly flexible (intensive: five daily 5-h sessions over 1 week; conventional, twelve weekly 1-h sessions; self-directed, ten 1-h lessons)	*Not specified*

Intervention	Detailed description	Brief description	Approach	Format	Suggested dosage	Suggested practice
Play and Language for Autistic Youngsters (PLAY project)	Solomon et al. (2014)	Improving parent-child interactions, social-emotional development, and other core symptoms of ASD using the DIR framework	Developmental	Group workshop and individual parent-child sessions	1-day introductory workshop or 2-h DVD; 3-h monthly parent-child sessions for 12 months	2 h/day
Preschool Autism Communication Trial (PACT; previously Child's Talk)	Green et al. (2010): supplemental materials	Targets social communication and interaction through modifications to parent's communication and interaction style	Developmental	Individual parent-child sessions	Biweekly 2-h sessions over 6 months and bi-monthly session for additional 6 months	30 min/day
Responsive teaching (RT)	Mahoney and MacDonald (2007)	Relationship-focused intervention to increase pivotal behaviors (such as initiation, affect, joint attention) through increased parental responsiveness	Developmental	Individual parent-child sessions	Weekly 1-h sessions over 12 months	*Not specified*
Joint Attention Mediated Learning (JAML)	Schertz (2005)	Developmentally grounded intervention to improve social competencies in toddlers through a focus on joint attention skills	Developmental	Individual parent-child sessions	15 weekly sessions of unknown length	30–60 min daily

Table 17.2 Evidence base for current parent-mediated social communication interventions for children with ASD

Intervention	Evidence base	Study design	Parent outcomes	Child outcomes	Parent fidelity posttreatment
ESI-PII	Wetherby et al. (2014)	RA: individual versus group ESI	*Not reported*	Increased social communication (CSBS), language (VABS and MSEL), daily living skills (VABS); no group differences in autism severity (ADOS), motor skills (VABS), or nonverbal cognition (MSEL)	*Not reported*
	Wetherby and Woods (2006)	QE: ESI versus TAU	*Not reported*	Increased nonverbal cognition (MSEL) adaptive skills (VABS); improved social signals, rate of communication, communicative functions, and understanding (CSBS-DP); no group difference in communicative means or actions to others (CSBS DP)	*Not reported*
FITT	Turner-Brown et al. (2016)	RA: FITT versus TAU	Decreased parental distress and overall stress (PSI); improved social functioning, role functioning, and vitality (RAND); no change in dysfunctional parent-child interactions or perception of child as difficult (PSI) or parent mental health (RAND)	Increased imitation (PIA-CV); no change in cognition (MSEL ELC), understanding, social reciprocity, nonverbal communication (PIA-CV)	Majority within 70–96% fidelity
	Welterlin, Turner-Brown, Harris, Mesibov, and Delmolino (2012)	QE: FITT versus TAU	*No change in parental stress (PSI)*	*Increase in overall cognition (MSEL), expressive language (SIB-R/MSEL), social interaction (SIB-R), and comprehension (SIB-R), but not different from waitlist control*	*Not reported*

Intervention	Evidence base	Study design	Parent outcomes	Child outcomes	Parent fidelity posttreatment
	Ozonoff and Cathcart (1998)	QE: FITT versus TAU	*Not reported*	Improved imitation, motor skills, overall cognition (PEP-R); no change in perception or verbal cognition (PEP-R)	*Not reported*
FPI	Siller, Swanson, Gerber, Hutman, and Sigman (2014)	*Additional analysis of Siller, Hutman* et al. *(2013)*	*Reported in Siller, Hutman* et al. *(2013)*	Increased perception (MPAC) and observation (average PCSB/AB) of child attachment; no data reported for cognition (MSEL) or social communication (ESCS)	*Not reported*
	Kasari, Siller et al. (2014)	RA: FPI versus social-emotional intervention (CSEFEL)	Increased parent responsivity (PCX observation coding); no moderation of parental responsiveness (PCX) on child outcomes (MSEL/ESCS)	*Improvement, but no group differences for overall cognition or subscales (MSEL), no change in joint attention (ESCS)*	*Not reported*
	Siller, Hutman et al. (2013)	RA: FPI and parent education (PAC) versus community services and parent education (PAC)	Increased maternal synchronization (PCX), effects moderated by maternal insightfulness (IA)	*Reported in* Siller et al. (2014)	*Not reported*
HMW	Carter et al. (2011)	RA: Hanen versus TAU	No significant change (but a large effect size) for parental responsivity (PCFP)	*Gains in child communication (PIA-CV) moderated by object interest (DPA); no change in child communication (PIA-CV) or joint attention (ESCS)*	*Not reported*
	Girolametto et al. (2007)	SS: baseline	Increased responsivity (PCX) and use of strategies (JAFA)	Increased vocabulary (CDI and observation coding), social engagement (PCX); mixed results for social initiation (PCX)	12.5–33 (max 36)

(continued)

Table 17.2 (continued)

Intervention	Evidence base	Study design	Parent outcomes	Child outcomes	Parent fidelity posttreatment
	McConachie et al. (2005)	RA: Hanen versus TAU	Increased use of facilitative strategies (JAFA); no change in parental stress (QRS-F) or adaptation (PFQ)	Increase in vocabulary size (MCDI); no change in child behavior problems (BSQ) or social communication (ADOS)	*Average not reported*
ImPACT	Ingersoll et al. (2016)	RA: self-directed versus therapist-assisted ImPACT	Increased use of strategies (fidelity); improvements, but no group difference in self-efficacy (PSOC) or stress (FIQ)	Increased language (PCX, MCDI); no change in adaptive skills (VABS)	3.39 (max 5)
	Stadnick, Stahmer, and Brookman-Frazee (2015)	RA: ImPACT versus TAU	Increased intervention adherence (parent fidelity of implementation); no change in parental stress (PSI) or depression (CES-D)	Increased child communication (VABS-II), increased socialization moderated by lower levels of parental stress (VABS)	4.0 (max 5)
	Ingersoll and Wainer (2013)	SS: baseline	Increased use of strategies (parent fidelity of implementation)	Increased spontaneous language (frequency count) moderated by parent's use of strategies (parent fidelity of implementation)	3.6 (max 5)
JAML	Schertz et al. (2013)	RA: JAML versus TAU	*Not reported*	Increased focus on faces, response to joint attention (PCX), receptive language (MSEL), and communication (VABS); no group differences in turn-taking, initiation of joint attention (PCX), expressive language (MSEL)	*Not reported*
	Schertz and Odom (2007)	SS: baseline	*Not reported*	Increased looks to face, turn-taking, response to joint attention, and initiation of joint attention (PCX)	*Not reported*

Intervention	Evidence base	Study design	Parent outcomes	Child outcomes	Parent fidelity posttreatment
MEHRIT	Casenhiser, Binns, McGill, Morderer, and Shanker (2015)	*Reanalysis of* Casenhiser et al. (2013)	*Reported in* Casenhiser et al. (2013)	Increased mean length utterances, frequency of communicative acts, response to questions, and contingent response (PCX); no change in response to comments (PCX)	*Reported in* Casenhiser et al., 2013
	Casenhiser et al. (2013)	RA: MEHRIT versus TAU	Increased use of strategies (MEHRIT Fidelity scale)	*Increased attention to activity, involvement, joint attention, and enjoyment in interaction (mCBRS); no group differences on language (PLS-IV, CASL) or compliance (mCBRS)*	*Average not reported*
P-ESDM	Vismara et al. (2016)	RA: P-ESDM telehealth versus TAU with information support	Increased use of strategies (P-ESDM parent fidelity tool)	Increased imitation (PCX); no change in joint attention or spontaneous language (PCX)	9 out of 14 parents met criteria
	Rogers, Estes et al. (2012)	RA: P-ESDM versus TAU	Stronger working alliance (WASIC); no group differences in parent use of strategies (P-ESDM parent fidelity tool)	Increased vocabulary (MCDI); no other group differences in child outcomes (ADOS, MSEL, VABS, SCL-90-R)	45.2 (max 60)
	Vismara, Colombi, and Rogers (2009)	SS: baseline	Increased use of strategies (P-ESDM Fidelity scale)	Increased imitation, spontaneous utterances (PCX), increased attention and social initiation (CBRS)	Seven out of eight parents met criteria of 85%
	Vismara and Rogers (2008)	SS: baseline	Increased use of strategies (P-ESDM Fidelity scale)	Increased imitation, spontaneous utterances (PCX), increased attention and social initiation (CBRS)	89– 96% fidelity
P-EMT	Kaiser and Roberts (2013)	RA: EMT parent and therapist versus EMT therapist only	Increased use of strategies (parent implementation tool)	Increased use of language target, length of utterances, and play activities (PCX); no other changes in language (PPVT, EVT, PLS, MCDI)	Average not reported

(continued)

Table 17.2 (continued)

Intervention	Evidence base	Study design	Parent outcomes	Child outcomes	Parent fidelity posttreatment
	Kaiser, Hancock, and Nietfeld (2000)	SS: baseline	Increased use of strategies (parent implementation tool)	Increased social communication (PCX); mixed results for improved language (SICD, PPVT, EOWPVT)	Five out of six parents met criteria
P-Jasper	Kasari et al. (2015)	RA: P-JASPER versus psychoeducation (PEI)	*No change stress related to parental functioning and reduction in child-related stress for control group (PSI)*	Increased time of joint engagement (PCX and classroom observation), more functional play (PCX); no group differences in initiation of joint attention, symbolic play (PCX), or language (Reynell)	*Not reported*
	Kasari, Lawton et al. (2014)	RA: P-JASPER individual versus parent-only group	*No group difference in adherence (diary) or involvement (CQI)*	Increased joint attention (PCX), increased initiation (ESCS); no change in play behaviors (SPA)	4.28 (max 5)
	Kasari et al. (2010)	RA: P-JASPER versus TAU	*Not reported*	More joint engagement, functional play acts, and response to joint attention (mediated by caregiver involvement quality), less object-focused play (PCX); no group difference in other engagement, initiation of joint attention, diversity of symbolic play (PCX)	Adherence 3.97 and competence 4.35 (max 5)
PRT	Brian, Smith, Zwaigenbaum, Roberts, and Bryson (2015)	QE: pre-post-comparison of adapted PRT for infants and toddlers	Increased provided language opportunities (PCX); no change in parent positive affect (PCX)	Increased language (MSEL), orienting to caregiver, responsivity, initiation, and functional verbal utterances (PCX); no change in positive affect (PCX)	84.3% fidelity
	Minjarez, Williams, Mercier, and Hardan (2011)	SS: baseline (group format)	Increased use of strategies (PCX)	Increased functional verbal utterances (PCX)	24.24 (max 30)

Intervention	Evidence base	Study design	Parent outcomes	Child outcomes	Parent fidelity posttreatment
	Coolican et al. (2010)	SS: baseline	Increased use of strategies (PCX); no change in perceived self-efficacy (PSES)	Increased functional and responsive utterances (PCX), decreased disruptive behavior (PCX); no change in language (PLS-4, PPVT-III)	Five out of eight parents met criteria of 75% fidelity
	Nefdt, Koegel, Singer, and Gerber (2010)	RA: self-directed PRT versus TAU	Increased use of strategies, provided language opportunities, and confidence (PCX)	Increased use of functional language (PCX)	75% fidelity
	Gillett and LeBlanc (2007)	SS: baseline	Increased use of strategies (PCX)	Increased prompted and spontaneous language (PCX), increased appropriate play (PCX); no change in inappropriate play (PCX)	95–100% fidelity
	Koegel, Symon, and Koegel (2002)	SS: baseline	Increased use of strategies, increased positive affect (PCX)	Increase language stage production (PCX)	80–100% fidelity
PLAY project	Solomon et al. (2014)	RA: PLAY versus TAU	Increased parent interaction (MBRS), decreased depression classification (CES-D); no group difference in parent stress (PSI)	Decreased symptom severity (ADOS-G), increased attention, initiation (CBRS), and social/pragmatic development (FEAS); no change in developmental level (MSEL) or language (MCDI)	*Not reported*
	Solomon, Necheles, Ferch, and Bruckman (2007)	QE: pre-post-comparison	*No change in parent social/pragmatic behavior (FEAS)*	Increased social/pragmatic development (FEAS) and functional development (FDL)	85% of families met criteria
PACT	Aldred et al. (2012)	*Mediational analysis of* Aldred et al. (2004)	Reported in Aldred et al. (2004)	Reduced symptom severity (ADOS) mediated by increased parental synchrony	*Not reported*

(continued)

Table 17.2 (continued)

Intervention	Evidence base	Study design	Parent outcomes	Child outcomes	Parent fidelity posttreatment
	Green et al. (2010)	RA: PACT versus TAU	Increased parental synchrony (PCX); no change in time spent in shared attention (PCX)	Increased child initiations (PCX), social communication (CSBS-DP), and language (MCDI); no group difference in symptom severity (ADOS-G) or adaptive functioning (VABS)	*Not reported*
	Aldred et al. (2004)	RA: PACT versus TAU	Increased parental synchrony (PCX); no change in parent stress (PSI)	Reduced symptom severity (ADOS), increased expressive language (MCDI), increased communicative acts (PCX); no group difference in adaptive behavior (VABS)	*Not reported*
RT	Baranek et al. (2015)	RA: adapted RT versus TAU with additional support	Less directive maternal interaction style (MBRS); no change on maternal responsiveness (MBRS)	Improved receptive language (MSEL), increased symbolic communication (CSBS-caregiver), decreased sensory hyporesponsivity (SEQ), increased hyperresponsivity (SEQ); increased socialization and communication (VABS); no change on expressive language (MSEL); sensory processing (SPA)	73–97% fidelity

Intervention	Evidence base	Study design	Parent outcomes	Child outcomes	Parent fidelity posttreatment
	Mahoney and Perales (2005)	QE: RT for ASD versus DD	Increased parental responsiveness and affect (MBRS); no group differences in directiveness or achievement orientation (MBRS)	Increased pivotal behaviors (CBRS), receptive language, object relations (TBPA), self-regulation (ITSEA), and temperament (TABS); no group differences in symbolic behavior, expressive language (TBPA), social competence, internalizing problems, externalizing problems (ITSEA), or hypersensitivity (TABS)	*Not reported*
	Mahoney and Perales (2003)	QE: pre-post-design	Increased parental responsiveness and affect (MBRS); no change in directiveness or achievement orientation (MBRS)	Improved social-emotional functioning (TABS, ITSEA) moderated by maternal responsiveness (MBRS)	

Study Design: RA random assignment, *QE* quasi-experimental, *SS* single-subject, *TAU* treatment as usual consequence of the interaction, meaning that the reinforcing item or activity is a logical response to the child's behavior, as opposed to being unrelated to the targeted response (Delprato, 2001). Treatment goals are socially meaningful and developmentally appropriate, targeting key foundation skills based on the individual's current developmental profile and trajectory as is common in developmental interventions. One of the greatest differences in developmental approaches and NDBIs is that developmental approaches do not include any direct prompting and, instead, interactions are wholly child driven. NDBIs attempt to balance adult-directed teaching opportunities with responsiveness and child-directed activities to increase motivation and learning; the primary difference across NDBIs is in how these components are balanced. NDBIs are particularly well suited for use by parents, especially those with young children, as they can be used to build a variety of skills, can be tailored to the individual parent and child context, and reflect many of the best practice guidelines for parent involvement in treatment.

The only intervention approach included in Table 17.1 that cannot be easily categorized according to the above guidelines is Family Implemented TEACCH for Toddlers (FITT; Turner-Brown et al., 2016). While FITT does have elements of behavioral, naturalistic, and developmental interventions, it is based on the traditional structured TEACCH model (Mesibov, Shea, & Schopler, 2005), which is an integrative approach designed originally for use in the classroom. Unlike the above models, TEACCH is not a curriculum that covers specific skills. Instead, it provides a framework of teaching techniques to support educational and therapeutic goals. A large portion of the focus is on organizing space and using visual materials to facilitate learning across topics. However, FITT does focus on early social communication skills, including language, play, and joint engagement as these are common core deficits in young children with ASD.

Despite strong theoretical support for each approach, the variations across these paradigms have a number of potential consequences to consider. Two such factors are related to the active ingredients and acceptability of each intervention paradigm. Active ingredients refer to the specific components of a treatment that are responsible for improvement in targeted skills. While parents and providers often agree about important guiding principles of intervention for children with ASD, such as individualized programming, collaboration, and the use of evidence-based strategies (e.g., Callahan, Henson, & Cowan, 2008), there has been little focus in autism intervention on identifying which particular techniques and strategies are responsible for change across a wide variety of comprehensive intervention packages (e.g., Pellecchia et al., 2015). This can make it difficult to make decisions between more complex, comprehensive interventions which have a number of potential active ingredients, versus those that choose to focus on a reduced number of techniques. Given the lack of consistent evidence in choosing intervention components, it may be more important to assess the fit of the individual components to family and child needs. Treatment components that are viewed as acceptable by parents are more likely to be used than components which are viewed as less acceptable (e.g., Bowker, D'Angelo, Hicks, & Wells, 2011; Calvert & McMahon, 1987). One potential solution to address active ingredients and treatment fit is to utilize a modular approach, which relies on breaking complex treatments down into their simpler parts (e.g., Chorpita, Daleiden, & Weisz, 2005; Chorpita & Weisz, 2009). A modular approach allows for testing of individual intervention components for active ingredients. Furthermore, selection of modules can be individualized based on child and family needs.

17.3.2 Intervention Targets and Measurement

Even within interventions targeting social communication, the way that social communication is defined varies widely. Social communication covers a broad range of abilities, including expressive and receptive language, joint attention, social imitation, engagement, and symbolic play.

While some interventions focus only on specific subtypes of social communication, such as joint attention (Joint Attention Mediated Learning; Schertz & Odom, 2007) or social imitation (Reciprocal Imitation Training; Ingersoll, 2008), other interventions take a more comprehensive approach, addressing multiple components of social communication throughout the program. For example, JASPER (Kasari et al., 2010), Project ImPACT (Ingersoll & Dvortcsak, 2010), and the Early Start Denver Model (Rogers, Dawson et al., 2012) all target engagement, communication, imitation, and play. However, it is unclear what skills are most important to target. For example, Reed (2016) reviewed the cognitive, communicative, and adaptive outcomes across a wide variety of PMI; he found that both comprehensive programs, such as ESDM and SCERTS, and specific programs, such as those focusing only on imitation, joint attention, or play, all related to strong and moderate child change across domains.

The way that outcomes are measured also has a significant impact on the conclusions that can be drawn regarding treatment effectiveness (Matson, 2007). While expressive and receptive language are the most consistent social communication variables used across intervention studies (Luyster, Kadlec, Carter, & Tager-Flusberg, 2008), this is not the case for other social communication skills, such as joint attention, engagement, play, and imitation (Fletcher-Watson & McConachie, 2015). While some studies of PMI utilize standardized observational assessments to assess social communication, such as the Early Social Communication Scales (ESCS; Mundy et al., 2003), most rely on semi-structured parent-child interactions and coding schemes developed specifically for that studyIt is important to note that studies that utilize standardized observational assessments are less likely to identify significant child change in social communication compared to those using a parent-child interaction, even within a single study. For example, Kaiser and Roberts (2013) found improvements in the use of language targets and utterance length during parent-child interactions, but did not find significant change on standardized assessments of language. This discrepancy in how outcomes are measured has led to more recent initiatives to develop consistent measures of social communication change to be used in intervention studies. One such initiative is the development of the Brief Observation of Social Communication Change (BOSCC; Grzadzinski et al., 2016), which is modeled off of the Autism Diagnostic Observation schedule (ADOS; Lord et al., 2012). It will be important for researchers to carefully consider measurement tools when designing intervention studies in order provide consistency in the literature.

17.3.3 Training Format and Intensity

The majority of PMIs in Table 17.1 are implemented in a one-on-one fashion with both the parent and child present for all sessions. Several intervention packages also have clear designs for both individual and group formats, including Early Social Interaction Parent-Implemented Intervention (ESI-PII; Wetherby et al., 2014), Improving Parents As Communication Teachers (Project ImPACT; Ingersoll & Dvortcsak, 2010), and Pivotal Response Training (PRT; Koegel et al., 2003). Only Hanen's More than Words (HMW, Sussman, 2012) is primarily designed to be group based. There are also differences in the intensity of the interventions. While most of the interventions shown in Table 17.1 take on a more traditional approach to therapy with weekly or biweekly sessions, others have greater variation in intensity. For example, Pivotal Response Training (PRT) offers up a large range of options for learning, including a 25-h intensive, 1-week intervention (Koegel et al., 2002); a brief, three-session intervention (Coolican et al., 2010); or completely self-directed intervention materials (Nefdt et al., 2010).

The way in which an intervention is conducted, in a group or one-on-one, is important to consider for both research and practice. For example, individual treatment may allow for a more tailored and intensive treatment experience that is more effective for certain families, while group treatments offer the opportunity to learn from others, build social supports, and are more cost effective, which may be beneficial for others (Holden, Lavigne, & Cameron, 1990; Lundahl, Risser, & Lovejoy, 2006). There are also differences in the core training components of individual and group parent training. Common components of parent training include didactics, in vivo and/or video modeling, role plays, immediate and/or delayed performance feedback, self-reflection, and discussion (Table 8.1 in Ruppert, Machalicek, Hansen, Raulston, & Frantz, 2016; Table 5 in Barton & Fettig, 2013). Group-based trainings rely more heavily on didactics, video modeling, role play, and discussion, while individual treatment relies most heavily on in vivo modeling and performance feedback, which is considered the most essential component in effective parent training (Barton & Fettig, 2013). Additionally, differences in intervention intensity have a strong influence on social communication gains (Virués-Ortega, 2010), but there are no studies that address this difference for PMI delivery models.

Despite the potential differences in outcomes between individual and group formats, few studies directly address this. Wetherby et al. (2014) found greater improvements in social, communication, and adaptive skills for individual coaching over groups, but there were no group differences in autism severity, motor skills, or nonverbal cognition. Kasari, Lawton, and colleagues (Kasari, Lawton et al., 2014) also saw greater effects for individual over group parent training models in joint attention and initiation; however, there were no group differences in treatment adherence or play behaviors. While individual coaching showed greater improvements compared to similar group-based treatments, both formats saw improvement in children's social communication skills.

17.3.4 Parent Variables Influencing Outcomes

Child characteristics, such as intellectual functioning, language level, and age, have often been examined as moderators of treatment effects in ASD intervention research (Reed, 2016). However, PMI requires additional consideration of variables that influence treatment outcomes. Meadan et al. (2009) describe research on PMIs as a "study-within-a-study" (p. 92), where the first study should assess parents' learning of the intervention techniques, while the second study focuses on how these techniques affect child outcomes. However, there is little focus on how well parents use intervention techniques, also known as intervention or treatment fidelity. Only half of the studies reported in Table 17.2 report any information regarding parent treatment fidelity. Even fewer directly explore how changes in parent behavior are related to child outcomes (e.g., Ingersoll & Wainer, 2013; Kasari, Siller et al., 2014; Siller, Hutman et al., 2013).

In addition to parent treatment fidelity, there is an increasing focus on how other parent variables, such as stress, well-being, or self-efficacy, affect child outcomes in early intervention for ASD (Karst & Van Hecke, 2012; Strauss et al., 2012; Wainer et al., 2016), given the reciprocal relationship between parent mental health and child development (Lecavalier et al., 2006). Wainer et al. (2016) reviewed a number of potentially valuable tools for assessing meaningful parent outcomes in PMI, drawing from broader literature in early intervention. However, few studies on social communication PMIs report parent outcomes which makes this potential relationship difficult to study; those that do assess parent outcomes have inconsistent findings. For example, Turner-Brown et al. (2016) found reductions in parent stress and improved social functioning. Solomon et al. (2014) found that fewer parents were classified as depressed. Others have found no changes in parenting stress (Aldred et al., 2004; Kasari et al., 2015; Welterlin et al., 2012), well-being (Stadnick et al., 2015), or self-efficacy (Coolican et al., 2010) after completing a PMI. Fewer studies assess how these differences in mental health impact intervention outcomes (Kasari, Siller et al., 2014; Siller, Hutman et al., 2013; Siller et al., 2014), despite evidence from the broader literature to suggest that it impacts the ability to effectively learn and implement PMI (see Reyno & McGrath, 2006, for review).

17.4 Recommendations for Choosing and Implementing Appropriate Intervention

Differences in the intervention approach taught to parents, the social communication skills targeted, the format and intensity of the parent training model, and parent variables that may influence treatment outcomes contribute to difficulties evaluating the evidence base for PMI. While parents are able to learn intervention strategies that improve child skills, it is unclear about how to best implement these interventions and what outcomes are important to assess. However, this should not discourage interested parents and practitioners from pursuing PMI as a component of a comprehensive family-wide intervention plan. In a continuing effort by researchers to address these concerns and to build a more solid evidence base for PMI, several workgroups have developed guidelines for both researchers and professionals (e.g., Lord et al., 2005; Siller & Morgan, 2013; Siller, Morgan et al., 2013; Smith et al., 2007). We direct researchers to methodological recommendations for designing and evaluating ASD interventions (Lord et al., 2005; Siller, Morgan et al., 2013; Smith et al., 2007). Recommendations for strategies to ensure the successful delivery of parent-mediated interventions for young children with ASD include improving collaboration between parents and professionals, increased focus on adult learning strategies, accommodating parents' needs through flexible implementation practices, valuing cultural and linguistic diversity, and developing professional, social, and emotional support networks for parents (ASTTN; Siller & Morgan, 2013).

PMIs serve as one way to improve collaboration between parents and professionals, as well as provide opportunities to individualize treatment to best fit the family and child's needs. Collaboration with parents in treatment planning helps to promote positive family and child outcomes by incorporating family values and routines into treatment (e.g., Buschbacher, Fox, & Clarke, 2004). The addition of these contextual factors has been shown to increase the success of comprehensive interventions for the management of challenging behaviors (Moes & Frea, 2002); there is also growing evidence of the importance of these components in the success of treatments targeting the core deficits of ASD (e.g., Brookman-Frazee, 2004). It will be important for parents and practitioners to explore how various treatment components fit with family values and beliefs when deciding on an intervention, as the acceptability of an intervention and its components is an important factor for parents when deciding with which treatments to engage (Nock, Ferriter, & Holmberg, 2007; Nock & Kazdin, 2001).

17.5 Future Directions

Despite best practice recommendations and the potential benefits of PMIs, PMIs are highly underutilized in community settings. While it is difficult to estimate community utilization of PMIs specifically, estimates for utilization of parent trainings more broadly have ranged from 8% (Pickard & Ingersoll, 2016; Thomas, Ellis, McLaurin, Daniels, & Morrissey, 2007) to 36% (Ruble & McGrew, 2007). However, families have ranked parent training as the most important and helpful component of their child's intervention services (Hume, Bellini, & Pratt, 2005; Mahoney & Filer, 1996) indicating that PMI is an unmet need in the community. There are a number of common barriers that may impede the successful dissemination and implementation of ASD interventions; as PMIs require more active involvement from the family, it can be expected that these barriers are especially relevant. At the family level, there are concrete barriers such as cost (Järbrink et al., 2003), transportation (Zeman et al., 2011), and time commitments (Montes & Halterman, 2008; Patterson & Smith, 2011), as well as cultural barriers that can impact treatment acceptability (Mandell & Novak, 2005; Tincani, Travers, & Boutot, 2009). At the provider level, barriers include providers' attitudes regarding the role of parents in their child's intervention service (e.g.,

Shapiro, Prinz, & Sanders, 2012), insufficient preparation in adult learning strategies to support parent coaching (e.g., Scheuermann, Webber, Boutot, & Goodwin, 2003), and a lack of proactive facilitation strategies, such as accessible trainer and parent manuals and data monitoring and collection strategies (e.g., Boardman, Argüelles, Vaughn, Hughes, & Klingner, 2005). At the system level, barriers can include the lack of fit between the structure of the parent-mediated intervention program and the structure of existing service delivery models and provider training models that are incompatible with the organizational training structures of many community programs (Schmidt & Taylor, 2002; Stahmer & Aarons, 2009). Thus, research is needed on strategies for increasing the successful dissemination and implementation of promising PMIs in community settings.

17.5.1 Development of Telehealth Models

One recent strategy has been to modify traditional PMI programs so that they can be delivered via the Internet. These programs have the potential to surmount many family-level barriers to access and may serve as a promising alternative service delivery model to increase access to evidence-based interventions for children with ASD, including PMI (Knutsen et al., 2016). Although still in its early stages, there is a growing literature demonstrating the feasibility, acceptability, and preliminary efficacy of both self-directed and therapist-assisted telehealth-based parent-mediated interventions for young children with ASD and their families (e.g., Ingersoll et al., 2016; Nefdt et al., 2010; Vismara et al., 2016; Wainer & Ingersoll, 2015). For example, a recent pilot RCT compared self-directed and therapist-assisted versions of ImPACT Online, an interactive, web application that teaches parents to promote their child's social communication within the context of play and daily routines. The content was modified from Project ImPACT, an evidence-based social communication PMI for young children with ASD (Ingersoll & Dvortcsak, 2010). Program engagement and treatment acceptability were high across both groups, although therapist assistance increased program engagement and led to slightly higher program satisfaction (Ingersoll & Berger, 2015). There were also positive effects on parent conceptual and procedural learning, stress and self-efficacy, and child social communication skills for both groups, although there was an added benefit of therapist assistance on some parent and child outcomes (Ingersoll et al., 2016; Pickard, Wainer, Bailey, & Ingersoll, 2016). There was also a significant positive relationship between program engagement and improvements in parent intervention knowledge and procedural fidelity, providing support for the role of the web application in parent learning (Ingersoll & Berger, 2015). Moving forward, larger-scale efficacy studies are needed to better understand the effects of such programs on parent and child outcomes, as well as to identify mediators and moderators of treatment. Despite the promise of telehealth for increasing access to PMI for families of children with ASD (Knutsen et al., 2016), it is not without its own barriers. These include limited Internet connectivity and access to the required technology in rural and underserved areas, concerns about confidentiality and service reimbursement by providers (Meadan et al., 2013), and limited reach and high rates of attrition of self-directed programs outside of research settings (Ingersoll, Shannon, Berger, Pickard, & Holtz, 2017). Research on the dissemination and implementation of telehealth and eHealth interventions from other fields can help identify ways to address these barriers moving forward.

17.5.2 Building Engagement in Under-resourced Communities

Even when PMIs are available in community settings, many low-resourced families experience barriers to accessing them. For example, lower-resourced parents are more likely than higher-resourced parents to spontaneously report PMIs an unmet healthcare need (Pickard & Ingersoll, 2016). In addition, although several studies have found that under-resourced families of children with ASD can benefit from parent-mediated intervention (Carr & Lord, 2016; Carr et al., 2015; Kasari, Lawton et al., 2014), they also reported high levels of parent attrition, even when supports were provided to reduce the transportation and time requirements of the intervention for parents. This suggests that there are many, yet undetermined, barriers to under-resourced families' ability to effectively engage in PMI and indicate a significant need for methods to improve the translation of evidence-based PMIs into under-resourced community settings (Stahmer & Pellecchia, 2015).

Research on parent engagement in interventions for children with conduct problems has identified several enhancements to behavioral parent training interventions that can increase parents' ability to implement and maintain parenting changes over time (Ingoldsby, 2010; Morrissey-Kane & Prinz, 1999). These interventions, which include early discussions of parent expectations and barriers to treatment, motivational interviewing, and enhancing family support and coping, have been shown to increase engagement and retention in parenting interventions among low-resourced and minority families (Ingoldsby, 2010). To date, there have been limited attempts to incorporate these types of engagement interventions into existing evidence-based PMIs for children with ASD and their families. One notable exception is Durand, Hieneman, Clarke, Wang, and Rinaldi's (2012) Positive Family Intervention which was designed to address psychological barriers to engagement in behavioral parent training for children with autism and other developmental disorders who exhibit severe challenging behavior. The intervention combined cognitive-behavioral strategies in which parents learned to challenge their own negative self-talk with parent training in positive behavior support (PBS) strategies. A randomized clinical trial comparing the enhanced intervention to PBS alone found greater improvements in the children's challenging behavior in the enhanced intervention group, and parents reported that they felt better able to handle their child's behaviors. However, there were no group differences in cancellations or attrition. This study suggests that engagement enhancement strategies can be easily incorporated into existing evidence-based PMIs and may lead to better outcomes. Future work should focus on the development and evaluation of enhanced PMIs as a method for increasing parent engagement, particularly among under-resourced families. Given the high rate of parenting stress experienced by parents of children with ASD (Baker-Ericzén et al., 2005; Davis & Carter, 2008), interventions that target stress and coping, such as mindfulness-based interventions, may be a particularly helpful strategy to enhance engagement in PMIs and while also improving parent well-being.

17.5.3 Increasing Acceptability through Community Partnerships and Cross-Cultural Adaptations

Another method to encourage community use of PMIs is to ensure that current evidence-based models are appropriate for use with diverse families. Many research studies outside of the ASD field have demonstrated the benefits of using community partnerships to adapt evidence-based parenting interventions in diverse settings. A recent meta-analysis of these studies suggests that culturally adapted parent-mediated programs appear to be equally efficacious but have greater perceived compatibility and parent retention rates when compared with their nonadapted counterparts (Baumann et al., 2015). This research suggests that using community partnership to adapt evidence-based PMIs may be one strategy to increase their fit and use within under-resourced community settings. To date, this approach has only recently been applied to PMIs for families of children with ASD. For example, Pickard, Kilgore, and Ingersoll (2016) conducted focus groups with Medicaid-eligible parents of children and ASD providers operating within a Medicaid system to identify potential adaptations to Project ImPACT, an evidence-based PMI. Across both stakeholder groups, themes emerged indicating the need to reduce the complexity of written materials, allow for a more flexible program delivery, ensure a strong parent-therapist alliance, involve the extended family, and help families practice the intervention within their preexisting routines.

In addition to implementation in community settings, there has been a recent increase in cross-cultural adaptations of PMI for use in other countries (see Mejia, Calam, & Sanders, 2012 for review). Divan and colleagues (Divan et al., 2015) used task shifting (i.e., delivery by nonexperts) and the Medical Research Council framework for development and adaptation of complex interventions to adapt PACT, an evidence-based PMI, for use in South Asia (PASS). This approach used qualitative studies, expert-led simplification of the manual, intervention adaptation workshops, and a case series delivered by specialists and nonspecialist workers in South Asia. A subsequent randomized controlled trial in South Asia indicated that nonspecialists were able to implement the adapted intervention with a high degree of fidelity and a positive effect of treatment on parent synchrony and child initiations (Rahman et al., 2016), similar to the original trial in the United Kingdom (UK; Green et al., 2010). At the same time, in contrast to the UK trial, the study also found a negative effect on length of time in shared attention and no effect on parent-reported measures of child language, which could indicate cultural differences in treatment response.

Future work using community partnerships and cultural adaptation frameworks is necessary to ensure that existing evidence-based PMIs can be successfully implemented in diverse settings. This strategy can also be used during the development process of novel PMIs in order to identify and address likely barriers to community implementation early in the development process and ensure that the models which undergo rigorous testing have the greatest chance of success in existing service delivery systems. In this process, it is important to consider family-, provider-, organization-, and system-level barriers.

References

Aldred, C. R., Green, J., & Adams, C. (2004). A new social communication intervention for children with autism: Pilot randomised controlled treatment study suggesting effectiveness. *Journal of Child Psychology and Psychiatry*, *45*, 1–11.

Aldred, C. R., Green, J., Emsley, R., & McConachie, H. (2012). Brief report: Mediation of treatment effect in a communication intervention for pre-school children with autism. *Journal of Autism and Developmental Disorders*, *42*(3), 447–454.

American Psychiatric Association. (2013). *Diagnostic and statistical manual of mental disorders* (5th ed.). Arlington, VA: American Psychiatric Publishing.

Baker-Ericzén, M. J., Brookman-Frazee, L., & Stahmer, A. (2005). Stress levels and adaptability in parents of toddlers with and without autism spectrum disorders. *Research and Practice for Persons with Severe Disabilities*, *30*(4), 194–204.

Baranek, G. T., Watson, L. R., Turner-Brown, L., Field, S. H., Crais, E. R., Wakeford, L., … Reznick, J. S. (2015). Preliminary efficacy of adapted responsive teaching for infants at risk of autism spectrum disorder in a community sample. *Autism Research and Treatment*. doi:10.1155/2015/386951

Barton, E. E., & Fettig, A. (2013). Parent-implemented interventions for young children with disabilities: A review of fidelity features. *Journal of Early Intervention*, *35*(2), 194–219.

Baumann, A. A., Powell, B. J., Kohl, P. L., Tabak, R. G., Penalba, V., Proctor, E. K., … Cabassa, L. J. (2015). Cultural adaptation and implementation of evidence-based parent-training: A systematic review and critique of guiding evidence. *Children and Youth Services Review*, *53*, 113–120.

Bearss, K., Burrell, T. L., Stewart, L., & Scahill, L. (2015). Parent training in autism spectrum disorder: What's in a name? *Clinical Child and Family Psychology Review*, *18*(2), 170–182.

Beaudoin, A. J., Sébire, G., & Couture, M. (2014). Parent training interventions for toddlers with autism spectrum disorder. *Autism Research and Treatment, 2014*, 1–15. http://dx.doi.org/10.1155/2014/839890

Bilaver, L. A., Cushing, L. S., & Cutler, A. T. (2016). Prevalence and correlates of educational intervention utilization among children with autism spectrum disorder. *Journal of Autism and Developmental Disorders*, *46*(2), 561–571.

Boardman, A. G., Argüelles, M. E., Vaughn, S., Hughes, M. T., & Klingner, J. (2005). Special education teachers' views of research-based practices. *The Journal of Special Education*, *39*(3), 168–180.

Bowker, A., D'Angelo, N. M., Hicks, R., & Wells, K. (2011). Treatments for autism: Parental choices and perceptions of change. *Journal of Autism and Developmental Disorders*, *41*(10), 1373–1382.

Brian, J. A., Smith, I. M., Zwaigenbaum, L., Roberts, W., & Bryson, S. E. (2015). The social ABCs caregiver-mediated intervention for toddlers with autism

spectrum disorder: Feasibility, acceptability, and evidence of promise from a multisite study. *Autism Research*, *9*, 899–912.
Brookman-Frazee, L. (2004). Using parent/clinician partnerships in parent education programs for children with autism. *Journal of Positive Behavior Interventions*, *6*(4), 195–213.
Bruner, J. (1983). Play, thought, and language. *Peabody Journal of Education*, *60*(3), 60–69.
Buschbacher, P., Fox, L., & Clarke, S. (2004). Recapturing desired family routines: A parent-professional behavioral collaboration. *Research and Practice for Persons with Severe Disabilities*, *29*(1), 25–39.
Callahan, K., Henson, R. K., & Cowan, A. K. (2008). Social validation of evidence-based practices in autism by parents, teachers, and administrators. *Journal of Autism and Developmental Disorders*, *38*(4), 678–692.
Calvert, S. C., & McMahon, R. J. (1987). The treatment acceptability of a behavioral parent training program and its components. *Behavior Therapy*, *18*(2), 165–179.
Carr, E. G., & Durand, V. M. (1985). Reducing behavior problems through functional communication training. *Journal of Applied Behavior Analysis*, *18*(2), 111–126.
Carr, T., & Lord, C. (2016). A pilot study promoting participation of families with limited resources in early autism intervention. *Research in Autism Spectrum Disorders*, *25*, 87–96.
Carr, T., Shih, W., Lawton, K., Lord, C., King, B., & Kasari, C. (2015). The relationship between treatment attendance, adherence, and outcome in a caregiver-mediated intervention for low-resourced families of young children with autism spectrum disorder. *Autism*, *20*(6), 643–652.
Carter, A. S., Messinger, D. S., Stone, W. L., Celimli, S., Nahmias, A. S., & Yoder, P. (2011). A randomized controlled trial of Hanen's 'More Than Words' in toddlers with early autism symptoms. *Journal of Child Psychology and Psychiatry*, *52*(7), 741–752.
Casenhiser, D. M., Binns, A., McGill, F., Morderer, O., & Shanker, S. G. (2015). Measuring and supporting language function for children with autism: Evidence from a randomized control trial of a social-interaction-based therapy. *Journal of Autism and Developmental Disorders*, *45*(3), 846–857.
Casenhiser, D. M., Shanker, S. G., & Stieben, J. (2013). Learning through interaction in children with autism: Preliminary data from a social-communication-based intervention. *Autism*, *17*(2), 220–241.
Chasson, G. S., Harris, G. E., & Neely, W. J. (2007). Cost comparison of early intensive behavioral intervention and special education for children with autism. *Journal of Child and Family Studies*, *16*(3), 401–413.
Chorpita, B. F., Daleiden, E. L., & Weisz, J. R. (2005). Modularity in the design and application of therapeutic interventions. *Applied and Preventive Psychology*, *11*(3), 141–156.
Chorpita, B. F., & Weisz, J. R. (2009). *MATCH-ADTC: Modular approach to therapy for children with anxiety, depression, trauma, or conduct problems.* Satellite Beach, FL: PracticeWise.
Coolican, J., Smith, I. M., & Bryson, S. (2010). Brief parent training in pivotal response treatment for preschoolers with autism. *Journal of Child Psychology and Psychiatry*, *51*(12), 1321–1330.
Davis, N. O., & Carter, A. S. (2008). Parenting stress in mothers and fathers of toddlers with autism spectrum disorders: Associations with child characteristics. *Journal of Autism and Developmental Disorders*, *38*(7), 1278–1291.
Dawson, G. (2008). Early behavioral intervention, brain plasticity, and the prevention of autism spectrum disorder. *Development and Psychopathology*, *20*(3), 775–803.
Delprato, D. J. (2001). Comparisons of discrete-trial and normalized behavioral intervention for young children with autism. *Journal of Autism and Developmental Disorders*, *31*(3), 315–325.
Divan, G., Hamdani, S. U., Vajartkar, V., Minhas, A., Taylor, C., Aldred, C., … Patel, V. (2015). Adapting an evidence-based intervention for autism spectrum disorder for scaling up in resource-constrained settings: The development of the PASS intervention in South Asia. *Global Health Action*, *8*. https://dx.doi.org/10.3402%2Fgha.v8.27278.
Durand, V. M., Hieneman, M., Clarke, S., Wang, M., & Rinaldi, M. L. (2012). Positive family intervention for severe challenging behavior: A multisite randomized clinical trial. *Journal of Positive Behavior Interventions*, *15*(3), 133–143.
Estes, A., Vismara, L., Mercado, C., Fitzpatrick, A., Elder, L., Greenson, J., … Dawson, G. (2014). The impact of parent-delivered intervention on parents of very young children with autism. *Journal of Autism and Developmental Disorders*, *44*(2), 353–365.
Fletcher-Watson, S., & McConachie, H. (2015). The search for an early intervention outcome measurement tool in autism. *Focus on Autism and Other Developmental Disabilities*. http://dx.doi.org/10.1177%2F1088357615583468
Gerber, S. (2003). A developmental perspective on language assessment and intervention for children on the autistic spectrum. *Topics in Language Disorders*, *23*(2), 74–94.
Gillett, J. N., & LeBlanc, L. A. (2007). Parent-implemented natural language paradigm to increase language and play in children with autism. *Research in Autism Spectrum Disorders*, *1*, 247–255.
Girolametto, L., Sussman, F., & Weitzman, E. (2007). Using case study methods to investigate the effects of interactive intervention for children with autism spectrum disorders. *Journal of Communication Disorders*, *40*(6), 470–492.
Green, J., Charman, T., McConachie, H., Aldred, C., Slonims, V., Howlin, P., … Barrett, B. (2010). Parent-mediated communication-focused treatment in children with autism (PACT): A randomised controlled trial. *The Lancet*, *375*(9732), 2152–2160.

Grzadzinski, R., Carr, T., Colombi, C., McGuire, K., Dufek, S., Pickles, A., & Lord, C. (2016). Measuring changes in social communication Behaviors: Preliminary development of the brief observation of social communication change (BOSCC). *Journal of Autism and Developmental Disorders, 46*(7), 2464–2479.

Herring, S., Gray, K., Taffe, J., Tonge, B., Sweeney, D., & Einfeld, S. (2006). Behaviour and emotional problems in toddlers with pervasive developmental disorders and developmental delay: Associations with parental mental health and family functioning. *Journal of Intellectual Disability Research, 50*(12), 874–882.

Holden, G. W., Lavigne, V. V., & Cameron, A. M. (1990). Probing the continuum of effectiveness in parent training: Characteristics of parents and preschoolers. *Journal of Clinical Child Psychology, 19*(1), 2–8.

Hoppes, K., & Harris, S. L. (1990). Perceptions of child attachment and maternal gratification in mothers of children with autism and down syndrome. *Journal of Clinical Child Psychology, 19*(4), 365–370.

Hume, K., Bellini, S., & Pratt, C. (2005). The usage and perceived outcomes of early intervention and early childhood programs for young children with autism spectrum disorder. *Topics in Early Childhood Special Education, 25*(4), 195–207.

Ingersoll, B. (2008). *Reciprocal imitation training.* Unpublished treatment manual.

Ingersoll, B., & Berger, N. I. (2015). Parent engagement with a telehealth-based parent-mediated intervention program for children with autism spectrum disorders: Predictors of program use and parent outcomes. *Journal of Medical Internet Research, 17*(10), e277.

Ingersoll, B., & Dvortcsak, A. (2010). *Teaching social communication to children with autism: A Practitioner's guide to parent training and a manual for parents*. New York: Guilford Press.

Ingersoll, B., Shannon, K., Berger, N., Pickard, K., & Holtz, B. (2017). Self-Directed Telehealth Parent-Mediated Intervention for Children With Autism Spectrum Disorder: Examination of the Potential Reach and Utilization in Community Settings. *Journal of Medical Internet Research, 19*(7), e248.

Ingersoll, B., & Wainer, A. (2013). Initial efficacy of project ImPACT: A parent-mediated social communication intervention for young children with ASD. *Journal of Autism and Developmental Disorders, 43*(12), 2943–2952.

Ingersoll, B., Wainer, A. L., Berger, N. I., Pickard, K. E., & Bonter, N. (2016). Comparison of a self-directed and therapist-assisted telehealth parent-mediated intervention for children with ASD: A pilot RCT. *Journal of Autism and Developmental Disorders,* 1–10. http://dx.doi.org/10.1007/s10803-016-2755-z

Ingoldsby, E. M. (2010). Review of interventions to improve family engagement and retention in parent and child mental health programs. *Journal of Child and Family Studies, 19*(5), 629–645.

Järbrink, K., Fombonne, E., & Knapp, M. (2003). Measuring the parental, service and cost impacts of children with autistic spectrum disorder: A pilot study. *Journal of Autism and Developmental Disorders, 33*(4), 395–402.

Kaiser, A. P., Hancock, T. B., & Nietfeld, J. P. (2000). The effects of parent-implemented enhanced milieu teaching on the social communication of children who have autism. *Early Education and Development, 11*, 423–446.

Kaiser, A. P., Hancock, T. B., & Trent, J. A. (2007). Teaching parents communication strategies. *Early Childhood Services: An Interdisciplinary Journal of Effectiveness, 1*, 107–136.

Kaiser, A. P., & Roberts, M. Y. (2013). Parent-implemented enhanced milieu teaching with preschool children who have intellectual disabilities. *Journal of Speech, Language, and Hearing Research, 56*(1), 295–309.

Karst, J. S., & Van Hecke, A. V. (2012). Parent and family impact of autism spectrum disorders: A review and proposed model for intervention evaluation. *Clinical Child and Family Psychology Review, 15*(3), 247–277.

Kasari, C., Gulsrud, A., Paparella, T., Hellemann, G., & Berry, K. (2015). Randomized comparative efficacy study of parent-mediated interventions for toddlers with autism. *Journal of Consulting and Clinical Psychology, 83*(3), 554–563.

Kasari, C., Gulsrud, A. C., Wong, C., Kwon, S., & Locke, J. (2010). Randomized controlled caregiver mediated joint engagement intervention for toddlers with autism. *Journal of Autism and Developmental Disorders, 40*(9), 1045–1056.

Kasari, C., Lawton, K., Shih, W., Barker, T. V., Landa, R., Lord, C., … Senturk, D. (2014). Caregiver-mediated intervention for low-resourced preschoolers with autism: An RCT. *Pediatrics, 134*(1), e72–e79.

Kasari, C., Siller, M., Huynh, L. N., Shih, W., Swanson, M., Hellemann, G. S., & Sugar, C. A. (2014). Randomized controlled trial of parental responsiveness intervention for toddlers at high risk for autism. *Infant Behavior & Development, 37*(4), 711–721.

Knutsen, J., Wolfe, A., Burke, B. L., Hepburn, S., Lindgren, S., & Coury, D. (2016). A systematic review of telemedicine in autism spectrum disorders. *Review Journal of Autism and Developmental Disorders, 3*(4), 330–344.

Koegel, L. K., Koegel, R. L., Bruinsma, Y., Brookman, L., & Fredeen, R. (2003). *Teaching first words to children with autism and communication delays using pivotal response training*. Santa Barbara, CA: University of California.

Koegel, R. L., Bimbela, A., & Schreibman, L. (1996). Collateral effects of parent training on family interactions. *Journal of Autism and Developmental Disorders, 26*(3), 347–359.

Koegel, R. L., Koegel, L. K., & Surratt, A. (1992). Language intervention and disruptive behavior in preschool children with autism. *Journal of Autism and Developmental Disorders, 22*(2), 141–153.

Koegel, R. L., Schreibman, L., Britten, K. R., Burke, J. C., & O'Neill, R. E. (1982). A comparison of parent training to direct child treatment. In R. L. Koegel, A. Rincover, & A. L. Egel (Eds.), *Educating and understanding autistic children*. San Diego, CA: College-Hill Press.

Koegel, R. L., Schreibman, L., Good, A., Cerniglia, L., Murphy, C., & Koegel, L. K. (1989). *How to teach pivotal behaviors to children with autism: A training manual*. Santa Barbara, CA/San Diego, CA: University of California.

Koegel, R. L., Symon, J. B., & Koegel, L. K. (2002). Parent education for families of children with autism living in geographically distant areas. *Journal of Positive Behavior Interventions*, *4*(2), 88–103.

Landa, R. J., Holman, K. C., & Garrett-Mayer, E. (2007). Social and communication development in toddlers with early and later diagnosis of autism spectrum disorders. *Archives of General Psychiatry*, *64*(7), 853–864.

Lang, R., Machalicek, W., Rispoli, M., & Regester, A. (2009). Training parents to implement communication interventions for children with autism spectrum disorders (ASD): A systematic review. *Evidence-Based Communication Assessment and Intervention*, *3*(3), 174–190.

Lecavalier, L., Leone, S., & Wiltz, J. (2006). The impact of behaviour problems on caregiver stress in young people with autism spectrum disorders. *Journal of Intellectual Disability Research*, *50*(3), 172–183.

Lord, C., Rutter, M., DiLavore, P. C., Risi, S., Gotham, K., & Bishop, S. (2012). *Autism diagnostic observation schedule, 2nd edition (ADOS-2)*. Torrance, CA: Western Psychological Services.

Lord, C., Wagner, A., Rogers, S., Szatmari, P., Aman, M., Charman, T., … Harris, S. (2005). Challenges in evaluating psychosocial interventions for autistic spectrum disorders. *Journal of Autism and Developmental Disorders*, *35*(6), 695–708.

Lovaas, O. I., Koegel, R., Simmons, J. Q., & Long, J. S. (1973). Some generalization and follow-up measures on autistic children in behavior therapy. *Journal of Applied Behavior Analysis*, *6*(1), 131–165.

Lundahl, B., Risser, H. J., & Lovejoy, M. C. (2006). A meta-analysis of parent training: Moderators and follow-up effects. *Clinical Psychology Review*, *26*(1), 86–104.

Luyster, R. J., Kadlec, M. B., Carter, A., & Tager-Flusberg, H. (2008). Language assessment and development in toddlers with autism spectrum disorders. *Journal of Autism and Developmental Disorders*, *38*(8), 1426–1438.

Maglione, M. A., Gans, D., Das, L., Timbie, J., & Kasari, C. (2012). Nonmedical interventions for children with ASD: Recommended guidelines and further research needs. *Pediatrics*, *130*(Supplement 2), S169–S178.

Mahoney, G., & Filer, J. (1996). How responsive is early intervention to the priorities and needs of families? *Topics in Early Childhood Special Education*, *16*(4), 437–457.

Mahoney, G., & MacDonald, J. (2007). *Autism and developmental delays in young children: The responsive teaching curriculum for parents and professionals*. Austin, TX: PRO-ED.

Mahoney, G., & Perales, F. (2003). Using relationship-focused intervention to enhance the social—Emotional functioning of young children with autism spectrum disorders. *Topics in Early Childhood Special Education*, *23*(2), 74–86.

Mahoney, G., & Perales, F. (2005). Relationship-focused early intervention with children with pervasive developmental disorders and other disabilities: A comparative study. *Journal of Developmental and Behavioral Pediatrics*, *26*(2), 77–85.

Mandell, D. S., & Novak, M. (2005). The role of culture in families' treatment decisions for children with autism spectrum disorders. *Mental Retardation and Developmental Disabilities Research Reviews*, *11*(2), 110–115.

Matson, J. L. (2007). Determining treatment outcome in early intervention programs for autism spectrum disorders: A critical analysis of measurement issues in learning based interventions. *Research in Developmental Disabilities*, *28*(2), 207–218.

McConachie, H., Randle, V., Hammal, D., & Le Couteur, A. (2005). A controlled trial of a training course for parents of children with suspected autism spectrum disorder. *The Journal of Pediatrics*, *147*(3), 335–340.

Meadan, H., Meyer, L. E., Snodgrass, M. R., & Halle, J. W. (2013). Coaching parents of young children with autism in rural areas using internet-based technologies: A pilot program. *Rural Special Education Quarterly*, *32*(3), 3–10.

Meadan, H., Ostrosky, M. M., Zaghlawan, H. Y., & Yu, S. (2009). Promoting the social and communicative behavior of young children with autism spectrum disorders: A review of parent-implemented intervention studies. *Topics in Early Childhood Special Education*, *29*(2), 90–104.

Mejia, A., Calam, R., & Sanders, M. R. (2012). A review of parenting programs in developing countries: Opportunities and challenges for preventing emotional and behavioral difficulties in children. *Clinical Child and Family Psychology Review*, *15*(2), 163–175.

Mesibov, G. B., Shea, V., & Schopler, E. (2005). *The TEACCH approach to autism spectrum disorders*. New York: Springer Science & Business Media.

Minjarez, M. B., Williams, S. E., Mercier, E. M., & Hardan, A. Y. (2011). Pivotal response group treatment program for parents of children with autism. *Journal of Autism and Developmental Disorders*, *41*(1), 92–101.

Moes, D. R., & Frea, W. D. (2002). Contextualized behavioral support in early intervention for children with autism and their families. *Journal of Autism and Developmental Disorders*, *32*(6), 519–533.

Montes, G., & Halterman, J. S. (2008). Association of childhood autism spectrum disorders and loss of family income. *Pediatrics*, *121*(4), e821–e826.

Morrissey-Kane, E., & Prinz, R. J. (1999). Engagement in child and adolescent treatment: The role of parental cognitions and attributions. *Clinical Child and Family Psychology Review*, *2*(3), 183–198.

Mundy, P., & Crowson, M. (1997). Joint attention and early social communication: Implications for research on intervention with autism. *Journal of Autism and Developmental Disorders*, *27*(6), 653–676.

Mundy, P., Delgado, C., Block, J., Venezia, M., Hogan, A., & Seibert, J. (2003). *Early social communication scales (ESCS)*. Coral Gables, FL: University of Miami.

Myers, S. M., & Johnson, C. P. (2007). Management of children with autism spectrum disorders. *Pediatrics*, *120*(5), 1162–1182.

National Research Council (NRC). (2001). *Educating children with autism*. Washington, DC: National Academic Press.

Nefdt, N., Koegel, R., Singer, G., & Gerber, M. (2010). The use of a self-directed learning program to provide introductory training in pivotal response treatment to parents of children with autism. *Journal of Positive Behavior Interventions*, *12*(1), 23–32.

Nock, M. K., Ferriter, C., & Holmberg, E. (2007). Parent beliefs about treatment credibility and effectiveness: Assessment and relation to subsequent treatment participation. *Journal of Child and Family Studies*, *16*(1), 27–38.

Nock, M. K., & Kazdin, A. E. (2001). Parent expectancies for child therapy: Assessment and relation to participation in treatment. *Journal of Child and Family Studies*, *10*(2), 155–180.

Oono, I. P., Honey, E. J., & McConachie, H. (2013). Parent-mediated early intervention for young children with autism spectrum disorders (ASD). *Evidence-Based Child Health: A Cochrane Review Journal*, *8*(6), 2380–2479.

Ozonoff, S., & Cathcart, K. (1998). Effectiveness of a home program intervention for young children with autism. *Journal of Autism and Developmental Disorders*, *28*(1), 25–32.

Patterson, S. Y., & Smith, V. (2011). The experience of parents of toddlers diagnosed with autism spectrum disorder in the More Than Words parent education program. *Infants & Young Children*, *24*(4), 329–343.

Patterson, S. Y., Smith, V., & Mirenda, P. (2012). A systematic review of training programs for parents of children with autism spectrum disorders: Single subject contributions. *Autism*, *16*(5), 498–522.

Pellecchia, M., Connell, J. E., Beidas, R. S., Xie, M., Marcus, S. C., & Mandell, D. S. (2015). Dismantling the active ingredients of an intervention for children with autism. *Journal of Autism and Developmental Disorders*, *45*(9), 2917–2927.

Pickard, K. E., & Ingersoll, B. R. (2016). Quality versus quantity: The role of socioeconomic status on parent-reported service knowledge, service use, unmet service needs, and barriers to service use. *Autism*, *20*(1), 106–115.

Pickard, K. E., Kilgore, A. N., & Ingersoll, B. R. (2016). Using community partnerships to better understand the barriers to using an evidence-based, parent-mediated intervention for autism spectrum disorder in a medicaid system. *American Journal of Community Psychology*, *57*(3–4), 391–403.

Pickard, K. E., Wainer, A. L., Bailey, K. M., & Ingersoll, B. R. (2016). A mixed-method evaluation of the feasibility and acceptability of a telehealth-based parent-mediated intervention for children with autism spectrum disorder. *Autism*, *20*(7), 845–855.

Prizant, B. M., & Wetherby, A. M. (1998). Understanding the continuum of discrete-trial traditional behavioral to social-pragmatic developmental approaches in communication enhancement for young children with autism/PDD. *Seminars in Speech and Language*, *19*(4), 329–353.

Rahman, A., Divan, G., Hamdani, S. U., Vajaratkar, V., Taylor, C., Leadbitter, K., … Patel, V. (2016). Effectiveness of the parent-mediated intervention for children with autism spectrum disorder in south Asia in India and Pakistan (PASS): A randomised controlled trial. *The Lancet Psychiatry*, *3*(2), 128–136.

Reed, P. (2016). Outcome-effectiveness for developmental and parent-mediated treatment models. In *Interventions for autism: Evidence for educational and clinical practice* (pp. 175–200). West Sussex, UK: John Wiley & Sons, Ltd..

Reyno, S. M., & McGrath, P. J. (2006). Predictors of parent training efficacy for child externalizing behavior problems–a meta-analytic review. *Journal of Child Psychology and Psychiatry*, *47*(1), 99–111.

Rogers, S. J., Dawson, G., & Vismara, L. A. (2012). *An early start for your child with autism: Using everyday activities to help kids connect, communicate, and learn*. New York: Guilford Press.

Rogers, S. J., Estes, A., Lord, C., Vismara, L., Winter, J., Fitzpatrick, A., … Dawson, G. (2012). Effects of a brief Early Start Denver Model (ESDM)–based parent intervention on toddlers at risk for autism spectrum disorders: A randomized controlled trial. *Journal of the American Academy of Child and Adolescent Psychiatry*, *51*(10), 1052–1065.

Ruble, L. A., & McGrew, J. H. (2007). Community services outcomes for families and children with autism spectrum disorders. *Research in Autism Spectrum Disorders*, *1*(4), 360–372.

Ruppert, T., Machalicek, W., Hansen, S. G., Raulston, T., & Frantz, R. (2016). Training parents to implement early interventions for children with autism spectrum disorders. In *Early intervention for young children with autism spectrum disorder* (pp. 219–256). Cham: Springer International Publishing.

Schertz, H. H. (2005). *Promoting joint attention in toddlers with autism: A parent-mediated developmental model* (Doctoral dissertation). Indiana University.

Schertz, H. H., & Odom, S. L. (2007). Promoting joint attention in toddlers with autism: A parent-mediated developmental model. *Journal of Autism and Developmental Disorders*, *37*(8), 1562–1575.

Schertz, H. H., Odom, S. L., Baggett, K. M., & Sideris, J. H. (2013). Effects of joint attention mediated learning for toddlers with autism spectrum disorders: An initial randomized controlled study. *Early Child Research Quarterly, 28*(2), 249–258.

Scheuermann, B., Webber, J., Boutot, E. A., & Goodwin, M. (2003). Problems with personnel preparation in autism spectrum disorders. *Focus on Autism and Other Developmental Disabilities, 18*(3), 197–206.

Schmidt, F., & Taylor, T. K. (2002). Putting empirically supported treatment into practice: Lessons learned in a children's mental health center. *Professional Psychology: Research and Practice, 33*(5), 483–489.

Schreibman, L., Dawson, G., Stahmer, A. C., Landa, R., Rogers, S. J., McGee, G. G., … McNerney, E. (2015). Naturalistic developmental behavioral interventions: Empirically validated treatments for autism spectrum disorder. *Journal of Autism and Developmental Disorders, 45*, 2411–2428.

Shapiro, C. J., Prinz, R. J., & Sanders, M. R. (2012). Facilitators and barriers to implementation of an evidence-based parenting intervention to prevent child maltreatment: The triple p-positive parenting program. *Child Maltreatment, 17*(1), 86–95.

Siller, M., Hutman, T., & Sigman, M. (2013). A parent-mediated intervention to increase responsive parental behaviors and child communication in children with ASD: A randomized clinical trial. *Journal of Autism and Developmental Disorders, 43*(3), 540–555.

Siller, M. & Morgan, L. (2013). *Making Parent-Mediated Interventions Work for Families: A roundtable hosted by the Autism Speaks Toddler Treatment Network on April 18, 2013 in Seattle, WA.* Retrieved from https://www.autismspeaks.org/science/research-initiatives/toddler-treatment-network/making-parent-mediated-interventions-work-fam

Siller, M., Morgan, L., Turner-Brown, L., Baggett, K. M., Baranek, G. T., Brian, J., … Kasari, C. (2013). Designing studies to evaluate parent-mediated interventions for toddlers with autism spectrum disorder. *Journal of Early Intervention, 35*(4), 355–377.

Siller, M., Swanson, M., Gerber, A., Hutman, T., & Sigman, M. (2014). A parent-mediated intervention that targets responsive parental behaviors increases attachment behaviors in children with ASD: Results from a randomized clinical trial. *Journal of Autism and Developmental Disorders, 44*(7), 1720–1732.

Smith, T., Scahill, L., Dawson, G., Guthrie, D., Lord, C., Odom, S., … Wagner, A. (2007). Designing research studies on psychosocial interventions in autism. *Journal of Autism and Developmental Disorders, 37*(2), 354–366.

Solomon, R., Necheles, J., Ferch, C., & Bruckman, D. (2007). Pilot study of a parent training program for young children with autism the PLAY Project Home Consultation program. *Autism, 11*(3), 205–224.

Solomon, R., Van Egeren, L. A., Mahoney, G., Huber, M. S. Q., & Zimmerman, P. (2014). PLAY Project Home Consultation intervention program for young children with autism spectrum disorders: A randomized controlled trial. *Journal of Developmental and Behavioral Pediatrics, 35*(8), 475–485.

Stadnick, N. A., Stahmer, A., & Brookman-Frazee, L. (2015). Preliminary effectiveness of project ImPACT: A parent-mediated intervention for children with autism spectrum disorder delivered in a community program. *Journal of Autism and Developmental Disorders, 45*(7), 2092–2104.

Stahmer, A. C., & Aarons, G. A. (2009). Attitudes toward adoption of evidence-based practices: A comparison of autism early intervention providers and children's mental health providers. *Psychological Services, 6*(3), 223.

Stahmer, A. C., & Pellecchia, M. (2015). Moving towards a more ecologically valid model of parent-implemented interventions in autism. *Autism, 19*(3), 259–261.

Strauss, K., Vicari, S., Valeri, G., D'Elia, L., Arima, S., & Fava, L. (2012). Parent inclusion in early intensive behavioral intervention: The influence of parental stress, parent treatment fidelity and parent-mediated generalization of behavior targets on child outcomes. *Research in Developmental Disabilities, 33*(2), 688–703.

Suppo, J., & Floyd, K. (2012). Parent training for families who have children with autism: A review of the literature. *Rural Special Education Quarterly, 31*(2), 12–26.

Sussman, F. (2012). *More Than Words: A guide to helping parents promote communication and social skills in children with autism spectrum disorder*. Toronto, ON, Canada: Hanen Centre.

Thomas, K. C., Ellis, A. R., McLaurin, C., Daniels, J., & Morrissey, J. P. (2007). Access to care for autism-related services. *Journal of Autism and Developmental Disorders, 37*(10), 1902–1912.

Tincani, M., Travers, J., & Boutot, A. (2009). Race, culture, and autism spectrum disorder: Understanding the role of diversity in successful educational interventions. *Research and Practice for Persons with Severe Disabilities, 34*(3–4), 81–90.

Turner-Brown, L., Hume, K., Boyd, B. A., & Kainz, K. (2016). Preliminary efficacy of family implemented TEACCH for toddlers: Effects on parents and their toddlers with autism spectrum disorder. *Journal of Autism and Developmental Disorders,* 1–14. http://dx.doi.org/10.1007/s10803-016-2812-7

Virués-Ortega, J. (2010). Applied behavior analytic intervention for autism in early childhood: Meta-analysis, meta-regression and dose–response meta-analysis of multiple outcomes. *Clinical Psychology Review, 30*(4), 387–399.

Vismara, L., McCormick, C., Wagner, A., Monlux, K., Nadhan, A., & Young, G. (2016). Telehealth parent training in the Early Start Denver Model: Results from a randomized controlled study. *Focus on Autism and Other Developmental Disabilities.* doi:10.1177/1088357616651064

Vismara, L. A., Colombi, C., & Rogers, S. J. (2009). Can one hour per week of therapy lead to lasting changes in young children with autism? *Autism, 13*(1), 93–115.

Vismara, L. A., & Rogers, S. J. (2008). The Early Start Denver Model: A case study of an innovative practice. *Journal of Early Intervention, 31*(1), 91–108.

Wainer, A. L., Hepburn, S., & Griffith, E. M. (2016). Remembering parents in parent-mediated early intervention: An approach to examining impact on parents and families. *Autism, 21*(1), 5–17.

Wainer, A. L., & Ingersoll, B. R. (2015). Increasing access to an ASD imitation intervention via a telehealth parent training program. *Journal of Autism and Developmental Disorders, 45*(12), 3877–3890.

Webster, A., Feiler, A., Webster, V., & Lovell, C. (2004). Parentl perspectives on early intensive intervention for children diagnosed with autistic spectrum disorder. *Journal of Early Childhood Research, 2*(1), 25–49.

Welterlin, A., Turner-Brown, L. M., Harris, S., Mesibov, G., & Delmolino, L. (2012). The home TEACCHing program for toddlers with autism. *Journal of Autism and Developmental Disorders, 42*(9), 1827–1835.

Werner, E., Dawson, G., Munson, J., & Osterling, J. (2005). Variation in early developmental course in autism and its relation with behavioral outcome at 3–4 years of age. *Journal of Autism and Developmental Disorders, 35*(3), 337–350.

Wetherby, A. M., Guthrie, W., Woods, J., Schatschneider, C., Holland, R. D., Morgan, L., & Lord, C. (2014). Parent-implemented social intervention for toddlers with autism: An RCT. *Pediatrics, 134*(6), 1084–1093.

Wetherby, A. M., & Woods, J. J. (2006). Early social interaction project for children with autism spectrum disorders beginning in the second year of life a preliminary study. *Topics in Early Childhood Special Education, 26*(2), 67–82.

Wilczynski, S., Green, G., Ricciardi, J., Boyd, B., Hume, A., Ladd, M., & Rue, H. (2009). *National standards report: The national standards project: Addressing the need for evidence-based practice guidelines for autism spectrum disorders*. National Autism Center: Randolph, MA.

Wong, C., Odom, S. L., Hume, K. A., Cox, A. W., Fettig, A., Kucharczyk, S., … Schultz, T. R. (2015). Evidence-based practices for children, youth, and young adults with autism spectrum disorder: A comprehensive review. *Journal of Autism and Developmental Disorders, 45*(7), 1951–1966.

Woods, J. J., & Wetherby, A. M. (2003). Early identification of and intervention for infants and toddlers who are at risk for autism spectrum disorder. *Language, Speech, and Hearing Services in Schools, 34*(3), 180–193.

Zeman, L. D., Swanke, J., & Doktor, J. (2011). Measurable successes for children with ASD: Perspectives from Mothers' virtual journals. *School Social Work Journal, 36*(1), 61–78.

Zwaigenbaum, L., Bauman, M. L., Choueiri, R., Kasari, C., Carter, A., Granpeesheh, D., … Pierce, K. (2015). Early intervention for children with autism spectrum disorder under 3 years of age: Recommendations for practice and research. *Pediatrics, 136*(Supplement 1), S60–S81.

Zwaigenbaum, L., Bryson, S., & Garon, N. (2013). Early identification of autism spectrum disorders. *Behavioural Brain Research, 251*, 133–146.

18 Using the Teaching Interaction Procedure to Teach Social Skills for Individuals Diagnosed with Autism Spectrum Disorder

Joseph H. Cihon, Sara M. Weinkauf, and Mitchell Taubman

18.1 Introduction

Autism spectrum disorder (ASD) is marked by qualitative impairments with social skills, communication, and restricted and/or repetitive behavior (American Psychiatric Association, 2013). Interventions based on the science of applied behavior analysis (ABA) have been designated as the only empirically supported interventions to address these areas of need (Smith, 2012). With respect to the development of social repertoires, one evidence-based intervention is the teaching interaction procedure (TIP; Leaf et al., 2015b; Phillips et al., 1968), which consists of a multistep, systematic teaching procedure. This chapter will provide an in-depth description of the TIP, a historical context, a summary of recent research as it applies to ASD and social skills, and a discussion of future directions and implications.

18.2 What Is the Teaching Interaction Procedure?

The term *teaching interaction* first appeared in print when Phillips and colleagues (1968) described the procedure in *The Teaching Family Handbook*. The TIP, specifically, was originally developed as a component of the Teaching Family Model (Phillips, 1968), which was designed as an ABA-based intervention approach to improve the lives and reduce the recidivism of pre-delinquent and delinquent youth. Lonnie and Elaine Phillips, who were the original Teaching Parents in the first Teaching Family Home (Kirigin, Braukmann, Atwater, & Wolf, 1982; Phillips, 1968; Wolf et al. 1976), furnished skill instruction to the program's court-adjudicated residents. Through videotape analyses, it was determined that the couple described and demonstrated necessary skills, provided reasons that the skills were important to the young residents' future success, and had the youth practice the skills while specific feedback was provided. Thus, the TIP was born and research into its effectiveness followed. Minkin et al. (1976) provided an early experimental analysis of using the TIP to teach social skills to pre-delinquent and delinquent girls (12–14 years of age). The girls who volunteered for the

J.H. Cihon (✉)
Autism Partnership Foundation,
Seal Beach, CA, USA

Endicott College, Beverly, MA, USA
e-mail: jcihon@autismpartnership.com

S.M. Weinkauf
JBA Institute, Torrance, CA, USA

M. Taubman
Autism Partnership Foundation,
Seal Beach, CA, USA

J.B. Leaf (ed.), *Handbook of Social Skills and Autism Spectrum Disorder*, Autism and Child Psychopathology Series, DOI 10.1007/978-3-319-62995-7_18

study demonstrated deficits in social communication skills with others. The researchers targeted asking appropriate conversational questions and providing positive conversational feedback. The results showed that the TIP was effective at increasing the use of the targeted conversational skills for all four girls.

Following the first description, coining of the term, and early research, the TIP was brought to the Young Autism Project at UCLA (Lovaas, 1987) by the third author (i.e., Mitchell Taubman) and implemented with individuals diagnosed with ASD, including those in residential facilities (Smith, Parker, Taubman, & Lovaas, 1992). Subsequently, the TIP has been included in curriculum books, such as *Crafting Connections* (Taubman, Leaf, & McEachin, 2011), and training manuals, such as *Effective Skills for Child-care Workers: A Training Manual from Boys Town* (Dowd, Czyz, O'Kane, & Elofson. 1994), and *The ASSET Manual* (Hazel, Schumaker, Sherman, & Sheldon-Wildgen, 1983). Although the steps of the TIP typically occur in the same order in these publications, as well as in practice, the order should be viewed as a guideline and the interventionist should remain flexible and modify as needed. What follows is a description of the common order found within the literature and curriculum guides as well as a visual representation of the common sequence outlined in Fig. 18.1.

18.2.1 Label and Identify

In the first step, the interventionist labels/identifies the skill that will be the target of the teaching interaction. The end of this step is typically marked by the learner repeating the skill to the interventionist. This step is used to ensure attending and that the learner can label the skill to be learned. As such, the interventionist should ensure that the label is clear and concise. The language used and length of the label (i.e., number of words or syllables used) should be appropriate for the learner's age and skill level.

18.2.2 Meaningful Rationales

The second step involves discussing meaningful rationales for why the skill is important. These rationales are meaningful in that they are important to the learner and are informed by the learner's experiences. For example, if talking to peers about superheroes is a preferred topic for the learner, but s/he does not maintain appropriate distance during the interaction which results in peers walking away, then learning this skill so peers stay close and talk about superheroes would potentially be meaningful for the learner. Furthermore, rationales should be comprised of potentially natural consequences for the behavior being taught. For instance, a rationale should not be "You should stay an arm's length away from your friends, so you don't get in trouble with your teacher," but, rather, "You should stay an arm's length away from your friends because it could make more friends want to stay by you and talk to you about superheroes." Therefore, rationales should not include external or artificial consequences (e.g., awarding of tokens) or potentially unrealistic outcomes (e.g., you will become the quarterback of your favorite NFL team). They are intended to introduce the student to salient, supportive consequences that will likely occur once the student learns and employs the skill being targeted. During the first session with the TIP, the interventionist may take a more active role in providing rationales and can then gradually fade so that the learner is providing the meaningful rationales in future TIPs (Braukmann, Ramp, Braukmann, Willner, & Wolf, 1983).

18.2.3 Description

Third, the interventionist breaks the skill down into its components or steps. These steps should be defined in a way that is clear to the learner. A description of the skill could be broken down into smaller steps similar to a task analysis or as a component of a larger social skill. No matter how the skill is broken down, it should be done prior to the teaching interaction so that the interven-

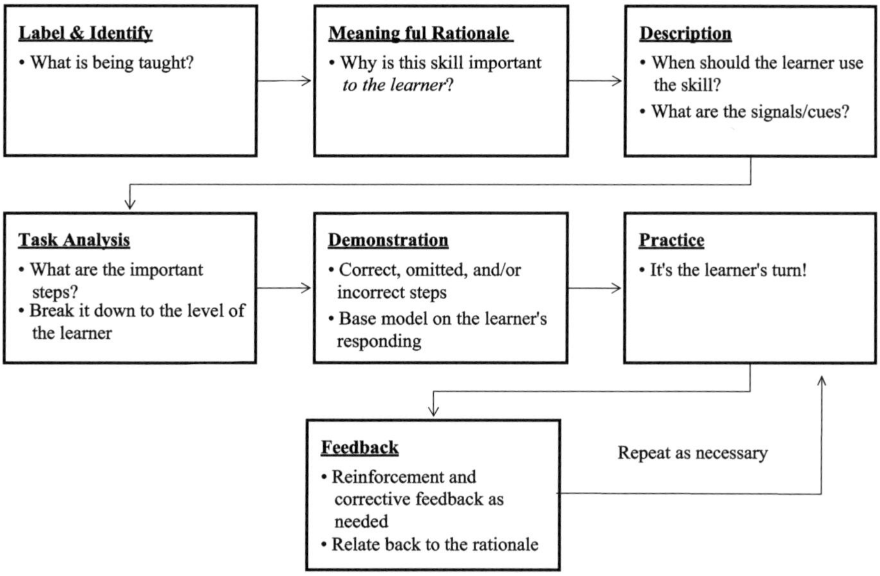

Fig. 18.1 A flowchart depicting the typical sequence for conducting a teaching interaction procedure (TIP). It should be noted this flowchart is provided as a guideline and should not be taken as the only way to conduct a TIP

tionist is prepared. Breaking down a complex social skill in vivo can be extremely difficult even for highly skilled and practiced interventionists. In addition, given the complex nature of social skills, the steps should include all relevant information. This often includes not only what *to* do but also *how* to do it (e.g., posture, tone, and gaze). This step is complete once the learner repeats or states the components or steps in the skill.

18.2.4 Demonstration

Following the description, or sometimes done concurrently, the interventionist models the skill for the learner. This is the fourth step of the TIP. The demonstration includes models of the correct and incorrect way to engage in the skill. This also sets the occasion for the learner to label if and why the demonstration was correct or incorrect. Modeling provides the interventionist with an opportunity to show the learner the exemplar performance and nonexemplar performance, ranging from more obvious examples to less obvious examples as the learner progresses. Furthermore, the interventionist can use the demonstration of the incorrect performance (sometimes referred to as "not-cool;" Leaf et al., 2016) to model the current way the learner responds in the social situation so that the learner can begin to identify that response as incorrect. Demonstrations can occur in vivo, written or pictorial, or via a recording, and should be selected based on what will be most beneficial for the learner. Regardless of the modality of the demonstration, the demonstration paired with the description should provide the learner with a complete representation of the targeted skill.

18.2.5 Practice

In the fifth, and perhaps most important, step, the learner practices/role-plays the skill with the interventionist or a peer. Practice takes the TIP beyond simply describing and demonstrating the skill for the learner and is an essential part of learning. In general, behavior must occur for it to be altered by consequences and practice provides this opportunity for the learner. The learner should have ample time to practice what has been modeled by the interventionist. Practice should be designed in a way that increases the likelihood that the learner will be successful. Over time, practice scenarios should be expanded to increase complexity, difficulty, and independence. Thus, practice begins to resemble the terminal environment in an effort to promote generalization (Stokes & Baer, 1977).

18.2.6 Feedback

Following practice/role-plays, the interventionist engages in the final step of the TIP, feedback. Practice in the absence of feedback will have a limited impact. If practice sets the occasion for the learner to engage in behavior, feedback is the set of consequences that will shape that behavior. Feedback should be specific and descriptive. Feedback can take the form of a potentially reinforcing event when the learner engages in the targeted step(s) of the skill correctly (e.g., verbal praise, access to a preferred event, a token). If the learner displays some or all of the steps incorrectly, feedback can take the form of corrective or instructive feedback (Werts, Wolery, & Holcombe, 1991). Role-plays and feedback continue until the learner meets a predetermined criterion for mastery selected by the interventionist (e.g., 100% of steps completed correctly across three consecutive role-plays).

18.3 Teaching Interaction Procedure and Behavioral Skills Training

Many teaching procedures based upon the principles of ABA have components of the TIP embedded into the procedures. The procedure that associates most closely with the TIP is behavioral skills training (BST; see Chap. 19). These two procedures sharing many common features have led to author commentaries discussing the similarities and differences of the two procedures (e.g., Leaf et al., 2015b). These commentaries have identified two primary features of the TIP that distinguish it from BST.

First, the TIP includes the provision of rationales. When developing and evaluating the TIP, the use of rationales was viewed as a critical component (Leaf et al., 2015b). It was hypothesized that meaningful rationales could result in faster fading of supplemental reinforcement (e.g., tokens). As noted previously, rationales typically include the description of naturally occurring contingencies. For example, losing graciously can result in your peers asking you to play more frequently, whereas being a "sore loser" can result in your peers asking you to play less often. Furthermore, it is speculated that the use of rationales can aide in developing the learner's understanding of cause and effect, as demonstrated by the learner providing potential outcomes based on the presentation of precipitating situations and desired choice making. In contrast, BST does not include meaningful rationales as a core component but, instead, focuses solely on the use of instructions, modeling, rehearsal, and feedback (Miltenberger, 2008) to achieve the desired change in behavior.

The second distinguishing feature is that the TIP includes a demonstration of the correct and incorrect way to engage in the targeted skill. Demonstrations of the incorrect response are often catered to the learner. That is, the interventionist models the features of the learner's current responding with respect to the targeted skill. This is done in an attempt to teach the learner the discrimination between her/his current performance and the desired performance. Conversely, demonstrations during BST include only the correct way to engage in the targeted skill.

18.4 The TIP, ASD, and Social Skills

Thirty-five years after the procedure first appeared in print and was initially used in treatment for persons diagnosed with autism, Leaf et al. (2009) provided the first empirical evaluation of the TIP with individuals diagnosed with ASD. Prior to this, Harchik et al. included the TIP in their 1992 study; however, the participants were adults diagnosed with mental retardation and not autism. Since Leaf et al., several other studies have also evaluated the effectiveness of the TIP for teaching individuals diagnosed with an ASD; many of which have targeted social skills. The focus of the remainder of this chapter is to provide a summary of the research exploring the effectiveness of the TIP to teach social skills to individuals diagnosed with ASD (for a full review of the use of the TIP, see Leaf et al., 2015b).

As previously mentioned, Leaf et al. (2009) provided the first empirical evaluation of the TIP with individuals diagnosed with an ASD. The researchers evaluated the effectiveness of the TIP to teach various social skills to children, ranging in age from 5 to 7 years old. Targeted social skills included following a peer, greeting a peer, including a peer in an activity, choosing a peer partner, changing the topic during a conversation, going with the flow of a conversation or game, giving a compliment, sharing, and making on-topic statements. The TIP was implemented within a one-to-one instructional format, and the effects were measured through naturalistic probes. These probes consisted of a confederate peer setting the occasion for the participant to engage in the targeted skill. For example, if the target skill was giving a compliment, the confederate peer would show the participant a piece of artwork s/he had completed. The confederate peers were not present throughout the course of intervention (i.e., while the skill was being taught to the participant via the steps of the TIP). The results of Leaf et al. (2009) demonstrated that the TIP was effective for teaching all three individuals the targeted social skills; however, no generalization measures were collected and maintenance measures were variable.

Leaf et al. (2010) examined the effectiveness of the TIP within group instruction for five individuals, ages ranging from 4 to 6 years old, diagnosed with ASD. Target skills included showing appreciation, giving a compliment, expressing or displaying empathy, and changing the game. The study took place over 5–7 months with sessions occurring twice a week for 1.5 h. Two typically developing peers served as models during teaching sessions. The results of a multiple probe design showed that the group TIP was effective for teaching the targeted skills for all of the participants. Furthermore, the skills maintained 8 weeks after intervention was completed, and social validity measures indicated that the intervention was satisfactory. In addition, generalization measures indicated variable levels of responding; however, these measures did not include the participants' typical learning or social environments (e.g., school).

Dotson et al. (2010) extended the use of the TIP within a group instructional format with five adolescents, aged 13 to 18 years old, diagnosed with ASD. The researchers used the TIP to teach the participants conversational basics, providing positive feedback to the speaker, and answering open-ended questions. These skills were broken down into smaller components, such as maintaining eye contact, using a positive voice tone, and listening from an appropriate distance. Four of the five participants reached the mastery criteria; however, the skills were maintained at variable rates across the five participants.

Leaf et al. (2012) compared the relative effectiveness of the TIP to Social Stories™ to teach six individuals, ages 5 to 13 years old, with ASD, social skills in a one-to-one instructional format. Three social skills were randomly selected for each condition (i.e., TIP and Social Stories™). Skills included losing or winning graciously, sportsmanship, giving compliments, cheering up a friend, showing appreciation, reciprocal compliments, maintaining an on-topic conversation, and changing the conversation. The results indicated that the TIP was more effective (i.e., participants mastered all skills taught using the TIP) than Social Stories™ (i.e., only four skills were mastered across all of the participants using Social Stories™). Furthermore, skills taught using the TIP were more likely to generalize and maintain after the intervention.

Oppenheim-Leaf et al. (2012a) used the TIP to teach two children with ASD, ages 5 and 7 years old, how to play three common games (Go Fish®, Uno®, and Yahtzee Junior®). Each of the components of the games was broken down into small steps and taught via the TIP. Both children participated in each TIP (i.e., a dyad instructional format). The rationale portion of the TIP also consisted of the purpose of the game. Both participants learned all three games with high levels of generalization.

Oppenheim-Leaf et al. (2012b) extended the literature in regard to the application of the TIP by examining the procedure's use in teaching typically developing children skills to promote social interactions with their siblings diagnosed with ASD. Participants included three siblings, ages 4 to 7 years old, who were taught within a small group format. Targeted skills were inviting a sibling to play, asking to share, providing play instructions, and choosing an activity. Skill acquisition was measured in three ways. The first was during role-plays within each TIP conducted with an adult. The second was during generalization probes with the participants' siblings (ages 4 to 5 years old) in which the researchers prompted the siblings with ASD to engage in behavior that would create an opportunity for the participants to display the targeted skills. And, finally, during free-play probes in which the participants and their siblings with ASD were instructed to "go play." Results from teaching and generalization probes indicated that the TIP was effective at teaching all three children the targeted skills; however, during free play probes, only one dyad demonstrated an increase in social interactions without additional support.

Kassardjian et al. (2013) examined the generalization of social skills taught using the TIP to a natural environment with four individuals diagnosed with ASD, ages ranging 4 to 13 years old. The researchers included a fifth participant as a control (i.e., no intervention). Targeted skills were taught in a one-to-one instructional format and consisted of expanding conversations, winning graciously, social initiations, greeting a peer, and joining on-going conversations. Unlike previous studies, the researchers implementing the TIP did not solely rely on predetermined mastery criterion but, rather, made in-the-moment assessments to modify the implementation of elements of the TIP based on participants' performance and progress (e.g., determining how many role-plays were conducted). Furthermore, the intervention was gradually faded out during stages of generalization. These stages consisted of (1) priming and tangible reinforcement, (2) tangible reinforcement without priming, (3) social praise without priming, and (4) no priming or programmed reinforcement. The results of a multiple baseline across participants design indicated that the flexible TIP was effective for teaching all four participants, the targeted social skills. Also, the skills generalized into naturally occurring settings, with additional peers, without the inclusion of supplemental reinforcement (Kassardjian et al., 2013).

Ferguson, Gillis, and Sevlever (2013) used the TIP with video games to teach six children diagnosed with ASD, ages 7 to 11 years old, team sportsmanship skills. These skills included giving compliments, taking turns, and making a positive post-game comment (e.g., "Good game!"). TIPs were conducted in a small group instructional format (i.e., $n < 6$), and intervention lasted 10 weeks. The results of the study showed an increase in the number of sportsmanship skills and a decrease in the number of negative comments. Generalization probes occurred in other settings or with other video games and indicated that the skills generalized to other contexts.

Kassardjian et al. (2014) replicated and extended Leaf et al. (2012). The extension consisted of using a group rather than a one-to-one instructional format, evaluating responding to peers rather than adults and an analysis of participant responding during each intervention. Three children, each 5 years old and diagnosed with ASD, participated in the study. One social skill was assigned to the TIP condition, the Social Stories™ condition, and a control condition (i.e., three skills in all). Changing the game when a friend is bored was selected as the target in the TIP condition, explaining a prior event in the Social Stories™ condition, and inviting a peer to play in the control condition. The results, which were similar to Leaf et al., indicated that the TIP was the most effective intervention (i.e., none of the participants reached the mastery criteria for skills in the control condition or the Social Stories™ condition). Data collected on responding during teaching indicated that both procedures resulted in accurate responses to comprehension questions, but this responding did not result in an increase in the percentage of correct steps displayed for the targeted skill. Furthermore, all of the skills maintained for at least 100 days following the TIP intervention.

Ng, Schulze, Rudrud, and Leaf (2016) examined the effectiveness of a modified TIP to teach social skills to four individuals, ages 9 to 15 years old, diagnosed with ASD. At the time of the study, each participant would have been considered *lower functioning* (i.e., an IQ score less than 75). Targeted skills included providing help, negotiating, giving a compliment, passing the phone, responding to offers of help, requesting without grabbing, and responding to comments. The TIP was utilized in a small group instructional format. Modifications to the TIP included the use of demonstrations of the rationales, picture prompts for identifying situations in which to engage in the skills, picture prompts to identify the steps of the skills, and only providing demonstrations of the correct way to engage in the targeted skill, as opposed to correct and incorrect, with the rationale of the final modification being to avoid the potential of imitating undesirable examples. The results indicated that the modified TIP was effective in teaching the targeted skills for all four participants; however, for one participant, a variable and increasing trend in baseline for the third skill limits the interpretation of the results with respect to a functional relation for that participant.

Peters, Tullis, and Gallagher (2016) extended Leaf et al. (2010) by evaluating the effectiveness of the TIP implemented in a group instructional format to improve social skills for four individuals, ages 8 to 10 years old, diagnosed with ASD. Peters et al. also assessed maintenance of the social skills targeted during the intervention (i.e., asking for help from an adult, ignoring classmates when they are distracting, joining activities that are already started, and responding appropriately when a game is changed). All sessions occurred in the individual's classrooms, and the TIP was conducted by the staff within each classroom. The results of a multiple-probe design indicated that the TIP was effective at teaching the targeted social skills for all four participants. Furthermore, maintenance checks showed that the skills were maintained at or near the mastery criterion level for all four participants, and social validity measures showed that the participants' parents were very satisfied with the intervention.

18.5 Future Areas of Research

There are several commonalities within the literature that has examined the use of the TIP to teach social skills to individuals diagnosed with ASD. First, the TIP has been empirically demonstrated to be an effective teaching procedure across many settings, participants, and skills. It has also been shown to be effective in both one-to-one and group instructional formats. Many of the studies have used a multiple baseline or multiple probe design to examine the effectiveness of the TIP, with the exception of Leaf et al. 2012, with skill acquisition commonly assessed through probes during teaching or in a more naturalistic setting. Another commonality found in the literature is that, for the majority of the studies to date, many of the participants would commonly be described as *high functioning*, with the exception of Ng et al. (2016). Finally, social validity measures taken throughout the TIP literature are limited. So, while the TIP has a respectable, emerging literature base for teaching social skills to individuals diagnosed with an ASD, there are still areas of research that require more investigation.

Although the TIP is a systematic procedure consisting of several components, no research to date has conducted a component analysis of the TIP; therefore, it remains unclear which components are necessary to ensure skill acquisition. A component analysis would allow researchers to explore the critical variables of the TIP and potentially improve efficiency if some components were deemed unnecessary. Furthermore, the two features that distinguish the TIP from BST are the inclusion of rationales and teacher modeling of correct and incorrect skill performance; therefore, a component analysis would allow for researchers to determine if these differing features result in specific short-term or long-term changes in learning or behavior that make the distinction necessary.

To date, the study by Ng et al. (2016) remains the only study to examine the use of the TIP to teach social skills to individuals with more severe cognitive impairments. The researchers modified some of the components of the TIP before teaching so the extent to which these modifications were necessary for the TIP to be effective remains unknown. Future research should continue to examine the use of the TIP to teach social skills to individuals diagnosed with ASD with a variety of skill levels. This research could examine what modifications or procedural components are necessary for which learners, which skills should be targeted with various populations, and what prerequisite skills are necessary for the TIP to be an effective teaching tool with a variety of populations.

Many studies have explored the use of the TIP within a group or one-to-one instructional format. The benefits of group instruction when teaching social skills has been well documented (e.g., Leaf et al., 2010). Nonetheless, research has yet to demonstrate the direct benefits of conducting the TIP in a group versus a one-to-one format. Some potential measures that could extend the literature base with respect to the benefits of conducting this procedure in a group format could include efficiency, observational learning repertoires, maintenance, and generalization. In addition to examining the potential benefits of conducting the TIP in a group format, research could also help determine the necessary prerequisite skills for a learner to benefit from a group TIP. For example, investigating if learners with less advanced observational learning repertoires would benefit as greatly from group TIPs as peers with more advanced observational learning repertoires.

Oppenheim-Leaf et al. (2012b) provided an innovative example of using the TIP to improve the social skills of children diagnosed with an ASD without direct intervention. The researchers taught specific social skills to siblings to improve their interactions with their brothers and sisters diagnosed with ASD. By teaching the siblings, these skills also resulted in improvements in the social skills of the children diagnosed with ASD. This research could be extended in several ways. For example, exploring what skills to target that would result in the largest collateral social improvements for their brothers and sisters diagnosed with ASD. Another possible extension could examine if similar skills, taught to parents, would result in similar effects. In addition, it may be beneficial to consider social validity measures to measure the children's satisfaction with the intervention as well as improvements in their overall relationship with their sibling with special needs.

To that end, the existence of social validity measures within the TIP literature is lacking, which is similar within much behavior analytic work in general (Carr, Austin, Britton, Kellum, & Bailey, 1999; Schwartz & Baer, 1991). The TIP is an effective tool to teach social skills; however, it remains unclear to what extent the skills taught, or the procedure itself, is socially acceptable or preferred. Effectiveness is not the only significant criterion when determining the appropriateness of a procedure or intervention approach. The procedure also needs to be socially acceptable and appropriate, with all stakeholders considered. Future TIP research and more behavior analytic work, in general, should include measures of social validity. These measures can include appropriateness of the procedure, skill selection, participant preference, and acceptability of levels of maintenance and generalization.

18.6 Recommendations for Practice

Social skills are complex phenomena and are often more difficult to teach than other skills typically targeted for individuals diagnosed with ASD (Taubman et al., 2011). There are an increasing number of procedures or techniques available to the interventionist to help teach these complex skills (the existence of this book is a perfect example of this increase). These procedures include but are not limited to, Social Stories™ (Gray, 2004), social scripts (e.g., Loveland & Tunali, 1991), TIP (Phillips et al., 1968), BST (Miltenberger, 2008), pivotal response training (PRT; Koegel et al., 1989), and video modeling (e.g., Charlop & Milstein, 1989). With this increase, it behooves the practitioner to evaluate the empirical literature base, or lack thereof, as well as the learner's current social repertoire and prerequisite skills before selecting the most appropriate procedure to use.

As discussed previously, the TIP has been empirically demonstrated to be an effective approach to developing meaningful social skills. The practitioner can be assured that when selecting the TIP to teach social skills, s/he is selecting a procedure with a strong evidence base. Furthermore, the frequent use of comparative designs when evaluating the TIP provides the practitioner with a guide for selecting the most efficacious procedure. For instance, if one is deciding between the use of Social Stories™ or the TIP, the current comparative evidence indicates that the TIP is the more desirable of the two procedures. Although there may be conditions under which Social Stories™ are more effective, the current literature base has yet to identify these conditions (Leaf et al., 2015a).

However, the TIP may not be well suited for all learners. Although the research is lacking in identifying which component skills are necessary for the TIP to be an effective teaching tool, some component skills should most likely be developed prior to using the TIP. First, given the exchanges that occur between the interventionist and the learner(s), some basic and/or intermediate conversation skills (e.g., commenting, responding to comments, answering open-ended questions; Leaf, & McEachin, 1999) and interaction skills (e.g., following the lead of another, social problem solving; Taubman et al., 2011) may be necessary. Second, even brief TIPs can require the learner to attend for rather long durations, so sustained attending may also be a necessary skill prior to using the TIP. Third, Taubman et al. (2011) discussed the need for a basic understanding of cause and effect relationships (e.g., turn the light off/the room is dark, drop an egg/the egg shell is broken; Leaf, & McEachin, 1999) as a prerequisite for the TIP. This understanding is demonstrated by the learner stating why an outcome occurred (e.g., "The egg is broken because it fell on the floor") and may be necessary for comprehending rationales as well as the relationships between role-play, employment of learned skills in everyday situations, and resultant changes in outcomes; therefore, this repertoire is also likely to be an important prerequisite before utilizing the TIP to teach social skills.

18.7 Conclusion

When addressing social skills deficits for individuals diagnosed with ASD, many procedures and approaches are available. Although there are still areas of research to investigate regarding different aspects of the TIP, it should be one of the prominent procedures selected for teaching social skills, especially over nonempirically based procedures, given its documented effectiveness, emerging literature base (Leaf et al., 2015b), and flexibility in teaching and targeted skills (Dotson et al., 2013; Kassardjian et al., 2013; Ng et al., 2016). Through continued research and investigation into this effective procedure, further improvements in the intervention strategies utilized to teach social skills to individuals with ASD can be achieved.

References

American Psychiatric Association. (2013). *Diagnostic and statistical manual of mental disorders* (5th ed.). Arlington, VA: American Psychiatric Publishing.

Braukmann, P. D., Ramp, K. K., Braukmann, C. J., Willner, A. G., & Wolf, M. M. (1983). The analysis and training of rationales for child care workers. *Children and Youth Services Review*, *5*(2), 177–194.

Carr, J. E., Austin, J. L., Britton, L. N., Kellum, K. K., & Bailey, J. S. (1999). An assessment of social validity trends in applied behavior analysis. *Behavioral Interventions*, *14*(4), 223–231.

Charlop, M. H., & Milstein, J. P. (1989). Teaching autistic children conversational speech using video modeling. *Journal of Applied Behavior Analysis*, *22*(3), 275–285.

Dotson, W. H., Leaf, J. B., Sheldon, J. B., & Sherman, J. A. (2010). Group teaching of conversational skills to adolescents on the autism spectrum. *Research in Autism Spectrum Disorders*, *4*(2), 199–209.

Dotson, W. H., Richman, D. M., Abby, L., Thompson, S., & Plotner, A. (2013). Teaching skills related to self-employment to adults with developmental disabilities: An analog analysis. *Research in Developmental Disabilities*, *34*(8), 2336–2350.

Dowd, T., Czyz, J. D., O'Kane, S. E., & Elofson, A. (1994). *Effective skills for child-care workers: a training manual from boys town*. Boys Town, NE: The Boys Town Press.

Ferguson, B. R., Gillis, J. M., & Sevlever, M. (2013). A brief group intervention using video games to teach sportsmanship skills to children with autism spectrum disorders. *Child & Family Behavior Therapy*, *35*(4), 293–306.

Gray, C. (2004). Social stories 10.0: The new defining criteria and guidelines. *Jension Autism Journal, 15*, 2–21.

Harchik, A. E., Sherman, J. A., Sheldon, J. B., & Strouse, M. C. (1992). Ongoing consultation as a method of improving performance of staff members in a group home. *Journal of Applied Behavior Analysis, 25*(3), 599–610.

Hazel, J. S., Schumaker, J. B., Sherman, J. A., & Sheldon-Wildgen, J. A. (1983). Social skills training with court-adjusted youths. In C. LeCroy (Ed.), *Social skills training for children and youth* (pp. 117–137). New York: Haworth Press.

Kassardjian, A., Leaf, J. B., Ravid, D., Leaf, J. A., Alcalay, A., Dale, S., … Oppeneheim-Leaf, M. L. (2014). Comparing the teaching interaction procedure to Social Stories: A replication study. *Journal of Autism and Developmental Disorders, 44*(9), 2329–2340.

Kassardjian, A., Rudrud, E., Taubman, M., Leaf, J. B., Edwards, A., Schulze, K., … Leaf, R. (2013). Utilizing teaching interactions to facilitate social skills in the natural environment. *Education and Training in Autism and Developmental Disabilities, 48*(2), 245–257.

Kirigin, K. A., Braukmann, C. J., Atwater, J. D., & Wolf, M. M. (1982). An evaluation of Teaching-Family (Achievement Place) group homes for juvenile offenders. *Journal of Applied Behavior Analysis, 15*(1), 1–16.

Koegel, R. L., Schreibman, L., Good, A., Cerniglia, L., Murphy, C., & Koegel, L. (1989). *How to teach pivotal behaviors to children with autism: A training manual*. Santa Barbara: University of California.

Leaf, J. B., Dotson, W. H., Oppeneheim, M. L., Sheldon, J. B., & Sherman, J. A. (2010). The effectiveness of a group teaching interaction procedure for teaching social skills to young children with a pervasive developmental disorder. *Research in Autism Spectrum Disorders, 4*(2), 186–198.

Leaf, R., & McEachin, J. (1999). *A work in progress: Behavior management strategies and a curriculum for intensive behavioral treatment of autism*. New York: DRL.

Leaf, J. B., Mitchell, E., Townley-Cochran, D., McEachin, J., Taubman, M., & Leaf, R. (2016). Comparing Social Stories™ to cool versus not cool. *Education and Treatment of Children, 39*(2), 173–186.

Leaf, J. B., Oppenheim-Leaf, M. L., Call, N. A., Sheldon, J. B., Sherman, J. A., Taubman, M., … Leaf, R. (2012). Comparing the teaching interaction procedure to social stories for people with autism. *Journal of Applied Behavior Analysis, 45*(2), 281–298.

Leaf, J. B., Oppenheim-Leaf, M. L., Leaf, R. B., Taubman, M., McEachin, J., Parker, T., … Mountjoy, T. (2015a). What is the proof? A methodological review of studies that have utilized social stories. *Education and Training in Autism and Developmental Disaibilities, 50*(2), 127–141.

Leaf, J. B., Taubman, M., Bloomfield, S., Palos-Rafuse, L., Leaf, R., McEachin, J., & Oppenheim, M. L. (2009). Increasing social skills and pro-social behavior for three children diagnosed with autism through the use of a teaching package. *Research in Autism Spectrum Disorders, 3*(1), 275–289.

Leaf, J. B., Townley-Cochran, D., Taubman, M., Cihon, J. H., Oppenheim-Leaf, M. L., Kassardjian, A., … Pentz, T. G. (2015b). The teaching interaction procedure and behavioral skills training for individuals diagnosed with autism spectrum disorder: A review and commentary. *Review Journal of Autism and Developmental Disorders, 2*(4), 402–413.

Lovaas, O. I. (1987). Behavioral treatment and normal educational and intellectual functioning in young autistic children. *Journal of Consulting and Clinical Psychology, 55*(1), 3–9.

Loveland, K. A., & Tunali, B. (1991). Social scripts for conversational interactions in autism and Down syndrome. *Journal of Autism and Developmental Disorders, 21*(2), 177–186.

Miltenberger, R. G. (2008). Behavioral skills training procedures. In R. G. Miltenberger (Ed.), *Behavior modification: Principles and procedures* (pp. 251–272). Belmont: Wadsworth.

Minkin, N., Braukmann, C. J., Minkin, B. L., Timbers, G. D., Timbers, B. J., Fixsen, D. L., … Wolf, M. M. (1976). The social validation and training of conversational skills. *Journal of Applied Behavior Analysis, 9*(2), 127–139.

Ng, A. H. S., Schulze, K., Rudrud, E., & Leaf, J. B. (2016). Using the teaching interactions procedure to teach social skills to children with autism and intellectual disability. *American Journal on Intellectual and Developmental Disabilities, 121*(6), 501–519.

Oppenheim-Leaf, M. L., Leaf, J. B., & Call, N. A. (2012a). Teaching board games to two children with an autism spectrum disorder. *Journal of Developmental and Physical Disabilities, 24*(4), 347–358.

Oppenheim-Leaf, M. L., Leaf, J. B., Dozier, C., Sheldon, J. B., & Sherman, J. A. (2012b). Teaching typically developing children to promote social play with their siblings with autism. *Research in Autism Spectrum Disorders, 6*(2), 777–791.

Peters, B., Tullis, C. A., & Gallagher, P. A. (2016). Effects of a group teaching interaction procedure on the social skills of students with autism spectrum disorders. *Education and Training in Autism and Developmental Disabilities, 51*(4), 421–433.

Phillips, E. L. (1968). Achievement Place: token reinforcement procedures in a home-style rehabilitation setting for "pre-delinquent" boys. *Journal of Applied Behavior Analysis, 1*(3), 213–223.

Schwartz, I. S., & Baer, D. M. (1991). Social validity assessments: Is current practice state of the art? *Journal of Applied Behavior Analysis, 24*(2), 189–204.

Smith, T. (2012). Evolution of research on interventions for individuals with autism spectrum disorder: implications for behavior analysts. *The Behavior Analyst Today, 35*(1), 101–113.

Smith, T., Parker, T., Taubman, M., & Lovaas, O. I. (1992). Transfer of staff training from workshops to group homes: A failure to generalize across settings. *Research in Developmental Disabilities, 13*(1), 57–71.

Stokes, T., & Baer, D. (1977). An implicit technology of generalization. *Journal of Applied Behavior Analysis, 10*(2), 349–367.

Taubman, M. T., Leaf, R. B., McEachin, J., & Driscoll, M. (2011). *Crafting connections: Contemporary applied behavior analysis for enriching the social lives of persons with autism spectrum disorder*. New York, NY: DRL Books.

Werts, M. G., Wolery, M., & Holcombe, A. (1991). *Instructive feedback: Increasing opportunities for learning through the addition of incidental information*. Pittsburgh, PA: Allegheny- Singer Research Institute.

Wolf, M. M., Phillips, E. L., Fixsen, D. L., Braukmann, C. J., Kirigin, K. A., Willner, A. G., & Schumaker, J. (1976). Achievement place: The teaching-family model. *Child Care Quarterly, 5*(2), 92–103.

19 Behavioral Skills Training to Promote Social Behavior of Individuals with Autism

Raymond G. Miltenberger, Heather M. Zerger, Marissa Novotny, and Cynthia P. Livingston

Behavioral skills training (BST) is a teaching method that consists of instructions, modeling, rehearsal, and feedback, utilized by a trainer in a role-play or simulation (Himle & Miltenberger, 2004; Miltenberger, 2016). In the role-play, the trainer simulates the discriminative stimulus (S^D) in the presence of which the target behavior should occur. When using BST to teach social behavior, the S^D presented in the role-play is the opportunity for a social interaction with another person. The use of role-play is important so that the learner can practice engaging in the correct response(s) when the S^D is present and receive feedback for correct and incorrect performance(s). BST is an ideal intervention for promoting social behavior because social contexts and social behavior of others can be simulated effectively in a role-play, and the learner can rehearse the social skills in the role-play context so the correct behavior can be reinforced and corrective feedback can be provided for incorrect behavior. The purpose of this chapter is to discuss the implementation of BST and review several applications of BST for promoting social behavior with individuals diagnosed with autism spectrum disorder (ASD).

R.G. Miltenberger (✉) • H.M. Zerger • M. Novotny • C.P. Livingston
University of South Florida, Tampa, FL, USA
e-mail: miltenbe@usf.edu

19.1 Components of BST

The components of BST are designed to prompt the correct response in the role-play context (instructions and modeling), provide an opportunity for execution of the correct response in the presence of the simulated S^D (rehearsal), and reinforce correct responses or provide further instruction to correct errors (feedback). BST utilizes the concept of the three-term contingency in repeated learning trials until the correct responses are executed fluently in the presence of all relevant S^Ds and no further prompting is required. For BST to be most successful, strategies must be implemented to increase the likelihood that the skills acquired in training will generalize to the natural context where they are expected to occur (Miltenberger, 2008, 2016). Each of the BST components is described next.

19.1.1 Instructions

Instructions give a detailed description of the correct behavior, or chain of behaviors in the correct sequence, and the context in which the behavior should occur (Miltenberger, 2016). For example, in teaching a child to respond safely to an abduction lure, the teacher would instruct the child to say "no" loudly, get away, and tell an adult. Additionally, the teacher would describe the types of abduction lures to which the child should

J.B. Leaf (ed.), *Handbook of Social Skills and Autism Spectrum Disorder*, Autism and Child Psychopathology Series, DOI 10.1007/978-3-319-62995-7_19

engage in the safety skills (e.g., when an adult asks the child to leave, asks the child for assistance, offers the child a reward for leaving, invokes authority when asking the child to leave). When developing instructions, one should consider a few factors. First, instructions should be delivered in terms that the learner can understand; therefore, the receptive language capabilities of the learner must be considered. Second, instructions must be given by someone who has an authority relationship with the learner, such as a parent or teacher. Third, instructions should only be delivered once the learner is paying attention. Fourth, the learner should be asked to repeat the instructions immediately after they are delivered. Finally, instructions should be delivered along with a model of the correct behavior so the learner sees the behavior after the teacher describes the behavior.

19.1.2 Modeling

Modeling involves a demonstration of the correct behavior in a simulation of the correct context for the learner. That is, the trainer presents the S^D and then exhibits the correct behavior in the presence of the S^D. For modeling to be effective, the learner must already have an imitative repertoire; the learner must be able to imitate the behavior of the model. The teacher can demonstrate the correct behavior through live modeling (i.e., demonstrating the behavior in real time for the learner) or symbolic modeling (i.e., demonstrating the behavior through video, audio, computer simulations, dolls, etc.). Live modeling is valuable because it offers the trainer the most flexibility to adjust aspects of the modeled behavior or context to fit the learner's needs. Symbolic modeling such as video modeling is valuable because it is consistent across iterations and it is more accessible to individuals across settings. For example, a video model can be made accessible through the internet and accessed by anyone for whom such a model is relevant to current training needs. A number of researchers incorporated video modeling into BST for teaching social skills (e.g., Plavnick, Kaid, & MacFarland, 2015; Plavnick, Sam, Hume, & Odom, 2013; Radley, Dart, Moore, Battaglia, & LeBrot, 2017; Radley et al., 2015; Radley, Ford, Battaglia, & McHugh, 2014a; Radley, Hanglein, & Arak, 2016).

Several factors that may influence the effectiveness of modeling should be considered. First, the model's behavior should be followed by favorable consequences so it appears the model's behavior is rewarded. Second, the model should have similar characteristics to the learner (e.g., a 7-year-old child who is being taught safety skills should be shown a model of a similar-age child) or should have a high status with the learner (e.g., teacher, parent, celebrity, etc.). Third, the modeled behavior should be appropriate for the learning ability of the learner. In other words, the modeled behavior must not be too lengthy or complex for the learner to imitate. Fourth, the learner should be oriented to the model before the model demonstrates the behavior. Fifth, modeling should take place in the appropriate situation (i.e., a simulation of the relevant S^D, as it would naturally occur). Finally, the model should be repeated as many times as necessary for the learner to correctly imitate the behavior and modeled in a variety of ways so that the behavior is more likely to occur in the variety of situations that are relevant for the learner. As the teacher provides the model, the teacher should also describe the important aspects of the model (e.g., "Did you see how Ray said 'no,' ran away, and told his mom about the man who asked him to get in the car."). It is also valuable to ask the learner to describe the model's behavior if the learner has the verbal skills to do so.

19.1.3 Rehearsal

Immediately following instructions and modeling, the learner should have the opportunity to practice the skill. Rehearsal allows the learner to practice the behavior in a simulation and allows the teacher to assess whether the behavior is being performed correctly and to provide reinforcement for correct responding and corrective feedback for incorrect responding. The learner should always practice the behavior in the appropriate context (in the presence of the simulated S^D), followed by immediate reinforcement for correct responding or corrective feedback for incorrect responding, and practice until the correct behavior has been emitted a few times. By rehearsing in a role-play that simulates the S^D, reinforcement for the correct behavior can be delivered in the presence of the S^D, and thus the behavior is more likely to generalize to the S^D that occurs in the natural environment.

19.1.4 Feedback

In BST, feedback involves the delivery of reinforcement contingent on correct responding and further instruction contingent on incorrect responding. Upon completion of the rehearsal, descriptive praise and/or some other reinforcers should be delivered immediately for some aspect of the behavior that was emitted correctly, regardless of whether the entire behavior was performed correctly. Corrective feedback should also be delivered immediately for incorrect responses. It is important to note that corrective feedback is not criticism or telling the learner what he or she did wrong. Corrective feedback is the provision of instruction for engaging in the correct behavior in the next rehearsal (Miltenberger, 2016). For example, if during abduction prevention skills training the learner said "no" to the abduction lure but failed to run away and tell, the trainer's feedback might be, "Sherry, you did a great job saying 'no' when the stranger asked you to leave. You said 'no' very loudly. Way to go! Now we are going to practice again, this time after the stranger asks you to get in his car, make sure to run into your house and tell your mom. Okay, let's try it again. Remember, as soon as the stranger asks you to leave, yell 'no' and then run away and tell your mom." If the learner's performance is correct, descriptive praise is provided. If some aspect of the behavior is incorrect, the trainer provides further instruction and perhaps another model. The learner then rehearses the behavior followed by delivery of the appropriate type of feedback until consistent, correct performance is observed across multiple rehearsals.

19.2 Promoting Generalization During BST

Because BST often consists of training in a classroom or another setting separate from the context in which the target behavior is expected to occur, the trainer must implement strategies to promote generalization. A number of strategies can be used to promote generalization (Miltenberger, 2008, 2016; Stokes & Baer, 1977; Stokes & Osnes, 1989). First, BST should incorporate multiple exemplars. That means the trainer should include multiple opportunities to rehearse the behavior in the presence of a variety of stimuli that sample the range of relevant stimuli in the natural environment (e.g., Radley et al., 2015). Incorporating multiple exemplars into training increases the likelihood that the individual will come into contact with stimuli in the natural environment to which he or she has already responded successfully in training. Second, the trainer can teach multiple variations of a social skill (i.e., a variety of functionally equivalent responses) to increase the likelihood that the social skill will result in reinforcing responses from communication partners (e.g., Peters & Thompson, 2015; Radley et al., 2017). Third, the trainer can incorporate common stimuli. By bringing stimuli from the natural environment into training, the learner is more likely to engage in the behavior successfully in the natural environment when those common stimuli are present. For example, when teaching social skills, incorporating a common stimulus might entail having a peer participate as a communication partner in training (e.g., Radley et al., 2014). Responding successfully to the peer in training increases the likelihood of responding successfully when that or another peer is present in the natural environment. Fourth, the target behaviors should be chosen so they are likely to contact reinforcement in the natural environment. That is, the social behavior the learner acquires during BST should be chosen so relevant individuals in the natural environment will likely react positively when the learner exhibits the behavior (e.g., Stewart, Carr & LeBlanc, 2007). For example, when teaching social skills to a child with autism, the targeted skills should be ones that are likely to evoke reciprocal social interactions from typical peers. Fifth, the trainer or others in the natural environment can reinforce instances of generalization. For example, a teacher might provide praise or other reinforcers when observing the target social behavior, or peers can be trained to respond favorably when the learner exhibits the social behavior with them (e.g., Barry et al., 2003). Finally, in situ training (described later) can be used to promote generalization.

19.3 In Situ Assessment and In Situ Training

After BST has been used to teach a skill, and the skill is demonstrated consistently in the training setting, it is important to assess the same skill in the natural environment in which it would be expected to occur (e.g., Radley et al., 2015). For example, a student might learn abduction prevention skills in the classroom, but the skills would be assessed when the student is alone in the community (e.g., at a bus stop) and approached by a stranger who presents a lure (e.g., Haseltine & Miltenberger, 1990; Poche, Yoder, & Miltenberger, 1988). This form of assessment, called an in situ assessment, takes place when the learner's skills are assessed in the natural environment and the learner does not know that an assessment is occurring (Miltenberger, 2016). Furthermore, the teacher or other adult who might exert stimulus control over the behavior is not present during an in situ assessment. In situ assessments are especially important to ensure that the skill will occur in the right context and that it will be exhibited without the influence of the trainer or other individuals who were present during training (Miltenberger, 2008). Because there are no programmed consequences for the behavior during in situ assessments, they demonstrate the occurrence of the behavior under the stimulus control of the naturally occurring context.

If the desired skill is not performed correctly in a natural context, in situ training can be conducted to promote generalization. In situ training (IST) takes place when the learner does not engage in the correct behavior during an in situ assessment and the trainer (or parent or teacher), who was unseen by the student, immediately enters the situation, provides feedback, and has the learner practice the skill a few times. For example, an in situ assessment might be used to assess a student's abduction prevention skills following safety skills training (e.g., Sanchez & Miltenberger, 2015). During the assessment, an adult unknown to the student presents a lure when the student is alone (e.g., the student is in the hallway while at school "running an errand," and the unknown adult walks up and asks the student to leave with him). If the student does not immediately run away and tell his teacher about the lure, the trainer would walk into the hallway at the moment the child failed to exhibit the safety skills and conduct training in the situation—thus, "in situ" training. In situ assessment is important for assessing the use of the skills in the natural environment without the stimulus control exerted by the presence of the trainer and in situ training is important for promoting generalization and maintenance of the skill taught during BST (Gatheridge et al., 2004; Miltenberger et al., 2004, 2005).

19.4 Applications of BST

BST has been used to teach a variety of skills to a variety of populations in a variety of settings (Gatheridge et al., 2004; Hanley, Heal, Tiger, & Ingvarsson, 2007; Johnson et al., 2005, 2006; Miltenberger, 2008; Palmen, Didden, & Arts, 2008; Rosales, Stone, & Rehfeldt, 2009). In the next section, we will review the application of BST to promote social behavior of individuals with ASD. Social behavior is defined broadly to include behavior required to interact successfully with others in a variety of contexts. In this section we focus on social skills, job skills, and safety skills. We also describe research on BST for teaching staff to deliver behavior-analytic procedures to clients who have been diagnosed with ASD.

19.4.1 Social Skills

The development of social skills is a crucial behavioral cusp (Rosales-Ruiz & Baer, 1997) allowing individuals to interact with others and establish relationships that can result in further development of communication and language skills and contact social reinforcement (Kornacki, Ringdahl, Sjostrom, & Nuernberger, 2013). One of the central characteristics of ASD is a deficit in social skills. Individuals with ASD often exhibit difficulties with the initiation and maintenance of conversations and may engage in inappropriate interactions. Social skills training research targets responses such as eye contact, greetings, asking questions, conversation skills, play skills (e.g., Barry et al., 2003; Peters & Thompson, 2015; Stewart et al., 2007) and interactions with others related to mutually reinforcing objects or activities (e.g., Gaylord-Ross, Haring, Breen, & Pitts-Conway, 1984). Researchers have also targeted skills to judge the interest of others in the conversational topic and varied responses to use in response to extinction of the original response by the listener (Peters & Thompson, 2015). Furthermore, the use of BST to improve social skills has been evaluated with not only children but also with adolescents and adults with ASD (e.g., Kornacki et al., 2013; Nuernberger, Ringdahl, Vargo, Crumpecker, & Gunnarsson, 2013; Palmen et al., 2008; Peters & Thompson, 2015; Stewart et al., 2007).

Nuernberger et al. (2013) assessed the effects of a BST package on teaching vocal and nonvocal communication skills to three young adults diagnosed with ASD. The training package included BST, in situ training, and reinforcer delivery implemented in a multiple baseline across participants design. During baseline, the experimenter prompted participants to choose a topic, start, and maintain a conversation with a peer about the chosen topic. Data were collected on the number of appropriate conversation skills the participants engaged in during their conversation. Each baseline session consisted of one conversation composed of at least three exchanges, lasting approximately 5 min. BST included providing participants written and vocal instructions, two experimenters modeling the conversation skills, participants rehearsing the conversation skills with one of the experimenters, and feedback provided for correct and incorrect responses. Once participants engaged in 100% of the conversation skills included in the task analysis, in situ training was implemented in the participants' living center. During in situ training, feedback was provided for conversation skills completed correctly and incorrectly. Additionally, 3-min access to preferred items was provided contingent on increases in correct responding. One or two weeks post-BST implementation, baseline sessions were conducted to assess maintenance of the conversation skills. Follow-up data were also collected for two of the three participants 6–8 weeks post-intervention, with procedures identical to baseline. The results indicated BST increased appropriate vocal and nonvocal communication skills. Additionally, skill maintenance was observed up to 8 weeks following completion of BST.

Kornacki et al. (2013) extended Nuernberger et al. (2013) by conducting a component analysis of the BST package to teach conversation skills to three young adults with ASD or intellectual disability. The BST package was broken into six components including—in order of implementation—instructions, modeling, rehearsal, rehearsal plus feedback, in situ training plus feedback in a contrived setting, and in situ training plus feedback and reinforcement. Following baseline sessions, each BST component was implemented cumulatively in sequential phases. That is, component 1 (i.e., instructions) was implemented first, and if the termination criterion of correct engagement in 80% of the conversation skills was not met, component 2 was added (i.e., instructions and modeling). If the termination criterion was not met, component 3 was added (i.e., instructions, modeling, and rehearsal). Components were sequentially implemented until the termination criterion was met or until all six components had been implemented. The results showed that different components of BST were required for each participant, suggesting no specific component was the key component responsible for acquisition of conversation skills.

These results indicate BST can be made more efficient for some individuals by eliminating unnecessary components, but, currently, the unnecessary components for any one individual can only be identified by assessment of that individual's responding to each component. Considering that the implementation of all four components of BST does not require substantial time, and the components make sense from a pedagogical perspective (i.e., all important components of a learning trial are present), the time required to evaluate which component(s) would be most effective for any one individual would not be more efficient than implementing the full BST procedure. Thus, it is our recommendation to include all components when teaching social skills, even if acquisition may occur for some individuals when fewer components are implemented.

Palmen et al. (2008) evaluated BST implemented in a small-group format to teach social skills to nine high-functioning adolescents with ASD. In this study, the target behavior was asking questions of a conversational partner. Training started with instructions and audiotaped modeling of conversation questions for the group. As the participants listened to the audiotape of a conversation, they rated whether the conversation questions in the audio were correct or incorrect and received feedback on their ratings. Each participant then participated in five individual role-plays during which he or she rehearsed question-asking and received feedback from the trainer. In addition, each of the other participants observed the rehearsal and used a flowchart to rate the participant's question-asking according to three criteria: (a) the question was about the conversation topic, (b) it occurred within 5 s of a pause, and (c) it started with a who, what, or when interrogative. In addition, training occurred in the context of a game in which the participants moved a pawn forward on the game board each time they responded correctly in the role-play or when evaluating the role-play performance. Results showed an increase in appropriate conversational questions for all participants during regularly scheduled tutorial conversations with their personal coaches.

Palmen et al. (2008) is an example of BST implemented in a group setting that included a number of positive features to complement the BST procedures. First, the flowchart was utilized as a cue that prompted the correct use of all three components of the skill and enhanced generalization of the conversational skill. Second, the use of the audio model with an active responding requirement helped the participants discriminate correct from incorrect questions in the audio. Third, by evaluating the performance of the individual engaging in rehearsal, all participants were actively engaged in the group training even when they, themselves, were not engaging in rehearsal. Finally, the game format provided a form of reinforcement for correct performance of all participants during training.

Radley and colleagues also evaluated BST implemented in a group training format for teaching social skills to preschoolers and young children with ASD (Radley et al., 2014a, 2014c, 2016, 2017). In each study, the researchers evaluated a manualized intervention called the Superheroes Social Skills program that included BST components. Although the program description varied slightly across studies, it consisted of a description of the skills and rationale presented via video, video modeling by the animated superhero and by typical peers, live modeling by typical peers, rehearsal of the skills with a typically developing peer, feedback from a facilitator consisting of praise and error correction, a social game in which the participant could use the skill and receive social reinforcement, and the use of a self-monitoring card to use during rehearsals. The participants received instructions to use the card to self-monitor the skills outside of the sessions. Radley et al. (2014a) evaluated the effects of the intervention on social engagement during recess with four 8–10-year-old children with ASD and showed improvements for all children. Radley et al. (2014c) evaluated the intervention with three 10–14-year-olds with ASD. They showed improvements in four social skills (i.e., participation, conversation, perspective taking, and problem-solving) in the training setting and in the generalization setting with different people and different stimuli. Radley et al. (2015) also showed increases in social skills in the training setting and during generalization assessments following training. Radley et al. (2016) evaluated the program with two 4-year-old children with ASD on four skills involved in playing appropriately with a peer (i.e., introduce self, get ready, participate, and body skills such as eye contact, facial expression, and tone of voice). They showed improvement in all four skills for both participants. Radley et al. (2017) evaluated the intervention with five 7–10-year-olds with ASD. They taught four social skills with the Superheroes program (i.e., responding to questions, maintaining a conversation, expressing wants and needs, and participation) and then implemented lag schedules of reinforcement to increase variability in responding following training. A lag schedule of reinforcement provides a reinforcer for a response that is different from the previous x number of responses. Participants showed increases in the targeted social skills and variability in responses.

Although BST has been shown to be effective when implemented in an individual and group format, it is most often implemented by researchers or other professionals. Stewart et al. (2007) evaluated the effectiveness of family-implemented BST for teaching social skills to a child with ASD. The researchers used BST to teach the mother and sister of a 10-year-old boy with Asperger's syndrome to implement BST to teach social skills (e.g., eye contact, appropriate conversation topics) that would help the boy interact more effectively with his peers. The researchers collected treatment integrity data and showed that the mother and sister implemented BST procedures with fidelity and that the boy's social skills improved following intervention. Laugeson, Frankel, Mogil, and Dillon (2009) and Radley, Jensen, Clarke, and O'Neill (2014b) also evaluated the effectiveness of teaching parents to conduct social skills training with their children with ASD. Laugeson et al. evaluated the PEERS program and Radley et al. evaluated the Superheroes Social Skills program; both programs are manualized interventions that include BST components. This research showed that parents can implement BST in the context of manualized interventions to produce improvements in their children's social skills.

Other researchers have evaluated interventions that included BST components for teaching social skills to children with ASD. For example, Leaf et al. (2012a) evaluated the "teaching interaction procedure" for teaching social skills to children with autism. Although not called BST, this procedure includes all of the components of BST. The teaching interaction procedure uses instructions, modeling, rehearsal, and feedback but places additional emphasis on providing a rationale for the behavior and having the participant describe the target behavior early in training. Leaf et al. compared the teaching interaction procedure to a Social Stories™ intervention and demonstrated the effectiveness of the teaching interaction procedure on 18 targeted social skills. Research by Leaf et al. (2009) and Leaf, Dotson, Oppenheim, Sheldon, and Sherman (2010) also demonstrated the effectiveness of the teaching interaction procedure for teaching social skills to children with ASD. In a similar vein, Leaf et al. (2012b) demonstrated the effectiveness of a cool versus not cool procedure with BST components for teaching social skills to children with ASD. In this study, the cool versus not cool procedure was used to teach children to discriminate examples and non-examples of appropriate social skills, similar to procedures used by Palmen et al. (2008). The researchers used this procedure in conjunction with modeling and role-plays that involved rehearsal of the skills with feedback.

Research has established the effectiveness of BST and procedures using BST components for teaching social skills to individuals with ASD in individual and group training formats. Although the research establishing the effectiveness of BST is robust, more research is needed to evaluate the relative merits of the component procedures. For example, many studies evaluated instructions and video modeling as components of the BST intervention. It would be valuable to investigate the effects of these antecedent components alone as they are more efficient than the entire BST intervention and would be more accessible as they could be delivered without an intervention agent. Although we believe interventionists should implement the full BST procedure as recommended earlier, knowing the conditions under which the instructions and modeling components can be effective is important because these components can be made widely accessible through various media (e.g., websites, training manuals). In addition further research should evaluate the need for ancillary procedures, such as self-management or the inclusion of games that have been included in some studies to see if they enhance the effectiveness of BST for teaching social skills. Finally, further research should continue to evaluate parent-implemented BST (e.g., Gross, Miltenberger, Knudson, Bosch, & Brower-Breitwieser, 2007; Jostad, Miltenberger, Kelso, & Knudson, 2008; Laugeson et al., 2009; Radley et al., 2014b; Stewart et al., 2007) as well as peer-implemented BST (Jostad et al., 2008) as strategies to make BST more accessible.

19.4.2 Job Skills

Individuals diagnosed with ASD often lack the skills necessary to obtain and maintain employment. Engstrom, Ekstrom, and Emilsson (2003) found only 2% of individuals with Asperger's syndrome or high-functioning autism were employed. Furthermore, Bellstedt, Gillberg, and Gillberg (2005) conducted a longitudinal study to assess the social and employment positions of individuals diagnosed with ASD, with results indicating 90% of the 120 participants were unemployed. One explanation for the low employment rate among individuals with ASD is their impairments in social and communicative functioning. These deficits can decrease the effectiveness of traditional job training programs and lead to poor performance on the job or failure to obtain a job. Although the research is limited, studies show that BST can be effective for teaching job skills to individuals with ASD.

Burke, Andersen, Bowen, Howard, and Allen (2010) assessed the effects of BST and a performance cue system (PCS) to teach social-vocation skills to six individuals with ASD. In study 1, participants were instructed to assist in a mock fire safety assembly as a firefighter mascot. During BST, participants received a training script containing information about the target behaviors and watched a training video that modeled the target behaviors. Participants could watch the video or review the script as many times as they wanted prior to practice sessions. Additionally, participants were given a practice log and instructed to record the date, start time, and end time of occasions in which they practiced the target behaviors outside of the scheduled training sessions. During training sessions, the participants performed the target skills and received praise for correct responses and corrective feedback for incorrect responses. Live modeling and additional rehearsal and feedback occurred when incorrect responses were performed. If participants did not engage in the correct responses at least 50% of the time by the second BST session, or did not meet the 80% termination criteria by the fifth BST session, PCS was implemented. The PCS included an iPhone application that displayed visual prompts for participants to engage in the target response. During the PCS phase, experimenters showed participants how the iPhone application worked and allowed them to practice responding to several prompts. The PCS was then put inside the mascot costume at participants' eye level, and participants were instructed to follow the instructions displayed on the screen. Study 2 was identical to study 1; however, PCS and BST were implemented in reverse order with new participants. The results of study 1 and 2 indicated BST alone was effective at teaching one participant the target social-vocational skills, PCS alone was effective for two participants, and BST and PCS were both required in teaching the remaining three participants.

In a similar study, Allen, Wallace, Greene, Bowen, and Burke (2010) evaluated video modeling (VM) with three young adults with ASD for promoting skills needed to entertain customers and promote products while wearing a mascot costume in a retail store. In this study, all participants carried out the job duties after watching the video model without the addition of the rehearsal and feedback components of BST. Although VM alone was a more efficient training approach than the implementation of BST, it is not clear under what circumstances VM alone will be effective or all components of BST will be required for skill acquisition. However, it appears the skills taught with VM by Allen et al. were less complex than the skills taught with BST and video prompting by Burke et al. (2010). More research is needed to compare VM versus BST for teaching job-related skills to individuals with ASD.

Task engagement has also been observed to be problematic with individuals with ASD in performing employment and academic tasks (e.g., Callahan & Rademacher, 1999). Palmen and Didden (2012) assessed the effects of BST implemented in a training setting on task engagement in a generalization setting (i.e., job training setting). Participants included six young adults at the treatment facility providing educational services and job-skills training to individuals with ASD. During baseline, data were collected on participants' off-task behaviors exhibited during the standard job training provided by the treatment facility. The BST package was implemented in a small-group setting, and data were again collected on participants' off-task behaviors exhibited during standard job training. The BST package included (a) an introduction, in which criteria for on-task behaviors were reviewed; (b) discrimination training, in which videos were shown to participants that included examples of on-task and off-task behaviors; (c) self-management training, in which participants were provided with written instructions for on-task behaviors in a flowchart format; and (d) rehearsal, in which participants practiced engaging in a specific target task with feedback provided for engagement in on- and off-task behaviors. Following the intervention, 6-week and 6-month follow-up observations were conducted to assess participants' off-task behaviors during standard job training in the absence of the intervention. Results indicated that BST decreased off-task engagement in the generalization setting for all six participants, with responding maintaining at the 6-week and 6-month follow-up assessments.

In further evaluations of BST to teach job skills, Lerman, Hawkins, Hoffman, and Caccavale (2013) and Lerman, Hawkins, Hillman, Shireman, and Nissen (2015) evaluated BST to train adults with ASD to conduct ABA procedures with young children with ASD. Lerman et al. (2015) used BST to train five adults to conduct mand training sessions through incidental teaching (IT) and discrete trial training (DTT) with eleven 3- to 7-year-old children enrolled in ABA services. In baseline, participants conducted the mand trials without any instruction. During BST, the researcher provided written and oral instructions, modeled the correct IT procedures, and answered questions. The participants rehearsed the procedures, and the researcher provided immediate feedback after each trial, consisting of a description of the steps performed correctly and incorrectly. The researcher modeled any steps performed incorrectly, and the trial was repeated until all of the response components were correctly performed. Once a participant reached 80% accuracy for two consecutive sessions during immediate feedback, delayed feedback was provided for the remainder of the training sessions. Monetary reinforcers were also earned contingent upon training session attendance, regardless of performance. Additional monetary reinforcers could be earned for each trial performed with 100% accuracy. Results of study 1 demonstrated that participants acquired the skills needed to implement mand training. Additionally, the mands exhibited by a majority of children increased from baseline to post-training.

In study 2, the same BST procedures were used to teach adults with ASD to implement DTT with children with ASD in the same setting. However, the adults were working at the same time with multiple children who engaged in problem behavior. Results of study 2 demonstrated that adult performance exceeded 90% correct responding on the targeted teaching skills. Further, these skills generalized to children who were not part of the adults' BST training. Similar findings were reported by Lerman et al. (2013) who used BST to teach five adults with ASD to use a DTT procedure to teach skills to children with ASD. In this study, the researchers used BST to teach the adults with ASD to conduct the procedures with researchers playing the role of children with ASD. After the adults with ASD demonstrated the teaching skills with the researchers, the researchers used in situ training to teach the adults with ASD to use the teaching skills with the children with ASD. Following training, the adults with ASD implemented the teaching procedures correctly, and the children with ASD exhibited improved skills following training.

These studies demonstrate the effectiveness of BST for increasing job skills for individuals diagnosed with ASD. Interestingly, additional procedures were implemented with BST, including performance cueing with a smartphone (Burke et al., 2010), self-management procedures (Palmen & Didden, 2012), and monetary reinforcement (Lerman et al., 2015). Although research on BST for teaching job skills shows promise, the research is limited, and more is needed to evaluate the effectiveness of BST with a larger variety of individuals with ASD and a larger variety of job-related skills. Furthermore, research should evaluate the need for ancillary procedures to enhance the effectiveness of BST.

19.4.3 Safety Skills

Another area in which BST has been used to promote social behavior is teaching safety skills. Such skills include pedestrian skills, responding appropriately to abduction and sexual abuse lures, and fire safety skills. However, the majority of research using BST to teach safety skills to individuals with autism and intellectual disabilities has focused on abduction prevention skills (Bergstrom, Najdowski, & Tarbox, 2014; Fisher, Burke, & Griffin, 2013; Gunby, Carr, & LeBlanc, 2010; Gunby & Rapp, 2014; Haseltine & Miltenberger, 1990; Sanchez & Miltenberger, 2015).

A number of studies have evaluated the effectiveness of BST and IST for teaching safety skills to typically developing children (Miltenberger, 2008). This research has focused on safety skills to prevent firearm injury (Gatheridge et al., 2004; Himle, Miltenberger, Flessner, & Gatheridge, 2004; Himle, Miltenberger, Gatheridge, & Flessner, 2004; Miltenberger et al., 2004, 2005, 2009) and abduction (Beck & Miltenberger, 2009; Johnson et al., 2005, 2006; Miltenberger et al., 2013; Poche, Brouwer, & Swearingen, 1981; Poche et al., 1988). Across these studies, safety skills were assessed before and after training using in situ assessments in which the children were exposed to an abduction lure from a research assistant or found a real, but disabled, firearm, and their responses were assessed without their knowledge that an assessment was taking place. A consistent finding across these studies is that BST produced generalized use of the safety skills with roughly half of the participants and IST was needed for correct responding during in situ assessments for half of the participants. Based on the results of these studies, it is recommended that teachers start safety skills training with BST, evaluate the effectiveness of the intervention with in situ assessments, and, if the children do not exhibit the safety skills, proceed to IST. The safety skills training research conducted with typically developing children has informed research on teaching safety skills to children and adolescents with ASD.

Bergstrom et al. (2014), Gunby et al. (2010), and Gunby and Rapp (2014) used BST and IST to teach children with autism how to respond when presented with an abduction lure by a stranger. During BST, participants were first given rules on what to do if a stranger were to approach them and ask them to leave (e.g., "Tell the person 'no,' run away, and then tell an adult."). Gunby et al. and Gunby and Rapp then used video modeling to show children responding correctly to abduction lures; Bergstrom et al. did not include a modeling component. During the rehearsal component, the experimenter presented the participant with an abduction lure and instructed the participant to engage in the safety skills. Correct responding to the lures resulted in praise and incorrect responding resulted in corrective feedback. In addition, Bergstrom et al. used a constant prompt-delay procedure to prompt the correct response when necessary. Following BST, in situ assessments were conducted in which strangers (i.e., research assistants) approached the participants and presented them with abduction lures. In addition, Gunby and Rapp added a high-p sequence prior to the abduction lure during in situ assessments to make it more challenging for the participants to refuse and engage in the safety skills (i.e., in the high-p procedure, the stranger made three high-probability requests to induce compliance before presenting the lure). During assessments, correct responding resulted in parents delivering praise, and incorrect responding resulted in corrective feedback consisting of additional instructions and rehearsals (i.e., in situ training). In situ assessments continued until the participant correctly engaged in all steps of the safety skill. Although BST resulted in correct safety skill engagement, some participants required further in situ training and, in one case, an incentive. However, all participants' correct responding maintained during follow-up assessments in each study.

Fisher et al. (2013) and Sanchez and Miltenberger (2015) used BST and IST to teach abduction prevention skills to young adults diagnosed with autism or developmental disabilities. The researchers taught participants to say "no," walk away from the stranger, and tell a trusted adult, and these responses were scored on a 0 to 4 scale (0 = agreed to leave with abductor, 1 = did not agree to leave, 2 = said "no," 3 = said "no" and got away, and 4 = said "no," got away, and told an adult). Modeling was provided live or via video. During in situ assessments following the BST intervention, if the participants did not respond correctly, IST was implemented in which the participants had to perform the skills during three consecutive rehearsals. All participants in Sanchez and Miltenberger's study scored at least a 3 out of 4, indicating that they said "no" to the stranger and walked away, but did not tell a trusted adult. Results of Fisher and colleagues' study were more variable, with some participants scoring only a 2 out of 4 after IST, indicating that they would say "no" to the stranger, but not walk away or tell an adult.

Teaching sexual abuse prevention is similar to teaching abduction prevention skills, given that the responses (e.g., saying "no," leaving the area, and telling someone) are similar. The difference is in the type of lure to which the participant must respond (i.e., abduction lures in which a stranger asks the child to leave versus sexual abuse lures in which a known individual asks the child to engage in inappropriate physical contact). Egemo-Helm et al. (2007) used BST to teach four women with intellectual disabilities how to respond when presented with sexual abuse lures. During BST, participants learned to discriminate sexual abuse situations from innocuous situations and the difference between appropriate and inappropriate relationships (e.g., a voluntary physical relationship with a peer is appropriate; sexual contact with a staff member or other authority figure is inappropriate). Trainers modeled correct responding in sexual abuse situations and had the participants engage in rehearsals in role-play scenarios, for which praise and corrective feedback were delivered. After training, in situ assessments were conducted in which a confederate posing as a staff member delivered a sexual abuse lure, and, if the participants did not engage in all of the correct behaviors, IST was implemented. All but one participant scored a 3 (i.e., they said "no" to the perpetrator and walked away) or a 4 (i.e., they said "no," walked away, and told a trusted adult) during in situ assessments. Similar results were reported by Miltenberger et al. (1999) who also demonstrated the effectiveness of BST and IST for teaching sexual abuse prevention skills to women with intellectual disabilities. Although the individuals in these studies had intellectual disabilities rather than ASD, it is likely that similar procedures would be successful for adolescents or adults with ASD. The success of BST and IST for teaching abduction prevention skills to individuals with ASD supports this assertion.

Pan-Skadden et al. (2009) used BST to teach three typically developing 4- to 6-year-old children how to ask for help if they were lost in a store. Participants were taught to recognize when they had been separated from their caregiver and walk to the front counter to report to an employee their name and that they were lost. The trainer provided instructions and modeled the correct responses in this situation live or with dolls, had participants practice the skills, and provided praise for correct responding and corrective feedback for incorrect responding. Following BST, in situ assessments were conducted in local stores, during which parents moved away from the child and the experimenter observed whether the child responded correctly. IST was conducted if the child engaged in incorrect responding during the assessments. For two participants, an incentive component was implemented contingent on correct responding during in situ assessments, resulting in correct performance observed during a 2-week follow-up assessment. Asking for help when lost is a skill that would be valuable for children and adolescents with ASD, and this study provides a model for how BST and IST may be applied to this skill and how an added incentive condition can enhance the effects of the intervention. This study illustrates the need for data-based decision making to determine when BST is not effective and IST or other interventions are needed.

Summers et al. (2011) used a modified version of BST to teach children with ASD how to safely respond to a doorbell and to finding household cleaning supplies in their home. To teach safety responses to a doorbell, the researchers instructed participants to not answer the door, go find an adult, and tell the adult someone was at the door. To teach safety responses to finding cleaning supplies, the researchers instructed participants to not touch the chemicals, get away, and tell an adult. The participants were then physically prompted to engage in the correct response if they did not do so independently (the authors did not mention whether praise or other reinforcers were delivered for correct responding during the prompted rehearsal). Following training, in situ assessments were arranged in which either a confederate rang the doorbell or the experimenter cleaned an item in the house and left the cleaning supply out for the child to see. Four out of six participants engaged in all of the correct behaviors during the assessments including telling an adult about the person at the door or the presence of the cleaning supplies.

BST has also been used to teach fire safety skills to children (e.g., Jones, Kazdin, & Haney, 1981) and adults with intellectual disabilities (Knudson et al., 2009). Houvouras and Harvey (2014) used two BST sessions to teach three 10-year-old boys how to respond when finding a lighter. They first told the boys about the dangers of handling a lighter and what to do if they found one. The experimenter then demonstrated the safety skills (i.e., not touching the lighter, leaving the room where the lighter was present, and telling an adult). After the experimenter modeled the skills, the participants practiced the skills and received feedback (i.e., praise for correct responses and further instruction for incorrect responses) until correct responding was achieved across three different sessions. In situ assessments were conducted in baseline and following training. In each assessment, the experimenters told participants to color a page from a coloring book in the guidance counselor's office and gave them a box of crayons which had a lighter inside. Following BST, the participants reached 100% correct performance, and results maintained during follow-up assessments. However, a limitation in this research is that the same location and scenario was utilized in every in situ assessment during baseline and following intervention (i.e., the child always found the lighter in a box of crayons in the counselor's office when sent there to do some coloring). Therefore, there is no evidence that the children would engage in the safety skills when encountering a lighter in any other location or in any other circumstance. To adequately assess any safety skill (e.g., fire safety, poison prevention, abduction prevention, sexual abuse prevention, firearm injury prevention), the in situ assessments must be carried out in a variety scenarios conducted in a variety of locations. Otherwise, the location and scenario, rather than the safety threat itself, might develop stimulus control over the use of the safety skills. One can imagine that the child knew he/she would find the same lighter in the same box of crayons each time he/she went to the counselor's office to color and that running out and telling an adult would get rewarded. It is possible, and perhaps likely, that the situation exerted more stimulus control over the execution of the safety skills than the presence of the lighter alone. Varied assessments would address this concern over unintended stimulus control.

Page, Iwata, and Neef (1976) used BST and a small-scale model to train pedestrian skills to adolescents with developmental disabilities. Page et al. built a small-scale model within the participants' classroom that included stoplights, stop signs, and other items found in the natural environment. During training, the experimenters instructed participants to move their doll to a specific area on the model so they had to demonstrate the pedestrian skill (e.g., moving the doll to a cross walk, moving the doll across the street when pedestrian light said "go"). As participants moved their dolls, they also described the safety skills the doll was demonstrating. Correct responding resulted in praise and incorrect responding resulted in repeating the trial with the experimenters modeling the correct response. Following training, street probes were conducted in which the participants were observed at a specific location in the community to evaluate the use of the pedestrian skills. No feedback was provided to the participants. By the end of training, all participants engaged in the pedestrian skills during both classroom and street probes. These results also maintained during a 3- and 6-week follow-up.

The use of BST in the context of small-scale simulation holds promise for teaching safety skills and possibly social skills to children and adolescents with ASD. The use of the model for training in the classroom made training more efficient. Components during training were instructions, modeling, engaging in the correct behavior with the doll in the model, and feedback from the experimenter as it would be delivered for an actual rehearsal of the safety skills. The researchers then used in situ assessments to evaluate generalization from the model to the natural environment. More research should evaluate BST implemented in small-scale simulations with other safety skills such as abduction prevention and sexual abuse prevention and for social skills more generally. If found to be effective, the use of BST in small-scale simulation training could be made widely accessible to teachers, parents, and others responsible for training individuals with ASD.

The research on BST and IST for teaching safety skills to children with ASD is small, but results are promising. Safety skills consist of important social behaviors, reporting the safety threat to a trusted adult and, in the case of a sexual abuse or abduction lure, engaging in an assertive response and refusing to comply with the requested behavior. Considering the greater number of studies showing the effectiveness of BST and IST for teaching safety skills to typically developing children, more research is needed to evaluate these procedures for a variety of safety skills with children and adolescents with ASD.

19.4.4 Applications of BST to Train Staff

In addition to the applications of BST for teaching social behavior to children with ASD, BST is also widely used to teach staff who work with children with ASD and other developmental disabilities.

Sarokoff and Sturmey (2004) taught three special education teachers to implement DTT with one child with ASD in the child's home. Teachers were trained to conduct a matching task and were scored for correct responding on ten components of the teaching sequence during trials. During BST, the experimenter provided a written form listing each component to be performed and provided graphical feedback based on responding in baseline. Rehearsal then took place in which the teacher practiced with the student, performed three discrete trials, and received immediate verbal feedback following the trials. Next, the experimenter modeled the correct responses with the child, and rehearsal and feedback were repeated. Teacher performance increased from moderate levels during baseline to 97–99% correct after BST.

Similarly, Noski, Willimas, Garrido, and Lee (2013) evaluated BST and computer-based instruction (CBI) to teach direct care staff at an adult day program to implement DTT. BST consisted of instructions delivered via a PowerPoint presentation, followed by modeling, in which the experimenter and a research assistant demonstrated the correct response to a correct response from the learner and to an incorrect response from the learner. Participants rehearsed with research assistants, followed by trials with clients in the natural environment once responding with the research assistants was stable. Feedback was provided after each DTT trial for the critical components that were not performed correctly. CBI consisted of the same PowerPoint delivered in the BST instruction, followed by video modeling scenarios that were the same as the live modeling scenarios in BST. Participants were instructed to watch a video scenario and use a checklist to identify the critical components that were performed correctly and incorrectly by the model in the video. The video provided feedback by showing which items on the checklist were correct and incorrect. Results indicated that BST was more effective than CBI in teaching DTT, with performances in the BST group generalizing to a novel problem and maintaining at increased levels during 6-week probes.

A number of other researchers used BST to teach adults how to implement teaching procedures with children with ASD. Miles and Wilder (2009) used BST to teach three caregivers to use guided compliance with children in a school or home setting. Following BST, participants performed a mean of 99% correct implementing the compliance procedure. Further, performance for each participant during the generalization probe was similar to the levels observed during post-training. Homlitas, Rosales, and Candel (2014) used BST to teach teachers to implement three of six phases of the picture exchange communication system with children with ASD. Following training in each of the phases, probes were conducted in the classroom with a student to evaluate whether the skills generalized to the natural environment. For all three participants correct responding increased from an average of 50–60% in baseline to above 90% correct responding after BST was implemented. Hogan, Knez, and Kahng (2015) evaluated the use of BST to improve staff members' implementation of behavior intervention plans (BIPs) in special education settings. Each BIP consisted of differential reinforcement of alternative behavior (DRA), noncontingent reinforcement, and extinction or signaled availability/unavailability of a reinforcer, DRA, and extinction. Following BST, participants increased correct performance in each component of the BIPs and maintained the improved performance during a post-training phase.

In summary, research demonstrates that BST is an effective procedure for teaching staff and teachers to implement behavioral procedures with children and adolescents with ASD. As an active learning approach, BST provides trainers the opportunity to teach correct responses, observe the learner's performance, and provide feedback until performance meets expectations. With the implementation of BST, the trainer can be confident the teacher or staff member has acquired the skills needed to work effectively with individuals with ASD.

19.5 Summary

The research presented in this chapter demonstrates how BST has been utilized to teach important social behaviors to children and adolescents with ASD and to train staff who work with individuals with ASD. Across the varied applications of BST, several steps are important for successful implementation. Below we offer some general guidelines for implementing BST.

1. Identify the target skill and provide a definition that clearly describes each component of the skill.
2. Identify all relevant contexts in which the social behavior will be used or is likely to occur. Furthermore, identify all the social responses of the communication partners (all relevant S^Ds) to which the learner must respond.
3. Before implementing BST, assess the learners' current skill level by creating the contexts in which the skill should occur (i.e., present the S^Ds as they would naturally occur) to see if the learner engages in the skills without instruction or feedback. The best form of assessment is an in situ assessment in which the learner is in the natural environment where the behavior should occur with no teacher or parent present to influence the behavior.

4. Initiate BST by providing instructions and modeling of the desired skill in the correct context. Begin training by targeting the easiest skills or situations in which the skill should occur. Have the learner repeat the instructions and describe the important aspects of the model's behavior.
5. Following instructions and modeling, have the learner practice the skill in a role-play. Rehearsal should take place in a context in which the skill is likely to be used (e.g., the learner will rehearse a social skill with a conversational partner in a simulated context).
6. After rehearsal, provide immediate feedback in the form of descriptive praise for correct responding and corrective feedback for incorrect responding consisting of instructions for improvement in the next rehearsal. Always praise some aspect of performance in the rehearsal to make participating in BST a reinforcing activity. Following the provision of feedback, have the learner immediately rehearse the same behavior and provide feedback. Continue until the behavior occurs unprompted.
7. Repeat steps 6–7 until correct performance has been exhibited multiple times.
8. Once correct performance occurs reliably in the initial training situation, introduce another situation. Repeat across all situations identified as relevant for the learner.

   Periodically role-play situations in which the learner has demonstrated mastery while incorporating new situations.
9. Program for generalization using multiple exemplars and common stimuli in training. Once the learner has demonstrated the skill across training situations, program for generalization using a variety of strategies including having the learner practice the skill in the natural environment, prompting or cueing the skills as needed in the natural environment, providing praise or other rewards for using the skills in the natural environment, and teaching caregivers to praise or otherwise reward the use of the skills in the natural environment.
10. Conduct post-training in situ assessments across a variety of relevant contexts to assess the generalized use of the skills. Provide in situ training as needed to promote generalization.

References

Allen, K. D., Wallace, D. P., Greene, D. J., Bowen, S. L., & Burke, R. V. (2010). Community-based vocational instruction using videotaped modeling for young adults with autism spectrum disorders performing in air-inflated mascots. *Focus on Autism and Other Developmental Disabilities*, *25*, 186–192.

Barry, T. D., Klinger, L. G., Lee, J. M., Palardy, N., Gilmore, T., & Bodin, S. D. (2003). Examining the effectiveness of an outpatient clinic–based social skills group for high-functioning children with autism. *Journal of Autism and Developmental Disorders*, *33*, 685–701.

Beck, K. V., & Miltenberger, R. G. (2009). Evaluation of a commercially available program and in situ training by parents to teach abduction-prevention skills to children. *Journal of Applied Behavior Analysis*, *42*(4), 761–772.

Bellstedt, E., Gillberg, C., & Gillberg, C. (2005). Autism after adolescence: Population-based 13- to 22-year follow-up study of 120 individuals with autism diagnosed in childhood. *Journal of Autism and Developmental Disorders*, *35*, 351–360.

Bergstrom, R., Najdowski, A. C., & Tarbon, J. (2014). A systematic replication of teaching children with autism to respond appropriately to lures from strangers. *Journal of Applied Behavior Analysis*, *47*, 1–5.

Burke, R. V., Andersen, M. N., Bowen, S. L., Howard, M. R., & Allen, K. D. (2010). Evaluation of two instruction methods to increase employment options for young adults with autism spectrum disorders. *Research in Developmental Disabilities*, *31*, 1223–1233.

Callahan, K., & Rademacher, J. A. (1999). Using self-management strategies to increase the on-task behavior of a student with autism. *Journal of Positive Behavior Interventions*, *1*, 117–122.

Egemo-Helm, K. R., Miltenberger, R. G., Knudson, P., Finstrom, N., Jostad, C., & Johnson, B. (2007). An evaluation of in situ training to teach sexual abuse prevention skills to women with mental retardation. *Behavioral Interventions*, *22*, 99–119.

Engstrom, I., Ekstrom, L., & Emilsson, B. (2003). Psychological functioning in a group of Swedish adults with Asperger syndrome or high-functioning autism. *Autism*, *7*, 99–110.

Fisher, M. H., Burke, M. M., & Griffin, M. M. (2013). Teaching young adults with disabilities to respond appropriately to lures from strangers. *Journal of Applied Behavior Analysis, 46*, 528–533.

Gatheridge, B. J., Miltenberger, R. G., Huneke, D. F., Satterlund, M. J., Mattern, A. R., Johnson, B. M., & Flessner, C. A. (2004). Comparison of two programs to teach firearm injury prevention skills to 6-and 7-year-old children. *Pediatrics, 114*, e294–e299.

Gaylord-Ross, R. J., Haring, T. G., Breen, C., & Pitts-Conway, V. (1984). The training and generalization of social interaction skills with autistic youth. *Journal of Applied Behavior Analysis, 17*, 229–247.

Gross, A., Miltenberger, R., Knudson, P., Bosch, A., & Breitwieser, C. B. (2007). Preliminary evaluation of a parent training program to prevent gun play. *Journal of Applied Behavior Analysis, 40*, 691–695.

Gunby, K. V., Carr, J. E., & LeBlanc, L. A. (2010). Teaching abduction-prevention skills to children with autism. *Journal of Applied Behavior Analysis, 43*, 107–112.

Gunby, K. V., & Rapp, J. T. (2014). The use of behavioral skills training and in situ feedback to protect children with autism from abduction lures. *Journal of Applied Behavior Analysis, 47*, 856–860.

Hanley, G. P., Heal, N. A., Tiger, J. H., & Ingvarsson, E. T. (2007). Evaluation of a classwide teaching program for developing preschool life skills. *Journal of Applied Behavior Analysis, 40*, 277–300.

Haseltine, B., & Miltenberger, R. (1990). Teaching self-protection skills to persons with mental retardation. *American Journal on Mental Retardation, 95*, 188–197.

Himle, M., & Miltenberger, R. (2004). Preventing unintentional firearm injury in children: The need for behavioral skills training. *Education and Treatment of Children, 27*, 161–177.

Himle, M. B., Miltenberger, R. G., Flessner, C., & Gatheridge, B. (2004a). Teaching safety skills to children to prevent gun play. *Journal of Applied Behavior Analysis, 37*, 1–9.

Himle, M. B., Miltenberger, R. G., Gatheridge, B. J., & Flessner, C. A. (2004b). An evaluation of two procedures for training skills to prevent gun play in children. *Pediatrics, 113*, 70–77.

Hogan, A., Knez, N., & Kahng, S. W. (2015). Evaluating the use of behavioral skills training to improve school staff's implementation of behavior intervention plans. *Journal of Behavioral Education, 24*, 242–254.

Homlitas, C., Rosales, R., & Candel, L. (2014). A further evaluation of behavioral skills training for implementation of the picture exchange communication system. *Journal of Applied Behavior Analysis, 47*, 198–203.

Houvouras, A. I., & Harvey, M. T. (2014). Establishing fire safety skills using behavioral skills training. *Journal of Applied Behavior Analysis, 47*, 420–424.

Johnson, B. M., Miltenberger, R. G., Egemo-Helm, K., Jostad, C. M., Flessner, C., & Gatheridge, B. (2005). Evaluation of behavioral skills training for teaching abduction-prevention skills to young children. *Journal of Applied Behavior Analysis, 38*, 67–78.

Johnson, B. M., Miltenberger, R. G., Knudson, P., Egemo-Helm, K., Kelso, P., Jostad, C., & Langley, L. (2006). A preliminary evaluation of two behavioral skills training procedures for teaching abduction-prevention skills to schoolchildren. *Journal of Applied Behavior Analysis, 39*, 25–34.

Jones, R. T., Kazdin, A. E., & Haney, J. I. (1981). Social validation and training of emergency fire safety skills for potential injury prevention and life saving. *Journal of Applied Behavior Analysis, 14*, 249–260.

Jostad, C. M., Miltenberger, R. G., Kelso, P., & Knudson, P. (2008). Peer tutoring to prevent firearm play: Acquisition, generalization, and long-term maintenance of safety skills. *Journal of Applied Behavior Analysis, 41*, 117–123.

Knudson, P., Miltenberger, R., Bosch, A., Gross, A., Brower-Breitwieser, C., & Tarasenko, M. (2009). Fire safety skills training for individuals with severe and profound mental retardation. *Journal of Developmental & Physical Disabilities, 21*, 523–535.

Kornacki, L. T., Ringdahl, J. E., Sjostrom, A., & Nuernberger, J. E. (2013). A component analysis of a behavioral skills training package used to teach conversation skills to young adults with autism spectrum and other developmental disorders. *Research in Autism Spectrum Disorders, 7*, 1370–1376.

Laugeson, E. A., Frankel, F., Mogil, C., & Dillon, A. R. (2009). Parent-assisted social skills training to improve friendships in teens with autism spectrum disorders. *Journal of Autism and Developmental Disorders, 39*, 596–606.

Leaf, J. B., Dotson, W. H., Oppenheim, M. L., Sheldon, J. B., & Sherman, J. A. (2010). The effectiveness of a group teaching interaction procedure for teaching social skills to young children with a pervasive developmental disorder. *Research in Autism Spectrum Disorders, 4*, 186–198.

Leaf, J. B., Oppenheim-Leaf, M. L., Call, N. A., Sheldon, J. B., Sherman, J. A., Taubman, M., … Leaf, R. (2012a). Comparing the teaching interaction procedure to social stories for people with autism. *Journal of Applied Behavior Analysis, 45*, 281–298.

Leaf, J. B., Taubman, M., Bloomfield, S., Palos-Rafuse, L. I., McEachin, J. J., Leaf, R. B., & Oppenheim, M. L. (2009). Increasing social skills and prosocial behavior for three children diagnosed with autism through the use of a teaching package. *Research in Autism Spectrum Disorders, 3*, 275–289.

Leaf, J. B., Tsuji, K. H., Griggs, B., Edwards, A., Taubman, M., McEachin, J., … Oppenheim-Leaf, M. L. (2012b). Teaching social skills to children with autism using the cool versus not cool procedure. *Educatbion and Training in Autism and Developmental Disabilities, 47*, 165–175.

Lerman, D. C., Hawkins, L., Hillman, C., Shireman, M., & Nissen, M. A. (2015). Adults with autism spectrum disorder as behavior technicians for young children with autism: Outcomes of a behavioral skills training program. *Journal of Applied Behavior Analysis, 48*, 233–256.

Lerman, D. C., Hawkins, L., Hoffman, R., & Caccavale, M. (2013). Training adults with an autism spectrum disorder to conduct discrete-trial training for young children with autism: A pilot study. *Journal of Applied Behavior Analysis*, *46*, 465–478.

Miles, N. I., & Wilder, D. A. (2009). The effects of behavioral skills training on caregiver implementation of guided compliance. *Journal of Applied Behavior Analysis*, *42*, 405–410.

Miltenberger, R. G. (2008). Teaching safety skills to children: Prevention of firearm injury as an exemplar of best practice in assessment, training, and generalization of safety skills. *Behavior Analysis in Practice*, *1*, 30.

Miltenberger, R. G. (2016). *Behavior modification: Principles and procedures* (6th ed.). Boston: Cengage Learning.

Miltenberger, R. G., Flessner, C., Gatheridge, B., Johnson, B., Satterlund, M., & Egemo, K. (2004). Evaluation of behavioral skills training procedures to prevent gun play in children. *Journal of Applied Behavior Analysis*, *37*, 513–516.

Miltenberger, R. G., Fogel, V. A., Beck, K. V., Koehler, S., Shayne, R., Noah, J., … Godish, D. (2013). Efficacy of the stranger safety abduction-prevention program and parent-conducted in situ training. *Journal of Applied Behavior Analysis*, *46*, 817–820.

Miltenberger, R. G., Gatheridge, B. J., Satterlund, M., Egemo-Helm, K. R., Johnson, B. M., Jostad, C., … Flessner, C. A. (2005). Teaching safety skills to prevent gun play: An evaluation of in situ training. *Journal of Applied Behavior Analysis*, *38*, 395–398.

Miltenberger, R., Gross, A., Knudson, P., Bosch, A., Jostad, C., & Breitwieser, C. B. (2009). Evaluating behavioral skills training with and without simulated in situ training for teaching safety skills to children. *Education and Treatment of Children*, *32*, 63–75.

Miltenberger, R. G., Roberts, J. A., Ellingson, S., Galensky, T., Rapp, J. T., Long, E. S., & Lumley, V. A. (1999). Training and generalization of sexual abuse prevention skills for women with mental retardation. *Journal of Applied Behavior Analysis*, *32*, 385–388.

Nosik, M. R., Williams, W. L., Garrido, N., & Lee, S. (2013). Comparison of computer based instruction to behavior skills training for teaching staff implementation of discrete-trial instruction with an adult with autism. *Research in Developmental Disabilities*, *34*, 461–468.

Nuernberger, J. E., Ringdahl, J. E., Vargo, K. K., Crumpecker, A. C., & Gunnarsson, K. F. (2013). Using a behavioral skills training package to teach conversation skills to young adults with autism spectrum disorders. *Research in Autism Spectrum Disorders*, *7*, 411–417.

Page, T. J., Iwata, B. A., & Neef, N. A. (1976). Teaching pedestrian skills to retarded persons: Generalization from the classroom to the natural environment. *Journal of Applied Behavior Analysis*, *9*, 433–444.

Palmen, A., & Didden, R. (2012). Task engagement in young adults with high-functioning autism spectrum disorders: Generalization effects of behavioral skills training. *Research in Autism Spectrum Disorders*, *6*, 1377–1388.

Palmen, A., Didden, R., & Arts, M. (2008). Improving question asking in high-functioning adolescents with autism spectrum disorders: Effectiveness of small-group training. *Autism*, *12*, 83–98.

Pan-Skadden, J., Wilder, D. A., Sparling, J., Severtson, E., Donaldson, J., Postma, N., … Neidert, P. (2009). The use of behavioral skills training and on-situ training to teach children to solicit help when lost: A preliminary investigation. *Education & Treatment of Children*, *32*, 359–370.

Peters, L. C., & Thompson, R. H. (2015). Teaching children with autism to respond to conversation partners' interest. *Journal of Applied Behavior Analysis*, *48*, 544–562.

Plavnick, J. B., Kaid, T., & MacFarland, M. C. (2015). Effects of a school-based social skills training program for adolescents with autism spectrum disorder and intellectual disabilities. *Journal of Autism and Developmental Disorders*, *45*, 2674–2690.

Plavnick, J. B., Sam, A., Hume, K., & Odom, S. L. (2013). Effects of video-based group instruction on the acquisition of social skills by adolescents with autism. *Exceptional Children*, *80*, 67–83.

Poche, C., Brouwer, R., & Swearingen, M. (1981). Teaching self-protection to young children. *Journal of Applied Behavior Analysis*, *14*, 169–175.

Poche, C., Yoder, P., & Miltenberger, R. (1988). Teaching self-protection skills to children using television techniques. *Journal of Applied Behavior Analysis*, *21*, 253–261.

Radley, K. C., Dart, E. H., Moore, J. W., Battaglia, A. A., & LaBrot, Z. C. (2017). Promoting accurate variability of social skills in children with autism spectrum disorder. *Behavior Modification*, *41*, 84–112.

Radley, K. C., Ford, W. B., Battaglia, A. A., & McHugh, M. B. (2014a). The effects of a social skills training package on social engagement of children with autism spectrum disorders in a generalized recess setting. *Focus on Autism and Other Developmental Disabilities*, *29*, 216–229.

Radley, K. C., Ford, W. B., McHugh, M. B., Dadakhodjaeva, K., O'Handley, R. D., Battaglia, A. A., & Lum, J. D. K. (2015). Brief report: Use of superheroes social skills to promote accurate social skill use in children with autism spectrum disorder. *Journal of Autism and Developmental Disorders*, *45*, 3048–3054.

Radley, K. C., Hanglein, J., & Arak, M. (2016). School-based social skills training for preschool age children with autism spectrum disorder. *Autism*, *20*, 938–951.

Radley, K., Jenson, W., Clark, E., & O'Neill, R. (2014b). The feasibility and effects of a parent- facilitated social skills training program on social engagement of children with autism spectrum disorder. *Psychology in the Schools*, *51*, 241–255.

Radley, K. C., O'Handley, R. D., Ness, E. J., Ford, W. B., Battaglia, A. A., McHugh, M. B., & McLemore, C. E. (2014c). Promoting social skill use and generalization in children with autism spectrum disorder. *Research in Autism Spectrum Disorders*, *8*, 669–680.

Rosales, R., Stone, K., & Rehfeldt, R. A. (2009). The effects of behavioral skills training on implementation of the picture exchange communication system. *Journal of Applied Behavior Analysis*, *42*, 541–549.

Rosales-Ruis, J., & Baer, D. M. (1997). Behavioral cusps: A developmental and pragmatic concept for behavior analysis. *Journal of Applied Behavior Analysis*, *30*, 533–544.

Sanchez, S., & Miltenberger, R. G. (2015). Evaluating the effectiveness of an abduction prevention program for young adults with intellectual disabilities. *Child & Family Behavior Therapy*, *37*, 197–207.

Sarokoff, R. A., & Sturmey, P. (2004). The effects of behavioral skills training on staff implementation of discrete-trial teaching. *Journal of Applied Behavior Analysis*, *37*, 535–538.

Stewart, K. K., Carr, J. E., & LeBlanc, L. A. (2007). Evaluation of family-implemented behavioral skills training for teaching social skills to a child with Asperger's disorder. *Clinical Case Studies*, *6*, 252–262.

Stokes, T. F., & Baer, D. M. (1977). An implicit technology of generalization. *Journal of Applied Behavior Analysis*, *10*, 349–367.

Stokes, T. F., & Osnes, P. G. (1989). An operant pursuit of generalization. *Behavior Therapy*, *20*, 337–355.

Summers, J., Tarbox, J., Findel-Pyles, R. S., Wilke, A. E., Bergstrom, R., & Williams, W. L. (2011). Teaching two household safety skills to children with autism. *Research in Autism Spectrum Disorders*, *5*, 629–632.

20 Evidence-Based Social Skills Groups for Individuals with Autism Spectrum Disorder Across the Lifespan

Ruth Ellingsen, Courtney Bolton, and Elizabeth Laugeson

20.1 Introduction

Deficits in social interaction and communication skills are the common impairment shared by all individuals with autism spectrum disorder (ASD), regardless of cognitive or language ability (Carter, Davis, Klin, & Volkmar, 2005). Broadly, social deficits often observed across the autism spectrum and throughout the lifespan include poor social communication and impaired social cognition. These social impairments do not appear to improve as a result of development or maturation; in fact, when left untreated, they can become more apparent during adolescence and adulthood with the increasing complexity and demands of social interactions (Laushey & Heflin, 2000; White, Keonig & Scahill, 2007; Schall & McDonough, 2010).

Consequences of impaired social functioning often manifest in the form of peer rejection, peer victimization, poor social support, and isolation. Individuals with ASD frequently report higher levels of loneliness and poorer quality of friendships than typically developing peers (Bauminger & Kasari, 2000; Capps, Sigman, & Yirmija, 1996; Humphrey & Symes, 2010), as well as elevated levels of anxiety, depression, and withdrawal (Sterling, Dawson, Estes & Greenson, 2008; Ghaziuddin, 2002; Kim, Szatmari, Bryson, Streiner, & Wilson, 2000). Thus, the importance of evidence-based interventions to address social development for individuals across the spectrum cannot be underestimated.

Despite the pervasiveness of social deficits and the negative consequences commonly experienced among individuals with ASD, social skills are comparatively much less studied than other aspects of ASD (Reichow & Volkmar, 2010). Fortunately, there is a steady growth of research on social skills interventions, many of which are conducted in group settings. Group instruction is an intuitive method for social skills training, as it allows for the opportunity to interact with and practice newly learned social skills with peers. By definition, a social skills group consists of three or more students that are simultaneously taught a variety of social behaviors. The research evidence to date suggests that social skills groups are a promising avenue for improving social competencies among individuals with ASD. And while most of these studies focus on childhood (Reichow & Volkmar, 2010), a growing body of research evidence suggests that this form of intervention can improve social functioning across the lifespan (Gantman, Kapp, Orenski, & Laugeson, 2012; Kasari & Patterson, 2012; Laugeson, Frankel, Gantman, Dillon, &

R. Ellingsen, PhD • C. Bolton, PhD • E. Laugeson, PsyD (✉)
University of California Los Angeles, Semel Insititute for Neuroscience, Department of Psychiatry & Biobehavioral Sciences,
300 Medical Plaza, Suite 1271, Los Angeles, CA 90095, USA
e-mail: elaugeson@mednet.ucla.edu

J.B. Leaf (ed.), *Handbook of Social Skills and Autism Spectrum Disorder*, Autism and Child Psychopathology Series, DOI 10.1007/978-3-319-62995-7_20

Mogil, 2012; Laugeson, Frankel, Mogil, & Dillon, 2009; Laugeson, Gantman, Kapp, Orenski, & Ellingsen, 2015; Leaf et al., 2017; Lerner & Mikami, 2012; Lopata, Thomeer, Volker, Nida, & Lee, 2008; Mandelberg et al., 2014; Minihan, Kinsella, & Honan, 2011; Vernon, Miller, Ko, & Wu, 2016; White et al., 2013).

20.2 Social Challenges for Individuals with ASD

Although deficits in social functioning are a pervasive and prominent feature of ASD, the social challenges experienced by individuals on the spectrum are broad and varied depending on developmental stage and level of cognitive and language ability. For example, in early childhood, preverbal social impairments are often exhibited, primarily in the domain of social attention. These deficits may include social orienting (i.e., failure to attend to social information in the environment), joint attention (i.e., shared attention to outside objects), and attention to the distress of others (Dawson, Meltzoff, Osterling, Rinaldi, & Brown, 1998; Klin, Lin, Gorrindo, Ramsay, Jones, 2009; Mundy, Sigman, Ungerer, & Sherman, 1986; Sigman, Kasari, Kwon, & Yirmiya, 1992). The considerable heterogeneity in the level of cognitive functioning among individuals with ASD also affects the presentation of social deficits. For example, Bauminger, Shulman, and Agam (2003) found that higher-functioning adolescents initiate social interaction with peers more frequently than do their lower-functioning peers. Yet, their interactions are often awkward and sometimes even intrusive or offensive. In fact, cognitively able adolescents may be no less affected by social deficits than those with cognitive limitations; rather, their heightened self-awareness and false appearance of being less impaired may actually increase the severity of their social limitations and motivation, perhaps increasing the likelihood of peer rejection and neglect.

Although the presentation of social deficits among individuals on the spectrum is varied, these social deficits are broadly observed in two areas: poor social communication and impaired social cognition. Poor social communication includes lack of reciprocity in conversation (i.e., having one-sided conversations), lack of attention to context and nuance in various social situations, and difficulty understanding nonverbal gestures (American Psychiatric Association, 2013). These pragmatic communication deficits within a social context appear to be universal for people with ASD. Specifically, inappropriate turn-taking in conversations, atypical prosody, pedantic manner of speaking, difficulty accounting for social context and setting, and challenges comprehending nonliteral language have been documented consistently through the research literature and have also been shown to influence social outcomes (Pijnacker, Hagoort, Buitelaar, Tuenisse, & Guerts, 2009). Individuals with ASD may perseverate on specific topics of personal interest and shift the conversation back to their preferred topic when their social partner transitions to a different subject (Ghaziuddin & Gerstein, 1996), often providing more information than necessary to illustrate a point (Elder, Caterino, Chao, Shacknai & De Simone, 2006). This inability to carry out a reciprocal bidirectional conversation makes it difficult for individuals with ASD to find common interests with social partners, limiting their likelihood of developing friendships, as friendships are often based upon common interests (Laugeson, 2013, 2014, 2017; Laugeson & Frankel, 2010). Therefore, enhancing two-way conversational skills might be considered an important element of training within social skills groups for individuals with ASD.

When providing excessive information on a topic of interest, youth with ASD frequently achieve the label of "little professor" for their extensive knowledge of a subject, as well as their "lecturing" style of conversing, characterized by a pedantic, or a formal and factual, style of speech (Ghaziuddin & Gerstein, 1996). Related to this pedantic style of speech, poor speech prosody, which includes the natural rising and falling of voice pitch and inflection that occurs during speech, has also been identified as a communication deficit in individuals with ASD (Starr, Szatmari, Bryson, & Zwaigenbaum, 2003). Individuals with ASD often demonstrate atypical rhythms and sounds in their speech which can lead to miscommunication, as it can make the person speaking sound annoyed, bored, or lethargic, and may possess a robotic or automated quality (Shriberg et al., 2001). Atypical prosody may be one of the most immediately recognizable social characteristics of ASD and also one of the most challenging characteristics to modify over the lifespan. While atypical patterns of speech might be more appropriately addressed through speech and language therapy, one might argue that remediation of hyper-verbosity and focus on restricted interests in conversations is an appropriate and necessary element of social skills groups for individuals with ASD.

Another deficit often experienced by individuals on the autism spectrum in the area of conversational skills is difficulty understanding and using humor appropriately (Winter, 2003). Specific challenges with humor include difficulty understanding punch lines to jokes (Emerich, Creaghead, Grether, Murray, & Grasha, 2003) or a tendency to tell jokes that are socially immature (Van Bourgondien & Mesibov, 1987), often with little regard to the reaction of the audience. Other forms of nonliteral language such as understanding sarcasm, analogies, metaphors, and figurative use of language have also been shown to be problematic for those with ASD, as they tend to think in very concrete and literal terms (Kerbel & Grunwell, 1998; Starr et al., 2003). Difficulty interpreting and using humor and other nonliteral language can impede one's ability to meaningfully participate in a social exchange (Dennis, Lazenby, & Lockyer, 2001; Emerich et al., 2003; Happé, 1995; Martin & McDonald, 2003). Therefore, social skills groups designed for individuals with ASD might address the appropriate use of humor, while avoiding the use of figurative language during instruction.

Social communication also includes nonverbal elements such as social touch, gestures, and eye contact. Individuals with ASD often have difficulty understanding the value and meaning of these nonverbal elements of social interaction (Griffin, Griffin, Fitch, Albera, & Gingras, 2006; Volkmar & Klin, 1998). Thus, nonverbal communication elements are also important to consider as a target of intervention in social skills groups for individuals with ASD.

Impaired social cognition, also known as theory of mind, is another area of social deficit among individuals on the autism spectrum. Individuals with ASD often experience difficulties in expressing emotions, understanding the feelings of others, and empathizing (Baron-Cohen, 1995; Frith, 2004; Klin & Volkmar, 2003; Krasny, Williams, Provencal, & Ozonoff, 2003; Travis & Sigman, 1998), as well as an overall lack of understanding of social causality (Baron-Cohen, Leslie, & Frith, 1985). Such deficits make it very difficult to make sense of or predict the behavior of others, as well as to know when it is appropriate to show comfort, express emotions, or take actions that convey empathy in a socially correct manner (Baron-Cohen, 1995; Klin & Volkmar, 2003; Krasny et al., 2003). Consequently, incorporating perspective taking into social skills groups is critical to improving social cognition.

20.3 Consequences of Social Challenges Common in ASD

Deficits in social communication and social cognition among individuals with ASD have significant consequences from early childhood throughout adulthood. Poor interpersonal skills are associated with rejection by peers, juvenile delinquency, early withdrawal from school, academic and occupational difficulties, and later mental health and adjustment problems (Buhrmester, 1990; Howlin & Goode, 1998; Myles, Bock, & Simpson, 2001; Tantam, 2003). Social engagement theory suggests that diminished social motivation and attention starting in early childhood may deprive a child with ASD of fundamental social learning opportunities during a critical developmental period and may lead to deficits in social cognition and ultimately social skills development (Chevallier, Kohls, Troiani, Brodkin & Schulz, 2012). The consequences of this lack of social attention and engagement typically become more apparent as children mature and begin engaging socially with peers. Individuals with ASD report less peer interaction, fewer friendships, lower friendship quality, higher rates of peer victimization, and greater loneliness than their typically developing peers (Baron-Cohen & Wheelwright, 2003; Bauminger & Kasari, 2000; Koegel, Vernon, Koegel, Koegel, & Paullin, 2012; Lasgaard, Nielsen, Eriksen, & Goossens, 2010). Consequently, individuals on the autism spectrum report elevated levels of anxiety and symptoms of depression (Bauminger et al., 2003; Shtayermann, 2007; Sze & Wood, 2007). These consequences of social challenges persist across the lifespan, and social challenges specific to ASD may even be greatest upon entering adulthood, possibly due to the greater salience and complexity of peer relationships, growing drive toward identity exploration, lack of availability and knowledge about appropriate services, and uncertainty about the balance of responsibility between individuals themselves and those who support them (Tantam, 2003). Research with adults has found that at least half of the adult population with ASD report not having friends or significant relationships with peers (Howlin, 2000; Orsmond, Krauss, & Seltzer, 2004). Furthermore, adults with ASD often desire romantic relationships, but only about 14% report being in an intimate relationship (Farley et al., 2009). Researchers have hypothesized that although the aspiration for a romantic relationship is consistent with typically developing peers, this lower than average rate of engagement in such relationships may be due to the lack of social competence and skills to initiate and maintain a romantic relationship (Henault & Attwood, 2002; Mezhabin & Stokes, 2011; Stokes & Kaur, 2005). This lack of social skills may manifest through higher levels of inappropriate bids or actions with a potential romantic partner that may even be perceived as stalking or harassment (Stokes, Newton, & Kaur, 2007).

Despite their apparent social difficulties, individuals with ASD often desire friendships and even express concern about the lack of closeness in their peer relationships (Church, Alisanski, & Amanullah, 2000). Given this desire for social relationships and concurrent lack of social proficiency, training in appropriate social skills is a logical and necessary approach. Moreover, increased levels of social competence and having at least one close friendship decrease the risk of depression, anxiety, loneliness, and peer victimization and may also indicate greater ability to form successful romantic relationships later in life (Buhrmester, 1990; Jennes-Coussens, Magill-Evans, & Konig, 2006; Stokes et al., 2007).

20.4 Group-Based Social Skills Interventions for Individuals with ASD

Although typically developing individuals often learn basic rules of social etiquette through observation of peers and/or through instruction from parents in nonclinical settings (Gralinski & Kopp, 1993; Rubin & Sloman, 1984), individuals with ASD often require additional support and assistance. Although social skills treatment programs for individuals with ASD are growing in availability, few of these intervention packages have shown significant improvement in social skills outcomes. However, certain empirically supported methods of treatment delivery have been identified, and in recent years, the emergence of evidence-based interventions has increased for group-based social skills interventions (Miller, Vernon, Wu & Russo, 2014). Targeting interventions to focus on common social deficits shared among individuals with ASD through the teaching of ecologically valid social skills within a group setting, while using evidence-based methods of social skills instruction, may make social skills interventions more effective with this population.

Just as social challenges experienced by individuals on the spectrum are largely varied depending on developmental stage, so too are the areas of focus for social skills group interventions for this population. For example, in early childhood, the treatment priorities often focus on developing joint attention and social orienting, given their importance as fundamental building blocks for deeper social communication and cognition. Additionally, social skills groups for preschool-aged children might place focus on play skills, as this is the primary form of socialization at this developmental stage. For example, topics of instruction might include sharing, asking for a turn, being a good sport, asking a friend to play, and body boundaries. Social skills groups for elementary school-aged children and adolescents tend to focus more on conversational skills and advanced social cognition, such as appropriate turn-taking in conversation, creating opportunities for social interaction, understanding of verbal and nonverbal social cues, ability to perspective-take, and competence at handling peer conflict (Laugeson & Ellingsen, 2014). Upon adulthood, dating etiquette might be added as a topic to social skills groups. Studies have shown that sexual development may mature at a slower rate for individuals with ASD, with an average 5-year delay in sexual maturation as compared to neurotypical peers (Stokes & Kaur, 2005; Volkmar, Carter, Sparrow, & Cicchetti, 1993). Thus, young adulthood, rather than adolescence, might be the most appropriate time for intervention and direct instruction regarding entering and maintaining romantic relationships.

These are just a few of the targeted areas in which social skills group instruction might be focused based on developmental stage. Importantly, the skills that are taught should be relevant to the population being served, including attention to developmental stage, level of functioning, as well as cognitive and language ability. Approaches to teach individuals with significant cognitive and verbal limitations may require simplified content, intensive repetition and instruction and prompting, augmentative communication devices, visually based teaching strategies, and tangible reinforcers. Approaches tailored to cognitively able individuals, on the other hand, will likely include verbally mediated strategies, instructor modeling (i.e., role-playing), and self-reinforcement. Above all, the content of social skills group interventions should be ecologically valid. Ecologically valid social skills are those behaviors that are exhibited by socially accepted individuals, rather than those gleaned from conventional wisdom (Laugeson, 2013, 2014, 2017; Laugeson & Frankel, 2010). One reason that the majority of social skills interventions used with individuals on the spectrum have not demonstrated strong outcomes may be that the skills being taught are those deemed appropriate by adults, clinicians, or researchers, rather than skills actually established by the dominant peer group. If the goal of social skills training is for the individual to be accepted by the dominant peer group, teaching the wrong set of social behaviors is futile and ineffective and could even increase levels of peer rejection. To illustrate this point, consider what many social skills interventions teach children and adolescents to do when they are being verbally bullied or teased. Most youths are told to ignore the person, walk away, or tell an adult (Laugeson, 2013). When asked whether those strategies work, most children and adults will say they are ineffective. For example, if you ignore the teaser, they will simply keep teasing you. If you walk away, they will follow you and keep teasing. If you tell an adult, they will likely want to retaliate. However, a more ecologically valid and effective tactic would be giving a short comeback that suggests what the teaser said did not bother you (Laugeson, 2013, 2014, 2017; Laugeson & Frankel, 2010). The individual being teased might respond by saying "Whatever" or "Anyway" or "Yeah, and?" or any other number of comments that show the teaser they were unaffected. This ecologically valid approach makes the teasing less enjoyable for the teaser, and thus, he or she will be less likely to target this individual after repeated failure to elicit the desired response. This is just one demonstration of the importance of teaching ecologically valid skills during social skills instruction. Instead of teaching a strategy (e.g., telling an adult) simply because it appears to be appropriate, teaching social skills naturally utilized by socially accepted individuals will be more likely to lead to improved social functioning and peer acceptance.

20.5 Effective Treatment Delivery Methods for Teaching Social Skills in a Group Setting

In addition to teaching developmentally appropriate and ecologically valid social skills, the treatment delivery methods for social skills groups should be research-based and empirically supported for use with individuals with ASD. Effective methods of instruction and treatment formats include:

- Evidence-based treatment manuals
- Didactic instruction
- Small group format
- Behavioral modeling
- Behavioral rehearsal
- Parent/caregiver social coaching
- Homework assignments
- School-based interventions
- Inclusion of typically developing peers

20.5.1 Evidence-Based Treatment Manuals

The use of evidence-based treatment manuals may help to ensure that individuals in community settings achieve comparable treatment gains as research participants upon which the evidence is based. Using treatment manuals may also help to standardize group interventions, although actual treatment delivery may still vary (Smith et al., 2007). Although there is a dearth of empirically supported social skills group interventions, a few publically available treatment manuals do exist (Frankel & Myatt, 2003; Laugeson, 2014, 2017; Laugeson & Frankel, 2010); yet, the extent to which these published manuals are used with fidelity is unknown. Unfortunately, measurements of treatment fidelity are underreported in ASD treatment research, but adherence to the original guidelines for delivering evidence-based group interventions may be particularly important for treatments delivered by parents or less experienced or credentialed professionals (Matson, 2007).

20.5.2 Didactic Instruction

The use of structured lesson plans to teach social skills using concrete rules and steps of social behavior is key to the development and successful implementation of an effective social skills group. Structured lesson plans ensure that a core set of skills will be taught. Some social skills programs attempt to teach social skills through "process groups" in which individuals are asked to give a recount of their week, while group leaders and other group members attempt to troubleshoot potential problems and brainstorm how to behave in a more socially constructive manner moving forward. The benefit of these types of process groups is unknown, but the risk of possibly failing to teach a core set of skills necessary to function adaptively in the social world may outweigh any benefits. The use of structured didactic lessons is recommended to ensure that some predetermined core set of ecologically valid skills is learned.

Additionally, when providing social skills instruction to individuals with ASD, it is important to consider the unique manner in which information is processed. Individuals with ASD tend to think in very concrete and literal terms and often struggle to comprehend metaphors, analogies, and other forms of figurative language (Kerbel & Grunwell, 1998; Starr et al., 2003). Therefore, didactic lessons presented using concrete rules and steps of social etiquette (and avoiding figurative use of language) will enhance comprehension of social skills instruction, even when presenting more complicated or abstract social behaviors. For example, consider how one might teach strategies for joining a conversation, a skill that can seem particularly complicated for individuals with ASD. By breaking down conversational entry into concrete steps, this complex social behavior becomes more manageable. There are three basic steps involved in conversational entry (Laugeson, 2014, 2017; Laugeson & Frankel, 2010). First, *watch and listen* to the conversation. This is the necessary first step to determine what the group is talking about and whether we share a common interest, while watching inconspicuously from a short distance and making periodic eye contact. Second, *wait for a pause*. Waiting for a brief pause in the conversation or some sign of receptiveness from the group helps us avoid being intrusive and allows for a more natural entrance into the conversation. Third, *say something on topic*. This last step involves joining the conversation and making a comment, asking a question, or giving a compliment that is on topic, so that we are adding to the conversation, rather than hijacking the conversation by being off-topic. While this sophisticated social behavior of peer entry might seem abstract at first, when broken down to its concrete parts, it becomes quite manageable for the individual with ASD and provides a good example of the necessity for teaching social skills using concrete rules and steps during didactic instruction.

20.5.3 Small Group Format

Social skills training in a small group format allows for the opportunity to practice newly learned social skills with peers, in addition to live performance feedback from group facilitators. Of course, there are several considerations that should be made before conducting social skills groups. First, group facilitators should have a shared understanding of each group member's history and current level of functioning, including language and cognitive ability, maturity level, as well as amount and degree of maladaptive social behavior. Heterogeneity of the group should be limited in order to aid learning and group cohesion (White, 2011). Even with these considerations, it is likely that the facilitator will have to deal with some disruption from group members. Therefore, a small group size (e.g., 8–10 group members) is ideal for being able to troubleshoot clinical issues when they arise. It is further suggested that social skills groups for adolescents and adults only include those members who are motivated to participate in the treatment (Laugeson, 2014, 2017; Laugeson & Frankel, 2010), thereby improving the likelihood of success and reducing the negative impact of treatment resistance and negative group contagion.

Another important consideration when forming social skills groups relates to the gender and age range of the group members. Although gender and age of group members ought to be considered when forming groups, it may be difficult to create groups with equal gender balance given that many more males than females are diagnosed with ASD. The interests of males and females can be very different – particularly during middle childhood and adolescence – and there is some evidence to suggest that being the only girl in a group of adolescents with ASD can be an uncomfortable and isolating experience (Barnhill, Cook, Tebbenkamp, & Myles, 2002). However, assuming the facilitator is mindful of gender differences, it may be useful to have a mixed-gender group, since this reflects the natural setting for most individuals outside of the treatment setting (White, 2011). It is also helpful to keep the age range of group members as homogeneous as possible, with particular attention paid to the context of the social setting. For example, segregating groups based on school or work setting (i.e., preschool, elementary school, middle school, high school, college, or work) would be more advantageous than creating groups based on a specific age range. For example, a 10-year-old boy in grade school and an 11-year-old boy in middle school may share less in common than 11- and 14-year-old boys both attending middle school.

Given the fact that many individuals with ASD have a history of peer rejection, an environment that provides support and care among group members and facilitators is particularly important for any social skills intervention for individuals with ASD (White, 2011) and another reason to teach social skills in a group format. Although it should be noted, a group format is not always the most appropriate setting for individuals who exhibit severe maladaptive behaviors (e.g., severe anxiety, unprovoked aggression) that could make interacting with group members aversive or unsafe (White, 2011).

20.5.4 Behavioral Modeling

A critical component to social skills groups is the use of behavioral modeling, or role-playing demonstrations, to act out certain targeted behaviors. This method of instruction in social skills groups is particularly important as it brings life to the lesson being taught, making concepts that might be viewed as theoretical or conceptual, more real and concrete. For example, individuals with ASD receiving instruction about having two-way conversations would more successfully synthesize this information by visually observing these tactics in action. In-person modeling by social coaches or watching a video demonstration (i.e., video modeling) is an effective observational learning format for elementary-aged children, adolescents, and adults. However, a more developmentally appropriate and engaging approach for young children might be to use puppets in role-playing demonstrations (Laugeson, Park, & Sanderson, 2016).

In contrast to video modeling, video self-modeling involves individuals observing themselves performing a targeted behavior successfully on video and then imitating the targeted behavior. While this method has demonstrated improvements in social skill acquisition, (Bellini, Akullian, & Hopf, 2007; Bernard-Ripoli, 2007; Boudreau & Harvey, 2013), the use of video self-modeling is only advisable in individual treatment settings and should be avoided in group settings in order to minimize shame and embarrassment when the targeted skills are not perfectly executed.

20.5.5 Behavioral Rehearsal

Another important approach to teaching social skills in a group setting involves the use of behavioral rehearsal (i.e., practice) with performance feedback through coaching (Laugeson et al., 2012; Laugeson, Ellingsen, Sanderson, Tucci, & Bates, 2014; Laugeson et al., 2015). It is recommended that individuals with ASD practice newly learned social skills with social coaches, peer mentors, or other group members before practicing these skills outside of the treatment setting. There are multiple benefits to in-group behavioral rehearsal. For one, the individual can practice the new skill in a comfortable and supportive environment, thus easing the initial anxiety of using the skill outside of the group setting. Also, it is important for group facilitators to witness the individual's understanding of and ability to implement the skills they have been taught to avoid misunderstanding or misuse of newly learned skills. Providing performance feedback through coaching during sessions is crucial to troubleshoot difficulty with acquisition and application of skills. Having multiple trainers or coaches in the group to prompt the individual and provide feedback is useful in ensuring that the individual does not become dependent on any one person to provide social cues (White, 2011). Given that individuals on the autism spectrum have likely experienced fewer successes in their social lives (particularly once they've entered adolescence or adulthood), it can also be helpful to set up behavioral rehearsals early in the intervention that will guarantee at least some degree of achievement (White, 2011).

20.5.6 Parent/Caregiver Social Coaching

Parents and caregivers (e.g., grandparents, aunts/uncles, adult siblings, job/life coaches) can have significant effects upon acquisition of social skills for individuals with ASD, both in terms of direct instruction and supervision and supporting the development of an appropriate peer network (Frankel et al., 2010; Gantman et al., 2012; Laugeson et al., 2012, 2015; Miller et al., 2014). The use of a parent-assisted (also known as parent-mediated) group model of social skills training was first introduced by Frankel and Myatt (2003) through the Children's Friendship Training Program (CFT), which has been shown to be effective in improving friendship skills for elementary-aged children with ASD (Frankel et al., 2010). The effectiveness of using parent/caregiver assistance has also been demonstrated for adolescents and young adults through the

Program for the Education and Enrichment of Relational Skills (PEERS: Laugeson, 2017; Laugeson & Frankel, 2010), an evidence-based social skills group intervention targeting friendship and relationship skills for individuals with ASD (Gantman et al., 2012; Karst et al., 2015; Laugeson et al., 2009, 2012, 2015; McVey et al., 2016; Schohl et al., 2014; Van Hecke et al., 2015; Yoo et al., 2014).

Parent or caregiver involvement in social skills groups may be crucial to help individuals with ASD improve their social skills, as these individuals are often quite dependent on their parents or other caregivers for support, even into their adolescent and adult years (Howlin & Moss, 2012). As an example, PEERS incorporates significant parental or caregiver involvement to ensure practice and generalization of social skills outside of the treatment setting. Parents and caregivers assist and monitor adolescents or adults in their completion of weekly homework assignments to practice the use of social skills taught during previous group sessions. Parents and caregivers are also taught to act as social coaches, when appropriate, in order to promote the generalization of skills to other settings such as the home and community. Involvement of parents and caregivers in the intervention is also critical to the expansion or enhancement of a peer social network. Parents and caregivers are taught to work with the adolescent or adult on identifying appropriate extracurricular activities and social hobbies where they might meet potential friends with common interests (Laugeson, 2017; Laugeson & Frankel, 2010). Findings from randomized controlled research trials with adolescents and young adults reveal significant gains in social skills across raters and settings, as well as increased frequency of social interactions in adolescent and adult participants (Gantman et al., 2012; Laugeson et al., 2009, 2012, 2015). Results of follow-up assessments further revealed maintenance of treatment gains 14 weeks after the completion of treatment (Laugeson et al., 2012) and as long as 1–5 years post-intervention (Mandelberg et al., 2014), strongly supporting the use of parents and caregivers within group treatment. Parents and caregivers are arguably the one factor that remains consistent across time, thereby enhancing generalization of social skills and maintenance of treatment gains across the lifespan.

20.5.7 Homework Assignments

Another treatment method to facilitate generalization of newly learned social skills is assignment of homework between sessions to practice the skills outside of the group. For example, in the case of joining a conversation, group members might be given a homework assignment to practice the steps for peer entry (i.e., watch and listen, wait for a pause, say something on topic) in a more natural environment like school or work. A portion of each group session (ideally at the beginning) should also be used to review the completion of homework assignments and troubleshoot any issues that may have come up. Homework review is also a nice opportunity to individualize the treatment within a group setting (Laugeson, 2014, 2017; Laugeson & Frankel, 2010); therefore, considerable time should be allotted for reviewing these assignments.

20.5.8 School-Based Social Skills Groups

The use of school-based interventions to improve social skills is not uncommon. In fact, many school districts require instruction on social skills through Individualized Education Plans (IEPs) for students with special needs, like those with ASD. Despite the widespread use of school-based social skills instruction, the effectiveness of this approach has been tested very little (White et al., 2007). Most social skills interventions provided in the schools are taught by speech and language pathologists, special education teachers, and school psychologists, many of whom develop their own programs based on an amalgam of existing interventions. Lack of adherence to evidence-based treatments is most likely due to short supply of empirically supported school-based curricula. However, the use of evidence-based social skills group interventions in the school setting has been studied to a limited extent and has been shown to be effective for middle and high school adolescents with ASD (Laugeson, 2014). The notion that teachers can effectively teach social skills in the classroom, much like teaching math or science, is a novel approach but is slowly gaining research evidence (Kaale, Smith, & Sponheim, 2012; Laugeson et al., 2014; Lawton & Kasari, 2012;). The use of teachers as social skills facilitators may be a nice alternative to traditional social skills groups as this method of treatment delivery has the capacity to reach a greater number of children and adolescents with ASD, while teaching social skills in a more natural social environment.

20.5.9 Inclusion of Typically Developing Peers

Inclusion of typically developing peers in social skills groups has gained popularity in recent years with promising results (Minihan et al., 2011; White et al., 2013). Socially competent peers are typically trained beforehand and then participate in the groups to teach, model, and reinforce appropriate social behavior. For example, White et al. (2013) included typically developing peer tutors in their social skills groups for adolescents with ASD. Before participating in a group, tutors met with the principal investigator to learn about ASD and the format of the group. They were given specific tasks for each session such as modeling the specific target behavior, being the first participant to practice in front of the group, or engaging another group member in the interaction.

20.6 Future Directions for Social Skills Groups

While social skills groups have increasingly become a popular method for helping individuals with ASD adapt to their social environment, with a growing body of evidence highlighting their effectiveness, there is still considerable work to be done to address limitations in our knowledge of what are the most effective group intervention strategies. As the field of social skills intervention moves forward, recommendations for future research include:

- An emphasis on older populations (including adolescents and adults)
- The use of randomized controlled trials as the standard for examining the efficacy and effectiveness of social skills group interventions
- Assessment of treatment outcome using a combination of standardized outcome measures and behavioral observations with multiple independent raters
- Group research designs with large sample sizes and well-characterized populations
- Long-term follow-up assessment to examine the maintenance of treatment gains over time

20.6.1 Adolescents and Adults

With emphasis on early intervention, most social skills treatment studies have targeted younger age groups on the autism spectrum, and research examining social skills interventions for adolescents and adults with ASD are especially rare. A meta-analysis conducted by Kasari and Patterson (2012) evaluated social skills interventions for individuals with ASD from early childhood through late adolescence. Out of 34 identified studies focused on social skills treatment, three reported on toddler interventions, 12 targeted preschoolers, 19 focused on school-aged children, and only two addressed adolescent social skill development. In a best evidence synthesis of 66 studies of social skills interventions for individuals with ASD published between 2001 and 2008, only three studies contained adolescent or adult participants (Reichow & Volkmar, 2010). Therefore, future research on social skills groups for individuals with ASD should focus on older age groups, including adolescents and particularly adults. To date, only two intervention studies for adults with ASD used a RCT design and found significant improvement in overall social and psychosocial functioning post-intervention; both of these interventions were conducted in a group setting (Gantman et al., 2012; Laugeson et al., 2015).

20.6.2 Randomized Controlled Trials

The use of RCTs is essential to testing the efficacy of an intervention. The key distinguishing feature of a RCT is that participants are randomly assigned to receive one or other of a particular treatment after being assessed for eligibility. After randomization, participants are treated in the same manner, the only difference being the treatment they receive. The benefit of using RCTs in the evaluation of treatment outcome is that they minimize selection bias, promote the comparison of equivalent groups, and allow the researcher to examine the true benefit of an intervention with fewer confounding variables. Within the ASD treatment literature, there is a particular need for more RCTs of social skills groups. A recent meta-analysis of group-based social skills interventions for adolescents with ASD revealed that only six of 44 studies reviewed implemented RCT methods to evaluate pre-post outcomes (Miller et al., 2014). These findings suggest the need for higher-quality research across the social skills treatment domain for individuals with ASD.

20.6.3 Assessing Treatment Outcome

One commonly cited issue in assessing social functioning in social skills research is the subjective nature of the measurements. The notion is that the assessment of social skills is difficult to measure accurately and without bias. To combat this criticism, future research should employ more objective methods of measurement, including observational behavior data taken by raters who are blind to the research conditions under investigation. The use of objective tests using standardized measures of social functioning that include norm-referenced scores would be a good start – allowing the researcher to compare the scores of a given participant to a larger population. Examples of well-regarded standardized measures of social functioning include the Social Skills Improvement System (SSIS; Gresham & Elliott, 2008) and the Social Responsiveness Scale-Second Edition (SRS-2; Constantino, 2012). Arguably, a good battery of social skills group treatment outcome measures should not only involve a combination of standardized ratings but should come from a variety of reporters, including independent raters who are blind to the conditions under investigation (i.e., do not know whether the individual is receiving treatment). When raters are blind to the treatment condition, there is a reduced chance of collecting biased ratings.

In some cases, it may not be feasible to have parents, caregivers, or teachers of individuals participating in social skills groups blind to the treatment condition. In that case, it would be advantageous for researchers to include behavioral ratings of social functioning. Behavioral ratings further enhance treatment outcomes by providing an even more objective rating of social behavior. For example, behavioral ratings might include observing targeted social behaviors, such as conversational skills, and then coding the behaviors of the participant and/or the responses of other individuals (e.g., peers) who observe the individual's social functioning. Behavioral ratings of social skills are underrepresented in the treatment literature but may characterize an unbiased and perhaps more accurate picture of the individual's social functioning, if raters are kept blind to the treatment conditions.

20.6.4 Generalization of Outcomes

Another factor that should be prioritized when conducting social skills group intervention research is generalizability of findings or the extent to which findings from a given study can be generalized to the larger population. Regrettably, most social skills intervention studies are limited in their ability to generalize research findings to other settings and other populations of individuals with ASD. Two of the biggest offenders to generalization are sample size and participant characteristics. Most research studies on social skills groups for individuals with ASD have small sample sizes, which may include a very heterogeneous group of individuals with developmental disabilities. While single subject designs offer good internal validity and may be useful as precursors to larger RCTs, they are difficult to use in a group intervention context. Future research would benefit from group research designs with larger sample sizes and well-characterized populations to better assess treatment efficacy and improve generalizability (Matson, Matson, & Rivet, 2007).

20.6.5 Maintenance of Treatment Gains

Whether or not targeted social skills are adequately maintained over time is another important consideration for social skills group intervention research. Assessment of maintenance of skill acquisition is rarely targeted in treatment studies or clinical programs, calling into question how beneficial these programs are over time. A recent study investigating the maintenance of treatment gains for high-functioning adolescents with ASD found that teens receiving the PEERS group intervention maintained positive outcomes in the areas of social responsiveness and social skills, frequency of peer interactions, and social skills knowledge 1–5 years posttreatment (Mandelberg et al., 2014). While these findings are promising for maintenance of treatment gains in a group intervention utilizing parent assistance, little is known about the social trajectories of individuals with ASD following other types of social skills treatment .

20.7 Conclusions

Despite the pervasiveness of social deficits affecting individuals across the spectrum and throughout the lifespan, social skills intervention research remains limited at this time, particularly for adolescents and adults. Fortunately, studies examining social skills interventions for individuals with ASD are steadily increasing, and a growing body of research evidence has identified several effective treatment elements and delivery methods for social skills groups. These include using a small group format, treatment manuals, didactic instruction, behavioral modeling, behavioral rehearsal, parent/caregiver involvement, homework assignments, school-based interventions, and involving typically developing peers. Perhaps most importantly, the social skills taught must be ecologically valid and relevant to the population being served, including attention to developmental stage, level of functioning, language ability, and cognitive aptitude. Suggestions for moving the field forward to address existing limitations in our knowledge base include greater attention to older age groups (particularly adults), higher-quality research designs (including RCTs), and the use of standardized outcome measures, behavioral observations, multiple independent raters, and long-term follow-up assessments. Taken in conjunction, these recommendations have the capacity to move the field forward in the development of more effective social skills group treatments to improve the social functioning of individuals with ASD.

References

American Psychiatric Association. (2013). *Diagnostic and statistical manual of mental disorders* (5th ed.). Washington, DC: APA.

Barnhill, G. P., Cook, K. T., Tebbenkanmp, K., & Myles, B. S. (2002). The effectiveness of social skills intervention targeting nonverbal communication for adolescents with Asperger syndrome and related pervasive developmental delays. *Focus on Autism and Other Developmental Disabilities*, *17*, 112–118.

Baron-Cohen, S. (1995). *Mindblindness: An essay on autism and theory of mind*. Cambridge, MA: The MIT Press.

Baron-Cohen, S., Leslie, A. M., & Frith, U. (1985). Does the autistic child have a "theory of mind"? *Cognition*, *21*, 37–46.

Baron-Cohen, S., & Wheelwright, S. (2003). The friendship questionnaire (FQ): An investigation of adults with Asperger syndrome or high functioning autism, and normal sex differences. *Journal of Autism and Developmental Disorders*, *33*, 509–517.

Bauminger, N., & Kasari, C. (2000). Loneliness and friendship in high-functioning children with autism. *Child Development, 71*, 447–456.

Bauminger, N., Shulman, C., & Agam, G. (2003). Peer interaction and loneliness in high functioning children with autism. *Journal of Autism and Developmental Disorders, 33*, 489–507.

Bellini, S., Akullian, J., & Hopf, A. (2007). Increasing social engagement in young children with autism spectrum disorders using video self-modeling. *School Psychology Review, 36*, 80–90.

Bernard-Ripoli, S. (2007). Using a self-as-model video combined with social stories to help a child with Asperger syndrome understand emotions. *Focus on Autism and Other Developmental Disabilities, 22*, 100–106.

Boudreau, J., & Harvey, M. T. (2013). Increasing recreational initiations for children who have ASD using video self modeling. *Education and Treatment of Children, 36*, 49–60.

Buhrmester, D. (1990). Intimacy of friendship, interpersonal competence, and adjustment during preadolescence and adolescence. *Child Development, 61*, 1101–1111.

Capps, L., Sigman, M., & Yirmija, N. (1996). Self-competence and emotional understanding in high-functioning children with autism. In M. E. Hertzig & E. A. Farber (Eds.), *Annual progress in child psychiatry and child development* (pp. 260–279). Hard, UK: Psychology Press.

Carter, A. S., Davis, N. O., Klin, A., & Volkmar, F. R. (2005). Social development in autism. In F. R. Volkmar, R. Paul, A. Klin, & D. Cohen (Eds.), *Handbook of autism and pervasive developmental disorders, Diagnosis, development, neurobiology, and behavior* (vol. 1, pp. 312–334). Hoboken, NJ: John Wiley & Sons.

Chevallier, C., Kohls, G., Troiani, V., Brodkin, E. S., & Schultz, R. T. (2012). The social motivation theory of autism. *Trends in Cognitive Sciences, 16*, 231–239.

Church, C., Alisanski, S., & Amanullah, S. (2000). The social, behavioral, and academic experiences of children with Asperger syndrome. *Focus on Autism and Other Developmental Disabilities, 15*, 12–20.

Constantino, J. N. (2012). *Social responsiveness scale* (2nd ed.). Los Angeles: Western Psychological Services.

Dawson, G., Meltzoff, A. N., Osterling, J., Rinaldi, J., & Brown, E. (1998). Children with autism fail to orient to naturally occurring social stimuli. *Journal of Autism and Developmental Disorders, 28*, 479–485.

Dennis, M., Lazenby, A. L., & Lockyer, L. (2001). Inferential language in high-functioning children with autism. *Journal of Autism and Developmental Disorders, 31*, 47–54.

Elder, L. M., Caterino, L. C., Chao, J., Shacknai, D., & De Simone, G. (2006). The efficacy of social skills treatment for children with Asperger syndrome. *Education & Treatment of Children, 29*, 635–663.

Emerich, D. M., Creaghead, N. A., Grether, S. M., Murray, D., & Grasha, C. (2003). The comprehension of humorous materials by adolescents with high-functioning autism and Asperger's syndrome. *Journal of Autism and Developmental Disorders, 33*, 253–257.

Farley, M. A., McMahon, W. M., Fombonne, E., Jenson, W. R., Miller, J., Gardner, M., … Coon, H. (2009). Twenty-year outcome for individuals with autism and average or near-average cognitive abilities. *Autism Research, 2*, 109–118.

Frankel, F., & Myatt, R. (2003). *Children's friendship training*. New York: Brunner-Routledge.

Frankel, F., Myatt, R., Sugar, C., Whitham, C., Gorospe, C. M., & Laugeson, E. A. (2010). A randomized controlled study of parent-assisted children's friendship training with children having autism spectrum disorders. *Journal of Autism and Developmental Disorders, 40*, 827–842.

Frith, U. (2004). Emanuel Miller lecture: Confusions and controversies about Asperger syndrome. *Journal of Child Psychology and Psychiatry, 45*, 672–686.

Gantman, A., Kapp, S. K., Orenski, K., & Laugeson, E. A. (2012). Social skills training for young adults with high-functioning autism spectrum disorders: A randomized controlled pilot study. *Journal of Autism and Developmental Disorders, 42*, 1094–1103.

Ghaziuddin, M. (2002). Asperger syndrome: Associated psychiatric and medical conditions. *Focus on Autism and Other Developmental Disabilities, 17*, 138–144.

Ghaziuddin, M., & Gerstein, L. (1996). Pedantic speaking style differentiates Asperger syndrome from high-functioning autism. *Journal of Autism and Developmental Disorders, 26*, 585–595.

Gralinski, J. H., & Kopp, C. (1993). Everyday rules for behavior: Mother's requests to young children. *Developmental Psychology, 29*, 573–584.

Gresham, F. M., & Elliott, S. N. (2008). *Social skills improvement system: Rating scales*. Bloomington, MH: Pearson Assessments.

Griffin, H. C., Griffin, L. W., Fitch, C. W., Albera, V., & Gingras, H. G. (2006). Educational interventions for individuals with Asperger syndrome. *Intervention in School and Clinic, 41*, 150–155.

Happé, F. (1995). Understanding minds and metaphors: Insights from the study of figurative language in autism. *Metaphor and Symbol, 4*, 275–295.

Henault, I., & Attwood, T. (2002). *The sexual profile of adults with Asperger's syndrome: The need for understanding, support and sex education* (pp. 10–14). Melbourne, Australia: Inaugural World Autism Congress.

Howlin, P., & Goode, S. (1998). Outcome in adult life for people with autism, Asperger syndrome. In F. R. Volkmar (Ed.), *Autism and pervasive developmental disorders* (pp. 209–241). New York: Cambridge University Press.

Howlin, P. (2000). Outcome in adult life for more able individuals with autism or Asperger syndrome. *Autism, 4*, 63–83.

Howlin, P., & Moss, P. (2012). Adults with autism spectrum disorders. *Canadian Journal of Psychiatry, 57*, 275–283.

Humphrey, N., & Symes, W. (2010). Perceptions of social support and experience of bullying among pupils with autistic spectrum disorders in mainstream secondary schools. *European Journal of Special Needs Education, 25*, 77–91.

Jennes-Coussens, M., Magill-Evans, J., & Koning, C. (2006). The quality of life of young men with Asperger syndrome: A brief report. *Autism, 10*, 511–524.

Kaale, A., Smith, L., & Sponheim, E. (2012). A randomized controlled trial of preschool-based joint attention intervention for children with autism. *Journal of Child Psychology and Psychiatry, 53*, 97–105.

Karst, J. S., Van Hecke, A. V., Carson, A. M., Stevens, S., Schohl, K., & Dolan, B. (2015). Parent and family outcomes of PEERS: A social skills intervention for adolescents with autism spectrum disorder. *Journal of Autism and Developmental Disorders, 45*(3), 752–765.

Kasari, C., & Patterson, S. (2012). Interventions addressing social impairment in autism. *Current Psychiatry Reports, 14*, 713–725.

Kerbel, D., & Grunwell, P. (1998). A study of idiom comprehension in children with semantic pragmatic difficulties. Part I: Task effects on the assessment of idiom comprehension in children. *International Journal of Language & Communication Disorders, 33*, 1–22.

Kim, J. A., Szatmari, P., Bryson, S. E., Streiner, D. L., & Wilson, F. J. (2000). The prevalence of anxiety and mood problems among children with autism and Asperger syndrome. *Autism, 4*, 117–132.

Klin, A., Lin, D. J., Gorrindo, P., Ramsay, G., & Jones, W. (2009). Two-year-olds with autism orient to nonsocial contingencies rather than biological motion. *Nature, 459*, 257–261.

Klin, A., & Volkmar, F. R. (2003). Asperger syndrome: Diagnosis and external validity. *Child and Adolescent Psychiatric Clinics of North America, 12*, 1–13.

Koegel, L. K., Vernon, T. W., Koegel, R. L., Koegel, B. L., & Paullin, A. W. (2012). Improving social engagement and initiations between children with autism spectrum disorder and their peers in inclusive settings. *Journal of Positive Behavior Interventions, 14*, 220–227.

Krasny, L., Williams, B. J., Provencal, S., & Ozonoff, S. (2003). Social skills interventions for the autism spectrum: Essential ingredients and a model curriculum. *Child and Adolescent Psychiatry Clinics of North America, 12*, 107–122.

Lasgaard, M., Nielson, A., Eriksen, M. E., & Goossens, L. (2010). Loneliness and social support in adolescent boys with autism spectrum disorders. *Journal of Autism and Developmental Disorders, 40*, 218–226.

Laugeson, E. A. (2013). *The science of making friends: Helping socially challenged teens and young adults*. San Francisco, CA: Jossey-Bass.

Laugeson, E. A. (2014). *The PEERS curriculum for school based professionals: Social skills training for adolescents with autism spectrum disorder*. New York: Routledge.

Laugeson, E. A. (2017). *PEERS® for young adults: Social skills training for adults with autism spectrum disorder and other social challenges*. New York: Routledge.

Laugeson, E. A., & Ellingsen, R. (2014). Social skills training for adolescents and adults with autism spectrum disorder. In F. R. Volkmar, B. Reichow, & J. C. McPartland (Eds.), *Adolescents and adults with autism spectrum disorders* (pp. 61–85). New York: Springer.

Laugeson, E. A., Ellingsen, R., Sanderson, J., Tucci, L., & Bates, S. (2014). The ABC's of teaching social skills to adolescents with autism spectrum disorder in the classroom: The UCLA PEERS program. *Journal of Autism and Developmental Disorders, 44*, 2244–2256.

Laugeson, E. A., & Frankel, F. (2010). *Social skills for teenagers with developmental and autism spectrum disorder: The PEERS treatment manual*. New York: Routledge.

Laugeson, E. A., Frankel, F., Gantman, A., Dillon, A. R., & Mogil, C. (2012). Evidence-based social skills training for adolescents with autism spectrum disorders: The UCLA PEERS program. *Journal of Autism and Developmental Disorders, 42*, 1025–1036.

Laugeson, E. A., Frankel, F., Mogil, C., & Dillon, A. R. (2009). Parent-assisted social skills training to improve friendships in teens with autism spectrum disorders. *Journal of Autism and Developmental Disorders, 39*, 596–606.

Laugeson, E. A., Gantman, A., Kapp, S. K., Orenski, K., & Ellingsen, R. (2015). A randomized controlled trial to improve social skills in young adults with autism spectrum disorder: The UCLA PEERS® program. *Journal of Autism and Developmental Disorders*, 1–12. doi: 10.1007/s10803-015-2504-8.

Laugeson, E. A., Park, M. N., & Sanderson, J. (2016). *PEERS® for preschoolers: Parent assisted social skills training for children with autism spectrum disorder*. Manuscript in preparation.

Laushey, K. M., & Heflin, L. J. (2000). Enhancing social skills of kindergarten children with autism through the training of multiple peers as tutors. *Journal of Autism and Related Disorders, 30*, 183–193.

Lawton, K., & Kasari, C. (2012). Teacher-implemented joint attention intervention: Pilot randomized controlled study for preschoolers with autism. *Journal of Consulting and Clinical Psychology, 80*, 687–693.

Leaf, J. B., Leaf, J. A., Milne, C., Taubman, M., Oppenheim-Leaf, M., Torres, N., et al. (2017). An evaluation of a behaviorally based social skills group for individuals diagnosed with autism spectrum disorder. *Journal of Autism and Developmental Disorders, 47*, 243–259.

Lerner, M. D., & Mikami, A. Y. (2012). A preliminary randomized controlled trial of two social skills interventions for youth with high-functioning autism spectrum disorders. *Focus on Autism and Other Developmental Disabilities, 27*, 147–157.

Lopata, C., Thomeer, M. L., Volker, M. A., Nida, R. E., & Lee, G. K. (2008). Effectiveness of a manualized summer social treatment program for high-functioning children with autism spectrum disorders. *Journal of Autism and Developmental Disorders, 38*, 890–904.

Mandelberg, J., Laugeson, E. A., Cunningham, T. D., Ellingsen, R., Bates, S., & Frankel, F. (2014). Long-term treatment outcomes for parent-assisted social skills training for adolescents with autism spectrum disorders: The UCLA PEERS program. *Journal of Mental Health Research in Intellectual Disabilities, 7*, 45–73.

Martin, I., & McDonald, S. (2003). Weak coherence, no theory of mind, or executive dysfunction? Solving the puzzle of pragmatic language disorders. *Brain and Language, 85*, 451–466.

Matson, J. L. (2007). Determining treatment outcome in early intervention programs for autism spectrum disorders: A critical analysis of measurement issues in learning based interventions. *Research in Developmental Disabilities, 28*, 207–218.

Matson, J. L., Matson, M. L., & Rivet, T. T. (2007). Social-skills treatments for children with autism spectrum disorders: An overview. *Behavior Modification, 31*, 682–707.

McVey, A. J., Dolan, B. K., Willar, K. S., Pleiss, S., Karst, J. S., Casnar, C. L., … Van Hecke, A. V. (2016). A replication and extension of the PEERS® for young adults social skills intervention: Examining effects on social skills and social anxiety in young adults with autism spectrum disorder. *Journal of Autism and Developmental Disorders, 46*, 1–16.

Mehzabin, P., & Stokes, M. A. (2011). Self-assessed sexuality in young adults with high-functioning autism. *Research in Autism Spectrum Disorders, 5*, 614–621.

Miller, A., Vernon, T., Wu, V., & Russo, K. (2014). Social skill group interventions for adolescents with autism spectrum disorders: A systematic review. *Review Journal of Autism and Developmental Disorders, 1*, 254–265.

Minihan, A., Kinsella, W., & Honan, R. (2011). Social skills training for adolescents with Asperger's syndrome using a consultation model. *Journal of Research in Special Educational Needs, 11*, 55–69.

Mundy, P., Sigman, M., Ungerer, J., & Sherman, T. (1986). Defining the social deficits of autism: The contribution of non-verbal communication measures. *Journal of Child Psychology and Psychiatry, 27*, 657–669.

Myles, B. S., Bock, S. J., & Simpson, R. L. (2001). *Asperger syndrome diagnostic scale*. Austin, TX: Pro-Ed.

Pijnacker, J., Hagoort, P., Buitelaar, J., Teunisse, J. P., & Geurts, B. (2009). Pragmatic inferences in high-functioning adults with autism and Asperger syndrome. *Journal of Autism and Developmental Disorders, 39*, 607–618.

Orsmond, G. I., Krauss, M. W., & Seltzer, M. M. (2004). Peer relationships and social and recreational activities among adolescents and adults with autism. *Journal of Autism and Developmental Disorders, 34*, 245–256.

Reichow, B., & Volkmar, F. R. (2010). Social skills interventions for individuals with autism: Evaluation for evidence-based practices within a best evidence synthesis framework. *Journal of Autism and Developmental Disorders, 40*, 149–166.

Rubin, Z., & Sloman, J. (1984). How parents influence their children's friendships. In M. Lewis (Ed.), *Beyond the dyad* (pp. 223–250). New York: Plenum.

Schall, C. M., & McDonough, J. T. (2010). Autism spectrum disorders in adolescence and early adulthood: Characteristics and issues. *Journal of Vocational Rehabilitation, 32*, 81–88.

Schohl, K. A., Van Hecke, A. V., Carson, A. M., Dolan, B., Karst, J., & Stevens, S. (2014). A replication and extension of the PEERS intervention: Examining effects on social skills and social anxiety in adolescents with autism spectrum disorders. *Journal of Autism and Developmental Disorders, 44*(3), 532–545.

Shriberg, L. D., Paul, R., McSweeny, J. L., Klin, A., Cohen, D. J., & Volkmar, F. R. (2001). Speech and prosody characteristics of adolescents and adults with high-functioning autism and Asperger syndrome. *Journal of Speech, Language, and Hearing Research, 44*, 1097–1115.

Shtayermann, O. (2007). Peer victimization in adolescents and young adults diagnosed with Asperger's syndrome: A link to depressive symptomatology, anxiety symptomatology and suicidal ideation. *Issues in Comprehensive Pediatric Nursing, 30*, 87–107.

Sigman, M. D., Kasari, C., Kwon, J. H., & Yirmiya, N. (1992). Responses to the negative emotions of others by autistic, mentally retarded, and normal children. *Child Development, 63*, 796–807.

Smith, T., Scahill, L., Dawson, G., Guthrie, D., Lord, C., Odom, S., et al. (2007). Designing research studies on psychosocial interventions in autism. *Journal of Autism and Developmental Disorders, 37*, 354–366.

Starr, E., Szatmari, P., Bryson, S., & Zwaigenbaum, L. (2003). Stability and change among high functioning children with pervasive developmental disorders: A 2-year outcome study. *Journal of Autism and Developmental Disorders, 33*, 15–22.

Sterling, L., Dawson, G., Estes, A., & Greenson, J. (2008). Characteristics associated with presence of depressive symptoms in adults with autism spectrum disorder. *Journal of Autism and Developmental Disorders, 38*, 1011–1018.

Stokes, M., & Kaur, A. (2005). High-functioning autism and sexuality: A parental perspective. *The International Journal of Research and Practice, 9*, 266–289.

Stokes, M., Newton, N., & Kaur, A. (2007). Stalking, and social and romantic functioning among adolescents and adults with autism spectrum disorder. *Journal of Autism and Developmental Disorders, 37*, 1969–1986.

Sze, K. M., & Wood, J. J. (2007). Cognitive behavioral treatment of comorbid anxiety disorders and social difficulties in children with high-functioning autism: A case report. *Journal of Contemporary Psychotherapy, 37*, 133–143.

Tantam, D. (2003). The challenge of adolescents and adults with Asperger syndrome. *Child and Adolescent Psychiatric Clinics of North America, 12*, 143–163.

Travis, L. L., & Sigman, M. (1998). Social deficits and interpersonal relationships in autism. *Mental Retardation and Developmental Disabilities Research Reviews, 4*, 65–72.

Van Bourgondien, M. E., & Mesibov, G. B. (1987). Humor in high-functioning autistic adults. *Journal of Autism and Developmental Disorders, 17*, 417–424.

Van Hecke, A. V., Stevens, S., Carson, A. M., Karst, J. S., Dolan, B., Schohl, K., … Brockman, S. (2015). Measuring the plasticity of social approach: A randomized controlled trial of the effects of the PEERS intervention on EEG asymmetry in adolescents with autism spectrum disorders. *Journal of Autism and Developmental Disorders, 45*(2), 316–335.

Vernon, T. W., Miller, A. R., Ko, J. A., & Wu, V. L. (2016). Social tools and rules for teens (the START program): Program description and preliminary outcomes of an experiential socialization intervention for adolescents with autism spectrum disorder. *Journal of Autism and Developmental Disorders, 46*, 1806–1823.

Volkmar, F. R., Carter, A., Sparrow, S. S., & Cicchetti, D. V. (1993). Quantifying social development in autism. *Journal of the American Academy of Child & Adolescent Psychiatry, 32*, 627–632.

Volkmar, F. R., & Klin, A. (1998). Asperger syndrome and nonverbal learning disabilities. In E. Schopler, G. B. Mesibov, & L. J. Kunce (Eds.), *Asperger syndrome or high functioning autism?* (pp. 107–121). New York: Plenum Press.

White, S. W. (2011). *Social skills training for children with Asperger syndrome and high-functioning autism.* New York: Guilford Press.

White, S. W., Keonig, K., & Scahill, L. (2007). Social skills development in children with autism spectrum disorders: A review of the intervention research. *Journal of Autism and Developmental Disorders, 37*, 1858–1868.

White, S. W., Ollendick, T., Alban, A. M., Oswald, D., Johnson, C., Southam-Gerow, M. A., et al. (2013). Randomized controlled trial: Multimodal anxiety and social skill intervention for adolescents with autism spectrum disorder. *Journal of Autism and Developmental Disorders, 43*(2), 382–394.

Winter, M. (2003). *Asperger syndrome: What teachers need to know*. London: Jessica Kingsley.

Yoo, H. J., Bahn, G., Cho, I. H., Kim, E. K., Kim, J. H., Min, J. W., … Laugeson, E. A. (2014). A randomized controlled trial of the Korean version of the PEERS® parent-assisted social skills training program for teens with ASD. *Autism Research, 7*, 145–161.

Matrix Training Procedures

21

Robert K. Ross

21.1 Introduction to and Rationale for Matrix Training

It is widely understood that children with autism spectrum disorder (ASD) and other intellectual disabilities often have significant challenges with the acquisition and generalized use of many aspects of language, social interaction, and play skills. These challenges result in many treatment programs and models focusing on the production and generalized use of language as an essential component of treatment. Models such as "the Lovaas Model" (Lovaas, 1987), Early Start Denver Model (Rogers & Dawson, 2009), Treatment and Education of Autistic and Communication related handicapped Children (TEACCH) (Ozonoff & Cathcart, 1998), Learning Experiences and Alternate Program for Preschoolers and their Parents (LEAP) (Strain & Cordisco, 1993), Pivotal Response Training (PRT) (Koegel, Koegel, Harrower, & Carter, 1996), and Verbal Behavior (VB) (Sundberg et al., 1979)-based treatment models all recognize that social language/communication skill deficits are a core diagnostic feature of children with ASD and make remediating these deficits an important aspect of treatment.

Instructional programming in the various treatment models noted previously targets a wide range and aspects of receptive and expressive language as well as play and social interaction. However, at this point it is clear to most researchers and clinicians that instruction for every single possible language target is inefficient, if not impossible (Curiel, Sainato, & Goldstein, 2016). As a result of recognizing this fundamental truth, researchers have sought to develop a range of procedures to support acquisition and generalized use of language. One such procedure is called *matrix training* (Goldstein, Angelo, & Mousetis, 1987). There are few more critical skills to the development of social relationships than having social language relevant to play; however, children with ASD often have significant difficulty in the acquisition and demonstration of language and play skills. In the words of Weiss and Harris (2001), they are "doubly challenged in learning the language of social skills" (p. 75). Children without appropriate play language are at risk for not developing the friendships and social relationships that undergird the development of more complex play and social behavior. For far too many parents of children with ASD, the lack of language skills and social play is often a significant barrier to their child developing

R.K. Ross (✉)
Beacon ABA Services, Inc, Milford, MA, USA
e-mail: bross@beaconservices.org

J.B. Leaf (ed.), *Handbook of Social Skills and Autism Spectrum Disorder*, Autism and Child Psychopathology Series, DOI 10.1007/978-3-319-62995-7_21

meaningful friendships. Overcoming this barrier requires a set of effective instructional practices, and matrix training procedures is one tool that has been shown to be effective in this domain. For those working with children with ASD, creating and implementing efficient instruction is critical to effective and timely treatment to address this critical area, and matrix training may be one of the more beneficial treatment procedures available for this purpose.

21.2 What Is Matrix Training?

Matrix training provides a structure for teaching and demonstrating specific combinations of responses (vocal and/or motor) which increases the probability that untrained combinations of those responses will emerge in the absence of explicit training. Matrix training refers to a set of procedures or instructional arrangements designed to support what is often referred to as *generative learning* or *recombinative generalization*. Suchowierska (2006) described generative learning as responding and producing "both receptive and expressive language that has never been directly taught, but is related to" (p. 515) what was directly taught. Recombinative generalization has been described as "the differential responding to novel combinations of stimulus components that have been included previously in other stimulus contexts" (Goldstein, 1983b, p. 281). These two terms are clearly related and overlap so closely that, at times, clinicians become confused as to how to describe matrix training outcomes. To understand matrix training, it is often best to understand how matrix training is conducted and how its formatting results in the performances that are often demonstrated when using matrix training procedures. In this chapter, multiple exemplars of the formatting and targeted performances will be reviewed to enable the reader to see how the initial performances are established and how the untrained performances are evoked.

21.3 A Brief Overview of Matrix Training and Its Applications

According to Curiel et al. (2016), matrix training was first applied by Esper in 1925 who called it a miniature linguistic system (MLS) in its initial development and use with undergraduates (Esper, 1925). Goldstein (1983a, 1983b), demonstrated how matrix training could be used to support development of generative language and generalization of lexical rules in typically developing children. While the development of matrix training comes out of the speech and language field, it has been adopted by the behavior analytic community in the service of a wide range of skill-teaching applications. Published studies in the behavior analytic literature using matrix training have largely focused on individuals with autism and intellectual disabilities (Curiel et al., 2016). The sections below provide demonstrations of the application of matrix training in clinical settings (Sect. 21.4.1) and demonstrations from the research literature (Sect. 21.4.2).

The adaptability of the matrix format in teaching widely disparate skills can be seen in the range of areas where matrix training has been implemented. Some notable applications of matrix training have included but are not limited to *language* (Curiel et al., 2016; Ezell & Goldstein, 1989; Goldstein & Brown, 1989; Goldstein & Mousetis, 1989; Mineo & Goldstein, 1990), preliteracy skills (Axe & Sainato, 2010; Saunders, O'Donnell, Vaidaya, & Williams, 2003), generative spelling (Kinney, Vedora, & Stromer, 2003; Tanji & Noro, 2011), and sociodramatic play (Dauphin, Kinney, & Stromer, 2004). Examples of how matrix training was used to teach basic play actions and simple language are detailed in Sect. 21.4.1 below, and Sect. 21.4.2 highlights the use of matrix training to establish receptive and expressive language performances. These examples provide a basic introduction to the structure and format of matrix training. Subsequent sections detail additional uses of matrix training.

21.4 Implementing Matrix Training

Matrix training procedures are best and most easily understood in the context of concrete examples. This section will explain how to implement matrix training by starting with some simple and then progressively more complex examples of how matrices are formatted and how instruction in the matrix format is conducted. The content is meant to provide a basic understanding of matrix training procedures within the context of basic instructional exemplars. It is by no means an exhaustive list of the possible applications and extensions that are possible using matrix training procedures. In fact, it is likely that the wide range of potential applications of matrix training have only begun to be explored.

21.4.1 Example 1: A 2 × 2 Matrix

In the first example, a simple sociodramatic play matrix (i.e., 2 × 2) is demonstrated. This matrix example was developed for use at Beacon ABA Services of Massachusetts as part of its staff training procedures on the use of matrix training. In this example, as in most matrices, the focus of teaching is on establishing discrete *Object Action Language* targets. This example helps highlight in a very simple and concrete way the clarity of what is meant by the phrase Object Action Language routines. For those new to matrix training or with little experience teaching play skills, it is extremely helpful to conceptualize play schemes to be taught in terms of these Object Action Language routines.

In this case, as in all similar play routines, we need to first define the routine. This requires prespecifying the objects, actions, and language. Each of these components is specified in the context of a table or matrix, hence the term matrix training (see Table 21.1).

The objects (i.e., motorcycle and car) are listed in the *horizontal axis*. The actions (i.e., push and roll) are noted along the *vertical axis*. The language (i.e., vroom-vroom and wheee) are also noted on the *vertical axis*. In this matrix, we are teaching language along with the motor action; however, it is not essential and could be omitted for a nonvocal child. By specifying each of these components in the context of the matrix, there is instructional clarity as to both orders of instruction and the conditions to be assessed for generalization.

Table 21.1 The 2 × 2 matrix described above should look like this

Action/Language	Target objects	
	Motorcycle	Car
Push (say vroom-vroom)	X	
Roll down ramp (say wheee)		X

To implement this matrix, the following materials are needed: toy car, toy motorcycle, and toy garage with a ramp to go down. The routine is taught sequentially as follows:

1. The learner is taught to push the motorcycle which is already in front of the garage:
   (a) With one hand, push the toy motorcycle in front of the garage (6–10 in of movement).
   (b) While pushing the motorcycle, the learner will say "vroom, vroom" (this typically requires instructional support such as in vivo modeling, peer modeling, video modeling, text prompts, etc.).

This routine should be explicitly taught to the learner using anyone of the specific teaching procedures noted in teaching methods section later in this chapter. Once this routine (i.e., both motor and vocal responses) is acquired and reliably demonstrated to the criteria specified by the instructor, the next step is to teach the second target (gray section of Table 21.1), car down the ramp of the garage.

1. Car down the ramp which is already in the garage near the ramp:
   (a) With one hand, roll the car down the ramp garage until at the end of the ramp

(b) While the car is rolling, the learner will say “wheee” (again instructional support is often required to support production of this targeted vocal response)

As you can see from the visual representation, the two performances taught are done sequentially (note the gray sections of the matrix in Table 21.1). This is referred to in matrix training, as *teaching along the diagonal*. Once the two target performances have been acquired (according to a mastery criteria set by the instructor), the car is now placed in front of the garage and the learner is expected to push the car and say “vroom-vroom.” If this performance emerges, it is reinforced. If it does not, it is directly taught. This process is repeated with the motorcycle placed on top of the garage, and the learner is expected to roll it down the ramp and say “wheee.” If successful, the learner would have demonstrated previously untaught combinations of vocal and motor performances (i.e., recombinative generalization or generative learning).

Moreover, an instructional context has been established where the point of the activity is for the learner to demonstrate previously taught responses with novel materials. This critical point, and advantage of matrix training procedures, cannot be overstated. The failure to demonstrate stimulus and response generalization is a significant concern for those teaching individuals on the autism spectrum. In matrix training procedures, once you have established and the learner has acquired several matrices, you have a set of instructional arrangements that signals to the learner that you will be expected to demonstrate all of the performances in the matrix with other materials and in other contexts. The routine of demonstrating existing language and motor actions with untrained materials is what the matrix training format establishes. The structure of matrix training is an explicit cue to “do that skill with other things,” which is a key point and the critical advantage of matrix training. For individuals whose strengths include learning routines but failing to demonstrate generalized performances of these routines, this structure is in many ways ideal. It capitalizes on the consistency of the routine while simultaneously establishing flexibility in the responses.

21.4.2 Example 2: A 3 × 3 Matrix

In this example, the model and targets specified in the 1989 Goldstein and Mousetis study are described, although the example below has been modified in some ways for instructional purposes. In this 3 × 3 matrix, the focus is on teaching known objects and location combinations as well as prepositions. The initial instructional target is to establish the routine of placing a series of known objects onto the target location. In this example, the participants are taught to place the button on the table. Once the initial response is established (see directly taught in Table 21.2), the performances that were not directly trained (a total of eight untrained responses) are tested.

The instructional sequence is as follows:

1. The instruction “put the button on the table” is given, and support for the production of that motor response is provided.
2. Once the initial response is established to the predetermined mastery criteria, the other responses are tested.
3. Those that are not demonstrated are directly taught as in the 2 × 2 matrix.

Table 21.2

Known Objects	Known Locations		
	Table	Bed	Couch
Button	Directly Taught	Tested for	Tested for
Paddle	Tested for	Tested for	Tested for
Comb	Tested for	Tested for	Tested for

The efficiency of using this format can be seen in the generalized demonstration of correct performance of responses not previously demonstrated by the participants. Goldstein and Mousetis (1989) noted that many of their participants demonstrate most or all of the untrained responses. Once they had demonstrated that novel combinations of responding emerged after instruction within the matrix above, Goldstein and Mousetis then took this model and format several steps further. They introduced/assessed additional language complexity. After they determined that the participants could follow the instruction to put the item in the correct location, they assessed if the participants could expressively answer the question "where is the button (paddle, comb)?" In some cases these performances emerged, and, where they did not, the same matrix process could be used to establish initial performances and support generalized demonstration of those newly acquired responses.

Goldstein and Mousetis (1989) then expanded the matrix by adding unknown object and locations as well as using the matrix with additional prepositions. The previous matrix was expanded as follows (Table 21.3).

Using the matrix displayed in Table 21.3, the participants were taught to place previously unknown objects on, and eventually in, under, etc., previously unknown locations. Once again, many of the participants demonstrated untrained receptive and expressive language performances within the context of the matrix.

For some participants, instruction in five target responses (i.e., T1–T5) resulted in the emergence of 44 untrained responses. The blank spaces in the matrix above reflect the 44 possible emergent responses. When considering the efficiency of this model compared with direct teaching of each instructional targets, the benefits are clear. Additionally, the model can be used across a range of categories of responding. The fact that Goldstein and Mousetis (1989) addressed receptive and expressive language performances in the context of gross/fine motor tasks is noteworthy and has immediate implications for teaching play skills as well as a wide range of other critical skill deficits for individuals with ASD and other intellectual disabilities.

As described above, other researchers have taken advantage of the format to address other areas of skill acquisition such as sociodramatic play (Dauphin et al., 2004) and literacy/preliter-

Table 21.3 Expanded matrix – (Adapted from Goldstein and Mousetis 1989)

Objects		Known Locations			Unknown Locations			
		Table	Bed	Couch	Dresser	Desk	Crib	Speaker
K	Button	T1						
N	Paddle							
O W N	Comb							
U	Barrette				T2			
N	Scale					T3		
K	Spool						T4	
O W N	Screw							T5

acy skills (Axe & Sainato, 2010; Kinney et al., 2003; Tanji & Noro, 2011).

21.5 Using Matrix Training to Teach Literacy Skills

Another application of matrix training procedures by Kinney et al. (2003) involved the teaching of generative spelling. In this study, the authors used matrix training in combination with video modeling and video rewards to create new words by placing a new consonant onto a targeted word ending (word beginnings were also targeted within the study). This was done using 3 × 3 matrices in the sequence described in Tables 21.4a, 21.4b, and 21.4c.

It is useful to note the results from the first matrix in this study. The shaded areas in Table 21.4a represent the targets that were directly taught, and the unshaded blocks were assessed for generalization. In the first matrix, the participant did not demonstrate generalized performances within the matrix. However, in subsequent matrices, the amount of teaching required and the amount of generative performances achieved increased. It is important to understand that not all learners will immediately demonstrate the untrained performances within matrix training. Some learners may require additional exposure to the format and effective histories of reinforcement for demonstrating untrained responses. These basic elements of instructional design need to be considered, and the procedures can only set the occasion for responding. The effective use of reinforcers will be necessary to establish response–consequence relations to support continued generative performances. Tables 21.4a, 21.4b, and 21.4c below shows the sequence and performances that Kinney and colleagues used in their 2003 study.

3 X 3 Matrix Adapted from Kinnet et al 2003

3 X 3 Matrix Adapted from Kinnet et al 2003

As can be seen from the tables, over the course of three matrices, the participants' performance within the matrix improved (i.e., less direct teaching was required to produce generative performances). Kinney et al. (2003) also taught word beginning and assessed for the targeted performances outside of the instructional condition in this study. The participants did acquire word beginnings and demonstrated target performances outside of the instructional conditions. This phenomenon of generalized performances being observed outside of the instructional conditions after matrix training has been reported by a number of authors (Axe & Sainato, 2010; Curiel et al., 2016; Goldstein & Mousetis, 1989).

21.6 Teaching Methods to Establish Performances in the Context of Matrix Training

It is important to understand that matrix training provides a format for supporting the generalized and generative production of responses established during instructional programming. These initial responses must still be established through some form of instructional practice. When using matrix training procedures, clinicians must also make decisions about what instructional procedures they will employ to establish the basic

Table 21.4a 3 × 3 Matrix (Adapted from Kinney et al. 2003)

Matrix 2	Word Endings		
	-ell	-est	-ook
b	Directly Taught	Generalization	Generalization
n	Directly Taught	Directly Taught	Generalization
t	Generalization	Directly Taught	Directly Taught

Table 21.4b 3 × 3 Matrix (Adapted from Kinney et al. 2003)

Matrix 3	Word Endings		
	-ack	-ad	-ap
p	Directly Taught	Generalization	No Generalization
r	Generalization	Directly Taught	Generalization
s	Generalization	Generalization	Directly Taught

Table 21.4c 3 × 3 Matrix (Adapted from Kinney et al. 2003)

Matrix 1	Word Endings		
	-ock	-ore	-op
l	Directly Taught	No Generalization	No Generalization
s	Directly Taught	Directly Taught	No Generalization
t	No Generalization	Directly Taught	Directly Taught

responses to be combined and supported to generalize as a function of matrix training. A critical step in this process is choosing between the variety of teaching methods that have been developed in the field of applied behavior analysis for teaching children with ASD. Many of these methods have strong empirical support in establishing a range of performances and can be readily implemented in the context of matrix training. For example, in order to get a child to engage in a target play action and use the language for that action, a clinician may choose to model the action and then reinforce the learner for imitating the response; they may also choose to simply verbally prompt the language and physically prompt the actions and use prompt fading procedures. These are just two examples of teaching procedures that may be used in the context of matrix training. Some of the teaching methods used in empirical studies include but are not limited to:

- *Video modeling* (Dauphin et al., 2004; Kinney et al., 2003): There are a range of variations to video modeling procedure and an extensive literature demonstrating the efficacy of video modeling with individuals with ASD and intellectual disabilities. Video modeling typically involves the presentation of a brief video of the target response(s) and is followed by an opportunity to imitate the modeled responses. Typically, correct performance is reinforced. A range of responses to errors can occur including hand over hand correction trials, repeating the video, and no programmed response (extinction). In matrix training the individual responses targeted are presented via video (on a screen), typically with only one set of the materials and target actions/language. Once the target performances are established, opportunities to perform the target skills with novel materials are provided absent the video model.
- In vivo/*peer modeling*: The correct target performance is modeled (by the experimenter or a peer), and then an opportunity is provided to imitate the observed responses. Typically, correct performance is reinforced. A range of responses to errors can occur including hand over hand correction trials, repeating the model, and no programmed response (extinction). In matrix training the individual responses targeted are modeled by a live

person, again typically with only one set of the materials and target actions/language. Once the target performances are established, opportunities to perform the target skills with novel materials are provided absent the model.
- *Physical prompting* (Axe & Sainato, 2010): In matrix training, the target performance is typically physically prompted (most to least or least to most can be used), and a form of prompt fading (e.g., graduated guidance, progressive time delay) is implemented until the target performance is independently demonstrated. This may or may not involve modeling prior to the prompting. It also typically involves the use of programmed reinforcement for correct responses. Once the target performances are established, opportunities to perform the target skills with novel materials are provided absent the prompting.

21.7 Summary

Matrix training is a potentially useful instructional format for establishing instructional control of target skills that also could lead to generalized performances of those targeted skills. With the number of published studies showing positive treatment effects across a range of skills, matrix training should be considered both an evidence-based practice and an essential component of programming for individuals on the autism spectrum. The clarity of the instructional formatting and the ability to maximize learning outcomes in a time- and resource-efficient manner make matrix training an important component of any Early Intensive Behavioral Intervention (EIBI) program. The fact that the core challenges for individuals with ASD and other intellectual disabilities (i.e., social language, social interactional, and play skills) are easily addressed within the context of matrix training further demonstrates the usefulness of these procedures. Finally, the ease of teaching the procedures to new staff and those with limited formal training in behavior analysis provides additional support for their use. For many staff and clinicians, the teaching of sociodramatic play and receptive and expressive language skill instruction are significant challenges. Taubman, Leaf, and McEachin (2011) noted that resistance to social and play skill instruction "may reflect just how difficult it is to generate curriculum for these behaviors" (p. 3). It is not unreasonable to suggest that the abstract and complex nature of such performances may result in avoidance of instruction in these areas or the use of practices that are not particularly effective. With matrix training procedures, these staff and clinicians have an evidence-based, highly efficient, and well-structured format for conducting such instruction.

Key Matrix Training Terms

Emergent Responding A synonym for generative learning and recombinative generalization, it refers to the fact that new responses or novel variations of trained responses "emerge" as a function of the instructional practices being used.

Generative Learning "Responding that has never been directly taught but is related to what (was) is taught" (Suchowierski, 2006, p. 515).

Recombinative Generalization Differential responding to novel combinations of stimulus components that have been included previously in other stimulus contexts (Goldstein, 1983b, p. 281). "... this occurs when stimulus components (such as words) that have been taught are rearranged with other stimulus components to create new untaught arrangements" (Curiel et al., 2016, p. 96).

Response Generalization The occurrence of a novel response or variation of a previously trained response(s) under stimulus conditions where a specific response was trained. The stimulus or stimulus conditions are the same; however, the response which occurs varies from the trained response.

Stimulus Generalization The occurrence or specific trained responses(s) under stimulus conditions other than those where the response was trained. The response that occurs is the same; however, the stimulus and/or stimulus conditions under which the performance occurs vary.

Teaching Along the Diagonal This refers to the process of teaching target responses within a matrix along the diagonal axis. It allows for the learner to be exposed to all target performances and all materials, without directly teaching the majority of possible combinations of materials and responses.

References

Axe, J. B., & Sainato, D. M. (2010). Matrix training of preliteracy skills with preschoolers with autism. *Journal of Applied Behavior Analysis*, *43*, 635–652.

Curiel, E. S. L., Sainato, D. D., & Goldstein, H. (2016). Matrix training of receptive language skills with a toddler with autism spectrum disorder: A case study. *Education and Treatment of Children*, *39*, 95–109.

Dauphin, M., Kinney, E. M., & Stromer, R. (2004). Using video-enhanced activity schedules and matrix training to teach socio-dramatic play to a child with autism. *Journal of Positive Behavior Interventions*, *6*, 238–250.

Esper, E. A. (1925). A technique for experimental investigation of associative interference in artificial linguistic material. *Language Monographs*, *1*, 5–47.

Ezell, H. K., & Goldstein, H. (1989). Effects of imitation on language comprehension and transfer of production in children with mental retardation. *Journal of Speech and Hearing Disorders*, *54*, 49–56.

Goldstein, H. (1983a). Training generative repertoires within agent-action-object miniature linguistic systems with children. *Journal of Speech and Hearing Research*, *26*, 76–89.

Goldstein, H. (1983b). Recombinative generalization: Relationships between environmental conditions and the linguistic repertoires of language learners. *Analysis and Interventions in Developmental Disabilities*, *3*, 279–293.

Goldstein, H., & Brown, W. H. (1989). Observational learning of receptive and expressive language by handicapped preschool children. *Education and Treatment of Children*, *12*, 5–37.

Goldstein, H., & Mousetis, L. (1989). Generalized language learning by children with severe mental retardation: Effects of peers' expressive modeling. *Journal of Applied Behavior Analysis*, *22*, 245–259.

Goldstein, H., Angelo, D., & Mousetis, L. (1987). Acquisition and extension of syntactic repertoires by severely mentally retarded youth. *Research in Developmental Disabilities*, *8*, 549–574.

Kinney, E. M., Vedora, J., & Stromer, R. (2003). Computer-presented video models to teach generative spelling to a child with autism spectrum disorder. *Journal of Positive Behavior Interventions*, *5*, 22–29.

Koegel, L. K., Koegel, J. K., Harrower, J. K., & Carter, C. M. (1996). Pivotal response intervention I: Overview of approach. *Journal of the Association for Persons with Severe Handicaps*, *24*(3), 174–185.

Lovaas, O. I. (1987). Behavioral treatment and normal educational and intellectual functioning in young autistic children. *Journal of Consulting and Clinical Psychology*, *55*, 3–9.

Mineo, B. A., & Goldstein, H. (1990). Generalized learning of receptive and expressive action-object responses by language delayed preschoolers. *Journal of Speech and Hearing Research*, *55*, 665–678.

Ozonoff, S., & Cathcart, K. (1998). Effectiveness of a home program intervention for young children with autism. *Journal of Autism and Developmental Disorders*, *28*, 25–32.

Rogers, S. J., & Dawson, G. (2009). *Play and engagement in early autism: The Early Start Denver Model. Volume I: The treatment*. New York: Guilford Press.

Saunders, K. J., O'Donnell, J., Vaidaya, M., & Williams, D. C. (2003). Recombinative generalization of within-syllable units of non-reading adults with mental retardation. *Journal of Applied Behavior Analysis*, *36*, 95–99.

Strain, P. S., & Cordisco, L. (1993). The LEAP preschool model. In S. Harris & J. Handleman (Eds.), *Preschool programs for children with autism* (pp. 115–126). Austin, TX: Pro-Ed.

Suchowierska, M. (2006). Recombinative generalization: Some theoretical and practical remarks. *International Journal of Psychology*, *41*, 514–522.

Sundberg, M. L., Ray, D. A., Braam, S. E., Stafford, M. W., Reuber, T. M., & Braam,C. A. (1979). *A manual for the use of B. F. Skinner's analysis of verbal behavior for language assessment and programming*. Western Michigan University Behavioral Monograph #9 , Western Michigan University, Kalamazoo, MI.

Tanji, T., & Noro, F. (2011). Matrix training for generative spelling in children with autism spectrum disorder. *Behavioral Interventions*, *26*, 326–339.

Taubman, M., Leaf, R., & McEachin, J. (2011). *Crafting connections; contemporary applied behavior analysis for enriching the social lives of persons with autism spectrum disorder*. New York, NY: DRL Books Inc.

Weiss, M. J., & Harris, S. L. (2001). *Reaching out and joining in: Teaching social skills to young children with autism*. Bethesda, MD: Woodbine House.

Social Stories™: A Cautionary Tale

22

Justin B. Leaf and Julia L. Ferguson

Social Stories™ are an intervention in which a teacher writes a brief text describing a target social behavior to be displayed, when the target behavior should be displayed, why the target behavior should be displayed, and how students can display the target social behavior correctly (Gray & Garand, 1993). In 1993, Gray and Garand first described Social Stories™ as a procedure that can be used to teach individuals diagnosed with autism spectrum disorder (ASD) a variety of behaviors, including social behavior. Since Gray and Garand's initial article, Social Stories™ have been evaluated in numerous empirical investigations (e.g., Adams, Gouvousis, VanLue, & Waldron, 2004; Barry & Burlew, 2004; Delano & Snell, 2006), have been described in several curriculum books (Gray, 2000; Gray, 2012), have been reviewed by professionals (e.g., Ali & Frederickson, 2006; Kokina & Kern, 2010; Leaf et al., 2015), are commonly implemented in clinical settings (Reynhout & Carter, 2009), and have been recommended as an effective and evidence-based procedure (National Autism Center, 2009, 2015). Despite Social Stories™ being widely investigated, implemented, and endorsed, there have been questions about the overall effectiveness and efficiency of Social Stories™ to teach social behaviors (e.g., Kokina & Kern, 2010; Leaf et al., 2015). The purpose of this chapter is to describe Social Stories™, the guidelines associated with Social Stories™, and the theoretical basis for Social Stories™, to review the research on Social Stories™, and to provide recommendations for future researchers and clinicians as it applies to teaching social behavior for individuals diagnosed with ASD.

J.B. Leaf (✉)
Director of Research, Autism Partnership Foundation, Seal Beach, CA, USA
e-mail: jblautpar@aol.com

J.L. Ferguson
Autism Partnership Foundation, Seal Beach, CA, USA

22.1 Gray and Garand 1993

In 1993, Gray and Garand were the first professionals to describe Social Stories™ as an intervention that can improve social behavior, and other behaviors, for individuals diagnosed with ASD. In this article, the authors stated that social behavior exhibited by others is often difficult for individuals diagnosed with ASD to interpret. The authors stated that in order for individuals with ASD to improve their social behaviors, they need to be able to answer questions about who, when, where, why, and what, with respect to the target behavior. Gray and Garand also stated that

J.B. Leaf (ed.), *Handbook of Social Skills and Autism Spectrum Disorder*, Autism and Child Psychopathology Series, DOI 10.1007/978-3-319-62995-7_22

traditional methods of teaching may be confusing for individuals diagnosed with ASD. As such, Gray and Garand recommend the use of Social Stories™ to teach social behaviors for this population.

In recommending the implementation of Social Stories™, Gray and Garand (1993) provided several guidelines, or recommendations, for their implementation. First the authors stated, "Social stories are most likely to benefit students functioning intellectually in the trainable mentally impaired range or higher who possess basic language skills" (Gray & Garand, 1993, p. 2). The authors recommended that Social Stories™ be written from the students' perspective, should be individualized to the student, and be written at the students' comprehension level. Gray and Garand stated that Social Stories™ should consist of three sentence types: (a) directive sentences, (b) descriptive sentences, and (c) prescriptive sentences (see Table 22.1 for a description of the sentence types). Another recommendation provided by Gray and Garand was that illustrations should not be used within a Social Story™, although Social Stories™ could be recorded either with video or audio devices. The authors recommended that the adult (e.g., parent or professional) first read the story aloud to the student while sitting next to them, and if the student is capable of reading, then the student should read the story to him or herself thereafter. Additionally, Gray and Garand recommended that the Social Story™ be read at least once per day. Finally, Gray and Garand claimed, "Experiences with social stories indicates that they are not effective for all students in all situations. In cases in which social stories are effective, results are often dramatic and apparent within one week" (p. 5). It should be noted that this first article on Social Stories™ was a description of the procedure and included no empirical evidence/data on the implementation of Social Stories™ for changing behavior of individuals diagnosed with ASD.

22.2 Defining Criterion

As Social Stories™ started to be implemented more frequently, it was important for the creators to define and clarify what constitutes a Social Story™.

Table 22.1 Sentence types

Sentence type	Definition	Year introduced
Descriptive	Describes the environmental events of the social behavior (e.g., where, why, and how)	Gray and Garand, 1993
Perspective	Describes the mental states others may feel if the student engages in the targeted behavior	Gray and Garand, 1993
Directive	Tells the student what behaviors to engage in	Gray and Garand, 1993
Control	Sentences written by the student explaining the story	Gray, 1994
Partial	Fill in the blank sentences that can be used for comprehension	Gray, 1994
Affirmative	Describes a commonly shared societal belief	Gray, 2000
Cooperative	Sentences that tell the student how others may help out the child	Gray, 2000

In 2004, Gray provided ten defining criteria of a Social Story™. First, Social Stories™ share meaningful social information, have a reassuring quality, and at least 50% of the story applauds achievements of the learner. Second, there are three parts of the Social Story™, (a) the introduction section, which identifies the topic; (b) the body, which explains the targeted social behavior; and (c) a conclusion that describes the importance of displaying the skill. Third, Social Stories™ answer "wh" questions (i.e., who, what, where, when, and why questions). Fourth, Social Stories™ should be written from a first or third person perspective. Fifth, Social Stories™ consist of positive language throughout the story (e.g., highlighting positive behaviors which the individual should display). Sixth, Social Stories™ always include descriptive sentences and should include the other sentence types (see Table 22.1 for list of type of sentences). Seventh, Social Stories™ should describe the target social behavior rather than directly instruct the student on what to do. Eighth, the adult should write the Social Story™ so that it is aligned with the abilities and interests of the student. Ninth, Social Stories™ can include meaningful illustrations, which was a change from the original recommendations (i.e., Gray & Garand, 1993). Tenth, the title of the Social Story™ should meet all appropriate Social Stories™ criteria.

22.3 Guidelines for Social Stories™

22.3.1 Sentence Types

Social Stories™ must use certain sentence types, which have evolved throughout the years of implementation of Social Stories™. When Gray and Garand (1993) first described Social Stories™ there were only three sentence types (i.e., directive, prescriptive, and descriptive). In 1994, Gray described two more sentence types: control and partial sentences (see Table 22.1) that can be used within Social Stories™. In 1998, Gray asserted that control and partial sentences were officially part of Social Stories™. In 2000, Gray created affirmative and cooperative sentences (see Table 22.1), which should be included as a part of Social Stories™. Today there are two types of Social Stories™ implemented for individuals diagnosed with ASD based on the types of sentences used within the Social Story™. The first type is a basic Social Story™, which only includes descriptive, affirmative, perspective, and directive sentences. The second type of Social Story™ is known as a complete Social Story™ in which all seven types of sentences are utilized (Reynhout & Carter, 2006).

It should be noted that the additional sentence types and the recommended changes of these sentence types did not occur through careful experimental evaluation or based upon empirical evidence, but rather were created based upon anecdotal experiences implementing Social Stories™. These ongoing and continual changes to sentence types may have led to a difficulty in second-party researchers adhering to the guidelines of how to write a Social Story™.

22.3.2 Ratio

Another important guideline of Social Stories™ is that the aforementioned sentences should be implemented in a specific order. Initially, therapists could write any type of Social Story™ as long as the correct types of sentences were utilized (Gray & Garand, 1993). If a therapist used more directive sentences within the story, it was known as a directive Social Story™; if a therapist used more descriptive sentences within the story, it was known as a descriptive Social Story™. In 1994, Gray provided the following recommendations of how the therapist should write a story, "A good formula to follow for most stories is to write a total of at least three to five descriptive, perspective, and/or control sentences for every directive sentence in a story" (p. 13–14). It was not until 1998 that this recommendation about the ratio of sentence types became a formal rule. In 2010, Gray added another recommendation stating that descriptive sentences should be written at least twice for every directive and control sentence. Similar to the changing criteria for the sentence types, the guidelines for the ratio of sentences has also evolved with no empirical evidence to support its change. Table 22.2 provides a list of the various recommendations in terms of ratio of sentences.

Table 22.2 Ratio guidelines

Publication	Guideline
Gray and Garand 1993	No ratio provided. Mostly directive stories
Gray, 1994	An optional ratio of one directive sentence for every three to five descriptive, perspective, or control sentences
Gray, 1995	The ratio provided from 1994 should be heavily considered
Gray, 1998	Required for every one directive sentence that there are at least two to five of the other sentence types
Gray, 2000	For every directive or control sentence, there should be two to five of the other sentence types
Gray, 2010	For every coaching sentence (i.e., those that gently guide behavior), there must be at least two descriptive, affirmative, or perspective sentences

22.3.3 Illustrations

In research and in practice, Social Stories™ have been implemented with illustrations (e.g., Brownell, 2002) and without illustrations (e.g., Kalyva & Agaliotis, 2009). When illustrations are used, they have included photographs of the learner (e.g., Barry & Burlew, 2004), cartoon illustrations (e.g., Leaf et al., 2012), and clip art (e.g., Leaf et al., 2012). Although illustrations have been used when implementing Social Stories™, the guidelines have also changed over time. Originally, Gray and Garand (1993) recommended, "With only a few exceptions, illustrations are not recommended; our experience indicates that they may be distracting, or a student may make an inaccurate interpretation of the situation based upon the illustration" (p. 4). However, without any supporting empirical data, these recommendations have changed, and now illustrations are encouraged when implementing Social Stories™ (Gray, 2010). As of today, Social Stories™ could or could not include illustrations as a supplement to the story. Table 22.3 provides a list of the various recommendations in terms of the use or nonuse of illustrations.

22.3.4 Other Guidelines

Other recommended guidelines for the implementation of Social Stories™ are that students should have basic language skills and be in the "trainable mentally impaired range" (Gray & Garand, 1993, p. 3). Although this is a guideline, researchers have implemented Social Stories™ with a wide range of individuals with varying intellectual capabilities (see Kokina & Kern, 2010). Another guideline is that the therapist should sit by the student's side while reading the Social Story™ (Gray & Garand, 1993). A final guideline is that Social Stories™ should be individualized for the learner (Gray & Garand, 1993). This is a recommended guideline; however, there are numerous curriculum books in which therapists can use prewritten generic Social Stories™ (Gray 2000, 2010, 2012), which may send a mixed message for the clinician, teacher, parent, etc. implementing the procedure.

Table 22.3 Illustration guidelines

Publication	Recommendation
Gray and Garand, 1993	No illustrations
Gray, 1994	Illustrations optional
Gray, 1995	Illustrations discouraged
Gray, 1998	Illustrations optional
Gray, 2010	Illustrations encouraged

22.4 Theoretical Basis

One of the main rationales for the use of Social Stories™ is that for students with ASD to change their social behavior, they must be able to understand their own social behavior. Therefore, in order for Social Stories™ to effectively teach social behavior, they must improve the learner's social cognition and teach the learner to read his or her own social behavior. Thus, one of the theoretical bases for Social Stories™ is that they address theory of mind (ToM; Baron-Cohen, 2001) for individuals diagnosed with ASD.

Another theoretical basis of Social Stories™ is that individuals diagnosed with ASD may not attend to the relevant components of their social behavior or to the environment around them, which influences social behavior. According to proponents of Social Stories™, the implementation of Social Stories™ may help individuals concentrate on the relevant components of social behavior by providing information visually (e.g., illustrations and text) (Gray, 2010). Visual information may be easier for individuals with ASD to understand (Wolfberg, 1995), and since Social Stories™ present information visually, it may be easier for individuals diagnosed with ASD to concentrate on what is being taught.

Researchers have also hypothesized that individuals diagnosed with ASD have impairments in planning, flexibility, and self-regulation (i.e., executive dysfunction; Ozonoff, 1998). It is believed that Social Stories™ may help improve this executive dysfunction, as Social Stories™ can provide individuals diagnosed with ASD clear rules and expectations to follow. Finally,

Gray and Garand (1993) claimed, "Considering that social interactions are difficult for students with autism, the use of traditional instruction to teach social behavior presents a student with a compound challenge…" (p. 2), and "Social Stories™ seek to minimize potentially confusing instructional interactions, to provide students with autism direct access to social information." (p. 2). Thus, according to Gray and Garand, the implementation of Social Stories™ may be more beneficial to teach social behavior than more traditional approaches such as video modeling (Charlop-Christy, Le, & Freeman, 2000), modeling and role-playing (Leaf et al., 2010), script fading (Krantz & McClannahan, 1993), and discrete trial teaching (Lovaas, 1987).

22.5 Research

There have been numerous studies that have evaluated Social Stories™ for individuals diagnosed with ASD (see Kokina & Kern, 2010 for a review). Some empirical research has evaluated Social Stories™ that target improving behaviors that are not social in nature, such as washing hands (e.g., Hagiwara & Myles, 1999) or reducing aberrant behavior (e.g., Lorimer, Simpson, Myles, & Ganz, 2002). The majority of research evaluating Social Stories™ has targeted social behavior (see Kokina & Kern, 2010). Researchers have evaluated the use of Social Stories™ to teach social behaviors such as gaining attention (Soenksen & Alper, 2006), increasing play (Barry & Burlew, 2004), verbal greetings (Reichow & Sabornie, 2009), social engagement (Delano & Snell, 2006), and game play (Quirmbach, Lincon, Feinberg-Gizzo, Ingersoll, & Andrews, 2009). There have been studies evaluating Social Stories™ utilizing a group design (e.g., Quirmbach et al., 2009), but the majority of evaluations have used single-subject research designs (e.g., Hanley-Hochdorfer, Bray, Kehle, & Elinoff, 2010). What follows is a description of several studies evaluating Social Stories™ as a stand-alone procedure (e.g., Swaggart et al., 1995), Social Stories™ combined with other procedures (e.g., Litras, Moore, and Anderson, 2010), and studies in which researchers have compared Social Stories™ to other procedures (e.g., Leaf et al., 2012).

22.5.1 Social Stories™ as a Stand-Alone Procedure

22.5.1.1 Social Communication

There are a few studies in which researchers evaluated the implementation of Social Stories™ to target deficits in social communication. Swaggart et al. (1995) conducted one of the earliest empirical evaluations of Social Stories™. In this study three participants diagnosed with autism were included. One participant, Danielle, was taught how to appropriately greet other individuals within her school environment. The authors wrote a Social Story™ that consisted of one descriptive sentence and four directive sentences. Each sentence was printed on one page with an icon depicting the appropriate action above the sentence. An appropriate greeting consisted of Danielle saying "hi" or waving her hand to the person and staying at least 3 ft away from the person. The authors used an AB case design (see Bailey & Burch, 2002 for an explanation of AB case design) to evaluate the effectiveness of the Social Story™ on the greeting behavior. The results showed an increase from greeting appropriately in 7% of opportunities during baseline to greeting appropriately in 74% of opportunities during intervention. The authors concluded that the study, "…provide[s] support for the use of social stories with children with autism" (p. 11). Although the authors reported positive findings, there are some serious methodological flaws, which include using an AB case design, not assessing maintenance, and starting intervention with an increasing trend during baseline.

In a more recent study, Hanley-Hochdorfer et al. (2010) evaluated the use of Social Stories™ targeted to increase social communicative behaviors of four individuals diagnosed with ASD. The authors targeted two forms of social communicative behavior; the first was verbal initiations, and the second was responding to peers. The Social Story™ followed the guidelines from Gray (2000) and Gray and Garand (1993) and included comprehension questions. The researchers read the Social Story™ no more than 15 min before lunch and evaluated the targeted social communication behaviors during lunchtime. The authors used a multiple baseline design across participants. Results of the evaluation showed no improvement in either initiations or responses from baseline, to intervention, and to maintenance for all four participants. The authors concluded, "Although evidence supports the use of social stories to decrease disruptive behaviors in students with ASD, practitioners should exercise caution when using social stories alone to increase social and communicative behaviors in students with ASD as outcomes may not be promising" (Hanley-Hochdorfer et al., 2010, p. 490).

22.5.1.2 Social Interaction

There are several studies in which researchers have evaluated the implementation of Social Stories™ to teach individuals diagnosed with ASD a variety of social behaviors, commonly referred to as a social interaction. One of the earliest studies to evaluate Social Stories™ on social interaction was conducted by Norris and Dattilo (1999). This study included one participant diagnosed with autism. Appropriate social interaction was defined as the student initiating or responding to a peer verbally, physically, or gesturally. The authors wrote three different Social Stories™ to target this behavior following Gray's (1997) guidelines. The authors used an AB case design to evaluate the estimated frequency of appropriate and inappropriate social interactions. The results showed no clear changes in behavior from baseline to the intervention condition. The study also had some methodological concerns which included no maintenance condition, using a preexperimental design, and no treatment fidelity data.

Scattone, Tingstrom, and Wilczynski (2006) conducted another analysis on the implementation of Social Stories™ to increase social interaction for three children diagnosed with autism. Appropriate social interaction was defined as (a) a verbal, physical, or gestural initiation or response to a peer, (b) a comment to the peer, (c) a question to the peer, (d) continued engagement in an activity, and/or (e) a physical gesture that could indicate disapproval or approval. Each participant received an individualized Social Story™. All Social Stories™ in this study followed Gray's (1998) guidelines. The authors used a multiple baseline design across participants, and the results showed no improvement for one participant and only minimal improvement for the other two participants. This study also had some methodological concerns including no maintenance condition, no specification of which behaviors improved, and starting intervention with one participant prior to behavior change for the other participant.

22.5.1.3 Other Social Behaviors

Researchers have also evaluated the implementation of Social Stories™ as a stand-alone procedure for increasing other specific social behaviors. Barry and Burlew (2004) taught two individuals diagnosed with autism how to appropriately play with peers. Appropriate play was defined as interacting with the materials and/or peers within a center in a way in which typically developing peers would interact with each other or the materials. The authors used a multiple baseline design that consisted of two legs. Each leg had multiple phases, which were (a) what was occurring already in the classroom (i.e., baseline), (b) the introduction of two Social Stories™ that focused on play and choice making, (c) the introduction of a Social Story™ on how to play appropriately, and (d) making the Social Stories™ available throughout the classroom. The researchers recorded the minutes of appropriate play, and the results of the study showed a positive increase. Despite the positive increase, there are serious methodological concerns which should be taken into consideration. These concerns include using a weak experimental design (i.e., a two-leg multiple baseline design) and no data on treatment fidelity.

In 2010, Okada, Ohtake, and Yanagihara evaluated the implementation of Social Stories™ on improving manners for one student diagnosed with ASD. The appropriate manners the authors targeted were elbow position and head position while eating meals. The authors used variations of Social Stories™ which included Social Stories™

with and without perspective sentences and the use of perspective sentences with a known or unknown person. The authors used an ABCDE design, and the results showed little change from the baseline condition across the other conditions.

22.5.1.4 Conclusions About Social Stories™ as a Stand-Alone Procedure

The aforementioned studies are a small representation of the literature in which Social Stories™ are evaluated as a solo intervention. Results of studies evaluating Social Stories™ as the only intervention have ranged from positive effects to no effects in changing behavior (Kokina & Kern, 2010). Additionally, many of the empirical studies have minor to serious methodological flaws which minimize the effectiveness of Social Stories™. The questionable effectiveness of Social Stories™ as a stand-alone procedure may be one of the reasons why Social Stories™ have been more frequently evaluated in conjunction with other procedures.

22.5.2 In Combination

22.5.2.1 Video Modeling

One of the more common procedures Social Stories™ are combined with is video modeling. Video modeling is an evidence-based procedure (see Chap. 14) which has been found to be effective in changing social behavior for numerous individuals diagnosed with ASD. In 2008, Scattone evaluated Social Stories™ combined with video modeling to improve three social behaviors for one child diagnosed with Asperger's syndrome. The three skills taught were appropriate eye contact, smiling, and initiating. Teaching started by the participant viewing a video that included the reading of a Social Story™ and two adults modeling the targeted social behavior. The results of the study showed that prior to intervention the participant rarely engaged in the targeted behaviors and during intervention the participant engaged in the targeted social behaviors in the majority of intervals. Thus, the study demonstrated that the combination of Social Stories™ and video modeling was effective.

Litras et al. (2010) also evaluated Social Stories™ combined with video modeling to increase three social behaviors for one individual diagnosed with autism. In this study, the authors taught the participant appropriate greetings, how to invite someone to play, and how to respond appropriately to a peer. The procedure consisted of two puppets reading a Social Story™ in a video followed by vignettes of the participant displaying the targeted behavior. The results of this study showed behavior increases in the targeted skills when intervention was implemented.

22.5.2.2 Prompts

Prompting is an effective way of increasing the likelihood that the participant is going to respond correctly (MacDuff, Krantz, & McClannahan, 2001). The implementation of Social Stories™ has been combined with prompts to improve the social behavior for individuals diagnosed with ASD. Crozier and Tincani (2007) evaluated the effects of Social Stories™ targeted to increase social behavior for three individuals diagnosed with ASD. Within this study, the authors evaluated Social Stories™ combined with verbal prompts to increase the frequency of talking to peers for one of the three participants. The study started with the implementation of a Social Story™ to increase talking to peers; however, when the Social Story™ alone did not increase talking to peers, the authors added vocal prompts to the Social Story™ condition. Using a reversal design, the authors clearly demonstrated that Social Stories™ plus vocal prompts increased the frequency of talking to peers for one participant.

22.5.2.3 Animal-Assisted Therapy

Using therapeutic dogs is an intervention that falls under the category of animal-assisted therapy, which has little to no empirical evidence to support its effectiveness (National Autism Center, 2009). Researchers have attempted to evaluate therapeutic dogs with the combination of Social Stories™ to assess the acquisition of social behaviors for individuals diagnosed with ASD (Grigore & Rusu, 2014). Grigore and Rusu (2014) evaluated the implementation of Social Stories™ combined with a therapy dog to increase appropriate social interaction and social initiation for three individuals diagnosed with ASD. The researchers used a Social Story™ following Gray's (2000) guidelines. During the condition in which the therapy dog was present, the researchers informed the participant that the dog was going to be in the room and then read the Social Story™ to the participant. The results showed that the participant engaged in higher rates of appropriate social behavior when the therapy dog was present. Although the results were positive, the authors moved between conditions prematurely (e.g., moving from the baseline condition to the intervention condition when the data was trending in the wrong direction).

22.5.2.4 Robot-Assisted Therapy

There has been a recent push to use robots as part of intervention as they may be less intimidating to individuals diagnosed with ASD (Diehl, Schmitt, Villano, & Crowell, 2012). As this has been a recommendation, researchers have begun to evaluate the use of robots implementing Social Stories™ (Vanderborght et al., 2012). Vanderborght and colleagues (2012) were one of the first to evaluate robots (i.e., Probo the robot) implementing Social Stories™ with four individuals diagnosed with ASD. The results of this study indicated that the participants made greater gains when the story was read by Probo the robot rather than when a human read the Social Story™. Pop et al. (2013) followed up on this study and utilized a group design to compare Social Stories™ implemented with a computer versus Social Stories™ implemented by a robot. Thirteen participants were included in the intervention groups (i.e., six individuals in the computer Social Story™ group and seven in the robot group). The main dependent variable was the level of prompting needed from a teacher for the participant to engage in the targeted social response. The results showed that the robot was superior to the computer. However, the study had a low number of participants for a group design and, therefore, had weak statistical power.

22.5.2.5 Intervention Packages

Comprehensive behavioral intervention usually includes multiple techniques implemented simultaneously within a teaching session. For example, during a given teaching session, a therapist might implement discrete trial teaching, shaping, and incidental teaching to improve behaviors for individuals diagnosed with ASD. As such, studies have evaluated the combination of various behavior analytic procedures for improving the lives of individuals diagnosed with ASD (e.g., Lovaas, 1987). Researchers have also evaluated Social Stories™ combined with multiple procedures.

Thiemann and Goldstein (2001) implemented Social Stories™, written text cues, and video feedback to improve the social communication for five individuals diagnosed with ASD. The authors followed Gray's (1995) guidelines on how to write a Social Story™. The intervention consisted of the authors reading the Social Story™ to the learner followed by comprehension questions. Next, the researcher presented a cue card to the participants. The cue card included textual and pictorial prompts, and the participants then practiced the target skill in the presence of the cue card. The researchers set up a 10 min social activity and provided prompts if the participants were not engaging in the targeted social behavior. Finally, following the social activity, the researchers provided video feedback based on the participant's social interactions during the social activity. Using a multiple baseline design across skills and replicated across participants, the results showed improvements from baseline levels.

22.5.2.6 Conclusions About Social Stories™ Combined with Other Procedures

The aforementioned studies are a small representation of the literature in which Social Stories™ are combined with other procedures. Studies that combine Social Stories™ with other procedures have shown more positive results than Social Stories™ implemented independently (see Leaf et al., 2015). This may lead to practitioners implementing Social Stories™ as part of a comprehensive intervention. Although studies have shown promising results, it is hard to determine if Social Stories™ were responsible for the behavior change, if the other procedures were responsible for the behavior change, or if the combination of procedures were responsible for the behavior change. Given that clinicians should implement the most parsimonious procedures possible (Etzel & LeBlanc, 1979), it would be advantageous for researchers to tease out which procedures are responsible for the behavior change (Cooper, Heron, & Heward, 2007).

22.5.3 Comparative Studies

Comparative studies allow clinicians and researchers to evaluate which procedures are more effective and efficient. Researchers have begun to compare Social Stories™ to other commonly implemented and empirically validated procedures (e.g., the teaching interaction procedure, video modeling, or cool versus not cool).

One of the first studies to compare Social Stories™ to another teaching procedure was done by Leaf et al. (2012). In this study, the authors compared Social Stories™ to a behaviorally based intervention known as the teaching interaction procedure (TIP; Phillips, 1968). This study included six participants diagnosed with ASD between the ages of 5 and 13 years. Each participant was taught six skills. Three skills were assigned to the Social Stories™ condition, and three skills were assigned to the TIP condition. A total of 18 skills were taught using Social Stories™, and 18 skills were taught using the TIP. In this study, the researchers used a basic Social Story™ (i.e., descriptive, directive, affirmative, and prescriptive sentence) written in book format, adhering to the recommended sentence ratio, and comprehension questions were administered after the story was read. The TIP consisted of seven steps: (1) labeling the target behavior, (2) providing a meaningful rationale of why displaying the target behavior is important, (3) describing cues for when the participant should display the behavior, (4) description of the skill in smaller components, (5) researcher demonstrating the target behavior, (6) student role-playing the behavior, and (7) the provision of feedback. The researchers used a token economy for correct responding, role-playing, and attending throughout both procedures.

The researchers measured skill acquisition through naturalistic probes, generalization probes with adults, and generalization probes with peers. Additionally, the researchers measured maintenance of the target behaviors after intervention. The results indicated that all six participants learned 100% of the skills assigned to the TIP condition but only learned 22.2% of the skills assigned to the Social Stories™ condition. The results also indicated participants displayed higher levels of generalization toward adults and peers for skills assigned to the TIP compared to skills assigned to Social Stories™. Finally, participants displayed higher levels of maintenance for skills assigned to the TIP condition compared to the Social Stories™ condition. Thus, the results of this study indicated that the TIP was more effective and efficient for teaching the target skills when compared to Social Stories™.

In 2014, Kassardjian and colleagues replicated and expanded the findings from Leaf et al. (2012), which compared Social Stories™ to the TIP. Kassardjian et al. (2014) compared a basic Social Story™ to the TIP to teach social behaviors for three children diagnosed with ASD, all who were 5 years of age. The two interventions (i.e., Social Stories™ and the TIP) were similar to the Leaf et al. (2012) procedures with the exception that both procedures were implemented in a group instructional format. Each participant was taught one skill with Social Stories™, one skill with the TIP, and one skill was assigned to a control condition where the researchers did not implement an intervention for that target behavior. In this study, the main dependent measure was participants displaying the target behaviors in a naturalistic probe with confederate peers. Additionally, the researchers measured each participant's correct responding during comprehension questions as part of the implementation of Social Stories™. In terms of displaying the target behaviors, the results indicated that participants reached the mastery criterion on the skill taught with the TIP. However, for the skill taught with

Social Stories™, all three participants did not show any improvements from baseline levels. Furthermore, all three participants demonstrated the control target behavior (i.e., the skill that received no intervention) more proficiently than the skill assigned to Social Stories™ during naturalistic probes. The results indicated that participants answered the majority of comprehension questions correctly in the Social Stories™ condition. Thus, showing that for these participants, Social Stories™ resulted in a failure of say-do correspondence (Rogers-Warren & Baer, 1976).

In 2015, Malmberg, Charlop, and Gershfeld conducted two experiments comparing Social Stories™ to other commonly implemented procedures (i.e., video modeling and prompting). In the first experiment, Social Stories™ were directly compared to video modeling to teach various social behaviors (e.g., sharing, social commenting, greetings, and turn taking) to four children diagnosed with ASD between the ages of 5 and 9 years old. Each participant was taught one target social behavior with Social Stories™ and one target behavior with video modeling. The Social Stories™ condition consisted of a basic Social Story™ format with comprehension questions, while the video modeling condition consisted of the participant watching a video of adults displaying the target social behavior. Using a multielement design, the researchers demonstrated that participants acquired skills taught with video modeling but showed little to no improvement for skills taught with Social Stories™. Thus, the results of the first experiment showed that video modeling was effective where as Social Stories™ were not.

In the second experiment, the researchers compared Social Stories™ to a time delay prompting procedure to teach various social behaviors (e.g., offering help, reciprocal comments, reciprocal questions, and empathy statements) for two children diagnosed with ASD (i.e., Malmberg, Charlop, & Gershfeld, 2015). In this experiment, the authors compared a basic Social Story™ with comprehension checks to a progressive time delay procedure. Each participant was taught two target social behaviors, one taught using progressive time delay and the second skill was taught using Social Stories™ and then followed by the progressive time delay procedure. Through the use of a multiple baseline design, the results indicated that the participants were able to demonstrate the first targeted skill following the implementation of the progressive time delay prompting procedure. For the second skill, the researchers demonstrated that participants did not improve responding with the implementation of the Social Story™ and only demonstrated the skill once the progressive time delay procedure was implemented. Thus, the results of this second experiment showed that the progressive time delay prompting procedure was more effective than Social Stories™.

In another study published in 2015, O'Handley, Radley, and Whipple compared Social Stories™ to video modeling to improve eye contact with six adolescents and adults diagnosed with ASD. The participants were divided into two groups. The researchers replicated Scattone's (2008) Social Stories™ procedure, which also included comprehension questions. The video modeling condition consisted of participants watching a video and answering comprehension questions. The researchers provided a rationale for displaying the targeted behavior in both teaching conditions. A multiple baseline design was used across all participants and groups. The order of conditions for the first group consisted of a baseline condition, followed by the Social Stories™ condition, and then Social Stories™ combined with video modeling condition. The order of conditions for the second group consisted of a baseline condition, followed by the video modeling condition, and then video modeling combined with Social Stories™ condition. The researchers measured eye contact during conversation with the primary researcher and had a generalization measure of eye contact during conversation with a novel communication partner. The results demonstrated that Social Stories™ implemented independently did not improve eye contact until Social Stories™ were combined with the video modeling procedure. The results also indicated that when video modeling was implemented independently, eye contact improved, and the addition of Social Stories™ with video modeling did not affect eye contact. Thus, the results of the study demonstrated that video modeling was more effective than Social Stories™ and that when the two interventions are combined, it is the video modeling procedure which is responsible for behavior change.

Social Stories™ have also been compared to the cool/not cool procedure (i.e., Leaf et al., 2016). Leaf et al. (2016) evaluated the two procedures with one high-functioning 7-year-old diagnosed with ASD. The researchers taught three skills using Social Stories™ and three skills using the cool/not cool procedure. These skills were measured through naturalistic probes (e.g., opportunities for the participant to respond to programmed events free from reinforcement or prompting) with an adult. The researcher used a Social Story™ that consisted of descriptive, perspective, affirmative, cooperative, control, and directive sentences. Comprehension questions and the provision of reinforcement were also used throughout the Social Stories™ condition. The cool/not cool procedure consisted of the researcher labeling the skill, the researcher modeling the target behavior correctly and incorrectly, the participant role-playing the behavior, and the provision of reinforcement. The researchers used an adapted alternating treatment design to compare the two teaching procedures. The participant reached the mastery criterion on all skills taught with the cool/not cool procedure. In the Social Stories™ condition, the participant displayed the targeted behaviors at levels similar to baseline. Thus, this study indicates that the cool/not cool procedure was more effective than Social Stories™ for this participant.

22.5.3.1 Conclusions About Social Stories™ Compared to Other Procedures

At the time of writing this chapter, Social Stories™ have been compared to the TIP, video modeling, prompting, and the cool/not cool procedure. The results across all of these studies have been fairly consistent demonstrating that Social Stories™ result in less improvement on social behaviors when compared to alternative procedures.

22.6 Reviews and Meta-Analysis

Professionals have also started to conduct reviews and meta-analyses on Social Stories™ (Kokina & Kern, 2010; Leaf et al., 2015; Sansosti, Powell-Smith, & Kincaid, 2004; Styles, 2011). Reviewers were specifically examining the methodological rigor implemented by different researchers and what effect the implementation of the Social Story™ had on changing behavior for the individuals diagnosed with ASD.

One of the earliest reviews on Social Stories™ was conducted by Sansosti et al. (2004). The authors reviewed eight studies that had evaluated Social Stories™. In this review, the authors described Social Stories™, the guidelines for Social Stories™, and the conceptual foundation of Social Stories™. The authors described eight studies that implemented Social Stories™. Based upon the review, the authors concluded, "Overall, the empirical foundation regarding the effectiveness of Social Stories is limited" (Sansosti et al., 2004, p. 200). Additionally, the authors stated, "…it may be premature based on the current literature, to suggest that Social Stories™ are an evidence-based approach when working with individuals with ASD" (Sansosti et al., 2004, p. 200). Based upon their review, the authors provided six recommendations for future researchers which included (1) more rigorous experimental control, (2) examining the components of Social Stories™, (3) evaluating treatment fidelity, (4) programming for both generalization and maintenance, (5) evaluating Social Stories™ for students who are mainstreamed into inclusive classrooms, and (6) comparing effects to typically developing children. Finally, the authors warned about implementing Social Stories™ as a stand-alone procedure.

In 2006, Ali and Frederickson reviewed 16 studies examining the effectiveness of Social Stories™ for individuals diagnosed with ASD. In the review, the authors evaluated the age of the participant, the experimental design used within the study, the dependent variable (i.e., targeted behavior), any special considerations within the study, and the reported results of the study. The authors noted that in the majority of studies evaluated, Social Stories™ were combined with other procedures, more rigorous control is needed, and more data should be taken on long-term maintenance and generalization of the learned skills. Despite these limitations, the authors concluded that Social Stories™ have promise, researchers should continue to evaluate the procedure, and Social Stories™ could be implemented with in clinical practice.

In 2010, Kokina and Kern reviewed 18 studies evaluating Social Stories™. Three of the studies evaluated by Kokina and Kern were doctoral dissertations (i.e., did not go through the peer-review process). In this meta-analysis, the authors reviewed characteristics of participants, the independent variables, the dependent variables, the research design, and other methodological characteristics (e.g., fidelity checks, social validity data, number of sessions) in each study. The main measure Kokina and Kern assessed was the percentage of nonoverlapping data (PND). PND is a method for determining effectiveness of an intervention by calculating the percentage of overlap between data taken prior to intervention (i.e., baseline) and data taken during intervention. Kokina and Kern found the mean PND score across studies evaluated to be 60% (range, 11–100%) indicating that the effectiveness of Social Stories™ falls into the low and questionable range of effectiveness.

In a more recent review, Leaf et al. (2015) reviewed 41 studies that used single-subject designs to evaluate the effectiveness of Social Stories™. Leaf and colleagues separated the studies evaluated into three categories based on the research design utilized: studies using an AB/case study design ($n = 9$), studies using a reversal design ($n = 13$), and studies using a multiple baseline design ($n = 19$). For each study, the authors evaluated a multitude of factors to determine the validity of the experimental design utilized. For example, in studies using a reversal design, the authors evaluated baseline levels for stability or data trends in the appropriate direction prior to the experimenters starting an intervention condition. After evaluation for factors influencing internal validity, the authors assigned studies to one of three categories: convincing, partially convincing, and no convincing evidence. The results of this analysis were that 7.3% of studies evaluated demonstrated convincing evidence, 41.5% demonstrated partially convincing evidence, and 51.2% demonstrated no convincing evidence that Social Stories™ were the cause of behavior change for participants. Therefore, Leaf and colleagues concluded, "… there is little empirical evidence to support that social stories are an effective procedure for children and adolescents with ASD" (p. 138). The authors further stated, "There appears to be little data to support the claim that social stories are a promising procedure" (p. 138).

The aforementioned articles were examples of reviews that have been published regarding Social Stories™. Across various reviews and meta-analyses on Social Stories™, there are several common limitations described by the reviewers. Some of these concerns are questionable effectiveness (Kokina & Kern, 2010), weak experimental control (Leaf et al., 2015), and Social Stories™ commonly being implemented along with other procedures (e.g., video modeling; Leaf et al., 2015).

There are several papers in which reviewers have provided recommendations for researchers to continue to evaluate Social Stories™ or for clinicians to continue to implement Social Stories™. For example, Ali and Frederickson (2006) noted that some Social Stories™ studies lacked experimental control and had weak treatment effects or confounding variables. However, Ali and Frederickson's overall recommendations were positive. Despite the previously mentioned limitations the authors stated, "We would suggest that the evidence base currently available indicates that the use of social stories with individual children who have ASD can be beneficial and that the use of the approach can be supported either alone, or in combination with other approaches…" (p. 373). In another example, Karkhaneh et al. (2010) reviewed six studies, all dissertations (i.e., non-peer-reviewed research), and stated, "Our findings support and highlight the effects of Social Stories™ for short term improvements of the social deficits among school-aged autistic children" (p. 658). Finally, Rhodes (2014) also noticed limitations with Social Stories™ but concluded, "…it would appear that Social Stories are a useful instrument, which causes no harm or stigma to the participant and is accepted by teachers and parents…" (p. 47).

There are also several examples where reviewers cautioned against the implementation of Social Stories™ (Leaf et al., 2015; Styles 2011; Reynhout & Carter, 2011). For example, Styles (2011) found limitations within research on Social Stories™ and stated, "There is also limitation of the effectiveness of Social Stories™ among their originally targeted population of individuals with HFA [High Functioning Autism] or AS [Asperger's Syndrome]…" (p. 425). This resulted in Styles stating that the limitations in Social Stories™ research would need to be addressed before Social Stories™ can be considered evidence based. Reynhout and Carter (2011) also found limitations in the research on Social Stories™ stating, "… given the limited potential for improvements, in many cases time may be better invested in more intensive interventions that are likely to yield more substantial gains" (p. 897). Leaf et al. (2015) were the most critical of the clinical implementation and research of Social Stories™. Leaf et al. stated, "Although social stories is an easy procedure to implement, at this point, clinicians should apply other empirically supported procedures (e.g., video modeling, script fading, behavioral skills training, the teaching interaction procedure) when trying to teach pro-social behavior or decrease aberrant behavior for children and adolescents diagnosed with autism" (p. 139). Table 22.4 summarizes the findings of each of the reviews on Social Stories™.

22.7 Future Directions and Conclusions

Social Stories™ are a commonly implemented procedure for individuals diagnosed with ASD and have been well evaluated in empirical research. Professionals have also proclaimed that Social Stories™ are evidence based and meet the standards to be an evidence-based practice (National Autism Center, 2009, 2015). Yet, there have been several professionals who have questioned the evidence behind Social Stories™ effectiveness (Leaf et al., 2015; Styles, 2011) and studies which have shown Social Stories™ to be less effective when compared to other commonly implemented procedures (Leaf et al., 2012; Kassardjian et al., 2014). Therefore, there are many questions about how researchers and practitioners should proceed.

Although there are numerous studies which have evaluated Social Stories™, more research is warranted. First and foremost, researchers need to ensure better experimental control in all future studies. This would include ensuring that the dependent variable is well defined, interobserver agreement data are collected, researchers measure treatment fidelity, researchers utilize stronger single-subject designs (e.g., multiple baseline designs, reversal designs, changing criterion designs), and these research designs are implemented appropriately. One of the major flaws within the body of research on Social Stories™ has been the lack of experimental rigor (Leaf et al., 2015). Ensuring that studies have strong internal validity will help professionals conclude the true effectiveness of Social Stories™. One goal of research should be to find the most effective and efficient procedures possible; therefore, more comparative studies should be conducted with a variety of procedures and with more individuals diagnosed with ASD. By conducting comparative studies, researchers may be able to discover which procedures are more effective and/or the conditions under which a procedure is more effective. Third, researchers should conduct component analyses when Social Stories™ are implemented with other procedures. Information found from a component analysis would allow consumers to know which part of the intervention is responsible for the behavior change. Fourth, researchers should evaluate all current recommendations and guidelines for Social Stories™ to determine if the recommended guidelines are pertinent to how Social Stories™ are written and implemented. Finally, there have been a limited number of group designs which have evaluated Social Stories™ compared to a no treatment

Table 22.4 Findings from reviews and meta-analysis on Social Stories™.

Publication	Number of studies evaluated	General findings (summarized by author of this chapter)
Ali & Frederickson, 2006	16	Limitations found in the research but Social Stories™ can be beneficial
Kokina& Kern, 2010	18*	Social Stories™ have low to questionable effectiveness with a percentage of nonoverlapping data (PND) score of 60
Leaf et al., 2015	41	Major limitations in the correct use of experimental design. Social Stories™ are not empirically based
Karkhaneh et al., 2010	6*	Has effective short-term improvements in social behavior
Mayton, Menendez, Wheeler, Carter, & Chitiyo, 2013	37	Findings indicated that on or above standard acceptability of evidence-based practice indicators
Reynhout & Carter, 2006	16*	Highly variable data but with a PND score of 43 indicating an ineffective procedure
Reynhout & Carter, 2011	62*	Social Stories™ are only mildly effective with PND scores of 56 for published articles and PND scores of 45 for dissertations. Time would be better spent on more intensive intervention
Rhodes, 2014	7	Social Stories™ are a useful instrument
Rust & Smith, 2006	8	Serious methodological concerns which minimize the overall effectiveness of Social Stories™
Sansosti et al., 2004	8	The overall empirical findings on Social Stories™ are limited
Styles 2011	51	Weakness in the literature precludes Social Stories™ from being considered evidence-based practices
Test, Richter, Knight, & Spooner, 2011	28	Numerous studies lacked strong methodological control causing Social Stories™ to not be considered evidence based at the current time of the review

*Denotes the inclusion of dissertations in the review or meta-analysis.

condition (i.e., a control condition) or another procedure (e.g., TIP). Group designs are important for determining the most efficacious procedures and allow for better external validity due to the larger number of participants (Campbell & Stanley, 1963); therefore, researchers should evaluate Social Stories™ utilizing these designs.

Future directions on the implementation of Social Stories™ for clinicians are a little less clear. While some professionals recommend Social Stories™ (e.g., Ali & Frederickson, 2006), others recommend exercising caution when implementing Social Stories™ (e.g., Reynhout & Carter, 2011), and others recommend against the implementation of Social Stories™ for individuals diagnosed with ASD (e.g., Leaf et al., 2015). We recommend that clinicians and parents working with individuals diagnosed with autism adhere to the following: (1) implement procedures that have been published in peer-reviewed journals, (2) carefully evaluate studies to ensure that they have a substantial amount of methodological rigor (e.g., the research design was implemented correctly) in order to determine if the behavior change was due to the implementation of the teaching procedure, (3) implement procedures which have been demonstrated to be effective, and (4) when faced with a choice between different evidence-based procedures, implement the most effective and efficient procedure possible.

References

Adams, L., Gouvousis, A., VanLue, M., & Waldron, C. (2004). Social story intervention: Improving communication skills in a child with an autism spectrum disorder. *Focus on Autism and Other Developmental Disabilities*, *19*, 87–94.

Ali, S., & Fredericskon, N. (2006). Investigating the evidence base of Social Stories. *Educational Psychology in Practice*, *22*, 355–377.

Bailey, J. S., & Burch, M. R. (2002). *Research methods in applied behavior analysis*. Thousand Oaks, California: Sage Publications.

Baron-Cohen, S. (2001). Theory of mind in normal development and autism. *Prisme*, *34*, 174–183.

Barry, L. M., & Burlew, S. B. (2004). Using social stories to teach choice and play skills to children with autism. *Focus on Autism and Other Develeopmental Disabilities*, *19*, 45–51.

Brownell, M. D. (2002). Musically adapted social stories to modify behaviours in students with autism: Four case studies. *Journal of Music Therapy, 39*, 117–144.

Campbell, D. T., & Stanley, J. C. (1963). *Experimental and quasi-experimental designs for research*. Boston, MA: Houghton Mifflin Company.

Charlop-Christy, M. H., Le, L., & Freeman, K. A. (2000). A comparison of video modeling for teaching children with autism. *Journal of Autism and Developmental Disorders*, *30*, 537–552.

Cooper, J. O., Heron, T. E., & Heward, W. L. (2007). *Applied behavior analysis* (2nd ed.). Upper Saddle River, NJ: Pearson.

Crozier, S., & Tincani, M. J. (2007). Effects of social stories on prosocial behavior of preschool children with autism spectrum disorders. *Journal of Autism and Developmental Disorders*, *37*, 1803–1814.

Delano, M., & Snell, M. E. (2006). The effects of social stories on the social engagement of children with autism. *Journal of Positive Behavior Interventions*, *8*, 29–42.

Diehl, J. J., Schmitt, L. M., Villano, M., & Crowell, C. R. (2012). The clinical use of robots for individuals with autism spectrum disorders: A critical review. *Research in Autism Spectrum Disorders*, *6*, 249–262.

Etzel, B. C., & LeBlanc, J. M. (1979). The simplest treatment alternative: The law of parsimony applied to choosing appropriate instructional control and errorless-learning procedures for the difficult-to-teach child. *Journal of Autism and Developmental Disorders*, *9*(4), 361–382. http://doi.org/10.1007/BF01531445

Gray, C. A., & Garand, J. D. (1993). Social stories: Improving responses of students with autism with accurate social information. *Focus on Autistic Behavior*, *8*, 1–10.

Gray, C. (1994). *Social stories*. Arlington, TX: Future Horizons.

Gray, C. A. (1995). *Social stories unlimited: Social stories and comic strip conversations*. Jenison, MI: Jenison Public Schools.

Gray, C. A. (1997). *Social stories and comic strip conversations: Teaching social understanding to students with autism spectrum disorder*. Paper presented at Building Bridges for a Better Tomorrow: 6th Annual Conference on Autism, Corpus Christi, TX.

Gray, C. (1998). Social Stories and comic strip conversations with students with Asperger syndrome and high-functioning autism. In E. Schopler, G. B. Mesibov, & L. J. Kunce (Eds.), *Asperger syndrome or high functioning autism?* (pp. 167–198). New York, NY: Plenum.

Gray, C. (2000). *The new Social Story™ book* (Illustrated ed.). Arlington, TX: Future Horizons.

Gray, C. (2004). Social Stories 10.0: The new defining criteria and guidelines. *Jenison Autism Journal*, *15*, 2–21.

Gray, C. (2010). *The new Social Story book: Revised and expanded* (10th anniversary ed.). Arlington, Texas: Future Horizons INC..

Gray, C. (2012). Carol Gray on Social Stories – An introduction and implications for the future. In N. C. Grove (Ed.), *Using storytelling to support children and adults with special needs*. London: Routledge.

Grigore, A. A., & Rusu, A. S. (2014). Interaction with a therapy dog enhances the effects of Social Story method in autistic children. *Society and Animals*, *22*, 241–261.

Hanley-Hocdorfer, K., Bray, M. A., Kehle, T. J., & Elinoff, M. J. (2010). Social stories to increase verbal initiation in children with autism and asperger's disorder. *School Psychology Review*, *39*, 484–492.

Hagiwara, T., & Myles, B. S. (1999). A multimedia Social Story intervention: Teaching skills to children with autism. *Focus on Autism and Other Developmental Disabilities*, *14*, 82–95.

Kalyva, E., & Agaliotis, I. (2009). Can Social Stories enhance the interpersonal conflict resolution skills of children with LD? *Research in Developmental Disabilities*, *30*, 192–202.

Karkhaneh, M., Clark, B., Ospina, M. B., Seida, J. C., Smith, V., & Hartling, L. (2010). Social Stories™ to improve social skills in children with autism spectrum disorder. *Autism*, *14*, 641–662.

Kassardjian, A., Leaf, J. B., Ravid, D., Leaf, J. A, Alcalay, A., Dale, S., …., Oppehneim-Leaf, M. L. (2014). Comparing the teaching interaction procedure to social stories: A replication study. Journal of Autism and Developmental Disorders, 44, 2329-2240.

Kokina, A., & Kern, L. (2010). Social story TM interventions for students with autism spectrum disorders: A meta-analysis. *Journal of Autism and Developmental Disorders*, *40*, 812–826.

Krantz, P. J., & McClannahan, L. E. (1993). Teaching children with autism to initiate to peers: Effects of a script-fading procedure. *Journal of Applied Behavior Analysis*, *26*, 121–132.

Leaf, J. B., Dotson, W. H., Oppeneheim, M. L., Sheldon, J. B., & Sherman, J. A. (2010). The effectiveness of a group teaching interaction procedure for teaching social skills to young children with a pervasive developmental disorder. *Research in Autism Spectrum Disorders*, *4*(2), 186–198.

Leaf, J. B., Oppenheim-Leaf, M. L., Call, N. A., Sheldon, J. B., Sherman, J. A., Taubman, M., … Leaf, R. (2012). Comparing the teaching interaction procedure to social stories for people with autism. *Journal of Applied Behavior Analysis*, *45*, 281–298.

Leaf, J. B., Oppenheim-Leaf, M. L., Leaf, R. B., Taubman, M., McEachin, J., Parker, T., … Mountjoy, T. (2015). What is the proof? A methodological review of studies that have utilized social stories. *Education and Training in Autism and Developmental Disabilities*, *50*, 127–141.

Leaf, J. B., Mitchell, E., Townley-Cochran, D., McEachin, J., Taubman, M., & Leaf, R. (2016). Comparing Social Stories™ to cool versus not cool. *Education and Treatment of Children*, *39*, 173–186.

Litras, S., Moore, D. W., & Anderson, A. (2010). Using video self-modelled Social Stories to teach social skills to a young child with autism. *Autism Research and Treatment*, *2010*, 1–9.

Lovaas, I. O. (1987). Behavioral treatment and normal educational and intellectual functioning in young autistic children. *Journal of Consulting and Clinical Psychology*, *55*, 3–9.

Lorimer, P. A., Simpson, R. L., Myles, B. S., & Ganz, J. B. (2002). The use of social stories as preventative behavioral intervention in a home setting with a child with autism. *Journal of Positive Behavior Interventions*, *4*, 53–60.

MacDuff, G. S., Krantz, P. J., & McClannahan, L. E. (2001). Prompts and prompt-fading strategies for people with autism. In C. Maurice, G. Green, & R. M. Foxx (Eds.), *Making a difference behavioral intervention for autism* (1st ed.pp. 37–50). Austin, TX: Pro Ed.

Malmberg, D., Charlop, M. H., & Gershfeld, S. J. (2015). A two experiment treatment comparison study: Teaching social skills to children with autism spectrum disorder. *Journal of Developmental and Physical Disabilities*, *27*, 375–392.

Mayton, M. R., Menendez, A. L., Wheeler, J. J., Carter, S. L., & Chitiyo, M. (2013). An analysis of Social Stories™ research using an evidence-based practice model. *Journal of Research in Special Educational Needs*, *13*, 208–217.

National Autism Center. (2009). *National standards project: findings and conclusions*. Randolph, MA: Author.

National Autism Center. (2015). *Findings and conclusions: National standards project phase 2*. Randolph, MA: Author.

Norris, C., & Dattilo, J. (1999). Evaluating effects of a social story intervention on a young girl with autism. *Focus on Autism and Other Developmental Disabilities*, *14*, 180–186.

O'Handley, R. D., Radley, K. C., & Whipple, H. M. (2015). The relative effects of social stories and video modeling toward increasing eye contract of adolescents with autism spectrum disorder. *Research in Autism Spectrum Disorders*, *11*, 101–111.

Okada, S., Ohtake, Y., & Yanagihara, M. (2010). Improving the manners of a student with autism: The effects of manipulating perspective holders in social stories™ – A pilot study. *International Journal of Disability, Development and Education*, *57*, 207–219.

Ozonoff, S. (1998). Assessment and remediation of executive dysfunction in autism and Asperger syndrome. In E. Schopler, G. B. Mesibove, & L. J. Kunce (Eds.), *Asperger syndrome or high-functioning autism?* New York, Plenum Press.

Phillips, E. L. (1968). Achievement place: Token reinforcement procedures in a home-style rehabilitation setting for "pre-delinquent" boys. *Journal of Applied Behavior Analysis*, *1*(3), 213–223.

Pop, C. A., Simut, R. E., Pineta, S., Saldien, J., Rusu, A. S., Vanderfaeillie, J., … Vanderborght, B. (2013). Social robots vs computer display: Does the way social stories are delivered make a difference for their effectiveness on ASD children? *Journal of Educational Computing Research*, *49*, 381–401.

Quirmbach, L. M., Lincoln, A. J., Feinberg-Gizzo, M. J., Ingersoll, B. R., & Andrews, S. M. (2009). Social Stories: Mechanisms of effectiveness in increasing game play skills in children diagnosed with autism spectrum disorder using a pretest posttest repeated measures of randomized control group design. *Journal of Autism and Developmental Disorders*, *39*, 299–321.

Reichow, B., & Sabornie, E. J. (2009). Brief report: Increasing verbal greeting initiations for a student with autism via a Social Story™ intervention. *Journal of Autism and Developmental Disorders*, *39*(12), 1740–1743.

Reynhout, G., & Carter, M. (2006). Social Stories™ for children with disabilities. *Journal of Autism and Developmental Disorders*, *40*, 149–166.

Reynhout, G., & Carter, M. (2009). The use of social stories by teachers and their perceived efficacy. *Research in Autism Spectrum Disorders*, *3*(1), 232–251.

Reynhout, G., & Carter, M. (2011). Evaluation of the efficacy of Social Stories™ using three single subject metrics. *Research in Autism Spectrum Disorders*, *36*, 445–469.

Rhodes, C. (2014). Do Social Stories help to decrease disruptive behaviour in children with autistic spectrum disorders? A review of the published literature. *Journal of Intellectual Disabilities*, *18*, 35–50.

Rogers-Warren, A., & Baer, D. M. (1976). Correspondence between saying and doing: Teaching children to share and praise. *Journal of Applied Behavior Analysis*, *9*(3), 335–354.

Rust, J., & Smith, A. (2006). How should the effectiveness of Social Stories to modify the behaviour of children on the autistic spectrum be tested? *Autism*, *10*, 125–138.

Sansosti, F. J., Powell-Smith, K. A., & Kincaid, D. (2004). A research synthesis of social story interventions for children with autism spectrum disorders. *Focus on Autism and Other Developmental Disabilities, 19*, 194–204.

Scattone, D., Tingstrom, D. H., & Wilczynski, S. M. (2006). Increasing appropriate social interactions of children with autism spectrum disorders using social stories™. *Focus on Autism and Other Developmental Disabilities, 21*, 211–222.

Scattone, D. (2008). Enhancing the conversation skills of a boy with asperger's disorder through social stories™ and video modeling. *Journal of Autism and Developmental Disorders, 38*, 395–400.

Soenksen, D., & Alper, S. (2006). Teaching a young child to appropriately gain attention of peers using a Social Story intervention. *Focus on Autism and Other Developmental Disabilities, 21*, 36–44.

Styles, A. (2011). Social Stories™: Does the research evidence support the popularity? *Educational Psychology in Practice, 27*, 415–436.

Swaggart, B. L., Gagnon, E., Bock, S. J., Earles, T. L., Quinn, C., Smith Myles, B., & Simpson, R. L. (1995). Using social stories to teach social and behavioral skills to children with autism. *Focus on Autism and Other Developmental Disabilities, 10*(1), 1–16.

Thiemann, K. S., & Goldstein, H. (2001). Social stories, written text cues, and video feedback: Effects on social communication of children with autism. *Journal of Applied Behavior Analysis, 34*, 425–446.

Test, D. W., Richter, S., Knight, V., & Spooner, F. (2011). A comprehensive review and meta-analysis of the Social Stories literature. *Focus on Autism and Other Developmental Disabilities, 26*, 49–62.

Vanderbroght, B., Simut, R., Saldien, J., Pop, C., Rusu, A. S., Pintea, S., … David, D. O. (2012). Using the social robot probo as a social story telling agent for children with ASD. *Interaction Studies, 13*, 348–372.

Wolfberg, P. (1995). Enhancing children's play. In K. A. Quill (Ed.), *Teaching children with autism: Strategies to enhance communication and vocalization*. Albany, NY: Delmar.

Emerging Social Skills Interventions for Individuals with Autism

23

Andrea Trubanova Wieckowski and Susan W. White

In addition to the evidence-based interventions discussed in this book, there are several interventions developed to improve social competence for individuals with autism spectrum disorder (ASD) that show promise. While the interventions we discuss in this chapter have one or more studies suggesting clinical benefit for individuals with ASD, by definition they are not well-established at this time, often because the research base lacks methodological rigor (e.g., large-scale controlled trials) and/or because the extant research is still fairly new. Further exploration of these emerging interventions, however, is crucial in order to gather evidence regarding effective interventions for individuals with ASD. In this chapter, we describe some of the emerging interventions targeting social skills for individuals with ASD, review the existing research on the use of the interventions, and highlight the clinical implications for these techniques.

As emphasized throughout this book, many evidence-based interventions have already been identified that target social skills in individuals with ASD. These interventions have established support for being beneficial in improving social skills for this population. Why is it therefore necessary to create and evaluate new interventions? While the evidence-based treatments have been shown to benefit children, adolescents, and adults with ASD, not every treatment significantly improves social skills for every individual. ASD is a heterogeneous condition, and every individual has different needs and learning styles. For example, while some individuals benefit from group social skills settings, others may find it difficult to participate or even attend such groups. This is especially a concern given the high comorbidity of conditions seen with this population. For an individual who is unable to leave the house or participate in existing interventions, other types of therapies (e.g., utilizing technology) might be beneficial. It is therefore necessary to create and evaluate these emerging interventions to provide interventions to those individuals for whom the current best practice treatments are not effective.

There are several published meta-analyses on social skills interventions for individuals with ASD (e.g., Bellini, Peters, Benner, & Hopf, 2007; Reichow & Volkmar, 2010; Wang, Parrila, & Cui, 2013), and even a National Professional Development Center (NPDC) dedicated to promoting the use of evidence-based practices with individuals with ASD. However, most of these reviews focus on evidence-based treatments only, and, therefore, the reviews on emerging interventions have

A.T. Wieckowski • S.W. White (✉)
Virginia Tech, Department of Psychology, Blacksburg, VA, USA
e-mail: sww@vt.edu

J.B. Leaf (ed.), *Handbook of Social Skills and Autism Spectrum Disorder*, Autism and Child Psychopathology Series, DOI 10.1007/978-3-319-62995-7_23

been left largely unexplored. A notable exception is the National Standards Project (NSP), an initiative of the National Autism Center in providing information regarding evidence-based guidelines and effective interventions for individuals with ASD. The main focus of NSP is to evaluate interventions for individuals with ASD, resulting in the categorization of interventions into established treatments, emerging treatments, and unestablished treatments. The reviewed treatments include any intervention for individuals with ASD including, but not limited to, interventions targeting social skills. In addition, the prior literature reviewing these interventions has not addressed the clinical implications of their use. Therefore, in this chapter, we expand on existing literature by providing full descriptions of the emerging interventions for targeting social skills in individuals with ASD, providing research highlighting the potential benefits of the intervention and the remaining aspects that need further exploration, and addressing the clinical implications for use of these emerging interventions.

When discussing emerging interventions, it is important to distinguish whether the discussed intervention is a specific program (i.e., a protocol) versus a broader technique or method used across different programs. In this chapter, we will describe the emerging interventions in terms of broader techniques used to improve social skills and highlight a few examples of specific programs within each broad categorization. The techniques and specific programs discussed in this chapter however are not exhaustive, as there are hundreds of interventions that show some support behind them. Instead, only selected examples are provided to give the reader an idea of how the technique can be implemented. The focus is on the research behind the technique (not a specific protocol), as the technique can be implemented in variety of ways. Given that there are many published studies exploring potential social skills interventions for individuals with ASD, in this chapter, we discuss intervention techniques that have sufficient support for their use and therefore would benefit from further exploration.

To provide an organizational heuristic, we review the research for each of the categories of social intervention across three main domains: (1) proximal vs. distal target of intervention, (2) taught vs. generalized skill, and (3) in-house vs. external evaluation. These categories provide basic information with which to make comparisons across a diverse set of intervention categories with respect to the development and maturity of the research base. While these categories are useful in this regard, they are not sufficient to make comparisons of relative efficacy. We focus on these domains in order to be able to make comparisons across diverse intervention approaches. Doing so permits a more nuanced perspective on the relative promise or efficacy of each approach, as they are at different stages of development and target separate, though related, processes related to social function. Proximal versus distal target refers to the question of whether the intervention targets the specific social skill or behavioral deficiency directly or indirectly. As highlighted by Yoder, Bottema-Beutel, Woynaroksi, Chandrasekhar, and Sandbank (2014), treatment effectiveness varies greatly depending on whether the skill is directly targeted or not, with much greater treatment effectiveness found for interventions targeting social communication directly (proximal outcome) compared to indirectly (distal outcome). Mechanism-focused interventions that evaluate proximal outcomes are important in order to understand the process, or drive, that leads to the change (cf, Lerner, White, & McPartland, 2012). However, as Yoder and colleagues note, to be able to conclude that treatment impacted the penultimate behavioral target (e.g., social skill), researchers should show change in behavior beyond the proximal target (e.g., facial recognition). Therefore, both proximal (mechanism-focused) and distal (outcome) interventions are necessary.

The second category, taught versus generalized skill, refers to the breadth of impact. In other words, is there change observed only in a discrete or tightly parameterized behavior (e.g., eye contact) or is change broader, extending beyond explicitly taught behaviors (e.g., initiations, social responsiveness, play)? This domain is related to the question of proximity, but highlights the task used to evaluate the treatment effectiveness and showing of the skills beyond the specific task. The importance of generalization in clinical intervention has been highlighted by multiple researchers throughout the years (e.g., Stokes & Baer, 1977). Many argue that generalization should not be treated as a passive phenomenon, such that one assumes generalization will occur organically; rather, researchers must actively promote generalization of the skills taught. Generalization is important when discussing treatment effectiveness as the aim of the intervention is to help individuals with ASD in everyday interactions, not just during treatment in a specific setting.

The third domain, in-house versus external evaluation, highlights the question of whether the approach or specific program has been evaluated by only one research team, usually the group that developed the approach, or whether the same program has been evaluated externally by another research team. This third domain has long been upheld as a variable in determining the rigor of evidence for the efficacy of treatment approaches. For instance, it is one of the criteria for empirically validated treatments put forth by Division 12 Task Force on Promotion and Dissemination of Psychological Procedures (Chambless et al., 1998). This criterion is important to avoid research bias as outcomes of certain therapies might or might not be reported based on self-serving interest of the researchers.

Of note, these three domains highlight only a few of the many parameters that need to be explored when establishing efficacy of an intervention. For this review, we focus on the general description of the intervention and the research behind the intervention type and, therefore, focus on three domains that are often noted as lacking in prior studies and reviews. The importance of exploration of mechanism-driven versus distal outcome interventions, generalizability, and replicability of studies has been established. While not exhaustive, all together, these three domains allow for an initial investigation of the research support behind the emerging interventions for social skills for individuals with ASD and in identifying gaps that need to be further explored.

23.1 Technology-Based Interventions

Technology-based interventions present instructional materials using the medium of technology, broadly defined as any tool, device, or procedure using electronics. There has been a recent increase in use of technology as an intervention tool, due to provision of speed, convenience, and accessibility. As highlighted in the meta-analysis by Grynszpan, Weiss, Perez-Diaz, and Gal (2014), several advantages of technology-based interventions for ASD have been identified, including consistency of a clearly defined task (Murray, 1997) and freedom from social demands that are often challenging for individuals with ASD (Moore, McGrath, & Thorpe, 2000; Murray, 1997). As highlighted by Grynszpan and colleagues, while technology-based interventions have been utilized for many years, they are still categorized as "emerging" (e.g., Wilczynski et al., 2009), as much of the published research focuses on the potential of its use (e.g., feasibility, acceptability) rather than assessment of treatment efficacy.

While all technology-based interventions utilize technology to deliver the treatment, it is important to emphasize the wide variety of interventions within this domain. Technology-based interventions include those run on computers, interventions run on mobile-based or handheld electronics that use wireless computing (e.g., phones, tablets), interventions utilizing virtual reality or computer-simulated reality which replicate an environment that can be interacted with, and interventions utilizing humanoid robots that directly interact with the participant. The technology-based interventions therefore span a wide variety of treatments that differ substantially. Distinguishing the type of technology-based intervention within this domain is therefore important in evaluating the evidence for the treatment's effectiveness. Among the different types of technology, computer-based training programs have attracted the most attention (Bölte, 2004), and, therefore, this section focuses on computer-based interventions.

Examples of technology-based interventions include *Let's Face It!* program (Tanaka et al., 2010), *Junior Detective Training Program*

(Beaumont & Sofronoff, 2008), and *Mind Reading: The Interactive Guide to Emotions* (Baron-Cohen, Golan, Wheelwright, & Hill, 2004). *Let's Face It!* program is a computer-based intervention comprised of interactive computer games targeting inattention to the eyes, impaired recognition of identity, and failure to perceive faces holistically, all aspects of social skills that have been found to be impaired with individuals with ASD. Specifically, the games reinforce attending to faces, recognition of facial identity and expression, and interpretation of facial cues in a social context through seven interactive computer games. Tanaka and colleagues evaluated the program and found that relative to the control group, children who completed the *Let's Face It!* program showed improvements in the recognition of mouth features and holistic recognition of a face.

Junior Detective Training Program (*JDTP*) is comprised of a group social skills training, parent training, teacher handouts, and a computer game. Therefore, as opposed to the *Let's Face It!* program, the technology is only one component as opposed to the entire intervention. The computer game aspect of the program focused on emotion recognition, emotion regulation, and social interaction skills. In the game, the user is a detective who specializes in decoding other's mental states. The computer system utilizes both human- and computer-animated characters to teach emotion recognition and social problem-solving. The game is tailored and individualized based on how the user progresses through the program. Results from the randomized controlled trial suggest that children who received the treatment significantly improved on their knowledge of emotion coping strategies, emotion recognition skills, as well as social skills as measured by parent report (Beaumont & Sofronoff, 2008). However, the study did not measure generalization of social skills to real-life social contexts.

Mind Reading: The Interactive Guide to Emotions is an interactive computer-based program developed to teach individuals with ASD about emotions and mental states. The program uses video, audio, and written text to teach emotions. Users are able to explore emotions through an interactive library, complete lessons and quizzes, and play games about emotions. Studies found that individuals who completed the intervention improved significantly on identifying emotions from faces and voices (Golan & Baron-Cohen, 2006). However, results found no difference between groups on a generalization task that used face and voice stimuli that were not included in the program.

Together, research across the technology-based interventions provides evidence for the usefulness of the interventions to address social skill deficits for individuals with ASD. The studies have found technology-based interventions to be feasible in changing targeted mechanisms and acceptable for individuals with ASD to use. Findings suggest that some studies have addressed mechanism-driven outcome (e.g., inattention to the eyes in the *Let's Face It!* program), but many technology-based studies have also evaluated more distal outcomes (e.g., emotion recognition). In terms of generalizability, the majority of the studies have not evaluated whether the skills generalize outside of the stimuli presented in the programs. Those that have attempted to explore generalization (e.g., *Mind Reading: The Interactive Guide to Emotions*) found that the results do not generalize to stimuli not presented in the program. Therefore, future research in the domain of technology-based interventions needs to address the lack of generalizability of the social skills taught. Lastly, across the interventions explored in this section, nearly all of the research has been conducted by the groups that developed the specific intervention. Replication studies need to be conducted outside of the parent lab in order to provide further evidence for the intervention's utility in augmenting social skills for individuals with ASD. Even though further evaluation needs to occur to address the gaps in generalization and the dearth of replication studies, the current state of research shows promise of utilizing technology-based interventions to increase social skills (e.g., emotion recognition) for individuals with ASD.

23.2 Cognitive-Behavioral Interventions

Cognitive-behavioral therapy (CBT) is an established treatment for many disorders, such as anxiety disorders (e.g., Hofmann & Smits, 2008; Olatunji, Cisler, & Deacon, 2010) and major depression (e.g., Hofmann, Asnaani, Vonk, Sawyer, & Fang, 2012). CBT-based approaches for a range of clinical problems have also been extended to youth with ASD, with considerable clinical promise (see Scarpa, White, & Attwood, 2013). In the context of social skill programs, interventions in this category share a dual focus on altering how the client acts and how she/he thinks or processes situations. Cognitive-behavioral interventions for socialization target both social skills, or behaviors, and the cognitive processes involved in social interaction, such as inferring others' unspoken intentions and anticipating the likely consequences of one's behaviors. Within this group of interventions, there is tremendous variability in the specific foci of protocols. For instance, some might focus primarily on cognitive skills such as perspective-taking or nonverbal emotion detection/interpretation and secondarily teach strategies for managing social situations.

The Secret Agent Society (*SAS*) is a cognitive-behavioral program that targets social-emotion skill development in children, ages 8–12, with ASD (Beaumont & Sofronoff, 2013). It is multi-component, in that the program employs an interactive computer game, weekly small-group meetings, parent sessions, and teacher training in the form of written "tip" sheets. The research to date on SAS suggests the program is helpful. A randomized controlled trial (RCT) in which SAS was compared to a wait list reported significant gains in both social skills and emotion regulation, and these gains were largely maintained 5 months following treatment (Beaumont & Sofronoff, 2008). The authors reported no significant gains in expression recognition, contrary to what was expected, given that recognition of emotion using facial expression and body posture was explicitly targeted in the intervention.

Lopata, Thomeer, Volker, and Lee (2013) developed a cognitive-behavioral social skills curriculum that is implemented in the context of a summer treatment program for higher functioning children with ASD. The program is delivered over the course of 5 weeks, 5 days per week, in a group format. The curriculum adapted *Skillstreaming* (McGinnis & Goldstein, 1997), a structured social skills training program to directly target multiple areas of social difficulty commonly seen in ASD, such as emotion recognition impairment (face-emotion recognition instruction), pragmatic communication (training in understanding nonliteral language), and skill generalization (parent training). Training is delivered in 20-min cycles throughout the day via the established stepwise procedure (e.g., define skill, model skill, role-play the skill). The summer treatment program also includes activities to promote social interaction and cooperative play among the youth. Four studies thus far have been published on the impact of this summer program, including a case study (Toomey, Lopata, Volker, & Thomeer, 2009) and three RCTs. Two of these RCTs did not include a no-treatment comparison group; rather, the comparator was the test intervention augmented with a response-cost behavior management system (Lopata, Thomeer, Volker, & Nida, 2006; Lopata, Thomeer, Volker, Nida, & Lee, 2008). The third RCT randomized the 36 participants to either the summer treatment program or wait-list control group, and results demonstrated significant improvement for the treatment group on most of the parent report and direct child-assessed outcome measures (Lopata et al., 2010). Collectively, this body of work suggests that the comprehensive, summer treatment program results in improved adaptability and social skills.

In addition, the *Cool* versus *Not Cool* procedure (Taubman, Leaf, & McEachin, 2011) similarly targets individuals' cognitions and behaviors. The *Cool* versus *Not Cool* procedure teaches individuals with ASD to understand the difference between cool behaviors (i.e., those that are socially appropriate) and those that are not cool (i.e., those that are not socially appropriate). Leaf et al. (2012) evaluated the effects of the procedure with three children diagnosed with ASD and found the procedure to be effective in teaching some social skills. In a recent study by Leaf, Mitchell, Townley-Cochran, McEachin, Taubman, and Leaf (2016) comparing *social stories* to *Cool* versus *Not Cool* procedure, they found the *Cool* versus *Not Cool* procedure to be more effective than the *social stories* procedure in terms of participants acquiring the skills taught. As authors note, however, generalization measures were limited, and therefore future research is needed in this domain.

The Cognitive-Behavioral-Ecological intervention (CBE; Bauminger-Zviely, 2013) is yet another promising curriculum. In addition to addressing how children think and feel in social interaction and what they do (i.e., behavior), CBE targets cognitive processes that may mediate behavioral-emotional responses in social interactions (e.g., misperceptions of social world). CBE can be delivered in a dyad format (Bauminger, 2002) or in groups (Bauminger, 2007) in schools, implemented by teachers (Bauminger-Zviely, 2013). CBE focuses on building basic and complex social-emotional understanding and skills training (e.g., social problem-solving). Several studies of CBE (both dyadic and group) have been conducted by Bauminger and her colleagues, the results of which are quite promising. CBE is associated with gains in the social-cognitive domain (e.g., emotion knowledge) and the behavioral domain, but limited generalization of skills to other contexts such as school recess (Bauminger, 2007). There is also evidence that CBE is associated with direct benefits (e.g., social-emotional understanding) and indirect, perhaps mediating, effects (e.g., theory of mind, executive function; Bauminger, 2007).

The majority of the published research has focused primarily on distal outcomes, although there has been emerging research on theorized proximal mechanisms of action (e.g., change in theory of mind). There has been little investigation on the generalization of learned skills. Finally, nearly all of the research in this domain has been conducted by the groups that developed them, with very little replication work or multisite study. Additionally, most CBT social skills interventions have been developed for, and exclusively evaluated within samples comprised of, youth with ASD with intact cognitive abilities. This is understandable given the demands on verbal reasoning and cognitive introspection associated with such programs. Nevertheless, consideration of the extant CBT-based social skills intervention research as a whole, including that on the aforementioned programs and other such interventions (e.g., Koning, Magill-Evans, Volden, & Dick, 2013), suggests that interventions in this category are promising and further study, especially multisite trials with sufficiently large samples, is warranted.

23.3 School-Based Interventions

There is a considerable amount of research examining interventions conducted in school settings, including several well-done qualitative and quantitative reviews. Most of these reviews have adopted the intervention categorization scheme initially used by McConnell (2002) in an early qualitative review of social interventions for young children with ASD, which groups strategies into five fairly broad categories: (1) environmental modifications (e.g., altering classroom to promote physical proximity to peers), (2) child-specific (e.g., direct skills training with the diagnosed student), (3) collateral skills (e.g., encouraging group play during recess), (4) peer-mediated (e.g., training typical peers to assist the student with ASD), and (5) comprehensive (e.g., combining at least two types of intervention). Given that the majority of this body of research has not focused on specific curricula, in this chapter we focus on these categories as well.

Bellini et al. (2007) conducted a meta-analysis of 55 single-subject school-based social interventions. In addition to finding that such interventions are "minimally effective" (p. 159), they also noted poor generalization of learned skills across settings and stimuli (Bellini et al., 2007). Recently, Whalon, Conroy, Martinez, and Werch (2015) conducted a meta-analysis of 37 single-subject, school-based interventions, implemented with preschool and elementary students, specifically targeting peer-related social competence. Using the same categorization scheme, Whalon et al. found the interventions to have moderate to high impact across the targeted behaviors of initiations toward peers, responses to peer initiations, interactions, and peer social engagement. Moreover, they found no evidence for difference across technique category (e.g., child-specific vs. collateral skills training).

The most common type of school-based social intervention is child-directed, encompassing a range of techniques such as video-modeling and social narratives (Whalon et al., 2015). One fairly common approach within the child-directed category is structured skills training delivered directly to the students with ASD. A common criticism levied against such skill-based approaches is that discrete skills (e.g., how to maintain a conversation) do not equate to social competence. In other words, learning the skill does not necessarily mean the student will use that skill when it is called for or in a socially appropriate way. To address this deficiency, some programs (e.g., *Superheroes Social Skills* program; Jenson et al., 2011) have been implemented in more generalized (e.g., non-pull-out) settings. The *Superheroes Social Skills* program includes strategies to directly promote generalization, and research on its efficacy when delivered during recess at school has shown positive effects on social engagement (Radley, Ford, Battaglia, & McHugh, 2014).

The extant research suggests that, regardless of type of intervention, utilization of peer-mediation (e.g., training typical peers to help reinforce taught skills) is helpful and should be considered an evidence-based practice (Reichow & Volkmar, 2010; Whalon et al., 2015). Watkins et al. (2015), based on a thorough review of peer-mediated interventions, concluded that the approach is promising not just for children but also for adolescents and young adults with ASD within inclusive settings. Peer-mediated interventions are diverse in structure, degree of training, and content ranging from giving peers direct, explicit instruction on how to prompt and reinforce social interaction for the student with ASD (e.g., Banda, Hart, & Lui-Gitz, 2010) to identifying mutual interests to incorporate into social activities (e.g., Koegel, Vernon, Koegel, Koegel, & Paullin, 2012).

In synthesizing the school-based intervention research, including the published reviews within this category, it is clear that much of the work in this area has focused on the observed, distal outcomes of interest (e.g., peer initiations). There has been little concerted effort to "move the needle" of targeted mechanisms of interest (e.g., social motivation or drive). This may be, at least partly, because these interventions are primarily behavioral in nature and, for the most part, not tethered to a particular theoretical framework. For example, in a cognitive framework, anticipatory fears may guide avoidance of a situation, and therefore targeting the cognitions (i.e., fears) under this framework may be more beneficial than targeting the behavior of avoidance alone. Additionally, in this category of social intervention research, there have been relatively few evaluations of specific programs or curricula, likely owing to the challenges inherent in intervention implementation within the school day (e.g., short periods, school absences, number of participants available in a given school or classroom). Perhaps more than any other type of intervention reviewed in this chapter, the generalizability of the effects of school-based social interventions has been well-studied. Although the quality of the data varies across studies, generalization across peers and settings has been explored. It is generally agreed, for example, that effects of peer-mediated interventions do generalize outside the confines of what is taught and where it is taught (e.g., Watkins et al., 2015). Finally, partly due to how interventions have been categorized (e.g., approaches such as "peer-mediated," rather than specific curricula), we see considerable external evaluation research.

23.4 Interventions Targeting Social Cognition

Social cognition refers to the cognitive mechanisms that influence social behavior. Under this umbrella, we often consider processes such as executive function, emotion recognition, perspective-taking, theory of mind, and social problem-solving or reasoning in ASD (see Mendelson, Gates, & Lerner, 2016). Several such processes have been targeted in social interventions. Herein we describe some interventions purported to address some of these social cognition processes.

In day-to-day social interaction, people rely on multiple cues (e.g., posture, facial expression, intonation, and gesture) to intuit the felt emotions of social partners. Of these nonverbal social-affective communication behaviors, facial emotion recognition (FER) has arguably been the most well-studied process within ASD. Although the research has not produced an entirely consistent picture, this is due at least in part to methodological variation (e.g., age range of sample, duration of stimuli) across studies (e.g., Harms, Martin, & Wallace, 2010), more so than actual ASD-related FER impairment or lack thereof. Additionally, recent research suggests that both motivational and perceptual processes are involved in observed FER impairments in ASD. Specifically, social motivation has been found to predict worse FER for youth with ASD and to partially mediate the relationship between early-stage face perception and FER (Garman et al., 2016). Two recent meta-analyses suggest that FER deficits are common in ASD and that the magnitude of deficiency (relative to similar-age peers) worsens with age (Lozier, Vanmeter, & Marsh, 2014; Uljarevic & Hamilton, 2013). These deficits are most apparent when using adult (as opposed to child) face stimuli, when the emotions are negatively valenced (e.g., anger), and when the emotions are expressed subtly (Lozier, Vanmeter, & Marsh, 2014; Uljarevic & Hamilton, 2013).

It is generally believed that recognizing and responding to others' emotional expressions is important for successful interpersonal relationships and that FER deficits likely contribute to the social disability that characterizes ASD (Ekman, 1992; Schultz et al., 2003). Although FER training has been extensively studied in ASD, this has primarily been within multicomponent intervention programs (e.g., Lopata et al., 2013). As such, it is not clear if remediation of FER impairment is sufficient to ultimately lead to observable improvement in social function. Golan and Baron-Cohen (2006) tested the effects of *Mind Reading* (Baron-Cohen, Golan, Wheelwright, & Hill, 2004), which targets emotion recognition using facial and vocal cues, in a small open trial. They found that the adult participants who received the intervention improved on close generalization tasks (recognizing emotion using stimuli included in the intervention) but not on more distant generalization tasks, such as recognizing emotions in characters from previously unseen film clips. There is, however, emerging support for a directional relationship between improved emotion recognition and social function. In a small RCT, Hopkins et al. (2011) showed that *FaceSay*, a computerized intervention that targets improved eye gaze, face processing, and FER, was associated with improved FER as well as better social functioning with peers in a sample of children with ASD.

It should be noted that there has not been clear discrimination within the treatment literature among the related constructs of social cognition, mind reading, theory of mind (ToM), and perspective-taking. In the last several years, interest in treatments targeting various aspects of social cognition has risen, due in part to questionable sustained and generalized impact for purely behavioral, skills-based intervention approaches (Howard & Renfrow, 2003). Although the research on ToM impairment in ASD has not uniformly revealed deficits relative to typical peers, it is generally accepted that perspective-taking is more universally and pervasively impaired for individuals with this disorder (Mendelson, Gates, & Lerner, 2016). In an RCT with 40 cognitively able youth with ASD, Begeer et al. (2011) found that participants who completed a ToM intervention showed significantly improved ToM conceptual skills, but no significant improvement in empathy or parent-reported social behavior, relative to controls.

Perspective-taking, which is closely related to ToM, involves appreciating another's cognitive or emotional experience and recognition that that experience is unique and different from one's own (e.g., Davis, 1983). The *Social Competence Intervention*, initially developed for adolescents (SCI-A; Stichter et al., 2010), was later modified for use with elementary-age youth (SCI-E). SCI targets a host of cognitive processes including impairments in ToM, emotion recognition, and executive functioning in order to effect positive change, ultimately, in social ability. Content includes training in FER, sharing ideas, and social problem-solving. An open trial of SCI-E with a modest size sample (n = 20) found significant improvements in parent-reported (unblended to treatment intent) executive function and social skills (Stichter, O'Connor, Herzog, Lierheimer, & McGhee, 2012). However, the study design did not permit examination of the mediating effect of the targeted social-cognitive processes. Crooke, Hendrix, and Rachman (2008) studied *Social Thinking* (Winner, 2000), a social intervention designed to target executive function impairments and teach the cognitive skills and knowledge underlying social discourse, rather than discrete skills (behaviors), in six children with ASD using a pre-post design (Crooke et al., 2008). Delivered over 8 weeks in hour-long sessions, the intervention primarily focuses on explaining the "why" (rationale) for social skills and that other people have independent thoughts (ToM and perspective-taking). Behavioral data indicated improvements in socially appropriate behaviors and decreases in unexpected or atypical behaviors, following intervention (Crooke et al., 2008).

Several curricula within this category target multiple aspects of social cognition. For instance, *Social Cognition and Interaction Training* (SCIT; Roberts, Penn, & Combs, 2004) targets emotion recognition, ToM, and attributions. Although originally developed for adult patients with psychosis, SCIT has been tested with adults with ASD (SCIT-A; Turner-Brown, Perry, Dichter, Bodfish, & Penn, 2008). In a small quasi-experimental treatment study, Turner-Brown and colleagues found that the participants who received SCIT-A showed improvements in ToM skills and a trend toward improved social communication skills (though not statistically significant). Another intervention initially developed for and tested among patients with schizophrenia that has since been adapted for individuals with ASD is *Cognitive Enhancement Therapy* (CET; Hogarty & Greenwald, 2006). In an open trial, Eack et al. (2013) tested CET with a sample of adults with ASD. Delivered over a course of 18 months, CET integrated computer-based neurocognitive training (targeting attention, memory, and problem-solving) with group sessions (targeting perspective-taking and social appraisal). Significant improvement was seen both for cognitive deficits and social behavior, with large effects (Eack et al., 2013).

Finally, *Unstuck and On Target* (UOT; Cannon, Kenworthy, Alexander, Werner, & Anthony, 2011) is a psychosocial treatment that targets executive function impairment for individuals with ASD, specifically cognitive flexibility (e.g., diminished insistence on sameness) and goal-directed behavior. In a rigorous RCT conducted by Kenworthy et al. (2014), UOT was implemented across contexts (i.e., school and home) and compared to a fairly structured social skills intervention. They found that the UOT group outperformed the comparator (i.e., social skills intervention) on measures of problem-solving, flexibility, and planning/organization. Moreover, the UOT participants made significantly greater improvement behaviorally in the classroom (e.g., rule-following, handling transitions) than the participants in the social intervention. However, there were no group differences in terms of improvement in social skills (Kenworthy et al., 2014).

There has been a tremendous upswing in research on interventions targeting the facets of social cognition in ASD in the last several years. Admittedly, we have reviewed just a small fraction of this treatment research. Although the majority of the studies in this category have assessed change in both proximal (e.g., ToM, FER) and distal (e.g., social competence) outcomes, the evidence for clinically significant improvement in the more manifest, distal outcomes remains sparse (exceptions include Eack et al., 2013 and Hopkins et al., 2011). Future clinical research in this area should continue to explore change at both levels in longitudinal, experimental designs in order to establish temporal precedence and causation. As a whole, this body of research has consistently explored variables of interest outside of those directly targeted in treatment (e.g., recognition of emotion using non-trained stimuli). Finally, this is a vast body of research that is still fairly young and being actively explored by multiple research teams. Understandably, therefore, most of this research has been conducted by teams that have developed the treatment protocols or modified preexisting protocols. In the future, we will need to focus efforts on replication and external site validation (e.g., trials conducted by nondevelopment sites).

23.5 Naturalistic Interventions

Naturalistic treatments address a major limitation of many existing interventions that are often highly structured in setting and delivery and therefore may impede generalization to the natural environment. Naturalistic behavioral treatments are specifically designed to address these limitations by incorporating techniques aimed to facilitate learning (e.g., multiple trials, shaping) with techniques to aid in generalization, including teaching during naturally occurring instances, using natural consequences, and by following the child's lead (Kaiser, Yoder, & Keetz, 1992). The distinctive features of naturalistic interventions include sessions that are less structured, lessons initiated and paced by the child, lessons taking place in variety of locations, and employment of a variety of stimuli and prompts (Cowan & Allen, 2007; Delprato, 2001). In addition, as noted by Delprato (2001), instead of functionally unrelated reinforcers (e.g., candy) which are often used in behavioral interventions, naturalistic treatments allow for child to select the desired object to serve as a natural reinforcer. Several of the naturalistic treatments have already been discussed in this book, including incidental teaching and pivotal response training. There are however several other interventions that fall in this category that are not yet established. We review a few examples of these in this section.

Enhanced Milieu Teaching (*EMT*) is a naturalistic, conversation-based teaching method that uses child's interest and initiations as opportunities to teach social communication (Kaiser, 1993). EMT takes a hybrid approach, incorporating behavioral and social interactionist approaches to intervention. Key components of EMT are (1) creating an environment that promotes engagement and communication, (2) responding to a child's interests and ability level to build conversational interaction, and (3) communicating in a way that promotes meaningful play and interaction (Hancock & Kaiser, 2009). Hancock, Ledbetter-Cho, Howell, and Lang (2016) reviewed the existing research on the effectiveness of EMT and found that overall, EMT implemented by therapists, teachers, and parents is an effective language intervention for preschool children with autism (e.g., Hancock & Kaiser, 2002) as well as other populations. As the authors noted, however, the research has been limited to preschool-age, Euro-American children who have significant language delays.

Multiple studies which have utilized imitation to increase social skills have suggested that repeated imitation results in an increase of social behaviors in children with ASD. While not always conducted in the naturalistic environment, some interventions utilizing imitation can be considered as a naturalistic intervention, as the child is not instructed to act a certain way, rather, the adult imitates the natural behaviors of the child. For example, Field, Field, Sanders, and Nadel (2001) explored the effects of adult repeated imitation with 20 nonverbal children with a diagnosis of ASD and found increases in looking, vocalizing, smiling, and engaging in reciprocal play. In addition, children who received the intervention showed several social behaviors, including being close to the adult, sitting next to the adult, and touching the adult following the intervention. Therefore, both distal and proximal social behaviors were augmented following the intervention. During the repeated imitation sessions, an adult imitated all of the child's natural behaviors (i.e., what the child was doing without any prompts) during the session. It was the action of the adult imitating these naturally occurring behaviors which resulted in change in social behavior. This study suggests the potential use of the imitative behavior by the adult in a naturalistic framework as an early intervention for children with ASD.

A specific example of a naturalistic imitation training is the *Reciprocal Imitation Training* (RIT; Ingersoll, 2008). RIT is a play-based, naturalistic intervention aimed at increasing imitation skills in children with ASD. RIT has been specifically designed for young children with autism, as they often show difficulty with imitation (see Rogers, 1999 for review). The goal of RIT is to teach imitation as a means of social interaction, in a naturalistic setting. It can be implemented during play inside and outdoors, as well as during daily routines. The technique incorporates several strategies, including contingent imitation, linguistic mapping (i.e., describing what the child is attending to or doing using simple language), following the child's lead, physical prompting, and contingent reinforcement (Ingersoll & Schreibman, 2006). Research suggests that RIT increases social communication skills, including social engagement and joint attention (Ingersoll, Lewis, & Kroman, 2007; Ingersoll & Schreibman, 2006). While this treatment approach has a substantial set of studies indicating efficacy for increasing variety of social skills (e.g., Ingersoll, 2010, 2012; Ingersoll & Lalonde, 2010; Ingersoll et al., 2007), most of this work has been conducted by the same research group.

Many naturalistic interventions (discussed in other chapters of this book) have a strong evidence base behind their effectiveness in augmenting social skills for individuals with ASD. The emerging naturalistic interventions discussed in this section (i.e., EMT, repeated imitation, RIT) show some evidence behind their utility; however, these emerging naturalistic interventions need further exploration. Although the majority of the research has been on distal targets of social skills, some beginning work on proximal factors is emerging with the repeated imitation intervention. A major strength of all naturalistic interventions, possibly more so than any other treatment category discussed in this chapter, is the work on generalizability of the results, since the programs have been specifically developed using techniques to aid in generalization (i.e., using natural environment to increase generalizability of skills). Lastly, in terms of replicability of results, while the specific protocols (i.e., RIT) have only been assessed using the team that developed the program, the general techniques discussed in this section have been replicated by multiple teams (e.g., repeated imitation has been explored by multiple teams). Therefore, the preliminary evidence suggests that these emerging naturalistic interventions show promise for augmenting social skills for individuals with ASD, and therefore further research into these techniques is required.

23.6 Theater-Based Interventions

Theatrical or drama-based interventions consist of interventions that use theater or dramatic training activities to practice areas of social skill deficits among individuals with ASD. These interventions address the limitations of several social skills interventions, including lack of generalization and posttreatment skill maintenance (e.g., White, Keonig, & Scahill, 2007). Drama-based interventions allow individuals with ASD to increase understanding of social narratives that arise from social interactions and help to increase imagination and sensitivity to others (Tytherleigh & Karkau, 2010). As highlighted by Corbett et al. (2014), acting teaches social awareness, cognition, communication, perception, and expression, and therefore, it holds promise as a tool to increase social skills for individuals with ASD. Prior research has shown that aspects of drama-based interventions, such as acting and role-play, increase empathy, ToM, and social skills for typically developing individuals (Goldstein, 2011; Goldstein & Cisar, 1992). Therefore, use of drama-based interventions holds promise to increase these social skills in children and adolescents with ASD.

Socio-dramatic affective-relational intervention (SDARI; Lerner, Mikami, Levine, 2010) is a group-based, six-week, manualized intervention for adolescents with ASD. The curriculum includes activities based on dramatic improvisation-based games that focus on training participants to attend to reciprocal interaction cues. The fun and interactive curriculum which incorporates games and humor provided participants an opportunity to practice the social skills within game-based instruction. The intervention includes three components: a performance-based social skills curriculum with improvisation games and dramatic training, focus on relationship building to reinforce social interaction, and employing age-appropriate motivators to promote the generalization of skills in other settings. Lerner et al. (2010) evaluated the intervention in a pilot study with individuals with ASD and found that individuals who participated in the intervention displayed gains in some social skills (e.g., social assertion and ability to detect emotions), but not others. The study also found evidence for generalization of the social skills and posttreatment maintenance.

Social Emotional NeuroScience Endocrinology Theatre (SENSE Theatre; Corbett et al., 2011) is an intervention program aimed at improving social and emotional functioning of children and adolescents. It uses behavioral intervention in combination with theatrical techniques to improve social skills for individuals with ASD. In the program, each child with ASD is paired with a typically developing child who serves as the peer model (Corbett et al., 2011). Corbett et al. (2011) investigated the efficacy of the intervention with eight individuals with ASD and found that in addition to reducing anxiety and stress among participants involved in the theater-based program, the program was also effective for improving the social perception skills of children with ASD. Corbett et al. (2014) further investigated the effectiveness of this drama-based peer-mediated intervention during a two-week summer camp and found further support for its use to improve social skill deficits among youth with ASD. Individuals with ASD significantly improved face perception skills (e.g., identify and remember facial stimuli, but not emotion recognition), even though participants did not receive direct instruction in face processing. In addition, improvements in social perception were observed outside of the treatment setting. Following the intervention, participants also demonstrated improvement in their ability to interpret the social meaning of engaging with others, and the amount of time they spend engaging with peers increased over the course of the intervention.

Theater-based interventions attempt to fill a gap of many social skills interventions in providing a fun, interactive, and motivating way for individuals with ASD to build social skills through group-based theater. Evidence suggests that through this modality, individuals with ASD learn multiple important skills for social interactions. However, large-scale studies looking at drama-based interventions, independent of a particular protocol, are lacking. Within the two reviewed protocols, the interventions have been focused primarily on distal outcomes of social skill improvement. Evaluation of proximal mechanisms behind the change (e.g., face memory), however, is emerging (Corbett et al., 2014). A strength of these interventions, however, is on the emerging investigation of the generalization of the skills, especially in regard to the SDARI model which was built upon existing social skills training taking into account recommendations to increase social motivation and skill generalization (Lerner et al., 2010). Further research on generalizability of the learned skills across these drama-based interventions is warranted. A noteworthy limitation of the current literature base on drama-based intervention, similar to other techniques discussed in this chapter, is the lack of replication of work by individuals outside of the groups that developed them. The promising emerging evidence regarding the improvement of some social skills with the use of drama-based interventions, however, suggests the need for further exploration and replication of these studies in larger samples.

23.7 Conclusions

In this chapter, we have provided a synopsis of the extant research on a vast array of emerging social skills interventions. Although the approaches reviewed herein are not yet considered well-established, they are considered *promising* based on the research published to date, and further evaluation of them is warranted. We reviewed emerging interventions across six fairly broad categories or foci: technology-based, cognitive-behavioral, school-based, social cognition, naturalistic, and theater-based. These categories are not mutually exclusive of one another; for instance, a treatment that targets social cognition might utilize technology.

It must also be noted that we have not conducted a comprehensive review of all social interventions that one might consider promising. Indeed, there are several curricula that have some research to suggest efficacy, which have not been included. Inclusion of all the relevant research is beyond the scope of a single chapter. Our goal was to provide a synthesis of the commonalities seen across different categories of intervention, in order to inform the field regarding future directions in this area.

In an attempt to draw conclusions across this diverse literature and offer suggestions for future research, we considered the following domains: (1) proximal vs. distal target of intervention, (2) taught vs. generalized skill, and (3) in-house vs. external evaluation. Most of the research to date has focused on either targeted mechanisms (proximal processes) or outcomes (distal processes). Few studies have attempted to examine both simultaneously. It is critical that clinical research examine both levels of change, in order to understand if and how effected change in the theoretical mechanisms leads to, or contributes to, change in more distal outcomes (e.g., use of social skills). Such questions call for sophisticated research designs that control for other possible change processes and establish temporal precedence in the candidate mechanism of action. Related to the second domain, there is terrific variability across categories of social intervention research. School-based research, for instance, in this area has closely examined the degree to which taught skills generalize to novel stimuli and settings. Other areas (e.g., cognitive-behavioral interventions) have dedicated less attention to generalization. Finally, with respect to the scope of external evaluation, most work on these interventions has been conducted by, or in close affiliation with, the labs that developed the interventions. This is not a criticism so much as a reflection of the nascency of much of this research. Replication and extension of existing programs (at nondevelopment sites), as well as multisite outcome evaluation studies, are needed.

In addition to these broader domains, the impact of much of the published research is hampered by methodological constraints such as small sample sizes and reliance of questionnaire data for outcome measurement. It should also be noted that many of the discussed interventions are multicomponent in nature (e.g., targeting discrete skills and FER), such that dismantling relative impact of the intervention's component parts is complicated.

Clinicians have many options from which to select, when targeting social impairment in clients with ASD. As discussed in this chapter, there are multiple available approaches which have an emerging research base to suggest efficacy. However, given that these approaches are not yet considered "established," clinicians must exercise caution and provide information about the limitations of the respective research base, as well as the relative and potential merits of the interventions to clients, in the interest of fully informed consent. Additionally, across the different categories of intervention reviewed herein, a multitude of outcome measures have been used. Selection of appropriate and clinically valid measures of change can be challenging, as we lack consensus on "gold standard" tools for many of the targets of intervention (e.g., FER, perspective-taking). Nevertheless, it is imperative that outcome monitoring be used to guide treatment planning and evaluation of progress with clients.

In conclusion, there are many exciting intervention avenues being actively explored. There is growing recognition that the social impairment that characterizes ASD is both profound and pervasive, regardless of the cognitive or verbal abilities of the client. Simultaneously, the nature of the social impairment is variable across affected individuals, as well as within a given person over the lifespan. As the field matures in knowledge base and research sophistication, it is likely that we will be able to provide research-based answers to the age-old questions of what works, when, and for whom.

References

Banda, D. R., Hart, S. L., & Liu-Gitz, L. (2010). Impact of training peers and children with autism on social skills during center time activities in inclusive classrooms. *Research in Autism Spectrum Disorders, 4*, 619–625.

Baron-Cohen, S., Golan, O., Wheelwright, S., & Hill, J. J. (2004). *Mind reading: The interactive guide to emotions*. London: Jessica Kingsley.

Bauminger, N. (2002). The facilitation of social-emotional understanding and social interaction in high-functioning children with autism: Intervention outcomes. *Journal of Autism and Developmental Disorders, 32*(4), 283–298.

Bauminger, N. (2007). Brief report: Group social-multimodal intervention for HFASD. *Journal of Autism and Developmental Disorders, 37*, 1605–1615. doi:10.1007/s10803-006-0246-3
Bauminger-Zviely, N. (2013). Cognitive-behavioral-ecological intervention to facilitate social-emotional understanding and social interaction in youth with high-functioning ASD. In A. Scarpa, S. W. White, & T. Attwood (Eds.), *CBT for children and adolescents with high-functioning autism spectrum disorders* (pp. 226–258). New York, NY: Guilford Publications.
Beaumont, R., & Sofronoff, K. (2008). A multi-component social skills intervention for children with asperger syndrome: The Junior Detective Training Program. *Journal of Child Psychology and Psychiatry, 49*(7), 743–753. doi:10.1111/j.1469-7610.2008.01920.x
Beaumont, R., & Sofronoff, K. (2013). Multimodal intervention for social skills training in students with high-functioning ASD: The Secret Agent Society. In A. Scarpa, S. W. White, & T. Attwood (Eds.), *CBT for children and adolescents with high-functioning autism spectrum disorders* (pp. 173–198). New York, NY: Guilford Publications.
Begeer, S., Gevers, C., Clifford, P., Verhoeve, M., Kat, K., Hoddenbach, E., & Boer, F. (2011). Theory of mind training in children with autism: A randomized controlled trial. *Journal of Autism and Developmental Disorders, 41*, 997–1006. doi:10.1007/s10803-010-1121-9
Bellini, S., Peters, J. K., Benner, L., & Hopf, A. (2007). A meta-analysis of school-based social skills interventions for children with autism spectrum disorders. *Remedial and Special Education, 28*(3), 153–162.
Bölte, S. (2004). Computer-based intervention in autism spectrum disorders. In O. T. Ryaskin (Ed.), *Focus on autism research* (pp. 247–260). New York, NY: Nova Biomedical.
Cannon, L., Kenworthy, L., Alexander, K. C., Werner, M. A., & Anthony, L. G. (2011). *Unstuck and on target!: An executive function curriculum to improve flexibility for children with autism spectrum disorders*. Baltimore, MD: Paul H. Brookes.
Chambless, D. L., Baker, M. J., Baucom, D. H., Beutler, L. E., Calhoun, K. S., Crits-Christoph, P., … Johnson, S. B. (1998). Update on empirically validated therapies, II. *The Clinical Psychologist, 51*(1), 3–16.
Corbett, B. A., Gunther, J. R., Comins, D., Price, J., Ryan, N., Simon, D., … Rios, T. (2011). Brief report: Theatre as therapy for children with autism spectrum disorder. *Journal of Autism and Developmental Disorders, 41*(4), 505–511.
Corbett, B. A., Swain, D. M., Coke, C., Simon, D., Newsom, C., Houchins-Juarez, N., … Song, Y. (2014). Improvement in social deficits in autism Spectrum disorders using a theatre-based, peer-mediated intervention. *Autism Research, 7*(1), 4–16.
Cowan, R. J., & Allen, K. D. (2007). Using naturalistic procedures to enhance learning in individuals with autism: A focus on generalized teaching within the school setting. *Psychology in the Schools, 44*(7), 701–715.
Crooke, P. J., Hendrix, R. E., & Rachman, J. Y. (2008). Brief report: Measuring the effectiveness of teaching social thinking to children with asperger syndrome (AS) and high functioning autism (HFA). *Journal of Autism and Developmental Disorders, 38*, 581–591. doi:10.1007/s10803-007-0466-1
Davis, M. H. (1983). Measuring individual differences in empathy: Evidence for a multidimensional approach. *Journal of Personality and Social Psychology, 44*, 113–126.
Delprato, D. J. (2001). Comparisons of discrete-trial and normalized behavioral language intervention for young children with autism. *Journal of Autism and Developmental Disorders, 31*(3), 315–325.
Eack, S. M., Greenwald, D. P., Hogarty, S. S., Bahorik, A. L., Litschge, M. Y., Mazefsky, C. A., & Minshew, N. J. (2013). Cognitive enhancement therapy for adults with autism spectrum disorder: Results from an 18-month feasibility study. *Journal of Autism and Developmental Disorders, 43*, 2866–2877. doi:10.1007/s10803-013-1834-7
Ekman, P. (1992). An argument for basic emotions. *Cognition and Emotion, 6*, 169–200. doi:10.1080/02699939208411068
Field, T., Field, T., Sanders, C., & Nadel, J. (2001). Children with autism display more social behaviors after repeated imitation sessions. *Autism, 5*(3), 317–323.
Garman, H. D., Spaulding, C. J., Webb, S. J., Mikami, A. Y., Morris, J. P., & Lerner, M. D. (2016). Wanting it too much: An inverse relation between social motivation and facial emotion recognition in autism spectrum disorder. *Child Psychiatry and Human Development*. Advance online publication. doi: 10.1007/210578-015-0620-5.
Golan, O., & Baron-Cohen, S. (2006). Systemizing empathy: Teaching adults with Asperger syndrome or high-functioning autism to recognize complex emotions using interactive multimedia. *Development and Psychopathology, 18*(02), 591–617.
Goldstein, H., & Cisar, C. L. (1992). Promoting interaction during sociodramatic play: Teaching scripts to typical preschoolers and classmates with disabilities. *Journal of Applied Behavior Analysis, 25*(2), 265–280.
Goldstein, T. R. (2011). Correlations among social-cognitive skills in adolescents involved in acting or arts classes. *Mind, Brain, and Education, 5*(2), 97–103.
Grynszpan, O., Weiss, P. L. T., Perez-Diaz, F., & Gal, E. (2014). Innovative technology-based interventions for autism spectrum disorders: A meta-analysis. *Autism, 18*(4), 346–361.
Hancock, T. B., & Kaiser, A. P. (2002). The effects of trainer-implemented enhanced milieu teaching on the social communication of children with autism. *Topics in Early Childhood Special Education, 22*, 39–54.
Hancock, T. B., & Kaiser, A. P. (2009). Enhanced milieu teaching. In R. McCauley & M. Fey (Eds.), *Treatment of language disorders in children*. Baltimore, MD: Paul Brookes.
Hancock, T. B., Ledbetter-Cho, K., Howell, A., & Lang, R. (2016). Enhanced milieu teaching. In *Early intervention for young children with autism spectrum disorder* (pp. 177–218). Springer International Publishing , Switzerland.
Harms, M. B., Martin, A., & Wallace, G. L. (2010). Facial emotion recognition in autism spectrum disorders:

A review of behavioral and neuroimaging studies. *Neuropsychology Review*, *20*, 290–322. doi:10.1007/s11065-010-9138-6

Hofmann, S. G., Asnani, A., Vonk, I. J. J., Sawyer, A. T., & Fang, A. (2012). The efficacy of cognitive behavioral therapy: A review of meta-analyses. *Cognitive Therapy and Research*, *36*, 427–440.

Hofmann, S. G., & Smits, J. A. J. (2008). Cognitive-behavioral therapy for adult anxiety disorders: A meta-analysis of randomized placebo-controlled trials. *Journal of Clinical Psychiatry*, *69*(4), 621–632.

Hogarty, G. E., & Greenwald, D. P. (2006). *Cognitive enhancement therapy: The training manual*. University of Pittsburgh Medical Center: Authors. Available through www.CognitiveEnhancementTherapy.com

Hopkins, I. M., Gower, M. W., Perez, T. A., Smith, D. S., Amthor, F. R., Wimsatt, F. C., & Biasini, F. J. (2011). Avatar assistant: Improving social skills in students with an ASD through a computer-based intervention. *Journal of Autism and Developmental Disorders*, *41*, 1543–1555. doi:10.1007/s10803-011-1179-z

Howard, J., & Renfrow, D. (2003). Social cognition. In J. Delamater (Ed.), *Handbook of social psychology* (pp. 259–281). New York, NY: Plenum.

Ingersoll, B. (2008). The social role of imitation in autism: Implications for the treatment of imitation deficits. *Infants & Young Children*, *21*(2), 107–119.

Ingersoll, B. (2010). Brief report: Pilot randomized controlled trial of reciprocal imitation training for teaching elicited and spontaneous imitation to children with autism. *Journal of Autism and Developmental Disorders*, *40*(9), 1154–1160.

Ingersoll, B. (2012). Brief report: Effect of a focused imitation intervention on social functioning in children with autism. *Journal of Autism and Developmental Disorders*, *42*(8), 1768–1773.

Ingersoll, B., & Lalonde, K. (2010). The impact of object and gesture imitation training on language use in children with autism spectrum disorder. *Journal of Speech, Language, and Hearing Research*, *53*(4), 1040–1051.

Ingersoll, B., Lewis, E., & Kroman, E. (2007). Teaching the imitation and spontaneous use of descriptive gestures in young children with autism using a naturalistic behavioral intervention. *Journal of Autism and Developmental Disorders*, *37*(8), 1446–1456.

Ingersoll, B., & Schreibman, L. (2006). Teaching reciprocal imitation skills to young children with autism using a naturalistic behavioral approach: Effects on language, pretend play, and joint attention. *Journal of Autism and Developmental Disorders*, *36*(4), 487–505.

Jenson, W., Bowen, J., Clark, E., Block, H., Gabriensen, T., Hood, J., … Springer, B. (2011). *Superheroes social skills*. Eugene, OR: Pacific Northwest.

Kaiser, A. (1993). Introduction: Enhancing children's social communication. In A. P. Kaiser & D. B. Gray (Eds.), *Enhancing children's communication: Research foundations for intervention* (pp. 3–9). Baltimore, MD: Brookes.

Kaiser, A. P., Yoder, P. J., & Keetz, A. (1992). Evaluating milieu teaching. In S. F. Warren & J. Reichle (Eds.), *Causes and effects in communication and language intervention* (pp. 9–48). Baltimore MD: Paul Brooks Publishing.

Kenworthy, L., Anthony, L. G., Naiman, D. Q., Cannon, L., Wills, M. C., Luong-Tran, C., … Wallace, G. L. (2014). Randomized controlled effectiveness trial of executive function intervention for children on the autism spectrum. *Journal of Child Psychology and Psychiatry*, *55*(4), 374–383. doi:10.1111/jcpp.12161

Koegel, L., Vernon, T., Koegel, R. L., Koegel, B., & Paullin, A. W. (2012). Improving socialization between children with autism spectrum disorder and their peers in inclusive settings. *Journal of Positive Behavioral Intervention*, *14*(4), 220–227.

Koning, C., Magill-Evans, J., Volden, J., & Dick, B. (2013). Efficacy of cognitive behavior therapy-based social skills intervention for school-age boys with autism spectrum disorders. *Research in Autism Spectrum Disorders*, *7*, 1282–1290. doi:10.1016/j.rasd.2011.07.011

Leaf, J. B., Mitchell, E., Townley-Cochran, D., McEachin, J., Taubman, M., & Leaf, R. (2016). Comparing Social Stories™ to Cool Versus Not Cool. *Education and Treatment of Children*, *39*(2), 173–185.

Leaf, J. B., Tsuji, K. H., Griggs, B., Edwards, A., Taubman, M., McEachin, J., … Oppenheim-Leaf, M. L. (2012). Teaching social skills to children with autism using the cool versus not cool procedure. *Education and Training in Autism and Developmental Disabilities*, 165–175.

Lerner, M. D., Mikami, A. Y., & Levine, K. (2010). Sociodramatic affective-relational intervention for adolescents with Asperger syndrome & high functioning autism: Pilot study. *Autism*, *1362361309353613*.

Lerner, M. D., White, S. W., & McPartland, J. C. (2012). Mechanisms of change in psychosocial interventions for autism spectrum disorders. *Dialogues in Clinical Neuroscience*, *14*(3), 307–318.

Lopata, C., Thomeer, M. L., Volker, M. A., & Lee, G. K. (2013). A manualized summer program for social skills in children with high-functioning ASD. In A. Scarpa, S. W. White, & T. Attwood (Eds.), *CBT for children and adolescents with high-functioning autism spectrum disorders* (pp. 199–225). New York, NY: Guilford Publications.

Lopata, C., Thomeer, M. L., Volker, M. A., & Nida, R. E. (2006). Effectiveness of a cognitive-behavioral treatment on the social behaviors of children with asperger disorder. *Focus on Autism and Other Developmental Disabilities*, *21*, 237–244.

Lopata, C., Thomeer, M. L., Volker, M. A., Nida, R. E., & Lee, G. K. (2008). Effectiveness of a manualized summer social treatment program for high-functioning children with autism spectrum disorders. *Journal of Autism and Developmental Disorders*, *38*(5), 890–904.

Lopata, C., Thomeer, M. L., Volker, M. A., Toomey, J. A., Nida, R. E., Lee, G. K., … Rodgers, J. D. (2010). RCT of a manualized social treatment for high-functioning autism spectrum disorders. *Journal of Autism and Developmental Disorders*, *40*, 1297–1310. doi:10.1007/s10803-010-0989-8

Lozier, L. M., Vanmeter, J. W., & Marsh, A. A. (2014). Impairments in facial affect recognition associated

with autism spectrum disorders: A meta-analysis. *Development and Psychopathology*, *26*, 933–945. doi:10.1017/S0954579414000479
McConnell, S. R. (2002). Interventions to facilitate social interaction for young children with autism: Review of available research and recommendations for educational intervention and future research. *Journal of Autism and Developmental Disorders*, *32*, 351–372.
McGinnis, E., & Goldstein, A. P. (1997). *Skillstreaming the elementary school child: New strategies and perspectives for teaching prosocial skills* (rev. ed.). Champaign, IL: Research Press.
Mendelson, J. L., Gates, J. A., & Lerner, M. D. (2016). Friendship in school-age boys with autism spectrum disorders: A meta-analytic summary and developmental, process-based model. *Psychological Bulletin*, *142*(6), 601–622. doi:10.1037/bul0000041
Moore, D., McGrath, P., & Thorpe, J. (2000). Computer-aided learning for people with autism – A framework for research and development. *Innovations in Education and Teaching International*, *37*(3), 218–228.
Murray, D. (1997). Autism and information technology: Therapy with computers. In S. Powell & R. Jordan (Eds.), *Autism and learning: A guide to good practice* (pp. 100–117). London: David Fulton Publishers.
Olatunji, P. J., Cisler, J. M., & Deacon, B. J. (2010). Efficacy of cognitive behavioral therapy for anxiety disorders: A review of meta-analytic findings. *Psychiatric Clinics of North America*, *33*, 557–577.
Radley, K. C., Ford, W. B., Battaglia, A. A., & McHugh, M. B. (2014). The effects of a social skills training package on social engagement of children with autism spectrum disorders in a generalized recess setting. *Focus on Autism and Other Developmental Disabilities*, *29*(4), 216–229. doi:10.1177/108835761452660
Reichow, B., & Volkmar, F. R. (2010). Social skills interventions for individuals with autism: Evaluation for evidence-based practices within a best evidence synthesis framework. *Journal of Autism and Developmental Disorders*, *40*(2), 149–166.
Roberts, D. L., Penn, D., & Combs, D. R. (2004). *Social cognition and interaction training: Unpublished treatment manual.*
Rogers, S. (1999). An examination of the imitation deficit in autism. In J. Nadel & G. Butterworth (Eds.), *Imitation in infancy* (pp. 254–279). Cambridge: Cambridge University Press.
Scarpa, A., White, S. W., & Attwood, T. (2013). *Cognitive-behavioral interventions for children and adolescents with high-functioning autism spectrum disorders.* New York, NY: Guilford Publications.
Schultz, R. T., Grelotti, D. J., Klin, A., Kleinman, J., Van der Gaag, C., Marois, R., & Skudlarski, P. (2003). The role of the fusiform face area in social cognition: Implications for the pathobiology of autism. *Philosophical Transactions of the Royal Society of London Series B: Biological Sciences*, *358*, 415–427. doi:10.1098/rstb.2002.1208
Stichter, J. P., Herzog, M. J., Visovsky, K., Schmidt, C., Randolph, J., Schultz, T., et al. (2010). Social competence intervention for youth with Asperger syndrome and high functioning autism: An initial investigation. *Journal of Autism and Developmental Disorders*, *40*, 1067–1079.
Stichter, J. P., O'Connor, K. V. O., Herzog, M. J., Lierheimer, K., & McGhee, S. D. (2012). Social competence intervention for elementary students with aspergers syndrome and high functioning autism. *Journal of Autism and Developmental Disorders*, *42*, 354–366. doi:10.1007/s10803-011-1249-2
Stokes, T. F., & Baer, D. M. (1977). An implicit technology of generalization. *Journal of Applied Behavior Analysis*, *10*(2), 349–367.
Tanaka, J. W., Wolf, J. M., Klaiman, C., Koenig, K., Cockburn, J., Herlihy, L., … Schultz, R. T. (2010). Using computerized games to teach face recognition skills to children with autism spectrum disorder: the Let's Face It! program. *Journal of Child Psychology and Psychiatry*, *51*(8), 944–952.
Taubman, M., Leaf, R., & McEachin, J. (2011). *Crafting connections: Contemporary applied behavior analysis for enriching the social lives of persons with autism spectrum disorder*. New York, NY: DRL Books, LLC.
Toomey, J. A., Lopata, C., Volker, M. A., & Thomeer, M. L. (2009). Comprehensive intervention for high-functioning autism spectrum disorders: An in-depth case study. In M. T. Burton (Ed.), *Special education in the 21st century* (pp. 95–118). Hauppauge, NY: Nova Science.
Turner-Brown, L. M., Perry, T. D., Dichter, G. S., Bodfish, J. W., & Penn, D. L. (2008). Brief report: Feasibility of social cognition and interaction training for adults with high functioning autism. *Journal of Autism and Developmental Disorders*, *38*, 1777–1784. doi:10.1007/s10803-008-0545-y
Tytherleigh, L., & Karkou, V. (2010). *Drama therapy, autism and relationship building: A case study. Arts therapies in schools: Research and practice* (pp. 197–216). Philadelphia, PA: Jessica Kingsley Publishers.
Uljarevic, M., & Hamilton, A. (2013). Recognition of emotions in autism: A formal meta-analysis. *Journal of Autism and Developmental Disorders*, *43*, 1517–1526. doi:10.1007/s10803-012-1695-5
Wang, S. Y., Parrila, R., & Cui, Y. (2013). Meta-analysis of social skills interventions of single-case research for individuals with autism spectrum disorders: Results from three-level HLM. *Journal of Autism and Developmental Disorders*, *43*(7), 1701–1716.
Watkins, L., O'Reilly, M., Kuhn, M., Gevarter, C., Lancioni, G. E., Sigafoos, J., & Lang, R. (2015). A review of peer-mediated social interaction interventions for students with autism in inclusive settings. *Journal of Autism and Developmental Disorders*, *45*, 1070–1083. doi:10.1007/s10803-014-2264-x
Whalon, K. J., Conroy, M. A., Martinez, J. R., & Werch, B. L. (2015). School-based peer-related social competence interventions for children with autism spectrum disorder: A meta-analysis and descriptive review of single case research design studies. *Journal of*

Autism and Developmental Disorders, 45, 1513–1531. doi:10.1007/s10803-015-2373-1

White, S. W., Keonig, K., & Scahill, L. (2007). Social skills development in children with autism spectrum disorders: A review of the intervention research. *Journal of Autism and Developmental Disorders, 37*(10), 1858–1868.

Wilczynski, S., Green, G., Ricciardi, J., Boyd, B., Hume, A., Ladd, M., & Rue, H. (2009). *National standards report: The national standards project: Addressing the need for evidence-based practice guidelines for autism spectrum disorders*. Randolph, MA: The National Autism Center.

Winner, M. G. (2000). *Inside out: What makes a person with social cognitive deficits tick?* San Jose, CA: Think Social Publishing.

Yoder, P. J., Bottema-Beutel, K., Woynaroski, T., Chandrasekhar, R., & Sandbank, M. (2014). Social communication intervention effects vary by dependent variable type in preschoolers with autism spectrum disorders. *Evidence-based communication assessment and intervention, 7*(4), 150–174.

Part IV

Future Directions

24 Future Research Directions as it Relates to Social Behavior for Individuals Diagnosed with Autism Spectrum Disorder

Justin B. Leaf, Misty Oppenheim-Leaf, and Mary Jane Weiss

In the last 20 years, there has been a drastic increase in the number of research articles evaluating various aspects of social behavior as it relates to individuals diagnosed with autism spectrum disorder (ASD) and/or developmental disabilities (Matson, Mastson, & Rivet, 2007). Research has expanded into identifying the social behaviors in which individuals with ASD engage (including strengths and deficits; Baron-Cohen & Wheelwright, 2004), the outcomes of developing or not developing appropriate social behavior (e.g., friendships, depressions, or suicidal ideation; Bauminger, Shulman, & Agam, 2003), and evaluating numerous interventions that can be used to improve social behavior for individuals diagnosed with ASD (e.g., Brodhed, Higbee, Gerncser, & Akers, 2016; Leaf et al., 2016c). This book is a representation of the expansion in research on this very important topic. The increase in research has resulted in more effective interventions and more socially valid clinical outcomes for individuals diagnosed with ASD. Although progress has been made in the area of social behavior, the amount of research pales in comparison with other commonly evaluated areas such as functional behavioral assessment/analysis (Hanley, Iwata, & McCord, 2003). Additionally, more research is needed on various aspects of social behavior so that we can better study social behavior as it pertains to individuals diagnosed with ASD.

The purpose of this chapter is to provide readers with some general themes of future research that would be valuable to individuals diagnosed with ASD, parents of individuals diagnosed with ASD, and professionals who work with individuals diagnosed with ASD. Throughout numerous chapters within this book, the authors describe areas of future research as it applies to the topic of their chapter. For example, Higbee and Sellers provided the chapter on visual learning strategies (e.g., activity schedules) to improve social behavior for individuals diagnosed with ASD (see Chap. 15). One of the authors' recommendations was that future researchers should evaluate ways to more effectively fade out activity schedules so that individuals diagnosed with ASD would not need these schedules to engage in appropriate social behavior. In the chapter on social assessment, authors Freeman and Cronin urged future researchers to evaluate different variables of checklists used to assess social behavior (see Chap. 6). Rather than rehash the areas of future

J.B. Leaf (✉)
Director of Research, Autism Partnership Foundation, Seal Beach, CA, USA
e-mail: jblautpar@aol.com

M. Oppenheim-Leaf
Autism Partnership Foundation, Seal Beach, CA, USA

M.J. Weiss
Endicott College, Beverly, MA, USA

J.B. Leaf (ed.), *Handbook of Social Skills and Autism Spectrum Disorder*, Autism and Child Psychopathology Series, DOI 10.1007/978-3-319-62995-7_24

research for specific interventions, assessments, or outcomes of engaging in social behavior, we are going to provide 11 large themes for the readers' consideration. These themes are going to cover components that should be included within future research as well as the type of studies that would be beneficial to the treatment of ASD.

24.1 Eleven Considerations for Future Research on Social Behavior

24.1.1 In Schools and the Community

Researchers have evaluated the social behavior of individuals diagnosed with ASD and interventions to improve social behaviors in multiple settings, including clinic-based centers (e.g., Leaf et al., 2016c), the individual's community (e.g., Cheung, Schulze, Leaf, & Rudrud, 2016), university settings (e.g., Leaf et al., 2012), camps (e.g., Walker, Barry, & Bader, 2010), home settings (e.g., Kassardjian et al., 2013), and school settings (e.g., Kamps et al., 1992). It is commendable that researchers are evaluating social behavior and interventions to improve social behavior in multiple settings; this should continue to occur in the future. However, one recommendation that should be seriously considered by future researchers is to increase the number of studies that evaluate social behavior and/or interventions to target social behavior within the school setting. In the case of research that evaluates interventions to improve social behavior (e.g., research improving social behavior using video modeling), researchers should have school personnel (e.g., teachers or paraprofessionals) implement the procedures as opposed to the researcher him or herself.

We feel it is important for there to be an increase in research conducted in school settings for several reasons. First, it is the case that the majority of formal education takes place within a school setting as opposed to clinic-based centers, university-based centers, or in the community. Therefore, it would be important for researchers to evaluate social behavior and interventions to improve social behavior within settings where individuals diagnosed with ASD spend a good portion of their day. Second, schools are a natural and convenient environment to address social skills deficits, as peers are readily available. By conducting research in these settings, we may increase the likelihood of generalization of targeted skills to peers, may increase the implementation of peer-mediated interventions (see Chap. 16), may reduce bullying (see Chap. 4), and may increase friendships (see Chap. 5). Given the promise of peer-mediated interventions and the prevalence of bullying, these are important outcomes. Third, by conducting research on the effectiveness of interventions for social behavior implemented within the school setting, we will strengthen the argument for more schools utilizing these interventions. In addition, school settings have natural extraneous/confounding variables (e.g., fire drills, sick days, lots of children present) that many practitioners face in the real world. By conducting research in these settings, we can examine how effective social intervention procedures are when these real-world extraneous variables are involved.

It is true that research conducted in school settings may result in a lower level of functional control, as a result of these extraneous variables; however, that should not deter researchers (Baer, Wolf, & Risley, 1968, 1987). As long as researchers obtain meaningful and believable results, implement systematic interventions with appropriate controls, and demonstrate functional relationships, the impact of researching these procedures in more natural environments should outweigh the lower functional control. We also feel it is important for school personnel to implement the interventions during the research study, as opposed to the trained researcher(s). If the independent variable is implemented by the researcher, that person typically has a long history of implementing the intervention procedure. This history and knowledge that the researcher may have for a given intervention probably results in higher fidelity of implementation, which is not representative of what may occur in "typical" school environments. Having a teacher or paraprofessional implement the intervention(s) will enhance the generality and face validity of any study; therefore, we encourage future researchers to not only conduct research in school settings but to have the intervention be implemented by school personnel. This might also indirectly assist the field in continuing to translate the science into protocols that can be simply and reliably implemented.

For older learners, the natural extension of this recommendation is to teach these skills in natural community-based settings. For adolescents and adults, this may include broad community settings and vocational settings. In fact, these are the places where these skills will need to be demonstrated. From an efficiency perspective, instruction in these settings makes practical sense and should reduce the need for generalization training to extend the effects of intervention.

24.1.2 Training Studies

In the previous section, we highlighted the need to conduct research in community settings and to have the interventions or assessments be implemented by school/community personnel. For this to occur, school/community personnel would need to receive training on how to conduct these assessments and how to implement these different procedures. Additionally, there has been an increasing growth in the number of professionals who are working with individuals diagnosed with ASD; they too will need advanced training on how to conduct assessments and how to implement various teaching procedures. This is an area that future researchers should continue to explore.

When conducting training studies, there are a number of meaningful contributions which could be made. First, we need to continue to evaluate what are the most efficacious methods to train staff on how to conduct assessments and implement teaching procedures. Right now, behavioral skills training is widely considered to be the best way to train new staff (see Chap. 19); although this may be the case, future researchers should evaluate and compare other methods (e.g., the teaching interaction procedure, video modeling, didactic instruction) to identify if they are just as effective or efficient. Second, future researchers should carefully analyze the amount of training it takes to master intervention procedures; mastery should involve implementing the procedure with a high degree of quality and fidelity, which then results in the student learning targeted behaviors. Too many studies simply measure whether the professional can perform the steps in the task analysis, but do not measure quality of intervention or student learning rates. This would provide important parameters for how long training might take and could inform policy makers deciding how much training is necessary before someone could be considered qualified.

Third, the main measure of training should be how well the professional can implement the assessment or procedure with his or her own student or child, as opposed to how well she or he can implement the procedure during role-play scenarios with another professional. Finally, future researchers should always measure both the behavior of the person that they are training as well as what effect they are having on their students or child. The readers of the manuscript can then determine if the training led to meaningful change for the individual(s) diagnosed with ASD. Although both measures should occur, it will be imperative for future researchers to utilize the behavior of the participant who they are serving as the main dependent variable that determines when condition changes within the experimental design occur.

24.1.3 Maintenance

One important goal when teaching any student, regardless of diagnosis, is that the student will continue to display the target skill when the teacher is no longer providing the intervention or when the teacher removes portions of the intervention.

Consider the hypothetical situation where a researcher designed a well-controlled study using any of the interventions described in this book to teach a child to share his toys when a peer asked to play with those toys. During the intervention condition, the student displayed sharing during 100% of sessions across three consecutive days. The researcher then decides to place the participant in a maintenance condition and evaluates the student's sharing behavior over a 15-day period. When the researcher evaluates sharing 15 days after the intervention, the participant never appropriately displays sharing. The question arises: did the student really learn the skill? If he did learn the skill, did the acquisition of the skill actually make a meaningful change in that student's life?

Now consider another hypothetical situation where a researcher designed a well-controlled study using any of the interventions described in this book to teach a child how to join into conversations with peers. During the intervention condition, the student displays joining into a conversation during 100% of opportunities across five consecutive days. Rather than evaluating long-term maintenance in the absence of the intervention, the researcher decides to end the study. Once again, the question arises: is this a meaningful change in the student's behavior? Another question is whether the study adequately demonstrated that the intervention was effective. These two issues highlight the importance of assessing maintenance of skills that have been taught to individuals diagnosed with ASD. It is critical to assess whether a student will display the behavior after the intervention has been terminated and to assess these behaviors over a long-term maintenance period; after all, how meaningful or effective is an intervention that only results in short-term behavior change?

24.1.3.1 Including a Maintenance Condition

One issue in the literature as it relates to maintenance are the inconsistencies of inclusion of a maintenance condition; some researchers include a maintenance condition (e.g., Leaf et al., 2016c) and some elect not to include a maintenance condition (e.g., Koegel & Frea, 1993). In an eloquent study conducted by Charlop-Christy, Le, and Freeman, (2000), the authors compared video modeling to in vivo modeling for teaching life skills (e.g., brushing teeth), social play (e.g., red rover), social communication (e.g., greetings), and social emotional skills (e.g., labeling of emotions) to five children diagnosed with ASD. Targeted skills were either assigned to a video modeling condition or to an in vivo modeling condition; the only difference between the two conditions was the presentation modality of the model (i.e., via video or in vivo). The authors evaluated skill acquisition of the targeted behaviors and generalization of these behaviors to different stimuli, peers, and settings. The findings suggested that video modeling was more effective than in vivo modeling in terms of skill acquisition and generalization for the participants within this study. Although this study was well designed and positive results were obtained, there was no measure of maintenance of the targets taught within this study; lack of maintenance data was a notable limitation of this study.

Nikopoulos and Kennan, (2004) also evaluated the impact of video modeling on increasing social initiation and play for three children diagnosed with ASD. The authors measured the latency for the participants to engage in social initiation (e.g., saying "Let's Play") and mean time engaged in play (i.e., playing with the toy and experimenter). The authors used a multiple baseline design across participants to evaluate the effects of video modeling. The results showed that latency times decreased for social initiations and play increased during the intervention condition. The authors implemented a 1- and 3-month assessment of maintenance condition; the results showed that duration of play was higher than in baseline and latency for social initiations was similar to the intervention condition.

The Charlop-Christy et al. (2000) and Nikopoulos and Kennan (2004) studies are just two examples of the range of inclusion of maintenance within the research. It is our contention that, going forward, all studies that evaluate procedures to improve social behavior *must* include a maintenance condition. Without a maintenance condition, it is impossible to know if the participants will still engage in the targeted behavior following conclusion of the intervention;

without this knowledge, it would be impossible to determine if a meaningful change actually occurred.

24.1.3.2 Duration of Maintenance

A second issue in the literature as it relates to maintenance is the timing of when maintenance data is collected. There is a wide range in terms of duration of maintenance observations, from 2 weeks after intervention was terminated (e.g., Leaf et al., 2016c) to several months following intervention (e.g., Chan & O' Reilly, 2008). Although we appreciate that there is a wide range of time frames when maintenance data is collected, we encourage future researchers to be more conservative when they evaluate maintenance. It is our belief that maintenance data should be taken at least 1 month after intervention and encourage even longer delays between the end of intervention and maintenance observations (e.g., 3 months). Evaluating more long-term maintenance will help ensure that participants have indeed learned the target skills long past the time when the intervention was implemented. When researchers evaluate maintenance a few days or a few weeks after intervention has been completed, it is impossible to know if the participants would continue engaging in the targeted behaviors.

Shorter evaluations of maintenance can also lead to overrepresentation of the effectiveness of a procedure. For example, if you were to implement the Cool versus Not Cool procedure (Leaf et al., 2016c) and the results showed that the students learned the targeted social behaviors during the intervention condition and maintained these behaviors a week after intervention, consumers could be under the impression that the procedure was effective and that the procedure resulted in long-lasting behavioral change. Although this may be the case, it could also be the case that the participants did not engage in the behavior a few weeks later. Thus, it could be the case that the procedure may not be highly effective. This highlights another rationale for why researchers should evaluate maintenance long after the intervention has been terminated.

24.1.4 Social Validity

An unfortunate recent trend in the behavior analytic research is the limited number of studies that include social validity measures (Carr, Austin, Britton, Kellum, & Bailey, 1999). Social validity can be defined as "…the extent to which target behaviors are appropriate, intervention procedures are acceptable, and important and significant changes in target and collateral behaviors are produced" (Cooper, Heron, & Heward, 2007, p. 704). In 1978, Montrose Wolf urged researchers to include measures of social validity within their research measures. Wolf suggested researchers measure social validity in three distinct ways. First, researchers should measure the significance of goals. Second, Wolf stated the need to measure the appropriateness of the interventions evaluated by ensuring that the consumers found the intervention procedure(s) to be acceptable. Finally, Wolf urged researchers to measure whether consumers were satisfied with the results of the study. Wolf felt that by collecting social validity measures and, thus, ensuring that procedures and outcomes were socially valid, that applied behavior analysis (ABA) would "find its heart." Although Wolf was discussing the importance of social validity in terms of ABA specifically, including social validity measures as part of any study would be critical regardless of philosophical orientation.

Although professionals have long discussed the importance of collecting social validity measures (e.g., Fawcett, 1991; Schwartz & Baer, 1991; Wolf, 1978), recent reviews have shown that these measures have not been prevalent, at least in the behavior analytic research (Carr et al., 1999). In 1999, Carr and colleagues reported an evaluation of the percentage of studies published in the *Journal of Applied Behavior Analysis* (*JABA*) that included social validity measures. In this study, the researchers evaluated social validity collected on treatment outcome and treatment acceptability for studies published in *JABA* from 1968 to 1998. The results showed that less than 13% of articles reported social validity measures on treatment outcomes and treatment acceptability measures.

This evaluation highlights that social validity data are not included in the majority of studies published in the flagship journal for behavior analytic research. These data do not give an indication of the level of social validity that is taken in all studies that evaluate social behaviors or increasing social behaviors for individuals diagnosed with autism; nor do the data give an indication on the level of social validity measures reported in studies outside of *JABA*. Although we cannot say with certainty the level of social validity measures reported within studies that have evaluated social behaviors or increasing social behaviors for individuals diagnosed with ASD, it is safe to presume that it is a relatively low level. Another recommendation for future researchers to consider is to include social validity measures in any study that evaluates assessments on social behavior or procedures to improve social behaviors. Doing so will allow the readers of the articles to know if participants and their families were satisfied with the goals, procedures, and outcomes. This information may lead to a greater acceptance and implementation of the various assessments or procedures. It also speaks to another issue related to social validity, that how a family perceives an intervention likely influences their future use of it. To better understand familial commitment and continuance of procedures, the assessment of social validity is vital.

24.1.5 Measures of Larger Outcomes

In the past 20 years, there has been a tremendous growth in the amount of research dedicated to social behavior as it relates to ASD (Matson et al., 2007). This increase in research has led to the development of social (see Chaps. 6 and 7) and curriculum assessments (see Chap. 8), which can help identify strengths and deficits of a student and guide clinicians in identification of social behavior skills to teach. Additionally, researchers have been able to demonstrate that a variety of interventions can teach critical skills to individuals diagnosed with ASD including but not limited to joint attention (e.g., Taylor & Hoch, 2008), observational learning (e.g., DeQuinzio & Taylor, 2015), joining in (e.g., Kassardjian et al., 2013), increasing play (e.g., Koegel, Firestone, Kramme, & Dunlap, 1974), and social communication (e.g., Leaf et al., 2016b). All of this research has led to positive outcomes for individuals diagnosed with ASD and their families, for those participants within the studies whose behavior was directly impacted and for individuals who were not part of the studies.

Although the increase of research has been positive, it is important that researchers also start to evaluate larger outcomes (e.g., increased friendships, increased engagement and interest, more rapid learning rates, better clinical outcomes) that may result from teaching new social behaviors to individuals with ASD, rather than only evaluating specific target behaviors taught within a study (e.g., joint attention, observational learning, social assessments). In most studies on social behavior, data collection has focused on the specific social behaviors being taught, and not on the larger or ancillary outcomes to which these new skills may lead. Thus, we are recommending that future researchers evaluate the "little" picture (i.e., targeted behaviors) *and* the "big" picture (i.e., ancillary measures).

There are numerous examples where researchers have conducted well-designed studies but have only looked at the little picture (i.e., specific skill acquisition) as opposed to looking to the little and big picture (i.e., global indices of social functioning.). One example of this in the research is the assessment of joint attention. Joint attention is considered an important early communication skill that greatly impacts overall social and language development (Murza, Schwartz, Hahs-Vaughn, & Nye, 2016). However, the research to date has mostly evaluated methods of assessing the presence of joint attention or ways to improve joint attention (e.g., Murza et al., 2016); the research has not measured the possible larger or long-term outcomes that may result from improved joint attention (e.g., language development or social development). Thus, future researchers should evaluate the effects of assessing and teaching joint attention but also evaluate the ancillary measures as well.

The need to evaluate ancillary measures does not just apply to joint attention, but to numerous social behaviors. We do not teach observational learning just so students with ASD can learn from a peer but rather to increase the rate of learning. Yet much of the research on observational learning has focused on the increase in observational learning as opposed to accelerating the efficiency of the learning process (Plavnick & Hume, 2014). We do not teach sharing to students so they can give up their favorite items or toys, but rather teach this important behavior as it might contribute to friendship development. Yet, most of the research on sharing has only focused on evaluating sharing behavior as opposed to evaluating if sharing leads to more peer engagement or friendship development. Finally, we do not evaluate social or curriculum assessments just to identify random behaviors to teach but to determine the most meaningful skills to teach within an appropriate order (e.g., teaching prerequisite or early learning skills prior to more advanced skills) to improve learning and improve social behaviors necessary for friendship development. Without extending our assessments into the realm of ultimate outcomes, we are preventing the identification of truly efficacious strategies that result in socially significant gains.

We understand the reason why the research on these larger outcomes are lacking. These types of behaviors are not as easy to directly measure; after all, how does one measure "friendships" or "engagement?" However, we encourage researchers to develop tools to identify and measure variables of these various larger outcomes. Measuring these outcomes may be more time-consuming or result in less functional control, but researchers should not be discouraged by these challenges. We must keep in mind that the end goal of teaching social behaviors to individuals diagnosed with ASD is to help them develop meaningful relationships, not so they can engage in isolated social behaviors. Finally, by measuring these "big picture" outcomes, we will increase acceptance of our teaching practices and goals, and be perceived as having teaching technologies that change lives.

24.1.6 Older Students

Since the seminal 1987 Lovaas study that showed the tremendous outcomes that individuals with ASD can make after receiving intensive behavioral services and the pivotal book *Let Me Hear Your Voice* (Maurice, 1994), there has been an increase in the demand for early and intensive intervention. This runs parallel with the research on social behavior for individuals diagnosed with ASD in two important ways. First, there has been a general increase in the amount of research and the need for clinical intervention in this area. Second, in clinical settings and within research, most clients/participants are younger. Thus, in the majority of research, we are not evaluating social assessment, social behavior, or interventions for teenagers or adults with ASD (Reichow & Volkmar, 2010). We appreciate the need for studies on social behavior for younger students and highly encourage researchers to continue these important lines of research; however, future researchers need to place a larger emphasis on evaluating social behavior, assessments, and interventions for teenagers and adults diagnosed with ASD.

It is important that this research be conducted because the skills that a young child needs to display are vastly different than the skills a high school student needs to display, which are both immensely different from the social behaviors that adults need to display. High school students diagnosed with ASD need to learn how to resist peer pressure, understand a wide range of pop culture knowledge, learn how to talk to their "crush," and learn how to successfully navigate the complexity of the social environment. Adults diagnosed with ASD need to learn how to live with roommates in an apartment or a group home, how to engage in different social situations in the work setting, how to handle the stressors that adulthood brings to any individual's life, how to avoid being victimized, how to ensure that they are not perceived as uncooperative or unstable, how to prevent clashes with the law resulting from behavior that frightens others, and learn how to maintain various relationships.

Although there are obviously certain social behaviors that overlap with younger age children, there are a great number of social behaviors that do not overlap and need to be directly taught to older adolescents and adults diagnosed with ASD. Thus, assessments, curriculum, and intervention procedures may need to specifically address this population. There are some professionals who have started to address curriculum, assessment, and intervention to teach this population. Great examples of this are the curriculum, assessment, and procedures from: Achievement Place (Phillips, Phillips, Fixsen, & Wolf, 1974), Boys and Girls Town Model (Dowd, Czyz, O'Kane, & Elfson, 1994), the PEERS Curriculum (e.g., Laugeson, 2014), and the work of Dr. Peter Gerhardt (Gerhardt, 2016).

Several resources have been specifically created for older learners diagnosed with ASD. McGreevy and Cornwall (2012) identified essential life skills for adults diagnosed with ASD, many of which are highly relevant to social functioning, including making requests, tolerating waiting, accepting no, sharing, and turn-taking. In addition, the Assessment of Functional Living Skills (AFLS ®, 2012) focuses on assessing skills relevant to adult independence. More research needs to be done to validate these instruments as assessments, curricular road maps, and outcome measures.

For several years, experts in the field have been voicing grave concerns over adult outcomes. The National Autism Indicators Project (2015) provided data that support these concerns. Approximately half of high school students diagnosed with ASD are bullied. In addition, one-quarter of individuals diagnosed with ASD receive no support after high school, and over one-quarter of individuals diagnosed with ASD in their 20s are entirely isolated, with a total absence of social connections. Almost 40% of individuals diagnosed with ASD in their 20s do not achieve gainful employment. Clearly, the interventions that are being provided are not successful in achieving the universally hoped for life-altering gains. The outcomes related to social variables (e.g., bullying and social connection) are dismal, indicating a failure to inoculate individuals from improper treatment by others and social isolation. It is imperative that researchers identify instructional procedures to alter these outcomes.

24.1.7 Impacted Students

Not only is the research for adults underrepresented but so is the research on more highly impacted students (e.g., students who have lower language, lower cognitive skills, and high rates of aberrant behavior) diagnosed with ASD (Reichow & Volkmar, 2010). Professionals have reported that 40 to 50% of individuals with ASD have cognitive deficits (Charman et al., 2010). In addition, the diagnostic criteria for ASD includes engagement in stereotypic behavior (American Psychiatric Association, 2013). Even with the best behavioral intervention possible, at least 50% of students will not become indistinguishable (Lovaas, 1987). Thus, a good majority of individuals diagnosed with autism may have impairments that slows rates of learning social behavior. Yet, the majority of research on social behavior tends to be for "mid-functioning" to "high-functioning" individuals diagnosed with ASD (Reichow & Volkmar, 2010). Unfortunately, this does not represent what the majority of clinicians, teachers, and parents encounter each day. Therefore, future researchers should start evaluating social assessments, the social behavior, and interventions to improve social behavior for more impacted individuals diagnosed with ASD. It is especially imperative that studies include individuals who are nonvocal communicators.

It is important that this research be conducted because the skills that more impacted individuals display may be vastly different than the skills that moderately impacted or higher functioning individuals diagnosed with ASD display. For moderately impacted or high-functioning individuals, assessment questions may ask about resolving conflicts with peers, joining into the conversation, or apologizing; therefore, interventions may focus on increasing such behaviors as changing the game when someone is bored, learning to play various age appropriate games, or even partaking in social skills groups. However, more impacted students may be working on more foundational social behaviors such as tolerating the presence of other peers, eye contact, or developing a robust mand repertoire. Due to the differences in the skills that the two populations may be displaying or learning, it is important for future researchers to start evaluating assessments and procedures aimed at improving social behavior for more impacted students.

In terms of assessments, this may mean including more basic skills within the assessment and excluding more advanced social behaviors. In terms of interventions, future researchers may need to develop new methods or modify existing interventions that have already been empirically evaluated with less impacted populations. Ng, Schulze, Rudrud, and Leaf, (2016) provide a good example of modifying procedures with positive outcomes. The researchers modified the teaching interaction procedure so that it could be implemented to students who were more impacted (for a detailed description of this study, see Chap. 18). Future researchers could modify and evaluate common procedures such as discrete trial teaching (Lovaas, 1987), social skills groups (Leaf et al., 2016b), and video modeling (Kourassanis, Jones, & Fienup, 2015), to name a few. One of our goals as researchers should be to increase our understanding of and ability to effectively teach social behaviors to all individuals diagnosed with ASD, regardless of level of impact.

24.1.8 Comparative Studies

This book highlighted the numerous assessments that exist to evaluate social behavior for individuals diagnosed with ASD (see Chaps. 6, 7, and 8) as well as the numerous interventions to improve social behavior (see Chaps. 10, 11, 12, 13, 14, 15, 16, 17, 18, 19, 20, 21, 22, and 23). This book also highlighted the many possible positive outcomes, such as friendship development, that may result from children engaging in appropriate social behavior (see Chap. 5) and the negative side effects (e.g., depression or bullying) when individuals diagnosed with ASD do not have appropriate social behavior (see Chaps. 3 and 4). Although there are numerous assessments and interventions researched and available that can be implemented for individuals diagnosed with ASD, it behooves researchers and professionals to identify the most effective and efficient assessments and interventions for individuals diagnosed with ASD.

To accomplish this goal, future researchers should continue to conduct comparative analyses, which is the only means of identifying the most effective and efficient assessments and procedures. This can be done in three meaningful ways. First, researchers should continue to conduct comparative analyses that evaluate variations of a given procedure. For example, past researchers have evaluated variations of video modeling (Wilson, 2013). Conducting these types of studies will help clinicians to determine the most effective ways to implement a given procedure or under which conditions a certain variation of a procedure is best to implement.

Second, researchers should continue to conduct comparative analysis of different procedures that have an abundant amount of isolated research (e.g., Social Stories™, video modeling, script fading) already published. Researchers have already conducted many of these studies, which have compared Social Stories™ to the teaching interaction procedure (Leaf et al., 2012), Social Stories™ to video modeling (Malmberg, Charlop, & Gershfeld, 2015), and discrete trial teaching to natural environmental teaching (Jennett, Harris, & Delmolino, 2008). We encourage future researchers not only to replicate previously conducted comparative analyses but also to expand comparative analysis research to procedures that have not yet been compared (e.g., script fading compared to behavioral skills training). Conducting these types of studies will help clinicians in three ways. First, they can demonstrate that one procedure is ineffective or less effective as compared to another and, therefore, should not be implemented clinically. Second, they could also demonstrate which procedures are more efficient; while multiple procedures may be effective in teaching social behavior to individuals, it is imperative we implement procedures that are most efficient in order to maximize learning. Finally, it may be the case that results of comparative studies are idiosyncratic dependent upon various participant or target skill characteristics; it is important that researchers identify these variables so that clinicians may better identify and tailor the best intervention to utilize given their particular clinical situation.

The third area of comparative research that future researchers should consider is to compare empirically supported procedures (e.g., discrete trial teaching, behavioral skills training, video modeling) to procedures that are not empirically supported (e.g., Social Thinking®). This type of research can help further demonstrate the effectiveness of the empirically supported procedure and will either provide evidence to the effectiveness of the nonempirically supported procedure, show that the nonempirically supported procedure is equal or superior to the empirically supported procedure, or further demonstrate that the nonempirically supported procedure is not effective or not as effective as the empirically supported procedure. This can help ensure that clinicians only implement interventions that are empirically supported, scientific in nature, and are evidence based (see Chap. 9 for more on this topic).

24.1.9 Group Designs

While there are some examples of research that have evaluated assessments, social behavior, and interventions using group experimental designs (e.g., Leaf et al., 2016b), the majority of current research has been conducted using single-subject methodology. While single-subject methodology does a nice job of controlling for the various threats to internal validity and can show how the individual participants perform, it usually demonstrates weaker external validity (Campbell & Stanley, 1963) and is not as widely accepted by the larger professional community (e.g., psychology and education). So, although we place great value in using single-subject methodology, we encourage researchers to also evaluate assessments, social behavior, and interventions using group design methodology. The utilization of group designs will increase the generality of the results of the study and the likelihood that the assessments, evaluations, and interventions will be more widely accepted by the general public. Other professionals have also recommended that single-subject studies be initially utilized to demonstrate effectiveness of procedures but that researchers should then follow up on those results by evaluating those procedures within group designs (Smith, 2012; Smith et al., 2007). We are in agreement with this natural path and encourage researchers to start implementing group designs to evaluate assessments and interventions aimed at improving social behavior.

24.1.10 Progressive Model

We have advocated for clinicians and researchers to move toward a progressive model when it comes to intervention for individuals diagnosed with ASD (Leaf et al., 2016a). A hallmark of this model is that clinicians and researchers do not adhere (i.e., respond) to rigid protocols but, instead, have the flexibility to make in-the-moment decisions, responding to the student's behavior (Leaf et al., 2016a). To make these decisions, the clinician(s) or researcher(s) use clinical judgment to determine what procedures to implement, when to implement a component of the procedure, and how to implement the procedure (Leaf et al., 2016a). Researchers have demonstrated that this progressive model can be effective in terms of prompting procedures (e.g., Soluaga, Leaf, Taubman, McEachin, & Leaf, 2008), identifying reinforcers (e.g., Leaf et al., 2015), and teaching social behavior (e.g., Leaf et al., 2016b). Researchers have also shown, in comparative studies, that the progressive model can be equal to, if not superior to, a more traditional model that adheres to rigid protocols (e.g., Soluaga et al., 2008).

Although our anecdotal evidence does suggest that clinicians are starting to use the progressive model in clinical teaching, the majority of research does not represent this trend toward a more progressive model of intervention. For instance, the majority of research studies on social interventions for individuals diagnosed with ASD have adhered to rigid protocols. This could be for several reasons. First, it could be that professionals believe in or prefer to implement interventions that are more protocol driven. Second, it could be that researchers are not aware of the progressive model or have not been trained to use this type of approach. Third, it could be harder to track how the independent variable is being implemented when not following a strict protocol. Fourth, it could be that it would be harder for replication to occur since there is no strict protocol to follow and decisions are individually determined by the research team. Fifth, it could be that clinical judgment and flexibility have not yet been adequately operationally defined. Finally, it could be due to the fact that the journals have generally accepted articles that have more experimental control/rigor. Using a progressive approach, by nature, would have less experimental control/rigor (Campbell & Stanley, 1963). It should be noted that many of the early studies in ABA utilized a flexible model, at least in part, prior to the shift toward more of an emphasis on methodological rigor. Maintaining rigor and control to levels that enable confidence in findings will be essential to the efforts to further evaluate the effectiveness of more flexible and dynamic instructional approaches.

A study that highlights the use of this progressive model was conducted by Leaf et al., (2016a) when they evaluated the effects of a behaviorally based social skills group for high-functioning children diagnosed with ASD. The authors used a randomized waitlist control group to evaluate the effects of the social skills group for 15 children diagnosed with ASD. Eight of the children were assigned to a treatment group, and seven of the children were assigned to a waitlist control group. Each group received 32 sessions of intervention, with each session lasting 2 h. A blind evaluator used the Social Skill Improvement System, the Social Responsiveness Scale, the Aberrant Behavior Checklist, and the Walker McConnell to determine the effects of the intervention as well as long-term maintenance (i.e., 16-week and 32-week maintenance). The results of the study showed highly significant results as both groups improved their social behavior and maintained their social behavior after intervention had concluded.

This group followed the progressive model, as the therapists were never given any specific protocols of what interventions to implement, were not provided with any protocols of what contingency systems to use, and were not given any specific rules of what to teach any of the participants. The therapists were simply instructed to implement the best intervention possible, to teach what skills they thought were important for each of the participants to learn, to work collaboratively with parents on determining social targets, and to use their clinical judgment throughout the study. Rather than predetermine how to teach or what to teach, the authors used a post hoc analysis to determine what interventions were implemented, the contingency systems used, and the specific social behaviors that were taught. This post hoc analysis showed that a variety of teaching procedures were implemented (e.g., the teaching interaction procedure, cool vs not cool, discrete trial teaching, incidental teaching) and showed that participant behavior was reinforced at a high and even rate across the two groups and that participants were taught over 100 social behaviors within each group. The authors believe that all of these variables, including the freedom to conduct an intervention based upon a progressive model, contributed to the highly significant findings of the study.

This study highlights how effective a progressive model can be within the context of a research study. This study remains consistent with previous large experimental studies that have demonstrated that a progressive model could result in life-altering changes (e.g., Leaf et al., 2016a; Lovaas, 1987). In addition, smaller experimental studies have shown that behaviors (e.g., receptive identification, play skills, and expressive learning) can be increased when the progressive model is implemented (e.g., Soluaga et al., 2008) and is similar to clinical data that have validated that a high percentage of children with ASD who are exposed to this progressive approach can become indistinguishable from their peers (Lovaas, 1987). So, it is our hope that researchers will embrace and implement a more progressive model, to further study its effects, particularly in comparison to more traditional approaches.

24.1.11 Quality of Life

Our final recommendation has to do with the quality of life for individuals diagnosed with ASD. It is our hope that professionals get into the field of ABA and/or ASD to make a meaningful and impactful difference in individuals' lives. Professionals are not only looking to improve specific behaviors for an individual but are looking to improve that individual's overall quality of life. We encourage researchers to take quality of life into account in all future research projects.

There are three areas that could be explored to better evaluate quality of life. The easiest route would be for researchers to utilize assessments that are already published and create a battery of assessments (e.g., SRS, Vineland, SSIS) that would quantify an individual's quality of life. A second route would be for researchers to create definitions of what constitutes a high quality, moderate quality, and low quality of life and compare how scores on various assessments (e.g., SRS, Vineland, SSIS) relate to those definitions of quality of life. The goal of this second option would be to determine whether scores on these various assessments are accurate predictors of quality of life. The hardest route would be for future researchers to create a new evaluation that measures quality of life; this would entail operationally defining various aspects of a high-quality life and empirically evaluating the resulting assessment. This option would also require the gathering of normative data, by which to compare results obtained when scoring individuals diagnosed with ASD. Although this final option is the most difficult, the resulting assessment would be the most influential in the field of ASD.

For future researchers who desire to further evaluate social behavior for individuals diagnosed with ASD, we encourage a focus on operationally defining components of a high quality life and then evaluating the percentage of individuals diagnosed with ASD that would meet the definition of "high-quality life." For example, future researchers should not just evaluate if a child is getting bullied but also include correlational measures to their quality of life; thus, researchers would then show that children who are bullied have a quantitatively lower quality of life than children who are not being bullied.

For future researchers who wish to evaluate interventions to improve social behavior, there are two are as that can be further explored. First, future researchers should start selecting only skills that are meaningful and that are going to improve the individual's overall quality of life. Researchers should no longer include non-meaningful social behaviors as their dependent variables; skills should be chosen based upon improving quality of life rather than ease of behavior change. Second, researchers should start incorporating quality of life measures as part of any intervention study to determine if the quality of life of an individual improves after the intervention.

Perhaps, and most importantly, quality of life improvement needs to be directly identified as a goal, particularly for adolescents and adults. Dimensions of quality of life need to be operationally defined, measured, and targeted for change with direct interventions. Bannerman, Sheldon, Sherman, and Harchik, (1990) identified a number of ways in which individuals with disabilities were prevented from the natural rights and experiences available to those without disabilities. These authors identified several goals that still remain elusive for most service recipients. For example, while choice has received more attention in programming and in service provision, there is a dearth of choice opportunities given to most individuals diagnosed with ASD. Furthermore, many learners diagnosed with ASD still lack choice making skills. Functionality, while discussed as a goal for decades, remains woefully uncommon and underrepresented in programs and instructional outcomes. Few goals are identified with next environments in mind, and interventionists are rarely considering the value of skills selected in the context of functionality. The list of questions outlined by Lou Brown (1979) to evaluate functionality remains a call to action for program planning and for the evaluation of success. Will the learner need someone to do this for them if they do not achieve independence with it? Will the skill contact reinforcement in the natural environment that will maintain it? Does the learner need the skill now and in the future? These are crucial considerations, not only for skill building in general, but especially for the all-important area of social competence.

24.2 Conclusions

We are highly encouraged with the increasing number of studies evaluating social behavior for individuals diagnosed with ASD. It is heartening that an entire book could be dedicated to the research of social behavior for individuals diagnosed with ASD. Although we are thrilled with the increase in research on social behavior as it relates to ASD, many challenges remain. Researchers should continue to evaluate new assessments, individuals' social behaviors, and various teaching methodologies. Much more research is needed in many areas if we are to truly achieve socially significant changes in learners diagnosed with ASD. The hallmark of science is that it continues to grow, adapt, and evolve (Leaf et al., 2016a). What is discovered through research today will most likely be different than what is explored through research in just a few years. Social skills instruction may be the most volatile target that researchers in the treatment of ASD select to address. In some ways, the field is just beginning to develop a nuanced understanding of how to define, study, and change these behaviors. In addition, the field is on the precipice of defining how to best measure changes in contexts that truly matter, such as impact on independence and quality of life.

Throughout the book, the authors of various chapters provided ideas of areas of future research as it applies to the chapter's topic. In this chapter, we provided *some* themes for future research as it applies to social behavior for individuals diagnosed with ASD as a whole. Our list is not all inclusive, as there are potentially many more themes and areas that future researchers should explore. Our hope is that the ideas provided in this chapter, as well as the ideas in other chapters, will lead to exceptional growth within the research. This growth will hopefully lead to better research, assessments, evaluations, and interventions for teaching social behavior for individuals diagnosed with ASD. Ultimately, this will lead to better outcomes for individuals diagnosed with ASD and for those who live, learn, and work with them.

References

American Psychiatric Association. (2013). *Diagnostic and statistical manual of mental disorders* (5th ed.). Arlington, VA: American Psychiatric Publishing.

Baer, D. M., Wolf, M. M., & Risley, T. R. (1968). Some current dimensions of applied behavior analysis. *Journal of Applied Behavior Analysis, 1*(1), 91–97.

Baer, D. M., Wolf, M. M., & Risley, T. R. (1987). Some still-current dimensions of applied behavior analysis. *Journal of Applied Behavior Analysis, 20*(4), 313–327.

Bannerman, D. J., Sheldon, J. B., Sherman, J. A., & Harchik, A. E. (1990). Balancing the right to habilitation with the right to personal liberties: The rights of people with developmental disabilities to eat too many doughnuts and take a nap. *Journal of Applied Behavior Analysis, 23*(1), 79–89.

Baron-Cohen, S., & Wheelwright, S. (2004). The empathy quotient: An investigation of adults with Asperger syndrome or high functioning autism, and normal sex differences. *Journal of Autism and Developmental Disorders, 34*(2), 163–175.

Bauminger, N., Shulman, C., & Agam, G. (2003). Peer interaction and loneliness in high-functioning children with autism. *Journal of Autism and Developmental Disorders, 33*(5), 489–507.

Brodhed, M. T., Higbee, T. S., Gerncser, K. R., & Akers, J. S. (2016). The use of a discrimination-training procedure to teach mand variability to children with autism. *Journal of Applied Behavior Analysis, 49*(1), 34–48.

Brown, L., Branston, M. B., Hamre-Nietupski, S., Pumpian, I., & Cetro, N. (1979). A strategy for developing chronological, age-appropriate, and functional curricular content for severely handicapped adolescents and young adults. *Journal of Special Education, 13*, 81–90.

Campbell, D. T., & Stanley, J. C. (1963). *Experimental and quasiexperimental designs for research*. Boston, MA: Houghton Mifflin Company.

Carr, J. E., Austin, J. L., Britton, L. N., Kellum, K. K., & Bailey, J. S. (1999). An assessment of social validity trends in applied behavior analysis. *Behavioral Interventions*, *14*(4), 223–231.

Chan, J. M., & O' Reilly, M. F. (2008). A social stories™ intervention package for students with autism in inclusive classroom settings. *Journal of Applied Behavior Analysis*, *41*(3), 405–409.

Charlop-Christy, M. H., Le, L., & Freeman, K. A. (2000). A comparison of video modeling with in vivo modeling for teaching children with autism. *Journal of Autism and Developmental Disorders*, *30*(6), 537–552.

Charman, T., Pickles, A., Simonoff, E., Chandler, S., Loucas, T., & Baird, G. (2010). IQ in children with autism spectrum disorders: Data from the special needs and autism project (SNAP). *Psychological Medicine*, *41*(03), 619–627.

Cheung, Y., Schulze, K. A., Leaf, J. B., & Rudrud, E. (2016). Teaching community skills to two young children with autism using a digital self-managed activity schedule. *Exceptionality*, *24*(4), 241–250.

Cooper, J. O., Heron, T. E., & Heward, W. L. (2007). *Applied behavior analysis* (2nd ed.). Upper Saddle River, NJ: Pearson.

DeQuinzio, J. A., & Taylor, B. A. (2015). Teaching children with autism to discriminate the reinforced and nonreinforced response of others: Implications for observational learning. *Journal of Applied Behavior Analysis*, *48*(1), 38–51.

Dowd, T., Czyz, J. D., O'Kane, S. E., & Elfson, A. (1994). *Effective skills for child-care workers: A training manual from Boys Town*. Boys Town, NE: Boys Town Press.

Fawcett, S. B. (1991). Social validity: A note on methodology. *Journal of Applied Behavior Analysis*, *24*(2), 235–239.

Gerhardt, P. F. (2016). *Is behavior analysis meeting our obligation to adults with ASD?* Invited Paper presented at the meeting of the California Association of Behavior Analysis, Santa Clara, CA.

Hanley, G. P., Iwata, B. A., & McCord, B. E. (2003). Functional analysis of problem behavior: A review. *Journal of Applied Behavior Analysis*, *36*(2), 147–185.

Jennett, H. K., Harris, S. L., & Delmolino, L. (2008). Discrete trial instruction vs mand training for teaching children with autism to make requests. *Analysis of Verbal Behavior*, *24*(1), 69–85.

Kamps, D. M., Leonard, B. R., Vernon, S., Dugan, E. P., Delquadri, J. C., Gershon, B., … Folk, L. (1992). Teaching social skills to students with autism to increase peer interactions in an integrated first-grade classroom. *Journal of Applied Behavior Analysis*, *25*(2), 281–288.

Kassardjian, A., Taubman, M., Rudrud, E., Leaf, J. B., Edwards, A., McEachin, J., … Schulze, K. (2013). Utilizing teaching interactions to facilitate social skills in the natural environment. *Education and Training in Autism and Developmental Disabilities*, *48*(2), 245–257.

Koegel, R. L., Firestone, P. B., Kramme, K. W., & Dunlap, G. (1974). Increasing spontaneous play by suppressing self-stimulation in autistic children. *Journal of Applied Behavior Analysis*, *7*(4), 521–528.

Koegel, R. L., & Frea, W. D. (1993). Treatment of social behavior in autism through the modification of pivotal social skills. *Journal of Applied Behavior Analysis*, *26*(3), 369–377.

Kourassanis, J., Jones, E. A., & Fienup, D. M. (2015). Peer-video modeling: Teaching chained social game behaviors to children with ASD. *Journal of Developmental and Physical Disabilities*, *27*(1), 25–36.

Laugeson, E. A. (2014). *The peers curriculum for school-based professionals: Social skills training for adolescents with autism spectrum disorder*. London: Routledge.

Leaf, J. B., Leaf, R., Alcalay, A., Leaf, J. A., Ravid, D., Dale, S., … Oppenheim-Leaf, M. (2015). Utility of formal preference assessments for individuals diagnosed with autism spectrum disorder. *Education and Training in Autism and Developmental Disabilities*, *50*(2), 199–212.

Leaf, J. B., Leaf, R., McEachin, J., Taubman, M., Ala'i-Rosales, S., Ross, R. K., … Weiss, M. J. (2016a). Applied behavior analysis is a science and, therefore, progressive. *Journal of Autism and Developmental Disorders*, *46*(2), 720–731.

Leaf, J. B., Leaf, J. A., Milne, C., Taubman, M., Oppenheim-Leaf, M., Torres, N., … Yoder, P. (2016b). An evaluation of a behaviorally based social skills group for individuals diagnosed with autism spectrum disorder. *Journal of Autism and Developmental Disorder*, *47*(2), 243–259.

Leaf, J. B., Mitchell, E., Townley-Cochran, D., McEachin, J., Taubman, M., & Leaf, R. (2016c). Comparing social stories™ to cool versus not cool. *Education and Treatment of Children*, *39*(2), 173–186.

Leaf, J. B., Oppenheim-Leaf, M. L., Call, N. A., Sheldon, J. B., Sherman, J. A., Taubman, M., … Leaf, R. (2012). Comparing the teaching interaction procedure to social stories for people with autism. *Journal of Applied Behavior Analysis*, *45*(2), 281–298.

Lovaas, O. I. (1987). Behavioral treatment and normal educational and intellectual functioning in young autistic children. *Journal of Consulting and Clinical Psychology*, *55*(1), 3–9.

Malmberg, D. B., Charlop, M. H., & Gershfeld, S. J. (2015). A two experiment treatment comparison study: Teaching social skills to children with autism spectrum disorder. *Journal of Developmental and Physical Disabilities*, *27*(3), 375–392.

Maurice, C. (1994). *Let me hear your voice: A family's triumph over autism*. New York, NY: Ballantine Books.

McGreevy, F., & Cornwall. (2012). *Essential for living: A communication, behavior, and functional skills assessment, curriculum, and teaching manual*. Orlando, FL: Pat McGreevy & Associates.

Matson, J. L., Mastson, M. L., & Rivet, T. T. (2007). Social-skills treatments for children with autism spectrum disorders: An overview. *Behavior Modification, 31*(5), 682–707.

Murza, K. A., Schwartz, J. B., Hahs-Vaughn, D. L., & Nye, C. (2016). Joint attention interventions for children with autism spectrum disorder: A systematic review and meta-analysis. *International Journal of Language and Communication Disorders, 51*(3), 236–251.

Ng, A. H. S., Schulze, K., Rudrud, E., & Leaf, J. B. (2016). Using the teaching interactions procedure to teach social skills to children with autism and intellectual disability. *American Journal on Intellectual and Developmental Disabilities, 121*(6), 501–519.

Nikopoulos, C. K., & Kennan, M. (2004). Effects of video modeling on social initiations by children with autism. *Journal of Applied Behavior Analysis, 37*(1), 93–96.

Phillips, E. L., Phillips, E. A., Fixsen, D. L., & Wolf, M. M. (1974). *The teaching-family handbook* (2nd ed.). Lawrence, KS: University Press of Kansas.

Plavnick, J. B., & Hume, K. A. (2014). Observational learning by individuals with autism: A review of teaching strategies. *Autism, 18*(4), 458–466.

Reichow, B., & Volkmar, F. R. (2010). Social skills interventions for individuals with autism: Evaluation for evidence-based practices within a best evidence synthesis framework. *Journal of Autism and Developmental Disorders, 40*(2), 149–166.

Schwartz, I. S., & Baer, D. M. (1991). Social validity assessments: Is current practice state of the art? *Journal of Applied Behavior Analysis, 24*(2), 215–230.

Smith, T. (2012). Evolution of research on interventions for individuals with autism spectrum disorder: Implications for behavior analysts. *The Behavior Analyst, 35*(1), 101–113.

Smith, T., Scahill, L., Dawson, G., Guthrie, D., Lord, C., Odom, S., … Wagner, A. (2007). Designing research studies on psychosocial interventions in autism. *Journal of Autism and Developmental Disorders, 37*(2), 354–366.

Soluaga, D., Leaf, J. B., Taubman, M., McEachin, J., & Leaf, R. (2008). A comparison of flexible prompt fading and constant time delay for five children with autism. *Research in Autism Spectrum Disorders, 2*(4), 753–765.

Taylor, B. A., & Hoch, H. (2008). Teaching children with autism to respond to an initiate bids for joint attention. *Journal of Applied Behavior Analysis, 41*(3), 377–391.

Walker, A. N., Barry, T. D., & Bader, S. H. (2010). Therapist and parent ratings of changes in adaptive social skills following a summer treatment camp for children with autism spectrum disorders: A preliminary study. *Child and Youth Care Forum, 39*(5), 305–322.

Wilson, K. P. (2013). Teaching social-communication skills to preschoolers with autism: Efficacy of video versus in vivo modeling in the classroom. *Journal of Autism and Developmental Disorders, 43*(8), 1819–1831.

Wolf, M. M. (1978). Social validity: The case for subjective measurement or how applied behavior analysis is finding its heart. *Journal of Applied Behavior Analysis, 11*(2), 203–214.

25 Future Directions for Clinical Social Skills Interventions

Mitchell Taubman and Julia L. Ferguson

It was not too long ago that the empirical and clinical social skill interventional landscape, for persons on the autism spectrum, was relatively barren (Matson, Matson, & Rivet, 2007; Taubman, Leaf, & McEachin, 2011). Social skills training or treatment practices with little empirical basis existed (e.g., Gray & Garand, 1993; Greenspan, 1992). However, in addition to these approaches having little empirical support for their effectiveness, lack of research often also meant that their clinical implementation lacked methodological consistency; they were variable in their approach to treatment and often heavily influenced by the prowess and style of the practitioner. Social skill groups for persons on the autism spectrum have been around for a long time (Mesibov, 1984; Williams, 1989). But, in clinical and educational practice, such groups mainly provide guided or led social lessons, opportunities, and experiences with little programming involved, and little research behind them (Kalyva & Avramidis, 2005; White, Keonig, & Scahill, 2007).

Research and practice of applied behavior analysis (ABA) in the social area was relatively limited as well. Research and intervention were typically focused on other areas (e.g., communication, behavior difficulties; Sundberg & Michael 2001; Iwata, Dorsey, Slifer, Bauman, & Richman, 1982/1994), and what did exist, treatment or training-wise, was often clunky and artificial. These ABA interventions typically focused on such social targets and protocols as eye contact (e.g., Foxx, 1977), handshakes (e.g., Tse, Strulovitch, Tagalaskis, Meng, & Fombonne, 2007), scripted conversations (e.g., Charlop & Milstein, 1989), and directed social initiations (e.g., Odom, Hoyson, Jamieson, & Strain, 1985).

In recent times, this has begun to change. The research covered in this book represents that change. Chapters within this work represent expansions in methodology (e.g., Cihon, Weinkauf, & Taubman, 2017; Ellingson, Bolton, & Laugeson, 2017; Weiss, Hilton, & Russo, 2017), broadening of social targets (e.g., Bauminger-Zviely & Kimhi, 2017), and results that represent meaningful social growth in naturalistic settings (e.g., Ala'i-Rosales, Toussaint & McGee, 2017; Ellingson et al., 2017; Vernon, 2017), all which demonstrate the field's progression in the area of social skills intervention for people diagnosed with autism spectrum disorder (ASD). With this growth, it is anticipated that similar progress will be witnessed in the clinical application arena. This chapter then, is focused on important matters for future inclusion and consideration in clinical interventions, and applied research for that matter, in the social area for persons on the autism spectrum. We will look

M. Taubman (✉) • J.L. Ferguson
Autism Partnership, Seal Beach, CA, USA
e-mail: mtautpar@aol.com

J.B. Leaf (ed.), *Handbook of Social Skills and Autism Spectrum Disorder*, Autism and Child Psychopathology Series, DOI 10.1007/978-3-319-62995-7_25

at the need for authenticity and meaningfulness in social skills work, focus upon social interest and desire, address the challenges of supporting friendship development, spend a little time on curricular issues, examine some issues pertaining to social skills groups, cover what may be the most important consideration of all in social skill clinical intervention, generalization (i.e., the transfer of learning from clinical arrangements to independent usage in natural everyday social situations), and finally consider the risks of unsupported interventions.

25.1 Authenticity

Interventionists in the field of ABA are rightly concerned that they deal with phenomena that can be objectively measured and with procedures that are empirically supported, replicable, and which can also be objectively assessed (Baer, Wolf, & Risley, 1968, 1987). Like much in the field of ABA, the absoluteness of these concerns and what this means in regard to actual practice is the subject of debate. That debate is beyond the scope of this chapter, but, suffice it to say that the issues involved are particularly relevant to the social domain in relation to ASD.

Social skills interventions that involve adherence to strict procedural protocols (as opposed to the use of clinical judgment, see below), targets that are largely selected because they can be easily objectified (as opposed to their social validity; that is, their meaningfulness and genuineness), and outcomes that are largely performance oriented (as opposed to the independent assimilation and employment of skills that are driven by social desire and intent) tend to result in limited social benefit (Wolf, 1978). Peers of individuals with autism have no difficulty identifying social behavior that is rigid, canned, and inauthentic (Cappadocia, Weiss, & Pepler, 2011; Hebron & Humphrey, 2014). Such responding impedes interactions, interferes with relationship development, and precludes the building of real friendships. Why teach social actions that, except for the most perfunctory of social situations, have little social benefit? And why direct individuals to engage in such social actions when there is little in the way of natural consequences for them? That is, when social behavior is largely just under instructional control in the absence of developing social desire and drive, then they will not be maintained by drive fulfillment, and are not likely to result in successful, maintaining true social outcomes.

Clinical interventions that involve rigid adherence to formulaic protocols, in the name of ABA science, tend to produce limited, rote, and stiff responding in the learners. In the social world, especially the young social world, in which flow, variability, and style are so prominent, such responding appears odd at best and paradoxically defeats the entire purpose of social skills intervention. On the other hand, much research now demonstrates the benefit of ABA intervention that includes clinical judgment; that is, assessment and decision-making in the moment (Leaf et al., 2016a; Leaf et al., 2016b; Leaf et al., 2017; Soluaga, Leaf, Tabuman, McEachin, & Leaf, 2008). Such work involves clinical finesse and training for the practitioner beyond the mere assimilation of ABA knowledge and learning of basic methodologies. However, that form of intervention is particularly suited to social skills treatment in all its variability and subtlety (e.g., Leaf et al., 2017).

Such flexible and progressive ABA also involves the development of social drive or interest (i.e., the building of the social reinforcement value of peers) and the infusing of social skills training with that social drive and intent. This means that skills that are meaningful and that will produce social benefit are taught. In addition, it means that they are taught in a manner that accentuates and will result in the achievement of that valued social benefit (Fawcett, 1991; Wolf, 1978). For example, in such a progressive approach, social initiations are not taught by directing the individual with ASD to ask a friend to play, but by establishing operations or social temptations (i.e., situations in which reinforcing activities are enhanced or enabled by the participation of a peer) much in the way independent communicative initiations and communicative intent are promoted by communication temptations (Leaf & McEachin, 1999, p. 199). With such an approach, not only would spontaneous social initiations be promoted but also social intent would be built as well. Although, also requiring additional effort and skill, complicated, nuanced, and genuine social skill targets can certainly be operationalized and objectively measured.

With a focus on meaningfulness and authenticity, future clinical interventions that are based on empirically supported principals and methodologies can provide social skills that will stand up to peer scrutiny and will provide the foundation for building relationships and genuine friendships. Such clinical intervention will also have the consumer appeal of other, nonempirically based approaches in that it will capture the social essence of interpersonal competencies. Other nonempirically based approaches to building social competencies do a good job of attempting to pursue social growth, that is in essence, social. They often have broad consumer appeal as a result. However, they lack the empirically supported methodologies that will result in actual success (National Autism Center, 2009, 2015). A progressive, yet systematic, ABA clinical approach, based on, but not conducted as if research, can be appealing and produce effective yet socially valid outcomes (Leaf et al., 2016c; Leaf, Dotson, Oppenheim-Leaf, Sherman, & Sheldon, 2012).

25.2 Social Desire

As noted previously, developing and promoting the reinforcing value of peers is often an essential part of clinical intervention for persons with ASD. Too often, such work is insufficiently addressed in clinical work. Some young people with ASD have some social interest in peers, whereas others may show interest in or affection for adults (other than relatives) but less for peers. Building social desire for peers typically cannot follow the same blueprint as establishing social desire for adults (e.g., through being sources of support, assistance, teaching, and direct reinforcement). Otherwise, peers become junior therapists, which is not a platform for developing typical social interaction skills or building reciprocal relationships. Appreciation for peers is a different matter. To have reinforcement value, peers need to be experienced as activity and situation (and ultimately life) enhancing. They must amplify the positive and diminish the negative. For some individuals with ASD that may mean something complicated and sophisticated (e.g., others seen as a source of camaraderie, companionship, affection, and intimate conversation). For others, it may mean something more simple (e.g., that leisure pursuit is enhanced by someone else's presence and participation). In either case, and in all cases in between, peers are valued and important.

Future clinical work, simultaneous to social and relationship skill development, will need to focus on the establishment of social drive and intent of individuals with ASD. As mentioned previously, similar to how establishing operation/communication temptation effort is intended to promote not only spontaneous communication but also communicative intent (Leaf & McEachin, 1999), work needs to be similarly directed at building independent, spontaneous social initiations, and social intent. Future clinical effort should be directed at building social interest through association of peers with reinforcing activities, pursuits, and experiences. It would also involve establishing the enhancing nature and/or essential necessity of peers' involvement in such experiences. Shared excitement, cooperative, competitive, and interactive types of highly pleasurable experiences have been effective in this regard and would certainly be feasible in clinical settings (e.g., Leaf et al., 2017).

With clinical work directed at building social desire, greater authenticity through natural drive is lent to social skills instruction. Social skills engaged in for social reasons feel, and are, genuine. Building social interest can be facilitative to motivational efforts and the reduction of aberrant responding, as concern for reputation can be an outgrowth. Social interest and desire can also be an important ingredient in the development of higher social capacities, such as genuine empathy, caring, and consideration (see below). Further, with social interest, relationship and friendship efforts can be genuinely pursued. Inclusion of systematic efforts directed at building social interest, just as with the inclusion of reinforcer development in any ABA clinical program is essential. Clinicians would be well advised to more heavily emphasize such efforts in the future.

25.3 Friendships

In the literature, much attention has been paid to speculation on the essential ingredients for friendship development. Factors that have been identified as important elements of friendships include common interests and activities, consistent contact, overlapping or shared enjoyment, experiences or knowledge, pleasant regard, emotional support, physical attraction, commitment, trust, desire for and anticipation of contact, opportunity for enhanced experience or personal growth, and, most consistently, reciprocity (Taubman, Rafuse, Leaf, & Leaf, 2011).

Too often, in clinical work, peer helpers, classroom acquaintances, guided confederates, and relatives are considered and referred to as friends. Unfortunately, such relationships, while of importance, do not provide the value obtained from friendships for persons on the autism spectrum. Research has illustrated the significance of genuine friendships in the lives of those with ASD (Bauminger & Kasari, 2000; Bauminger, Solomon, & Rogers, 2010) as well as the risks associated with the absence of these significant relationships (Cappadocia, Weiss, & Pepler, 2011; Hebron & Humphrey, 2014). Future clinical work will need to emphasize specific skills necessary for authentic friendship development as well as strategies and processes for facilitating the emergence of such reciprocal relationships.

The attributes and nature of the parties involved in a friendship often determine the skills necessary for the friendship to build and maintain. However, some of the following skills, in addition to the general building of social competencies and desire, represent abilities on a continuum from basic to sophisticated that are often helpful to such relationships. These include listening, acknowledging, and being responsive to the other person; knowing and anticipating the other's likes, choices, and preferences; some level of reciprocal and open communication; gestures and actions that appropriately convey respect and appreciation and, in more complex friendships, thoughtfulness; abilities necessary to engage in common or shared interests and activities; capacity and skills for compromise; assertion skills; and for some more sophisticated friendships, higher order capacities, such as caring, consideration, empathy, and altruism (Berndt, 2002; Taubman et al., 2011). Given the capabilities of the learner and the potential complexity of his or her future friendships, future clinical interventions will need to increasingly focus on some of these skills, or others as indicated, and at fitting levels of sophistication.

In addition to individual skill development, future clinical directions will need to include the development of resources for bringing individuals on the autism spectrum together. These might be clubs and groups (beyond social skills groups) that have interest, leisure, and/or recreational components but also include elements of systematic interventional effort. With such resources, opportunities will be increased for possible matches and candidates for potential reciprocal relationships. In such arrangements, repeated exposure and contact, at times necessary for friendships to build, will also be furnished. Further, chances for instructional and facilitative work for skill and relationship development in dyad and group contexts will also be enhanced. In future clinical work, interventionists will do well to remember that relationships generally cannot be forced, and that development of friendships requires a balance of orchestration on the one hand, and on the other hand, respect for the need for the process to play out on its own.

25.4 Curricula

Though several social skills curricula for persons with ASD are currently available (e.g., Rogers & Dawson, 2010; Laugeson, 2014; Taubman et al., 2011; Prizant, Wetherby, Rubin,

Laurent, & Rydell, 2006), they are still relatively limited in number. It would be hoped that in the future, clinicians will develop and share curricula that have been successfully employed. Until such curricula can be empirically validated, compiled, and published, online accumulations of such material would be extremely useful for clinical intervention. Though instructional content in the social area often needs to be distinctly individualized, the larger the amount of curricular material amassed, the more likely that, at least, a similar curriculum will have already been developed. Further, the larger the number of curricula in the compilation, the greater the exemplars.

Future social curricula, no matter the nature or form, will need to address the extremely broad range of social needs found in ASD. And as noted above, it will need to include meaningful, natural, and authentic targets (Brown et al., 1979). Clinically oriented curricula should also include guidance on facilitating higher order social capacities, such as caring, consideration, altruism, and empathy. Clinical settings are perfect for work, which may be less traditionally instructional in nature and designed more for fostering such capacities. Respondent oriented strategies are well suited for such settings and could result in genuine capacity growth, as affect is so centrally and critically involved.

25.5 Social Skills Groups

Recent research has shown the power of programmatic ABA social skills groups for persons with ASD (Laugeson, Gantman, Kapp, Orenski, & Ellingson, 2015; Leaf et al., 2017). This would contrast with the customary educational or clinical social skills groups, which typically provides whole group lessons on social topics (often discussions or worksheets), mere facilitation of social behaviors, and exposure to adult-guided social experiences (e.g., Koning, Magill-Evans, Volden, & Dick, 2013). A major challenge for social groups for persons with ASD in the future will be to ensure that they consist of systematic instructional efforts. This would mean that assessments of individual social needs are conducted, individualized and group curricula and lessons are developed, and teaching on the instructional content proceeds in a deliberate, progressive manner. Only in this way will clinical social skills groups do more than just look and seem social, and instead will actually provide effective instruction in social competencies (Leaf et al., 2016c).

Further, another future challenge to social skills groups is that they find their balance. For example, groups must be part fun and part program, part planned and part capturing teachable moments, part behavior problem oriented and part socially focused, part about group goals and part concerned with differentiated instruction, and part facilitator led and part limited adult involvement. In the future, clinicians should look to more thoroughly examining and assessing the individual social needs of the participants in order to determine the proportions of the various parts that will form the content and individual personality of any group. Such analysis will also shape the individual and overall objectives of the group. The clinical assessment should be an ongoing matter as the group evolves as a cohort and with the social growth of its participants.

It is also hoped that some social skills groups will be tailored to the common needs of participants. This would mean greater growth of specialized clinical groups, such as social awareness and observational learning groups for more heavily impacted individuals, friendship groups, dating groups, and interacting with coworker groups. Appropriately, social skills groups are the main vehicles for clinical social skills work for persons with ASD. Increasing their clinical substance and focus will only add to service delivery in this critical area.

25.6 Generalization

Generalization is perhaps the greatest challenge for intervention in the social skills domain for persons with ASD, clinical, or otherwise. ABA is by nature about changing environments to teach and support adaptive behaviors (Bear et al., 1968, 1987). Through structure, behavior programming, and formalized instructional techniques, learning and growth occur (Lovaas, 1987; Lovaas, Koegel, Simmons, & Long, 1973; Wolf, Risley, & Mees, 1964). Paradoxically, the more structured, formal, and precise the technique and approach, the more the intervention is removed from what occurs naturally. This is particularly problematic in the social skills area, in which the independent employment of skills in everyday natural environments is essentially everything. Too often, in the clinical world, it is noted that an individual does well in one-to-one social intervention or has shown great growth in controlled social skills groups, but that such improvements are much less evident outside of those settings (Strain & Fox, 1981). Too often, the solution devised by clinicians is getting the outside environment (e.g., home, play dates) to include as much structure and program, like the intervention, as possible. This helps transfer some of the changes to some circumstances outside of therapy, but does little to move change to natural, unprogrammed social situations.

Certainly, by following some of the recommendations in this chapter, generalization will be facilitated for the clinician. That is, by focusing on the development of consumers' social interest and desire, individualizing curriculum, addressing independent performance of meaningful targets, and promoting authenticity, generalization will be promoted. However, this will likely not be enough. Future clinical work must be directed at bringing skills into the natural environment in a systematic manner (Stokes & Baer, 1977). This does not only mean insuring that change occurs in multiple environments or across different people. It means that overtime, intervention becomes looser, less structured, and less formal. It means that personal and programmatic stimulus control, which had been so painstakingly built, has to be gradually faded and eliminated. This would include the fading of small but discriminable differences between interventions, including groups and natural social situations. It will also mean that external motivation arrangements are faded as natural consequences are experienced (e.g., through the acquisition of social success promoting competencies and the enhancement of their reinforcing value through social interest development). Such efforts at gradually blurring the many distinctions between interventional arrangements and the natural social world need to be as systematic as the instructional efforts themselves. Otherwise, social skills growth will largely remain the exclusive province of the environments that produce them, namely interventional arrangements and settings.

25.7 A Final Word about Social Skill Clinical Interventions

As noted at the beginning of this chapter, there is more attention being paid to intervention in the social skills area then has previously been the case. This means that a variety of approaches are currently available (e.g., Ala'i-Rosales et al., 2017; Ayres, Traves, Shepley, & Cagliani, 2017; Cassagrande & Ingersoll, 2017; Cihon et al., 2017; Ellingson et al., 2017; Higbee & Sellers, 2017; Kamps, Mason, & Heitzman-Powell, 2017; Miltenberger, Zerger, Novotny, & Livingston, 2017; Rogers, Vivanti, & Rocha, 2017; Ross, 2017; Vernon, 2017; Weiss et al., 2017), and others are likely to arise in the future. As noted previously, many have little to no empirical support (Freeman, 2008; National Autism Center, 2009, 2015), and, typically, limited logic or common sense behind them. That is, often there is little reason, including empirically supported reasons, to believe that anyone, let alone someone with ASD with his or her challenges in the area, could acquire social skills in such a manner. What these approaches have, and will likely have in the future, is curb appeal. They often present straightforward, easy to use, relatively brief procedures that are often fun and attractive to consumers. They also conceptualize social skills and capture social phenomena in a manner that feels authentically social. As mentioned previously, this is often lacking in stiff, limited ABA social interventions. However, like miracle cures for weight loss or chemical addiction, there are currently no easy or magical treatments for social skill deficits for individuals with ASD. Any product, device, or approach that appears to be such should be treated with immediate skepticism.

We have witnessed many ABA clinical providers utilizing these unsupported approaches. This is surprising, not only because of the lack of empirical evidence behind the interventions but also because the approaches are at odds with the principles of learning and human behavior underlying ABA. They are also inconsistent with the procedural foundations of ABA as we have come to know them; that is, painstakingly careful, systematic instructional and programmatic effort is necessary for people with ASD to learn and grow. There are indications that behavior interventionists may offer such unsupported services only as long as they make it clear they are not doing so under the auspices of their certification. To us, this would make as much sense as a licensed practitioner trained in the medical sciences deciding to offer voodoo on "Witch Doctor" Thursdays. ABA is not only a set of procedures. It is a set of underlying principles, a concept base, and an ideology of human behavior, human development, intervention, and treatment.

We heavily recommend that those clinicians who desire to provide effective social skills intervention for those with ASD avoid unsupported approaches. This book provides many empirically based and supported interventions. Utilizing a behavior analytic approach in clinical practice, that is authenticity driven, and infused with meaningful goals that are purposefully transferred to independent usage in everyday life, will satisfy clients and consumers and most importantly, effectively enhance the social lives and relationships of persons with ASD.

References

Ala'i-Rosales, S., Toussaint, K. A., & McGee, G. (2017). Incidental teaching: Happy progress. In J. B. Leaf (Ed.), *The handbook of social skills and autism spectrum disorder: Assessment, curricula, and intervention* (pp. 360–396). New York, NY: Springer.

Ayres, K. M., Travers, J., Shepley, S. B., & Cagliani, R. (2017). Video based instruction for learners with autism. In J. B. Leaf (Ed.), *The handbook of social skills and autism spectrum disorder: Assessment, curricula, and intervention* (pp. 480–519). New York, NY: Springer.

Baer, D. M., Wolf, M. M., & Risley, T. R. (1968). Some current dimensions of applied behavior analysis. *Journal of Applied Behavior Analysis, 1*(1), 91–97.

Baer, D. M., Wolf, M. M., & Risley, T. R. (1987). Some still current dimensions of applied behavior analysis. *Journal of Applied Behavior Analysis, 20*(4), 313–327.

Bauminger, N., & Kasari, C. (2000). Loneliness and friendship in high-functioning children with autism. *Child Development, 71*(2), 447–456.

Bauminger, N., Solomon, M., & Rogers, S. J. (2010). Predicting friendship quality in autism spectrum disorders and typical development. *Journal of Autism and Developmental Disorders, 40*(6), 751–761.

Bauminger-Zviely, N., & Kimhi, Y. (2017). Friendship in ASD. In J. B. Leaf (Ed.), *The handbook of social skills and autism spectrum disorder: Assessment, curricula, and intervention* (pp. 147–176). New York City: Springer.

Berndt, T. J. (2002). Friendship quality and social development. *Current Directions in Psychological Science, 11*(1), 7–10.

Brown, L., Branston-McClean, M. B., Baumgart, D., Vincent, L., Falvey, M., & Schroeder, J. (1979). Using the characteristics of current and subsequent least restrictive environments in the development of curricular content for severely handicapped students. *Research and Practice for Persons with Severe Disabilities, 4*(4), 407–424.

Cappadocia, M. C., Weiss, J. A., & Pepler, D. (2011). Bullying experiences among children and youth with autism spectrum disorders. *Journal of Autism and Developmental Disorders, 42*(2), 266–277.

Casagrande, K. A., & Ingersoll, B. R. (2017). Parent-mediated interventions for social communication in young children with ASD. In J. B. Leaf (Ed.), *The handbook of social skills and autism spectrum disorder: Assessment, curricula, and intervention* (pp. 611–663). New York City: Springer.

Charlop, M. H., & Milstein, J. P. (1989). Teaching autistic children conversational speech using video modeling. *Journal of Applied Behavior Analysis, 22*(3), 275–285.

Cihon, J. H., Weinkauf, S. M., & Taubman, M. T. (2017). The teaching interaction procedure. In J. B. Leaf (Ed.), *The handbook of social skills and autism spectrum disorder: Assessment, curricula, and intervention* (pp. 664–687). New York, NY: Springer.

Ellingson, R., Bolton, C., & Laugeson, E. (2017). Evidence-based social skills groups for individuals with autism spectrum disorder across the lifespan. In J. B. Leaf (Ed.), *The handbook of social skills and autism spectrum disorder: Assessment, curricula, and intervention* (pp. 729–766). New York, NY: Springer.

Fawcett, S. B. (1991). Social validity: A note on methodology. *Journal of Applied Behavior Analysis, 24*(2), 235–239.

Foxx, R. M. (1977). Attention training: The use of overcorrection avoidance to incresase the eye contact of autistic and retarded children. *Journal of Applied Behavior Analysis, 10*(3), 489–499.

Freeman, B. J. (2008). Alternative treatments for autism spectrum disorders: What is the science? In R. Leaf, M. Taubman, & J. McEachin (Eds.), *Sense and nonsense in the behavioral treatment of autism: It has to be said* (pp. 63–104). New York: DRL Books.

Gray, C. A., & Garand, J. D. (1993). Social stories: Improving responses of students with autismwith accurate social information. *Focus on Autistic Behavior, 8*, 1–10.

Greenspan, S. I. (1992). *Infancy and early childhood: The practice of clinical assessment and intervention with emotional and developmental challenges*. Madison, CT: International Universities Press.

Hebron, J., & Humphrey, N. (2014). Exposure to bullying among students with autism spectrum conditions: A multi-informant analysis of risk and protective factors. *Autism, 18*(6), 618–630.

Higbee, T. S., & Sellers, T. P. (2017). Visual learning strategies to promote independence and appropriate social behavior. In J. B. Leaf (Ed.), *The handbook of social skills and autism spectrum disorder: Assessment, curricula, and intervention* (pp. 520–556). New York, NY: Springer.

Iwata, B. A., Dorsey, M. F., Slifer, K. J., Bauman, K. E., & Richman, G. S. (1982). Toward a functional analysis of self-injury. *Analysis and Intervention in Developmental Disabilities, 2*(1), 3–20.

Iwata, B. A., Dorsey, M. F., Slifer, K. J., Bauman, K. E., & Richman, G. S. (1994). Toward a functional analysis of self-injury. *Journal of Applied Behavior Analysis, 27*(2), 197–209.

Kalyva, E., & Avramidis, E. (2005). Improving communication between children with autism and their peers through the 'circle of friends': A small-scale intervention study. *Journal of Applied Research in Intellectual Disabilities, 18*(3), 253–261.

Kamps, D. M., Mason, R., & Heitzman-Powell, L. (2017). Peer mediation interventions to imporve social and communication skills for children and youth with autism spectrum disorders. In J. B. Leaf (Ed.), *The handbook of social skills and autism spectrum disorder: Assessment, curricula, and intervention* (pp. 557–610). New York, NY: Springer.

Koning, C., Magill-Evans, J., Volden, J., & Dick, B. (2013). Efficacy of cognitive behavior therapy-based social skills intervention for school-aged boys with autism spectrum disorders. *Research in Autism Spectrum Disorders, 7*(10), 1282–1290.

Laugeson, E. A. (2014). *The PEERS curriculum for school based professionals: Social skills training for adolescents with autism spectrum disorder*. New York: Routledge.

Laugeson, E. A., Gantman, A., Kapp, S. K., Orenski, K., & Ellingsen, R. (2015). A randomized controlled trial to improve social skills in young adults with autism spectrum disorder: The UCLA PEERS® program. *Journal of Autism and Developmental Disorders, 45*(12), 1–12.

Leaf, J. B., Dotson, W. H., Oppenheim-Leaf, M. L., Sherman, J. A., & Sheldon, J. B. (2012). A programmatic description of a social skills group for young children with autism. *Topics in Early Childhood Special Education, 32*(2), 111–121.

Leaf, J. B., Leaf, J. A., Alcalay, A., Kassardjian, A., Tsuji, K., … Leaf, R. (2016a). Comparison of most-to-least prompting to flexible prompt fading for children with autism spectrum disorder. *Exceptionality, 24*(2), 109–122.

Leaf, J. B., Leaf, R., Leaf, J. A., Alcalay, A., Ravid, D., Dale, S., … Oppenheim-Leaf, M. L. (2016b). *Comparing paired-stimulus preference assessments with in-the-moment reinforcer analysis on skill acquisition: A preliminary investigation.* Focus on Autism and Other Developmental Disabilities. Advance online publication.

Leaf, J. B., Leaf, R., McEachin, J., Taubman, M., Ala'i-Rosales, S., Ross, R. K., … Weiss, M. J. (2016c). Applied behavior analysis is a science and, therefore, progressive. *Journal of Autism and Developmental Disorders, 46*(2), 720–731.

Leaf, J. B., Leaf, J. A., Milne, C., Taubman, M., Oppenheim-Leaf, M., Torres, N., … Yoder, P. (2017). An evaluation of a behaviorally based social skills group for individuals diagnosed with autism spectrum disorder. *Journal of Autism and Developmental Disorders, 47*(2), 243–259.

Leaf, R., & McEachin, J. (1999). *A work in progress: Behavior management strategies and a curriculum for intensive behavioral treatment of autism*. New York: DRL.

Lovaas, O. I. (1987). Behavioral treatment and normal educational and intellectual functioning in young autistic children. *Journal of Consulting and Clinical Psychology, 55*(1), 3–9.

Lovaas, O. I., Koegel, R., Simmons, J. Q., & Long, J. S. (1973). Some generalization and follow-up measures on autistic children in behavior therapy. *Journal of Applied Behavior Analysis, 6*(1), 131–165.

Matson, J. L., Matson, M. L., & Rivet, T. T. (2007). Social-skills treatments for children with autism spectrum disorders: An overview. *Behavior Modification, 31*(5), 682–707.

Mesibov, G. B. (1984). Social skills training with verbal autistic adolescents and adults: A program model. *Journal of Autism and Developmental Disorders, 14*(4), 395–404.

Miltenberger, R. G., Zerger, H. M., Novotny, M., & Livingston, C. P. (2017). Behavior skills training to promote social behavior of individuals with autism. In J. B. Leaf (Ed.), *The handbook of social skills and autism spectrum disorder: Assessment, curricula, and intervention* (pp. 688–728). New York, NY: Springer.

National Autism Center. (2009). *National Standards Project: Findings and conclusions*. Randolph, MA: Author.

National AutismCenter. (2015). *National Standards Project, phase 2: Findings and conclusions. Addressing the need for evidence-based practice guidelines for autism spectrum disorder*. Randolph, MA: Author.

Odom, S. L., Hoyson, M., Jamieson, B., & Strain, P. S. (1985). Increasing handicapped preschoolers' peer social interactions: Cross-setting and component analysis. *Journal of Applied Behavior Analysis, 18*(1), 3–16.

Prizant, B. M., Wetherby, A. M., Rubin, E., Laurent, A. C., & Rydell, P. J. (2006). *The SCERTS model: A comprehensive educational approach for children with autism spectrum disorders (volume 1)*. Baltimore, MD: Brookes Publishing.

Rogers, S. J., & Dawson, G. (2010). *Early start Denver model for young children with ASD: Promoting language, learning, and engagement*. New York: Guilford Press.

Rogers, S. J., Vivanti, G., & Rocha, M. (2017). Helping young children with autism spectrum disorder develop social ability: The early start Denver model approach In J. B. Leaf (Ed.), *The handbook of social skills and autism spectrum disorder: Assessment, curricula, and intervention* (pp. 420–480). New York, NY: Springer.

Ross, R. K. (2017). Matrix training procedures. In J. B. Leaf (Ed.), *The handbook of social skills and autism spectrum disorder: Assessment, curricula, and intervention* (pp. 767–790). New York City: Springer.

Soluaga, D., Leaf, J. B., Taubman, M., McEachin, J., & Leaf, R. (2008). A comparison of flexible prompt fading and constant time delay for five children with autism. *Research in Autism Spectrum Disorders, 2*(4), 753–765.

Stokes, T. F., & Baer, D. M. (1977). An implicit technology of generalization. *Journal of Applied Behavior Analysis, 10*(2), 349–367.

Strain, P. S., & Fox, J. J. (1981). Peer social initiations and the modification of social withdrawal: A review and future perspective. *Journal of Pediatric Psychology, 6*(4), 417–433.

Sundberg, M. L., & Michael, J. (2001). The benefits of Skinner's analysis of verbal behavior for children with autism. *Behavior Modification, 25*(5), 698–724.

Taubman, M., Leaf, R., & McEachin, J. (2011). *Crafting connections: Contemporary applied behavior analysis for enriching the social lives of persons with autism spectrum disorder*. New York: DRL Books.

Taubman, M., Rafuse, J., Leaf, J., & Leaf, R. (2011). True friendships. In M. Taubman, R. Leaf, & J. McEachin (Eds.), *Crafting connections: Contemporary applied behavior analysis for enriching the social lives of persons with autism spectrum disorder* (pp. 51–57). New York: DRL Books.

Tse, J., Strulovitch, J., Tagalakis, V., Meng, L., & Fombonne, E. (2007). Social skills training for adolescents with Asperger syndrome and high-functioning autism. *Journal of Autism and Developmental Disorders, 37*(10), 1960–1968.

Vernon, T. (2017). Pivotal response treatment: Empirically supported strategies to target social competencies and motivation in individuals with ASD. In J. B. Leaf (Eds.)., *The handbook of social skills and autism spectrum disorder: Assessment, curricula, and intervention* (pp. 397–419). New York, NY: Springer.

Weiss, M. J., Hilton, J., & Russo, S. (2017). Don't throw the baby out with the bathwater. In J. B. Leaf (Eds.)., *The handbook of social skills and autism spectrum disorder: Assessment, curricula, and intervention* (pp. 327–359). New York, NY: Springer.

White, S. W., Keonig, K., & Scahill, L. (2007). Social skills development in children with autism spectrum disorders: A review of the intervention research. *Journal of Autism and Developmental Disorders, 37*(10), 1858–1868.

Williams, T. I. (1989). A social skills group for autistic children. *Journal of Autism and Developmental Disorders, 19*(1), 143–155.

Wolf, M. M. (1978). Social validity: The case for subjective measurement or how applied behavior analysis is finding its heart. *Journal of Applied Behavior Analysis, 11*(2), 203–214.

Wolf, M., Risley, T., & Mees, H. (1964). Application of operant conditioning procedures to the behavior problems of an autistic child. *Behaviour Research and Therapy, 1*, 305–312.

Index

J.B. Leaf (ed.), *Handbook of Social Skills and Autism Spectrum Disorder*, Autism and Child Psychopathology Series, DOI 10.1007/978-3-319-62995-7

D

O

P